Recent Advances in Gestational Diabetes Mellitus

Recent Advances in Gestational Diabetes Mellitus

Editor

Katrien Benhalima

MDPI • Basel • Beijing • Wuhan • Barcelona • Belgrade • Manchester • Tokyo • Cluj • Tianjin

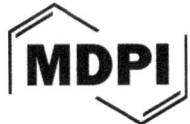

Editor
Katrien Benhalima
Endocrinology
University Hospital
Gasthuisberg, KU Leuven
Leuven
Belgium

Editorial Office
MDPI
St. Alban-Anlage 66
4052 Basel, Switzerland

This is a reprint of articles from the Special Issue published online in the open access journal *Journal of Clinical Medicine* (ISSN 2077-0383) (available at: www.mdpi.com/journal/jcm/special_issues/Gestational_Diabetes_Mellitus).

For citation purposes, cite each article independently as indicated on the article page online and as indicated below:

LastName, A.A.; LastName, B.B.; LastName, C.C. Article Title. *Journal Name* **Year**, *Volume Number*, Page Range.

ISBN 978-3-0365-1394-2 (Hbk)
ISBN 978-3-0365-1393-5 (PDF)

© 2021 by the authors. Articles in this book are Open Access and distributed under the Creative Commons Attribution (CC BY) license, which allows users to download, copy and build upon published articles, as long as the author and publisher are properly credited, which ensures maximum dissemination and a wider impact of our publications.

The book as a whole is distributed by MDPI under the terms and conditions of the Creative Commons license CC BY-NC-ND.

Contents

About the Editor vii

Preface to "Recent Advances in Gestational Diabetes Mellitus" ix

Katrien Benhalima
Recent Advances in Gestational Diabetes Mellitus
Reprinted from: *Journal of Clinical Medicine* **2021**, *10*, 2202, doi:10.3390/jcm10102202 1

Agnieszka Zawiejska, Katarzyna Wróblewska-Seniuk, Paweł Gutaj, Urszula Mantaj, Anna Gomulska, Joanna Kippen and Ewa Wender-Ozegowska
Early Screening for Gestational Diabetes Using IADPSG Criteria May Be a Useful Predictor for Congenital Anomalies: Preliminary Data from a High-Risk Population
Reprinted from: *Journal of Clinical Medicine* **2020**, *9*, 3553, doi:10.3390/jcm9113553 5

Xinglei Xie, Jiaming Liu, Isabel Pujol, Alicia López, María José Martínez, Apolonia García-Patterson, Juan M. Adelantado, Gemma Ginovart and Rosa Corcoy
Inadequate Weight Gain According to the Institute of Medicine 2009 Guidelines in Women with Gestational Diabetes: Frequency, Clinical Predictors, and the Association with Pregnancy Outcomes
Reprinted from: *Journal of Clinical Medicine* **2020**, *9*, 3343, doi:10.3390/jcm9103343 17

Maria-Christina Antoniou, Leah Gilbert, Justine Gross, Jean-Benoît Rossel, Céline Julie Fischer Fumeaux, Yvan Vial and Jardena Jacqueline Puder
Main Fetal Predictors of Adverse Neonatal Outcomes in Pregnancies with Gestational Diabetes Mellitus
Reprinted from: *Journal of Clinical Medicine* **2020**, *9*, 2409, doi:10.3390/jcm9082409 33

Caro Minschart, Kelly Amuli, Anouk Delameillieure, Peggy Calewaert, Chantal Mathieu and Katrien Benhalima
Multidisciplinary Group Education for Gestational Diabetes Mellitus: A Prospective Observational Cohort Study
Reprinted from: *Journal of Clinical Medicine* **2020**, *9*, 509, doi:10.3390/jcm9020509 45

Delia Bogdanet, Paula O'Shea, Claire Lyons, Amir Shafat and Fidelma Dunne
The Oral Glucose Tolerance Test—Is It Time for a Change?—A Literature Review with an Emphasis on Pregnancy
Reprinted from: *Journal of Clinical Medicine* **2020**, *9*, 3451, doi:10.3390/jcm9113451 63

Delia Bogdanet, Catriona Reddin, Dearbhla Murphy, Helen C. Doheny, Jose A. Halperin, Fidelma Dunne and Paula M. O'Shea
Emerging Protein Biomarkers for the Diagnosis or Prediction of Gestational Diabetes—A Scoping Review
Reprinted from: *Journal of Clinical Medicine* **2021**, *10*, 1533, doi:10.3390/jcm10071533 85

Lore Raets, Kaat Beunen and Katrien Benhalima
Screening for Gestational Diabetes Mellitus in Early Pregnancy: What Is the Evidence?
Reprinted from: *Journal of Clinical Medicine* **2021**, *10*, 1257, doi:10.3390/jcm10061257 125

Ellen Deleus, Bart Van der Schueren, Roland Devlieger, Matthias Lannoo and Katrien Benhalima
Glucose Homeostasis, Fetal Growth and Gestational Diabetes Mellitus in Pregnancy after Bariatric Surgery: A Scoping Review
Reprinted from: *Journal of Clinical Medicine* 2020, 9, 2732, doi:10.3390/jcm9092732 141

Charlotte Nachtergaele, Eric Vicaut, Sopio Tatulashvili, Sara Pinto, Hélène Bihan, Meriem Sal, Narimane Berkane, Lucie Allard, Camille Baudry, Jean-Jacques Portal, Lionel Carbillon and Emmanuel Cosson
Limiting the Use of Oral Glucose Tolerance Tests to Screen for Hyperglycemia in Pregnancy during Pandemics
Reprinted from: *Journal of Clinical Medicine* 2021, 10, 397, doi:10.3390/jcm10030397 161

Aoife M. Egan, Elizabeth Ann L. Enninga, Layan Alrahmani, Amy L. Weaver, Michael P. Sarras and Rodrigo Ruano
Recurrent Gestational Diabetes Mellitus: A Narrative Review and Single-Center Experience
Reprinted from: *Journal of Clinical Medicine* 2021, 10, 569, doi:10.3390/jcm10040569 175

Carola Deischinger, Jürgen Harreiter, Karoline Leitner, Dagmar Bancher-Todesca, Sabina Baumgartner-Parzer and Alexandra Kautzky-Willer
Secretagogin is Related to Insulin Secretion but Unrelated to Gestational Diabetes Mellitus Status in Pregnancy
Reprinted from: *Journal of Clinical Medicine* 2020, 9, 2277, doi:10.3390/jcm9072277 187

Anoush Kdekian, Maaike Sietzema, Sicco A. Scherjon, Helen Lutgers and Eline M. van der Beek
Pregnancy Outcomes and Maternal Insulin Sensitivity: Design and Rationale of a Multi-Center Longitudinal Study in Mother and Offspring (PROMIS)
Reprinted from: *Journal of Clinical Medicine* 2021, 10, 976, doi:10.3390/jcm10050976 199

Lucia Gortazar, Juana Antonia Flores-Le Roux, David Benaiges, Eugènia Sarsanedas, Humberto Navarro, Antonio Payà, Laura Mañé, Juan Pedro-Botet and Albert Goday
Trends in Prevalence of Diabetes among Twin Pregnancies and Perinatal Outcomes in Catalonia between 2006 and 2015: The DIAGESTCAT Study
Reprinted from: *Journal of Clinical Medicine* 2021, 10, 1937, doi:10.3390/jcm10091937 211

Caro Minschart, Toon Maes, Christophe De Block, Inge Van Pottelbergh, Nele Myngheer, Pascale Abrams, Wouter Vinck, Liesbeth Leuridan, Chantal Mathieu, Jaak Billen, Christophe Matthys, Babs Weyn, Annouschka Laenen, Annick Bogaerts and Katrien Benhalima
Mobile-Based Lifestyle Intervention in Women with Glucose Intolerance after Gestational Diabetes Mellitus (MELINDA), A Multicenter Randomized Controlled Trial: Methodology and Design
Reprinted from: *Journal of Clinical Medicine* 2020, 9, 2635, doi:10.3390/jcm9082635 225

Verónica Melero, Carla Assaf-Balut, Nuria García de la Torre, Inés Jiménez, Elena Bordiú, Laura del Valle, Johanna Valerio, Cristina Familiar, Alejandra Durán, Isabelle Runkle, María Paz de Miguel, Carmen Montañez, Ana Barabash, Martín Cuesta, Miguel A. Herraiz, Nuria Izquierdo, Miguel A. Rubio and Alfonso L. Calle-Pascual
Benefits of Adhering to a Mediterranean Diet Supplemented with Extra Virgin Olive Oil and Pistachios in Pregnancy on the Health of Offspring at 2 Years of Age. Results of the San Carlos Gestational Diabetes Mellitus Prevention Study.
Reprinted from: *Journal of Clinical Medicine* 2020, 9, 1454, doi:10.3390/jcm9051454 239

Hannah Nijs and Katrien Benhalima
Gestational Diabetes Mellitus and the Long-Term Risk for Glucose Intolerance and Overweight in the Offspring: A Narrative Review
Reprinted from: *Journal of Clinical Medicine* **2020**, *9*, 599, doi:10.3390/jcm9020599 . . . . **253**

About the Editor

Katrien Benhalima

K. Benhalima is a clinical scientist and clinician in endocrinology. Since 2019, she has been an assistant professor at KU Leuven (Belgium), and she is a senior clinical research fellow with the Flemish Research Council. She is an expert in the field of gestational diabetes mellitus (GDM). In addition, her research includes pregestational diabetes and pregnancy, type 2 diabetes in young adults, and early diagnosis and prevention of type 2 diabetes. K. Benhalima has 50 publications in international journals, with a current H-index of 20. She is actively involved in the 'Diabetic Pregnancy Study Group'(DPSG) associated with EASD. She won several awards for her research, such as the rising star researcher award by Primary Care Diabetes Europe in 2018, and the Belgium Novo Nordisk award for Diabetetology and the Dr. Karel-LodewVerleysen award of the 'Royal Academy of Medicine of Belgium'in 2020.

Preface to "Recent Advances in Gestational Diabetes Mellitus"

This is a Special Issue dedicated to recent advances in the field of gestational diabetes mellitus (GDM). The prevalence of GDM is rising globally, and GDM is an important modifiable risk factor for pregnancy outcomes and long-term metabolic risk in mothers and offspring. The papers included in this issue vary from research on pregnancy outcomes to screening and diagnosis of GDM, the use of new biomarkers, and the evaluation of long-term metabolic risk and intervention strategies postpartum in mothers and offspring. This work is therefore of interest to all health care professionals dealing with women with GDM during pregnancy or dealing with long-term follow-up after pregnancy. We thank all of the authors for their valuable contributions to this Special Issue.

Katrien Benhalima
Editor

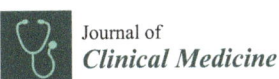

Editorial

Recent Advances in Gestational Diabetes Mellitus

Katrien Benhalima

Department of Endocrinology, University Hospital Gasthuisberg, KU Leuven, Herestraat 49, 3000 Leuven, Belgium; katrien.benhalima@uzleuven.be

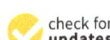

Citation: Benhalima, K. Recent Advances in Gestational Diabetes Mellitus. *J. Clin. Med.* **2021**, *10*, 2202. https://doi.org/10.3390/jcm10102202

Received: 6 May 2021
Accepted: 11 May 2021
Published: 19 May 2021

Publisher's Note: MDPI stays neutral with regard to jurisdictional claims in published maps and institutional affiliations.

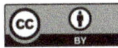

Copyright: © 2021 by the author. Licensee MDPI, Basel, Switzerland. This article is an open access article distributed under the terms and conditions of the Creative Commons Attribution (CC BY) license (https://creativecommons.org/licenses/by/4.0/).

The incidence of gestational diabetes mellitus (GDM) and overt diabetes in pregnancy is rising globally. GDM leads to increased risks for maternal and neonatal adverse pregnancy outcomes. In addition, GDM is also associated with an increased long-term metabolic risk in mothers and offspring [1]. Although much is known about GDM, evidence gaps persist. For instance, more research is needed on how to prevent GDM, on whether screening and treatment of GDM in early pregnancy are beneficial, on non-fasting biomarkers to screen for GDM, on new biomarkers to predict pregnancy complications, and on how to reduce the long-term metabolic risk in mothers and infants after delivery. To address this important health issue, the present Special Issue in the Journal of Clinical Medicine was dedicated to recent advances in the field of GDM. This Special Issue published 16 articles on this topic. The issues evaluated in these papers varied from research on pregnancy outcomes to screening and diagnosis of GDM, use of new biomarkers, and evaluation of long-term metabolic risk and intervention strategies postpartum in mothers and offspring.

This Special Issue includes various important findings. For example, Zawiejska et al. show that in high-risk women, early screening for GDM using the IADPSG criteria may be a useful predictor of congenital anomalies [2]. Another study showed that inadequate gestational weight gain was very common in a large cohort of GDM with a lower risk for adverse pregnancy outcomes in women with insufficient gestational weight gain [3]. Another study demonstrated that third-trimester fetal anthropometric parameters such as fetal weight centile can be used to predict adverse neonatal outcomes beyond the classical maternal risk factors [4]. The ELENA study showed that multidisciplinary group education might help to better manage the increasing workload and is also positively evaluated by women with GDM [5].

There has long been controversy on how to screen and diagnose GDM. Bogdanet et al. provide an extensive narrative review on the several factors that can influence the results of an oral glucose tolerance test (OGTT) in pregnancy and negatively impact patient care [6]. Another review discusses emerging biomarkers to simplify screening for GDM without the need for an OGTT [7]. Raets, L. et al. reviewed the current evidence and controversies on screening for GDM in early pregnancy [8]. Another important evidence gap is how to screen and diagnose GDM in pregnant women with a history of bariatric surgery. Deleus, E. et al. reviewed the challenges of using an OGTT in pregnancy after bariatric surgery and discussed potential alternatives to screen for GDM in this high-risk population. In addition, the evidence on the association between hypoglycemia and glycemic variability with adverse pregnancy outcomes in this population was reviewed [9]. A large retrospective French study evaluated different screening strategies for hyperglycemia in pregnancy to limit the number of OGTTs during pandemics [10]. Egan, A.M. et al. from the Mayo Clinic provided an extensive narrative review on the recurrence of GDM in a second pregnancy and presented the experience from their center [11].

Deischinger, C. et al. evaluated secretagogin (SCGN) in pregnancy, which is a calcium-binding protein related to insulin release in the pancreas. They showed that SCGN is related to insulin secretion but is unrelated to the diagnosis of GDM [12]. The study design and rationale were presented of the PROMIS study, a Dutch multi-center longitudinal study to evaluate insulin sensitivity and glucose metabolism in overweight pregnant women and the impact on pregnancy outcomes, including early growth of the offspring [13]. In addition, a population-based study evaluated the evolution in the prevalence of diabetes among twin pregnancies and pregnancy complications in Catalonia [14].

Long-term follow-up after pregnancy with GDM is important to timely prevent metabolic complications in mothers and offspring. The study protocol of the Melinda trial was presented. This is an ongoing RCT comparing a telephone- and mobile-based lifestyle intervention with standard of care in women with prediabetes after GDM [15]. Two-year follow-up data of offspring of the San Carlos GDM Prevention Study showed that a Mediterranean diet during pregnancy was associated with a reduction in hospitalizations with antibiotic and corticosteroid treatment, and fewer hospitalizations due to asthma/bronchiolitis [16]. A review with extensive scope on the long-term metabolic risk in the offspring showed that the prevalence of overweight/obesity and glucose disorders is higher in offspring exposed to GDM compared to unexposed offspring. Importantly, overall, this association remained significant after correction for maternal overweight [17].

Conflicts of Interest: The author declares no conflict of interest.

References

1. McIntyre, H.D.; Catalano, P.; Zhang, C.; Desoye, G.; Mathiesen, E.R.; Damm, P. Gestational diabetes mellitus. *Nat. Rev. Dis. Primers* **2019**, *5*, 47. [CrossRef] [PubMed]
2. Zawiejska, A.; Wroblewska-Seniuk, K.; Gutaj, P.; Mantaj, U.; Gomulska, A.; Kippen, J.; Wender-Ozegowska, E. Early Screening for Gestational Diabetes Using IADPSG Criteria May Be a Useful Predictor for Congenital Anomalies: Preliminary Data from a High-Risk Population. *J. Clin. Med.* **2020**, *9*, 3553. [CrossRef] [PubMed]
3. Xie, X.; Liu, J.; Pujol, I.; Lopez, A.; Martinez, M.J.; Garcia-Patterson, A.; Adelantado, J.M.; Ginovart, G.; Corcoy, R. Inadequate Weight Gain According to the Institute of Medicine 2009 Guidelines in Women with Gestational Diabetes: Frequency, Clinical Predictors, and the Association with Pregnancy Outcomes. *J. Clin. Med.* **2020**, *9*, 3343. [CrossRef] [PubMed]
4. Antoniou, M.C.; Gilbert, L.; Gross, J.; Rossel, J.B.; Fumeaux, C.J.F.; Vial, Y.; Puder, J.J. Main Fetal Predictors of Adverse Neonatal Outcomes in Pregnancies with Gestational Diabetes Mellitus. *J. Clin. Med.* **2020**, *9*, 2409. [CrossRef] [PubMed]
5. Minschart, C.; Amuli, K.; Delameillieure, A.; Calewaert, P.; Mathieu, C.; Benhalima, K. Multidisciplinary Group Education for Gestational Diabetes Mellitus: A Prospective Observational Cohort Study. *J. Clin. Med.* **2020**, *9*, 509. [CrossRef] [PubMed]
6. Bogdanet, D.; O'Shea, P.; Lyons, C.; Shafat, A.; Dunne, F. The Oral Glucose Tolerance Test-Is It Time for a Change?—A Literature Review with an Emphasis on Pregnancy. *J. Clin. Med.* **2020**, *9*, 3451. [CrossRef] [PubMed]
7. Bogdanet, D.; Reddin, C.; Murphy, D.; Doheny, H.C.; Halperin, J.A.; Dunne, F.; O'Shea, P.M. Emerging Protein Biomarkers for the Diagnosis or Prediction of Gestational Diabetes—A Scoping Review. *J. Clin. Med.* **2021**, *10*, 1533. [CrossRef]
8. Raets, L.; Beunen, K.; Benhalima, K. Screening for Gestational Diabetes Mellitus in Early Pregnancy: What Is the Evidence? *J. Clin. Med.* **2021**, *10*, 1257. [CrossRef]
9. Deleus, E.; van der Schueren, B.; Devlieger, R.; Lannoo, M.; Benhalima, K. Glucose Homeostasis, Fetal Growth and Gestational Diabetes Mellitus in Pregnancy after Bariatric Surgery: A Scoping Review. *J. Clin. Med.* **2020**, *9*, 2732. [CrossRef] [PubMed]
10. Nachtergaele, C.; Vicaut, E.; Tatulashvili, S.; Pinto, S.; Bihan, H.; Sal, M.; Berkane, N.; Allard, L.; Baudry, C.; Portal, J.J.; et al. Limiting the Use of Oral Glucose Tolerance Tests to Screen for Hyperglycemia in Pregnancy during Pandemics. *J. Clin. Med.* **2021**, *10*, 397. [CrossRef]
11. Egan, A.M.; Enninga, E.A.L.; Alrahmani, L.; Weaver, A.L.; Sarras, M.P.; Ruano, R. Recurrent Gestational Diabetes Mellitus: A Narrative Review and Single-Center Experience. *J. Clin. Med.* **2021**, *10*, 569. [CrossRef]
12. Deischinger, C.; Harreiter, J.; Leitner, K.; Bancher-Todesca, D.; Baumgartner-Parzer, S.; Kautzky-Willer, A. Secretagogin is Related to Insulin Secretion but Unrelated to Gestational Diabetes Mellitus Status in Pregnancy. *J. Clin. Med.* **2020**, *9*, 2277. [CrossRef] [PubMed]
13. Kdekian, A.; Sietzema, M.; Scherjon, S.A.; Lutgers, H.; van der Beek, E.M. Pregnancy Outcomes and Maternal Insulin Sensitivity: Design and Rationale of a Multi-Center Longitudinal Study in Mother and Offspring (PROMIS). *J. Clin. Med.* **2021**, *10*, 976. [CrossRef]
14. Gortazar, L.; Flores-Le Roux, J.A.; Benaiges, D.; Sarsanedas, E.; Navarro, H.; Paya, A.; Mane, L.; Pedro-Botet, J.; Goday, A. Trends in Prevalence of Diabetes among Twin Pregnancies and Perinatal Outcomes in Catalonia between 2006 and 2015: The DIAGESTCAT Study. *J. Clin. Med.* **2021**, *10*, 1937. [CrossRef]
15. Minschart, C.; Maes, T.; De Block, C.; Van Pottelbergh, I.; Myngheer, N.; Abrams, P.; Vinck, W.; Leuridan, L.; Mathieu, C.; Billen, J.; et al. Mobile-Based Lifestyle Intervention in Women with Glucose Intolerance after Gestational Diabetes Mellitus (MELINDA), A Multicenter Randomized Controlled Trial: Methodology and Design. *J. Clin. Med.* **2020**, *9*, 2635. [CrossRef] [PubMed]

16. Melero, V.; Assaf-Balut, C.; Torre, N.G.; Jimenez, I.; Bordiu, E.; Valle, L.D.; Valerio, J.; Familiar, C.; Duran, A.; Runkle, I.; et al. Benefits of Adhering to a Mediterranean Diet Supplemented with Extra Virgin Olive Oil and Pistachios in Pregnancy on the Health of Offspring at 2 Years of Age. Results of the San Carlos Gestational Diabetes Mellitus Prevention Study. *J. Clin. Med.* **2020**, *9*, 1454. [CrossRef] [PubMed]
17. Nijs, H.; Benhalima, K. Gestational Diabetes Mellitus and the Long-Term Risk for Glucose Intolerance and Overweight in the Offspring: A Narrative Review. *J. Clin. Med.* **2020**, *9*, 599. [CrossRef] [PubMed]

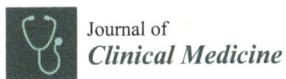

Article

Early Screening for Gestational Diabetes Using IADPSG Criteria May Be a Useful Predictor for Congenital Anomalies: Preliminary Data from a High-Risk Population

Agnieszka Zawiejska [1,*], Katarzyna Wróblewska-Seniuk [2], Paweł Gutaj [1], Urszula Mantaj [1], Anna Gomulska [3], Joanna Kippen [3] and Ewa Wender-Ozegowska [1]

[1] Department of Reproduction, Poznan University of Medical Sciences, 60-512 Poznan, Poland; pgutaj@o2.pl (P.G.); urszula.mantaj@gmail.com (U.M.); eozegow@ump.edu.pl (E.W.-O.)
[2] Department of Newborns' Infectious Diseases, Poznan University of Medical Sciences, 60-512 Poznan, Poland; kwroblewska@post.pl
[3] Student Scientific Society—Student Research Group, Department of Reproduction, Poznan University of Medical Sciences, 60-512 Poznan, Poland; anagomulska@gmail.com (A.G.); joannakippen@gmail.com (J.K.)
* Correspondence: azawiejska@ump.edu.pl

Received: 30 September 2020; Accepted: 2 November 2020; Published: 4 November 2020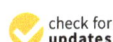

Abstract: Background: Our aim was to investigate whether the International Association of the Diabetes and Pregnancy Study Groups (IADPSG) glycemic thresholds used for detecting hyperglycemia in pregnancy can be predictive for malformations in women with hyperglycemia detected in early pregnancy. Methods: a single-center, retrospective observational trial of 125 mother-infant pairs from singleton pregnancies with hyperglycemia according to the IADPSG criteria diagnosed at the gestational age below 16 weeks. Glucose values obtained from 75-g OGTT (oral glucose tolerance test) were investigated as predictors for congenital malformations in newborns. Results: Characteristics of the cohort: maternal age: 31.5 ± 5.2, pre-pregnancy body mass index (BMI) ≥ 30 kg/m^2: 42.0%, gestational age at diagnosis (weeks): 12.0 ± 4.0, and newborns with congenital malformations: 8.8%. Fasting blood glycemia (FBG) and HbA1c (Haemoglobin A1c) at baseline significantly predicted the outcome (expB: 1.06 (1.02–1.1), $p = 0.007$ and expB: 2.05 (1.24–3.38), $p = 0.005$, respectively). Both the fasting blood glucose (FBG) value of 5.1 mmol/dL (diagnostic for gestational diabetes mellitus (GDM)) and 5.5 mmol/dL (upper limit for normoglycemia in the general population) significantly increased the likelihood ratio (LR) for fetal malformations: 1.3 (1.1; 1.4) and 1.5 (1.0; 2.4), respectively. Conclusions: (1) Fasting glycemia diagnostic for GDM measured in early pregnancy is associated with a significantly elevated risk for congenital malformations. (2) Our data suggest that women at elevated risks of GDM/diabetes in pregnancy (DiP) should have their fasting blood glucose assessed before becoming pregnant, and the optimization of glycemic control should be considered if the FBG exceeds 5.1 mmol/dL.

Keywords: hyperglycemia in pregnancy; early gestational diabetes; fetal malformations

1. Introduction

Maternal hyperglycemia is a well-studied risk factor for fetal abnormalities. Clinical studies on diabetic pregnancies consistently report an increased proportion of fetal malformations in type 1 or type 2 diabetes-complicated pregnancies [1,2]. There is a common consensus—supported by data from animal models on the mechanism of teratogenic action of maternal hyperglycemia—that clinically relevant hyperglycemia increases the risk of embryonic and fetal maldevelopment [3,4]. Therefore, preconception counselling in the diabetic population focuses mainly on achieving blood glucose levels as close as possible to those seen in nonpregnant, normoglycemic women, provided that such an intensification of metabolic control does not put a woman at risk of hypoglycemic complications.

Unfortunately, elevated blood glucose is a continuous risk factor without a clear cut-off value discriminating low-risk individuals from those at high risk. Thus, despite the considerable improvement in metabolic control and treatment, the proportion of early pregnancy complications still remains elevated in women with pregestational diabetes who achieve a good level of metabolic control before their pregnancies [5,6]. The disease remains associated with an elevated risk of fetal malformations, even if novel therapies or glycemic surveillance methods are used [7,8].

However, as fasting glucose measurements at the first visit during pregnancy became a part of the standard antenatal care offered for the general population in many countries, we are now facing a new clinical problem of hyperglycemia detected in early pregnancy in women without a history of diabetes mellitus or prediabetes [9]. The question as to whether this biochemical finding is clinically relevant raises several controversies, as we still lack a consensus on normal blood glucose in early pregnancy [10,11]. The Hyperglycemia and Adverse Pregnancy Outcome (HAPO) study linked mid-pregnancy glucose levels in 75-g OGTT to the risk of certain maternal or neonatal complications and recommended diagnostic thresholds for gestational diabetes mellitus, later adopted by an international consensus [12,13]. However, these cut-off points were identified at the gestational ages of 24–28 weeks for the specific adverse outcomes typically resulting from hyperglycemia in the second half of pregnancy. There is the paucity of data validating the use of the International Association of the Diabetes and Pregnancy Study Groups (IADPSG) criteria in early pregnancy for predicting gestational diabetes mellitus (GDM) in late-pregnancy or reducing adverse neonatal outcomes [6,14,15]. Hormonal alterations that are typical of pregnancy change the glycemic response throughout gestation. Therefore, some researchers suggested that thresholds identified for the early third trimester of pregnancy are inappropriate to use in early pregnancy [16–18].

Standards of the Polish Society of Obstetrician and Gynaecologists (PSOG) adopted in 2014 recommend testing for GDM according to the IADPSG protocols and criteria not only in the third trimester for all pregnant women without pregestational (type 1 or type 2) diabetes mellitus but, also, in early pregnancy, for (1) normoglycemic women who are at elevated risk of GDM (positive for at least one from the following: body mass index (BMI) $\geq$ 30 kg/m^2, history of GDM/macrosomia in previous pregnancies, history of polycystic ovary syndrome (PCOS), or insulin resistance) or (2) pregnant women presenting with fasting glycemia above 5.1 mmol/dL at the first trimester antenatal visit [19]. Moreover, previous PSOG recommendations, issued in 2011, also confirmed using fasting glycemia routinely measured in the general pregnant population in the first trimester of pregnancy as a screening test: women with a fasting glycemia > 5.5 mmol/dL should be offered a single-step procedure of a diagnostic 75-g OGTT performed in early pregnancy [20]. Therefore, we were able to design an observational study linking the blood glucose levels in early pregnancy to neonatal complications specifically resulting from maternal hyperglycemia in the periconceptional period.

We hypothesized that IADPSG criteria used in early pregnancy are suitable to identify women at elevated risk of congenital malformations, which are severe fetal complications caused by maternal hyperglycemia in early pregnancy and the periconceptual period.

2. Experimental Section

2.1. Inclusion and Exclusion Criteria

To test our hypothesis, we designed a retrospective observational trial. All pregnant women in singleton pregnancies referred to our tertiary level of care unit dealing with pregnancy and diabetes (a department within the University Obstetrical and Gynaecological Hospital at the Poznan University of Medical Sciences Poznan, Poland, which serves a population of ca. 4 million of citizen, with ca 7500 deliveries per year) between 2007 and 2017 for further treatment because of hyperglycemia detected before a gestational age of 20 weeks were considered eligible for the study. We reviewed maternal and neonatal records and used the following exclusion criteria: multiple pregnancies, lacking maternal/neonatal data, miscarriage, late intrauterine death, and did not give birth in our hospital. Finally, we identified 125 mother-newborn pairs.

2.2. Patients' Enrolment and Data Collection

Patients enrolled into the study had 75-g OGTT done in the first trimester of pregnancy, because they were qualified as having a high risk for GDM/diabetes in pregnancy (DiP) or presented for their first antenatal visit with a fasting glycemia above 5.1 mmol/dL if diagnosed following the IADPSG criteria (adopted in Poland in 2014) or above 5.5 mmol/dL if diagnosed before 2014. The patients were subsequently referred to our unit if the diagnostic 75-g OGTT was found abnormal, i.e., at least one value was above the thresholds: 100-(180—measurement not mandatory)-140 mg/dL for women diagnosed until 2014 or 92-180-153 mg/dl for women diagnosed after 2014. During the whole study period, women with no history of pregestational diabetes mellitus who presented with a fasting glycemia above 7.0 mmol/dL or with a random glucose level above 11.1 mmol/dL were immediately referred to our department with a diagnosis of hyperglycemia in early pregnancy, without the 75-g OGTT.

For purposes of our study, we defined gestational diabetes mellitus (GDM) or diabetes in pregnancy (DiP) using IADPSG criteria in the whole cohort [13].

Pre-pregnancy bodyweight and glycemic values during 75-g OGTT were retrieved from patients' pregnancy charts during their first admission to the department and transferred to the hospital documentation and, thus, were available for the researchers reviewing the records. The same applied to the gestational age, which was confirmed with the first ultrasound scan available in patients' documentation and also transferred to the documentation upon admission for the baseline hospitalization. All participants had their scan for genetic risk assessment done between the 11th and 13th gestational weeks, and none of them required invasive diagnostic procedures due to an increased risk of trisomies. In the mid-trimester scan, four women were diagnosed with fetal malformations, none of which were lethal. None of the patients opted for pregnancy termination.

HbA1c and lipids were measured at the first admission to our unit (at the baseline) in the central laboratory of the academic hospital, holding certificates of quality management ISO 9000. To get some information on the average maternal daily glucose, which allows for gestational age as a modulator of the maternal glycemic profile, we calculated the pregnancy-specific estimated average glucose (PeAG) using the formula provided by Law et al. [21] from the daily glycemic profile collected during the baseline hospitalization. During this admission, pregnant women participated in the training, which addressed specific issues concerning general and diabetic dietary requirements in pregnancy, glucose self-monitoring, and lifestyle interventions. If glucose readings exceeded the targets, we added a basal-bolus insulin treatment, and these patients received further training on insulin therapy.

From the neonatal records, we obtained data on neonatal outcomes concerning congenital malformations confirmed postpartum. The postpartum assessment of each newborn was performed by a pediatrician—a neonatologist, including a postpartum cardiac echocardiographic scan.

The Bioethics Committee at the Poznan University of Medical Sciences confirmed that our research was not a medical experiment, therefore exempting our study from the need to obtain the committee's approval (decision No 1321/18).

2.3. Statisticala Analysis

We used SPSS 14.0 for Windows (SPSS Inc. Chicago, IL, USA) and Medcalc 19.0 (Medcalc Software, Mariakerke, Belgium) to perform the statistical analysis. Variables were tested for normality with the D'Agostino-Pearson test—all variables, apart from maternal age, were not normally distributed. We used the chi-square test to compare the categorical variables. ROC (receiver operating characteristic) curve analysis was used to calculate the diagnostic power of the predictors for congenital malformations in the offspring. Descriptive variables are presented as mean ± standard deviation, unless stated otherwise. Two-sided $p < 0.05$ was considered statistically significant.

Logistic regression models with malformation status yes/no as a dependent variable were built to identify predictors of congenital malformations in the study group. We then used a forward selection to build models, including maternal characteristics known as risk factors for neonatal malformations, as confounders. Testing for the goodness of fit of a logistic regression model was performed with the Hosmer-Lemeshow test.

We used the chi-square test to calculate the likelihood ratios and 95% confidence intervals for particular glycemic thresholds used in the general or pregnant population and the risk of fetal malformations.

To verify, whether the small size of our cohort would allow for statistically sound observations, we performed a post-hoc analysis using Medcalc 19.0 (Medcalc Software, Mariakerke, Belgium) The analysis revealed that, with a proportion of malformations of 8.8% detected in our cohort, a minimum sample size of 75 would be needed to detect a difference in the proportions of fetal malformations compared to the general European population (2.5%, according to the European network of population-based registries for the epidemiological surveillance of congenital anomalies, EUROCAT), with an alpha of 0.05 and power of 0.8 [22]. We also performed a sample size estimation based on data regarding the prevalence of congenital malformations (3.33%) available for the whole cohort of N = 8055 neonates born or referred to the hospital in 2017. With an alpha of 0.5 and power of 0.8, a minimum sample size of 120 participants would be needed to detect a difference in the proportions.

We also confirmed that our study was powered to find a statistically significant difference in the outcome for the fasting glucose above 6.6 mmol/dL (post-hoc power: 96.2%) and 2-h glucose above 11.7 mmol/dL (post-hoc power: 94.2%). The post-hoc power for HbA1c above 5.7% was 73.3%.

3. Results

Characteristics of the study group are summarized in Table 1.

Table 1. Characteristics of the study group (N = 125 mother-infant pairs); non-normally distributed variables are presented as medians (interquartile range) or %. BMI: body mass index, IADPSG: International Association of the Diabetes and Pregnancy Study Groups, and DiP: diabetes in pregnancy; IDF: International Diabetes Federation.

Maternal age (years)	31.5 ± 5.2
Pre-pregnancy body weight (kg)	81.1 ± 19.6
Pre-pregnancy BMI (kg/m^2)	29.1 ± 6.5
% of women with pre-pregnancy BMI ≥ 30 kg/m^2	42.0%
Gestational age at diagnosis (weeks)	12.0 ± 4.0
75-g OGTT fasting glycemia (mg/dL)/(mmol/dL)	101.0 (94.0; 112.5)/ 5.6 (3.5; 6.2)
75-g OGTT 120′ glycemia (mg/dL)/(mmol/dL) available for 91 participants	160.0 (135.0; 188.0)/ 8.9 (7.5; 10.4)
75-g OGTT 60′ glycemia (mg/dL)/(mmol/dL) available for 42 participants	168.0 (141.0; 192.0)/ 9.3 (7.8; 10.7)
% of women with DiP according to the IADPSG criteria [10]	21.5%
HbA1c (%) at baseline	5.5 (5.1; 6.0)
HDL cholesterol (mg/dL) at baseline	64.0 (54.7; 79.0)
% of women on diet and insulin	60.0%
% of women with Hba1c ≥ 6.5% at admission time	14.4%

Table 1. Cont.

% of women with chronic hypertension	11.2%
% of women meeting criteria of metabolic syndrome according to the IDF criteria at the baseline	17.6%
% of newborns with congenital malformations in the cohort	8.8%
% of healthy newborns with persistent foramen ovale	6.1%
Gestational age at delivery	38 (38; 39)
% of premature deliveries (delivery before 37th gestational age completed)	9.5%
Birth weight (g)	3420 (3080; 3756)
Birth weight > 4000 g (%)	12.8%

The participants were mostly referred for early GDM testing by their obstetricians because of pre-pregnancy obesity (39.6%), hyperglycemia, defined as fasting blood glucose above 5.1 mmol/dL in the cohort tested according to IADPSG/5.5 mmol/dL in the cohort tested before the IADPSG criteria came into use (76.9%), and either/or GDM in a past pregnancy (24.6% of women who had delivered at least once). In 18.6% of patients, 75-g OGTT was skipped, because fasting glycemia exceeded the threshold for overt diabetes in the general population, according to the WHO (7.0 mmol/dL). The cohort consisted of similar proportions of women diagnosed with GDM before IADPSG criteria were recommended (49.1%) and after that (50.9%). These two subgroups did not differ significantly regarding maternal BMI or maternal age.

Eleven out of 125 women delivered newborns with congenital malformations (8.8%). Three of them were minor, i.e., two cases of cryptorchism and one case of a syndactylia of the second and third finger. We confirmed cardiac malformations in six, genitourinary defects in two and skeletal defects in two out of these eleven cases. In one newborn, we diagnosed multiple defects of the skeletal and central nervous system and gastrointestinal tract. Women who gave birth to affected infants did not differ from those who delivered healthy newborns in terms of pregnancy-specific estimated average glucose, maternal age, pre-pregnancy body weight, pre-pregnancy BMI, parity, or the prevalence of chronic hypertension. The prevalence of congenital malformation in the subgroup treated with a diet (8.5%) was similar to the proportion found in women who required insulin treatment (9.3%, $p = 0.852$). Additionally, newborns with malformations did not differ from healthy infants in terms of gestational age at the delivery and birth weight. No statistically significant difference in the proportion of congenital malformations was found between participants diagnosed according to the earlier criteria (until 2014) and those diagnosed according of the IADPSG criteria (5.7% vs. 9.8%, $p = 0.483$)

In seven out of 114 healthy newborns (6.1%), a neonatal cardiac assessment done postpartum found an open foramen ovale. However, this feature was not classified as a malformation. In a separate analysis, we found no differences comparing maternal anthropometric, metabolic, or glycemic characteristics between women who gave birth to healthy newborns with vs. without this cardio-sonographic finding.

None of the available maternal anthropometrics, i.e., maternal age, pre-pregnancy body weight, or pre-pregnancy BMI, were associated with an increased risk of fetal malformations.

Maternal lipids in the first trimester of pregnancy were not associated with an elevated risk of fetal malformations, except low HDL (high-density lipoprotein) cholesterol levels: the relative risk for congenital malformations was significantly higher in women with HDL ≤ 45 mg/dL (likelihood ratio (LR): 3.2 95% CI: 1.1–9.8).

Comparing glycemic parameters between women who gave birth to affected vs. healthy newborns, we found a significant difference between the groups in blood glucose levels during 75-g OGTT and HbA1c measured at the first admission to the referral unit (for fasting glucose: 8.8 ± 3.5 vs. 5.6 ± 0.8 mmol/dL, $p = 0.001$, for 2-h glucose: 13.0 ± 6.6 vs. 8.9 ± 2.4, $p = 0.034$ mmol/dL, and for HbA1c at the baseline: 6.6 ± 1.9 vs. 5.7 ± 1.0, $p = 0.023$). In the multiple logistic regression models, we were able to confirm that fasting glycemia in 75-g OGTT and HbA1c at the baseline remained statistically significant predictors of birth defects in the cohort and when other maternal parameters, known as risk factors for congenital malformations in the general population (maternal age and BMI), were included in the models (Table 2).

Table 2. Predictors for congenital malformations—data from multivariate logistic regression models.

Parameter	expB	95% CI for expB	p	R2 (Nagelkerke)
75-g OGTT fasting (mg/dL)	1.06	1.02–1.10	0.007	0.412
75-g OGTT 2 h (mg/dL)	1.02	0.99–1.04	0.09	0.197
HbA1c at baseline	2.05	1.24–3.38	0.005	0.191

After adjustment for maternal age, the pre-pregnancy body weight, pre-pregnancy BMI, and parity and gestational age at diagnosis.

Being aware of the specific nature of maternal glycemia as a continuous risk factor for neonatal complications, we obtained cut-off points with an optimal specificity and sensitivity for our cohort from ROC curves (Table 3). We then calculated the relative risk for congenital malformations for different values used as diagnostic thresholds in the general or pregnant population. To define the thresholds that could be clinically useful for a risk assessment in early pregnancy in our cohort, we used the approach described by the HAPO group, i.e., calculated the glycemic thresholds related to the 75% increase in the risk for the outcome [12]. We also estimated the highest glycemic values, for which the risk for congenital malformations remained close to 1.00, i.e., it was similar to the unaffected subgroup (Table 4).

Table 3. ROC curves for predictors of congenital malformations in the cohort. AUC: area under the curve and FBG: fasting blood glycemia.

Parameter	AUC	p	Sensitivity	Specificity
75-g OGTT FBG > 6.6 mmol/dL	0.82	0.002	77.8	90.1
HbA1c > 5.7%	0.72	0.035	80.0	71.2
75-g OGTT 2-h > 11.7 mmol/dL	0.73	0.093	62.5	94.0

Table 4. The risk for congenital malformations for different diagnostic thresholds; the risk is computed from glycemic data collected for our cohort; the thresholds are linked to the likelihood ratio (LR) (95% CI).

	75-g OGTT Fasting	75-g OGTT 2-h	HbA1c
Cut-off values from ROC curves constructed for our cohort;	6.6 mmol/dL (LR) 7.9 (3.9–16.0)	11.7 mmol. dL 10.4 (3.8–28.3)	5.7% 2.8 (1.8–4.2)
The upper limit for normal fasting glycemia in the general population	5.5 mmol/dL (LR) 1.5 (1.0–2.3)	–	–
Diagnostic thresholds for GDM according to 2013 the WHO/IADPSG criteria	5.1 mmol/dL (LR) 1.3 (1.1–1.4)	8.5 mmol/dL 1.4 (0.9–2.2)	–
Diagnostic thresholds for DiP according to the WHO/IADPSG criteria	7.0 mmol/dL (LR) 12.1 (4.6–32.0)	11.1 mmol/dL 7.4 (3.0–18.0)	6.5% * 4.0 (1.6–10.4)
The HAPO Study approach—glycemic thresholds nearest to the OR of 1.75 in our cohort (approximated)	5.6 mmol/dL (LR) 1.73 (1.1–2.6)	9.2 mmol/dL 1.73 (1.1–2.8)	5.5% ** 1.78 (1.2–2.6)

Table 4. *Cont.*

	75-g OGTT Fasting	75-g OGTT 2-h	HbA1c
Glycemic thresholds nearest to the OR of 1.0 in our cohort (approximated)	4.2 mmol/dL	6.1 mmol/dL	4.9%
	(LR) 1.05 (1.00–1.09)	0.99 (0.76–1.31)	1.03 (0.83–1.28)

* According to the ADA (American Diabetes Association), HbA1c ≥ 6.5% can be used as a diagnostic for overt diabetes in the general population; 75-g OGTT 1-h glycemia was not used for calculations, because this value was available only in a small number of patients. ** The Hyperglycemia and Adverse Pregnancy Outcome (HAPO) study did not provide odds ratios (ORs) for the HbA1c levels. GDM: gestational diabetes mellitus.

4. Discussion

Our study provides data from a specific population. Our cohort is heterogeneous: it is comprised of women qualified as being at high risk of carbohydrate intolerance due to obesity/other risk factors for hyperglycemia present before pregnancy, or women without pre-pregnancy risk factors but with elevated fasting glucose diagnosed in early pregnancy. Regarding both indications, we can expect this population of pregnant women to increase mainly due to an increased prevalence of overweightness/obesity and advanced procreation age [23].

We confirmed maternal glycemia as a preventable risk factor for a severe fetal condition in the group of pregnant women without a diagnosis of hyperglycemia before pregnancy. From our data, we concluded that a fasting glycemia diagnostic for GDM according to the IADPSG criteria is associated with a significantly increased risk of congenital anomalies if used in pregnant women tested for gestational hyperglycemia in early pregnancy. Considering the ongoing discussion about whether these criteria are useful outside the gestational age at which they were used in the HAPO study, our research supports the use of IADPSG criteria also in early pregnancy to assess the risk of complications characteristic of maternal hyperglycemia in early pregnancy/periconception.

By adopting a more rigid threshold for normoglycemia for women attempting to conceive, we could likely further reduce the risk of severe neonatal complications in women without a history of pregestational diabetes mellitus but meeting the criteria of the high risk for the GDM population. From our data, we believe that reducing maternal glycemia would allow the management of fetal risk in our societies, characterized by women of childbearing age becoming older and heavier, which means an increasing prevalence of fetal anomalies in clinically normoglycemic individuals [24–26]. Adopting more stringent criteria for fasting glycemia would improve the neonatal prognosis in an epidemiological milieu of increased maternal age, which is an unmodifiable risk factor for adverse perinatal outcomes, and excessive maternal body weight, which is extremely difficult to treat in a short-term perspective necessary to adopt in a woman of a more advanced procreative age. Moreover, aiming at stricter fasting glycemia to protect from congenital malformation would also reflect a natural decrease in maternal glycemia typical of normal early pregnancy [10]. Moreover, a recent meta-analysis from Parnell et al. confirmed that the elevated risk for congenital malformations was seen only in women with GDM and obesity [27]. The authors emphasized that glycemic derangement typical of pre-pregnancy obesity, which remains undiagnosed until pregnancy, might be an actual driving factor behind this association.

In our cohort, we also noted a birth weight distribution similar to that seen in the normal population. This striking observation supports the notion that improved glycemic control resulting from the early treatment of GDM is likely to mitigate a late-pregnancy metabolic risk arising from mild maternal hyperglycemia in the second half of pregnancy, but the teratogenic impact of hyperglycemia evidently occurs before a diagnosis is made and any treatment can be commenced. However, the normal birth weight in our cohort might raise some concerns, suggesting that what we actually see is also a suboptimal growth (a number of LGA (large for gestational age)/macrosomia cases smaller than expected for such a dysmetabolic cohort) reflecting a subclinical placental dysfunction in women with severe insulin resistance (metabolic syndrome) or asymptomatic dysglycemia undiagnosed until pregnancy. Moreover, over 10% of our cohort suffered from arterial hypertension, which is a well-known disease affecting placental function. From our data we concluded that women at an elevated risk of gestational hyperglycemia should be identified in the general population and offered preconceptional counseling, similar to that offered to women with pregestational diabetes mellitus. Our results suggest that women with a high risk for GDM/DiP could be encouraged to start lifestyle interventions that aim at lowering fasting blood glycemia. More large-scale research is necessary to define the target, but our calculations indicate an optimal value even below 4.4 mmol/dL. We believe that a threshold of 5.1 mmol/dL can be safely used before more refined data from adequately powered studies are available. Discussing fetomaternal safety given future procreation plans could also prompt testing for all components of the metabolic syndrome and initiate a medical treatment of insulin resistance, if present.

Our study has some limitations. Due to the retrospective nature of our research, we had no data to check for hyperinsulinemia or insulin resistance, which seems to be another risk factor for fetal malformations [28,29]. Data from other studies suggest that the prevalence of this condition is currently increasing among young women [30,31]. This metabolic trait could be a driving force behind the coexistence of high-normal glucose levels and congenital malformations, which we noted in our cohort. This hypothesis is supported by our observation of a low HDL level, which is also a marker of metabolic syndrome, as a predictor of congenital malformations.

Another limitation comes from both the retrospective nature of our study and a specific setting in which our research was performed. We sampled the high-risk population of patients referred to the tertiary level of care unit. A proportion of malformations recorded for our hospital in 2017 was 3.3%—which is significantly larger than for a general population and reflects the specific nature of a large, referral academic center taking care for high-risk pregnancies. To appropriately assess an actual proportion of excess congenital malformations, prospective studies would be necessary with a specifically designed high-risk control group, i.e., pregnant women at the high risk for hyperglycemia in pregnancy but who were tested negative for GDM/DiP in early pregnancy.

As we mentioned above, our cohort is heterogeneous; it is comprised of women screened for GDM/DiP in early pregnancy because of their high-risk profiles known before pregnancy but, also, of women who did not present with any risk factors for GDM/DiP but were referred for further tests because of the elevated fasting glycemia found in early pregnancy. Such a biochemical finding can be noted in a healthy pregnancy as a result of prolonged overnight fasting. However, our study confirmed that the fasting glycemia was the only predictor for congenital malformations; maternal body weight/BMI itself did not increase the risk of birth defects in this very specific cohort. This suggests that a "high-normal" fasting blood glucose has a predictive value both in women with a pre-pregnancy high-risk profile and a low-risk profile concerning the GDM/DiP risk.

Elevated fasting glycemia in a pregnant woman not otherwise qualifying for early GDM/DiP testing can indicate an early stage of an autoimmune process against pancreatic beta cells or MODY (Maturity-onset diabetes of the young). Data on the prevalence of anty-islet antibodies among women with gestational diabetes are inconsistent: numbers reported for different populations vary from 6% to as high as 44% [32–34]. Our study provides another reason for such tests to be carried out in women with hyperglycemia detected in early pregnancy, especially if they meet the criteria of DIP. Even if intensive treatment and surveillance throughout pregnancy mitigate a short-term fetomaternal risk, such information is critical for planning future care and discussing prognosis with a patient.

We confirm that even "normal" fasting glycemia might be a reason for a "background rate" of congenital malformations. Due to a poor prognosis and the seriousness of this entity, every attempt should be made to avert as many cases of birth defects as possible. Although our center covers a large population of ca 4 million people, multicenter, large-scale studies are necessary to investigate the glycemic thresholds for particular BMI and ages, because a combination of these two risks can have an impact on the actual glycemic level necessary to optimize the risk. Additionally, from such studies, one could obtain information about a high-normal glycemia as an additional risk for early pregnancy loss.

The question as to whether women at low risk for GDM/DiP and a high-normal fasting glycemia should also be offered any pre-pregnancy intervention for further reducing their blood glucose, remains open. Although we can expect health benefits in women at high-risk for gestational hyperglycemia because their metabolic traits also increase the risk for premature cardiovascular morbidity, no such data is available for women of low cardiometabolic risk. However, these women could benefit from early testing towards anti-islet autoimmunity.

Data from our cohort suggest that fasting glycemia should be measured routinely in women who wish to get pregnant, mainly in populations with an increased prevalence of overweightness/obesity. Interventions to optimize fasting glycemia could then be initiated for women with fasting blood glucose above 5.1 mg/dL to reduce the risk of congenital malformations. Further, large-scale studies are warranted to investigate an optimal age- and BMI-specific fasting glycemia in view of the risk of congenital malformations and any specific pre-pregnancy interventions.

Author Contributions: All authors have contributed significantly to the manuscript, according to the latest guidelines of the International Committee of Medical Journal Editors, as follows: A.Z.—conception and design of the study, analysis, and interpretation of the data and the draft of the paper; K.W.-S.—acquisition of the data and revising the manuscript critically for important intellectual content; P.G.—conception and design of the study and revising the manuscript critically for important intellectual content; U.M.—analysis and interpretation of the data and revising the manuscript critically for important intellectual content; A.G.—acquisition of the data and drafting the paper; J.K.—acquisition of the data and drafting the paper; and E.W.-O.—conception and design of the study and revising the manuscript critically for important intellectual content. All authors have read and agreed to the published version of the manuscript.

Funding: This research received no external funding.

Conflicts of Interest: The authors declare no conflict of interest.

Abbreviations

ADA—American Diabetes Association, AUC—area under curve, DiP—diabetes in pregnancy, HbA1c—haemoglobin A1c (glycated haemoglobin), GDM—gestational diabetes mellitus, FBG—fasting blood glycemia, HAPO Study—Hyperglycemia and Adverse Pregnancy Outcome Study, HDL—high-density lipoprotein, IADPSG—International Association of the Diabetes and Pregnancy Study Groups, IDF—International Diabetes Federation, LGA—large for gestational age, LR—likelihood ratio, MODY—Maturity-onset diabetes of the young, OGTT—oral glucose tolerance test; PCOS—polycystic ovary syndrome, and PeAG—pregnancy-specific estimated average glucose, ROC curve—receiver operating characteristic curve.

References

1. Wender-Ozegowska, E.; Wroblewska, K.; Zawiejska, A.; Pietryga, M.; Szczapa, J.; Biczysko, R. Threshold values of maternal blood glucose in early diabetic pregnancy—Prediction of fetal malformations. *Acta Obstet. Gynecol. Scand.* **2005**, *84*, 17–25. [CrossRef] [PubMed]
2. Gabbay-Benziv, R.; Reece, E.A.; Wang, F.; Yang, P. Birth defects in pregestational diabetes: Diabetes range, glycemic thresholds and pathogenesis. *World J. Diabetes* **2015**, *6*, 481–488. [CrossRef] [PubMed]
3. Mills, J.L. Malformations in Infants of Diabetic Mothers. *Birth Defects Res. A Clin. Mol. Teratol.* **2010**, *88*, 769–778. [CrossRef] [PubMed]
4. Ornoy, A.; Reece, E.A.; Pavlinkova, G.; Kappen, C.; Miller, R.K. Effect of maternal diabetes on the embryo, fetus, and children: Congenital anomalies, genetic and epigenetic changes and developmental outcomes. *Birth Defects Res. C Embryo Today* **2015**, *105*, 53–72. [CrossRef]
5. Schaefer-Graf, U.; Napoli, A.; Nolan, C.J.; Diabetic Pregnancy Study Group. Diabetes in pregnancy: A new decade of challenges ahead. *Diabetologia* **2018**, *61*, 1012–1021. [CrossRef] [PubMed]
6. Ringholm, L.; Damm, P.; Mathiesen, E.R. Improving pregnancy outcomes in women with diabetes mellitus: Modern management. *Nat. Rev. Endocrinol.* **2019**, *15*, 406–416. [CrossRef]
7. De Jong, J.; Garne, E.; Wender-Ożegowska, E.; Morgan, M.; Berg, L.D.J.-V.D.; Wang, H. Insulin analogues in pregnancy and specific congenital anomalies: A literature review. *Diabetes Metab. Res. Rev.* **2016**, *32*, 366–375. [CrossRef]

8. Wang, H.; Wender-Ozegowska, E.; Garne, E.; Morgan, M.; Loane, M.; Morris, J.K.; Bakker, M.K.; Gatt, M.; De Walle, H.; Jordan, S.; et al. Insulin analogues use in pregnancy among women with pregestational diabetes mellitus and risk of congenital anomaly: A retrospective population-based cohort study. *BMJ Open* **2018**, *8*, e014972. [CrossRef]
9. Sweeting, A.N.; Ross, G.P.; Hyett, J.; Molyneaux, L.; Constantino, M.; Harding, A.J.; Wong, J. Gestational Diabetes Mellitus in Early Pregnancy: Evidence for Poor Pregnancy Outcomes Despite Treatment. *Diabetes Care* **2016**, *39*, 75–81. [CrossRef]
10. Mills, J.L.; Jovanovic, L.; Knopp, R.; Aarons, J.; Conley, M.; Park, E.; Lee, Y.; Holmes, L.; Simpson, J.L.; Metzger, B. Physiological reduction in fasting plasma glucose concentration in the first trimester of normal pregnancy: The diabetes in early pregnancy study. *Metabolism* **1998**, *47*, 1140–1144. [CrossRef]
11. Cosson, E.; Carbillon, L.; Valensi, P. High Fasting Plasma Glucose during Early Pregnancy: A Review about Early Gestational Diabetes Mellitus. *J. Diabetes Res.* **2017**, *2017*, 8921712. [CrossRef]
12. HAPO Study Cooperative Research Group; Metzger, B.E.; Lowe, L.P.; Dyar, A.R.; Trimble, E.R.; Chaovarindr, U.; Coustan, D.R.; Hadden, D.R.; McCance, D.R.; Hod, M.; et al. Hyperglycemia and adverse pregnancy outcomes. *N. Engl. J. Med.* **2008**, *358*, 1991–2002. [CrossRef]
13. International Association of Diabetes and Pregnancy Study Groups Consensus Panel. International Association of Diabetes and Pregnancy Study Groups Recommendations on the Diagnosis and Classification of Hyperglycemia in Pregnancy. *Diabetes Care* **2010**, *33*, 676–682. [CrossRef]
14. Corrado, F.; D'Anna, R.; Cannata, M.L.; Interdonato, M.L.; Pintaudi, B.; Di Benedetto, A. Correspondence between first-trimester fasting glycaemia and oral glucose tolerance test in gestational diabetes mellitus. *Diabetes Metab.* **2012**, *38*, 458–461. [CrossRef]
15. Zhu, W.-W.; Yang, H.-X.; Wei, Y.-M.; Yan, J.; Wang, Z.-L.; Li, X.-L.; Wu, H.-R.; Li, N.; Zhang, M.-H.; Liu, X.-H.; et al. Evaluation of the Value of Fasting Plasma Glucose in the First Prenatal Visit to Diagnose Gestational Diabetes Mellitus in China. *Diabetes Care* **2013**, *36*, 586–590. [CrossRef]
16. Bhavadharini, B.; Uma, R.; Saravanan, P.; Mohan, V. Screening and diagnosis of gestational diabetes mellitus—Relevance to low and middle income countries. *Clin. Diabetes Endocrinol.* **2016**, *2*, 1–8. [CrossRef]
17. Huhn, E.A.; Rossi, S.W.; Hoesli, I.; Göbl, C.S. Controversies in Screening and Diagnostic Criteria for Gestational Diabetes in Early and Late Pregnancy. *Front. Endocrinol.* **2018**, *9*, 696. [CrossRef]
18. Agarwal, M.M. Consensus in Gestational Diabetes MELLITUS: Looking for the Holy Grail. *J. Clin. Med.* **2018**, *7*, 123. [CrossRef]
19. Wender-Ozegowska, E.; Bomba-Opon, D.; Brązert, J.; Celewicz, Z.; Czajkowski, K.; Gutaj, P.; Malinowska-Polubiec, A.; Zawiejska, A.; Wielgoś, M. Standards of Polish Society of Gynaecologists and Obstetricians in management of women with diabetes. *Ginekologia Polska* **2018**, *89*, 341–350. [CrossRef]
20. Wender-Ozegowska, E.; Bomba-Opoń, D.; Brązert, J.; Celewicz, Z.; Czajkowski, K.; Karowicz-Bilińska, A.; Malinowska-Polubiec, A.; Męczekalski, B.; Zawiejska, A. Polish Gynecological Society standards for medical care in management of women with diabetes. *Ginekologia Polska* **2011**, *82*, 474–479. [PubMed]
21. Law, G.R.; Gilthorpe, M.S.; Secher, A.L.; Temple, R.; Bilous, R.; Mathiesen, E.R.; Murphy, H.R.; Scott, E.M. Translating HbA1c measurements into estimated average glucose values in pregnant women with diabetes. *Diabetologia* **2017**, *60*, 618–624. [CrossRef] [PubMed]
22. European Network of Population-Based Registries for the Epidemiological Surveillance of Congenital Anomalies (EUROCAT). Available online: eu-rd-platform.jrc.ec.europa.eu (accessed on 24 October 2020).
23. Cho, N.H.; Shaw, J.E.; Karuanga, S.; Huang, Y.; da Rocha Fernandes, J.D.; Ohlrogge, A.W.; Malanda, B. IDF Diabetes Atlas: Global estimates of diabetes prevalence for 2017 and projections for 2045. *Diabetes Res. Clin. Pract.* **2018**, *138*, 271–281. [CrossRef] [PubMed]
24. Morris, J.K.; Springett, A.L.; Greenlees, R.; Loane, M.; Addor, M.-C.; Arriola, L.; Barisic, I.; Bergman, J.E.H.; Csaky-Szunyogh, M.; Dias, C.; et al. Trends in congenital anomalies in Europe from 1980 to 2012. *PLoS ONE* **2013**, *13*, 0194986. [CrossRef]
25. Biggio, J.R., Jr.; Chapman, V.; Neely, C.; Cliver, S.P.; Rouse, D.J. Fetal Anomalies in Obese Women: The Contribution of Diabetes. *Obstet. Gynecol.* **2010**, *115*, 290–296. [CrossRef]
26. Persson, M.; Cnattingius, S.; Villamor, E.; Söderling, J.; Pasternak, B.; Stephansson, O.; Neovius, M. Risk of major congenital malformations in relation to maternal overweight and obesity severity: Cohort study of 1.2 million singletons. *BMJ* **2017**, *357*, j2563. [CrossRef]

27. Parnell, A.S.; Correa, A.; Reece, E.A. Pre-pregnancy Obesity as a Modifier of Gestational Diabetes and Birth Defects Associations: A Systematic Review. *Matern. Child Health J.* **2017**, *21*, 1105–1120. [CrossRef]
28. Chi, M.M.; Schlein, A.L.; Moley, K.H. High insulin-like growth factor 1(IGF-1) and insulin concentrations trigger apoptosis in the mouse blastocyst via down-regulation of the IGF-1 receptor. *Endocrinology* **2000**, *141*, 4784–4792. [CrossRef]
29. Lupo, P.J.; Mitchell, L.E.; Canfield, M.A.; Shaw, G.M.; Olshan, A.F.; Finnell, R.H.; Zhu, H. Maternal–fetal metabolic gene–gene interactions and risk of neural tube defects. *Mol. Genet. Metab.* **2014**, *111*, 46–51. [CrossRef]
30. Black, R.E.; Victoria, C.G.; Walker, S.P.; Bhutta, Z.A.; Christian, P.; De Onis, M.; Ezzati, M.; Grantham-McGregor, S.; Katz, J.; Martorell, R.; et al. Maternal and child undernutrition and overweight in low-income and middle-income countries. *Lancet* **2013**, *382*, 427–451. [CrossRef]
31. NCD Risk Factors Collaboration. Trends in adult body-mass index in 200 countries from 1975 to 2014: A pooled analysis of 1698 population-based measurement studies with 19.2 million participants. *Lancet* **2016**, *387*, 1377–1396. [CrossRef]
32. Fuchtenbusch, M.; Ferber, K.; Standl, E.; Ziegler, A.G. Prediction of type 1 diabetes postpartum in patients with gestational diabetes mellitus by combined cell autoantibody screening: A prospective multicenter study. *Diabetes* **1997**, *46*, 1459–1467. [CrossRef]
33. Nilsson, C.; Ursing, D.; Åberg, A.; Landin-Olsson, M.; Törn, C. Presence of GAD Antibodies During Gestational Diabetes Mellitus Predicts Type 1 Diabetes. *Diabetes Care* **2007**, *30*, 1968–1971. [CrossRef] [PubMed]
34. Amer, H.M.; El Baky, R.S.A.; Nasr, M.S.; Hendawy, L.M.; Ibrahim, W.A.; Taha, M.O. Anti-islet Cell Antibodies in a Sample of Egyptian Females with Gestational Diabetes and its Relation to Development of Type 1 Diabetes Mellitus. *Curr. Diabetes Rev.* **2018**, *14*, 389–394. [CrossRef]

Publisher's Note: MDPI stays neutral with regard to jurisdictional claims in published maps and institutional affiliations.

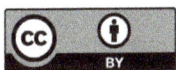

© 2020 by the authors. Licensee MDPI, Basel, Switzerland. This article is an open access article distributed under the terms and conditions of the Creative Commons Attribution (CC BY) license (http://creativecommons.org/licenses/by/4.0/).

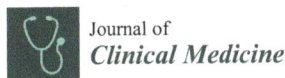

Article

Inadequate Weight Gain According to the Institute of Medicine 2009 Guidelines in Women with Gestational Diabetes: Frequency, Clinical Predictors, and the Association with Pregnancy Outcomes

Xinglei Xie [1], Jiaming Liu [1], Isabel Pujol [2], Alicia López [2], María José Martínez [2], Apolonia García-Patterson [3], Juan M. Adelantado [4], Gemma Ginovart [5] and Rosa Corcoy [1,2,3,6,*]

1. Departament de Medicina, Universitat Autònoma de Barcelona, Bellaterra, 08193 Barcelona, Spain; xxienglei@santpau.cat (X.X.); ljiaming@santpau.cat (J.L.)
2. Servei d'Endocrinologia i Nutrició, Hospital de la Santa Creu i Sant Pau, 08041 Barcelona, Spain; ipujol@santpau.cat (I.P.); alopezar@santpau.cat (A.L.); mmartinezr@santpau.cat (M.J.M.)
3. Institut de Recerca, Hospital de la Santa Creu i Sant Pau, 08041 Barcelona, Spain; 31178agp@comb.cat
4. Servei de Ginecologia i Obstetricia, Hospital de la Santa Creu i Sant Pau, 08041 Barcelona, Spain; adelantadojm@gmail.com
5. Servei de Pediatria, Hospital de la Santa Creu i Sant Pau, 08041 Barcelona, Spain; gginovart.germanstrias@gencat.cat
6. CIBER-BBN, 28029 Madrid, Spain
* Correspondence: rcorcoy@santpau.cat; Tel.: +349-3556-5661

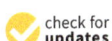

Received: 21 September 2020; Accepted: 14 October 2020; Published: 18 October 2020

Abstract: Background: In the care of women with gestational diabetes mellitus (GDM), more attention is put on glycemic control than in factors such as gestational weight gain (GWG). We aimed to evaluate the rate of inadequate GWG in women with GDM, its clinical predictors and the association with pregnancy outcomes. Methods: Cohort retrospective analysis. Outcome variables: GWG according to Institute of Medicine 2009 and 18 pregnancy outcomes. Clinical characteristics were considered both as GWG predictors and as covariates in outcome prediction. Statistics: descriptive, multinomial and logistic regression. Results: We assessed 2842 women diagnosed with GDM in the 1985–2011 period. GWG was insufficient (iGWG) in 50.3%, adequate in 31.6% and excessive (eGWG) in 18.1%; length of follow-up for GDM was positively associated with iGWG. Overall pregnancy outcomes were satisfactory. GWG was associated with pregnancy-induced hypertension, preeclampsia, cesarean delivery and birthweight-related outcomes. Essentially, the direction of the association was towards a higher risk with eGWG and lower risk with iGWG (i.e., with Cesarean delivery and excessive growth). Conclusions: In this cohort of women with GDM, inadequate GWG was very common at the expense of iGWG. The associations with pregnancy outcomes were mainly towards a higher risk with eGWG and lower risk with iGWG.

Keywords: gestational diabetes mellitus; Institute of Medicine; weight gain; length of follow-up; pregnancy outcome

1. Introduction

Gestational diabetes mellitus (GDM) entails risks for the mother and the newborn, both at short and long-term [1,2]. Among others, it increases the risk of preeclampsia, caesarean section, and future type 2 diabetes for the mother [3,4] and for the baby it increases the risk of diabetic fetopathy at short term and metabolic syndrome at long term [5]. In turn, high pre-pregnancy body mass index (BMI) is associated with higher risks of gestational hypertension and GDM [6] as well as with unfavorable pregnancy outcomes [7,8]. Likewise, gestational weight gain (GWG) is related to adverse pregnancy outcomes. In the general obstetric population, excessive GWG (eGWG) is associated with a higher risk of hypertensive disorders of pregnancy, GDM, caesarean section, postpartum weight retention, large for gestational age (LGA) and macrosomic newborns [9,10]. In turn, insufficient GWG (iGWG) is associated with a higher risk of preterm birth and small for gestational babies (SGA) [11–13]. In 2009, the Institute of Medicine (IOM) provided specific guidelines regarding the recommended GWG according to BMI categories to optimize pregnancy outcome [14].

In diabetic pregnancy, inadequate GWG is prevalent both in women with GDM and those with pregestational diabetes [13,15,16] and has also been related to perinatal outcome. In a meta-analysis on GWG and pregnancy outcomes in women with GDM, eGWG was associated with a higher frequency of pregnancy-induced hypertension (PIH), cesarean delivery, LGA newborns and macrosomia in relation to an adequate GWG (aGWG) whereas iGWG was associated with a lower risk of LGA and macrosomia. The risk of LGA was ≃double with eGWG and ≃0.70 with iGWG [13]. Articles addressing this point in our background are limited [17–19] and, therefore, we aimed to evaluate the frequency of inadequate GWG in women with GDM attended in our center, its clinical predictors and the association with pregnancy outcomes.

2. Materials and Methods

2.1. Study Design

The present study is a retrospective analysis of data collected prospectively in the database of the Endocrinology and Pregnancy Clinic at Hospital de la Santa Creu i Sant Pau. All patients provided written informed consent for inclusion in the database and the study has been approved by the Ethics Committee of the Institut de Recerca de l'Hospital de la Santa Creu i Sant Pau and has been performed in accordance with the Declaration of Helsinki. We evaluated patients with GDM who were attended in our center between 1 January 1985 and 31 December 2011. Throughout this period, GDM has been diagnosed after National Diabetes Data Group Criteria, continued after an evaluation of the potential impact of Carpenter and Coustan criteria [20,21]. Treatment approach has essentially kept constant: normocaloric diet (usually ranging from 1800 to 2200 calories per day), self-monitoring of ketonuria (aiming at its absence) and of blood glucose (aiming at fasting/preprandial <90 mg/dL and 1 h postprandial <120 mg/dL unless fetal growth is <10th centile).

2.2. Variables Collected

Adequacy of GWG was categorized according to IOM 2009 into insufficient, adequate (reference category) and excessive weight gain. GWG was calculated as the difference between the last weight available during pregnancy and prepregnancy (see Appendix A Table A1). As potential independent variables, we have considered maternal ethnicity (non-Caucasian), age at the beginning of pregnancy, maternal anthropometry (height and prepregnancy BMI category), family history of diabetes, prior history of abnormal glucose tolerance (GDM/impaired fasting glucose/glucose intolerance), prior pregnancy, unfavorable obstetric history (macrosomia, pregnancy-induced hypertension, recurrent miscarriage, non-syndromic malformation, unexplained fetal death, polyhydramnios, pyelonephritis), multiple pregnancy, smoking habit during pregnancy (non-smoker at the beginning of pregnancy, quitter or active smoker during pregnancy), characteristics of GDM diagnosis (gestational age at diagnosis, season, glycemic values, number of abnormal glucose values, autoimmunity against beta cell), gestational age at delivery and length of specific follow-up at the Diabetes and Pregnancy Clinic.

We addressed 4 maternal and 14 neonatal outcomes, defined as follows: PIH (blood pressure ≥ 140/90 mmHg, ×2 times separated ≥ 6 h, starting at a gestational age ≥ 20 weeks or worsening chronic hypertension), preeclampsia (PIH, accompanied by proteinuria), insulin treatment, cesarean delivery (total), fetal scalp blood pH < 7.25 [22], preterm birth (defined as a gestational age at birth less than 37 complete weeks), Apgar 5 min < 7 [23], arterial pH < 7.10 [24], significant obstetric trauma,

LGA newborn (birth weight >90% centile for the same gestational age and sex [25], macrosomia (defined as a birth weight ≥ 4000 g), small for gestational age (SGA) newborn (birth weight <10% centile for the same gestational age and sex) [25], neonatal hypoglycemia (Cornblath criteria applied to capillary blood) [26], neonatal jaundice requiring treatment [27], neonatal respiratory requiring treatment distress [28], neonatal hypocalcemia [29], polycythemia [30] and perinatal mortality (intrauterine or until 28 days postpartum taking into account fetal viability: before 1991, <28 completed weeks; 1991–1994, <26 completed weeks; 1995–1999, <24 completed weeks and from 2000 onwards, <23 completed weeks). As potential independent variables for pregnancy outcomes in addition to GWG, we considered the following characteristics: maternal ethnicity, age at the beginning of pregnancy, maternal anthropometry (height and pre-pregnancy BMI category), prior pregnancy, multiple pregnancy, smoking habit during pregnancy (non-smoker at the beginning of pregnancy, quitter or active smoker during pregnancy), characteristics of GDM diagnosis (gestational age at diagnosis, glycemic values), delay between diagnosis and initiation of specific follow-up, first HbA1c after diagnosis, average HbA1c in the third trimester) and fetal sex. In multiple pregnancies, a variable of concordant fetal sex was computed to be used in the analysis of fetal outcomes; for maternal outcomes, the sex of the fetus with higher risk was used. The variables above were used for the adjusted analysis of all outcomes with the exception of average HbA1c in the third trimester that was excluded for the adjusted analysis of insulin treatment. Over the years, different methods have been used to determine glycated hemoglobin. Currently, it is measured in whole blood using cation exchange HPLC (Variant II Turbo HbA1c, Bio-Rad Laboratories, Hercules, CA, USA). The results obtained with the different methods have been collected as SD around the mean and translated into values referred to DCCT.

2.3. Statistical Analysis

Statistical analyses were performed using the SPSS version 26.0 software package. Descriptive results are expressed as mean and standard deviation (SD) or P50 (P25–P75) for continuous variables according to their normal or non-normal distribution. Categorical variables are expressed as percentages. We compared characteristics between the GWG categories using a Chi-square test or a Kruskal–Wallis test as appropriate (the variable being categorical or quantitative, non-normally distributed). Imputations were not used to deal with missing data.

To address the clinical characteristics associated with GWG according to IOM, we performed a multivariate multinomial logistic regression analysis with a forward method using as dependent variable weight gain according to IOM (reference category: aGWG) and using as potential predictors the variables with a p value <0.100 in the bivariate analysis.

To determine the association of GWG according to IOM with pregnancy outcomes, we performed a logistic regression analysis (forward method) using aGWG as the reference category. Results were expressed as non-adjusted odds ratios (OR) and adjusted odds ratios (aOR) and 95% confidence intervals (95% CI). For the adjusted analysis, we fed in the model all the potential predictors indicated above.

A p value <0.05 was used as the cut-off for significance in the multivariate analysis. All p values were two-sided.

3. Results

A total of 2842 pregnant women with GDM were attended during the period and information regarding GWG according to IOM and potential predictors was available in 2700 (2594 with singleton pregnancies, 106 with multiple pregnancies, 95.0% of the target population), with analyses being performed in this group. A total of 2818 babies were born from these mothers (2594 from singleton, 224 from multiple pregnancies). Figure 1 displays the flowchart of patient inclusion. Results on preeclampsia are limited to the last period when information on proteinuria was included in the database (N = 377).

Table 1 shows the characteristics of these women. Main characteristics are as follows: most women had a normal prepregnancy BMI, 62.3% women had been pregnant before, GDM was diagnosed at a gestational age of 29 weeks and length of specific follow-up was 7 weeks. Median GWG was 10.2 kg. The distribution of GWG according to IOM was: 50.3% insufficient, 31.6% adequate and 18.1% excessive (Figure 2). In the bivariate analysis, 13 out of the 20 characteristics considered as potential independent variables had a *p* value <0.100 among the three groups of women. Among these variables, prepregnancy overweight/obesity and smoking habit at the beginning of pregnancy (women quitting smoking/active smokers during pregnancy) increased throughout the categories of GWG. The length of follow-up for GDM was negatively associated with GWG (Table 1, Appendix B, Figure A1).

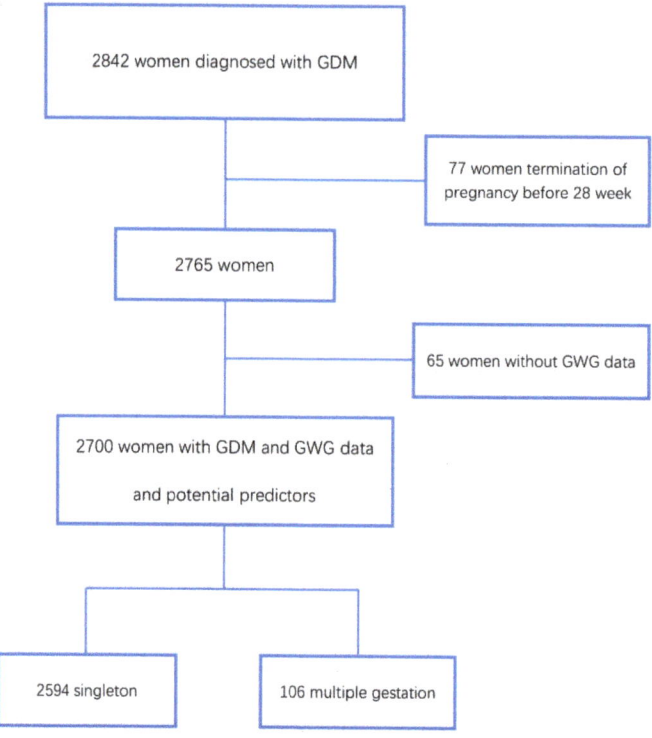

Figure 1. Flowchart of inclusion of patients in the study. GDM: Gestation Diabetes Mellitus. GWG: Gestational Weight Gain.

Results of the multinomial logistic regression are presented in Table 2 with seven characteristics being significantly associated with categories of GWG after IOM: non-Caucasian ethnicity, height, prepregnancy BMI category, unfavorable obstetric history, smoking habit, gestational age at delivery and length of follow-up.

For iGWG, independent variables were maternal height, prepregnancy overweight/obesity, unfavourable obstetric history, smoking habit (active smoker and quitter during pregnancy), gestational age at delivery and length of follow-up, all of them negatively associated with the exception of length of follow-up (OR 1.035 per week; 95% CI 1.018–1.052). For eGWG, independent variables were non-Caucasian ethnicity, prepregnancy overweight/obesity and smoking habit (active smoker and quitter during pregnancy), all of them positively associated with eGWG. The length of follow-up was negatively associated with borderline significance.

According to the recommendations of Institute of Medicine 2009, approximately 50% of women with gestational diabetes had insufficient weight gain during pregnancy, 18% excessive weight gain and 32% adequate weight gain.

Table 1. Characteristics of the study participants, both overall and according to category of weight gain after Institute of Medicine 2009.

Characteristic	Overall	% or P50 (P25, P75) in Each Weight Gain Category			p within IOM Categories *
		Weight Gain < IOM	Weight Gain within IOM	Weight Gain > IOM	
Non-Caucasian ethnicity (%)	5.5	4.4	3.8	11.3	<0.001
Age (years)	33.0 (29.0; 36.0)	33.0 (29.0; 36.0)	33.0 (30.0; 36.0)	33.0 (29.0; 36.0)	0.694
Height (cm)	160 (155; 164)	159 (155; 163)	160 (156; 164)	160 (156; 164)	0.002
Prepregnancy BMI category (%)					<0.001
• Underweight	2.6	2.7	3.4	1.0	
• Normal weight	63.1	77.9	58.5	30.1	
• Overweight	23.5	12.3	28.8	45.5	
• Obesity	10.7	7.1	9.3	23.4	
Family history of diabetes (%)	56.4	54.4	57.7	59.8	0.083
Prior history of abnormal glucose tolerance/gestational diabetes mellitus (%)	13.7	13.5	13.5	14.7	0.783
Prior pregnancy (%)	62.3	60.0	64.6	65.0	0.041
Unfavorable obstetric history (%)	12.8	9.3	15.3	18.4	<0.001
Multiple pregnancy (%)	3.9	5.7	2.3	1.6	<0.001
Smoking habit during pregnancy					<0.001
• quitter (%)	11.5	9.5	12.2	15.8	
• active smokers (%)	23.4	20.8	24.7	28.2	
Season at gestational diabetes mellitus diagnosis					0.681
• summer	31.0	30.6	30.7	32.4	
• autumn	25.2	24.6	26.7	24.2	
• winter	19.3	20.1	17.6	20.1	
Gestational age at diagnosis of gestational diabetes mellitus (weeks)	29 (26; 33)	29 (25; 33)	30 (26; 33)	29 (26; 34)	0.008
Glycemic values (mmol/L) at diagnosis					
• Glucose 0 h	4.7 (4.3; 5.1)	4.6 (4.3; 5.0)	4.7 (4.3; 5.1)	4.9 (4.5; 5.4)	<0.001
• Glucose 1 h	11.6 (10.9; 12.5)	11.6 (10.9; 12.5)	11.6 (10.8; 12.4)	11.5 (10.9; 12.6)	0.562
• Glucose 2 h	10.2 (9.6; 11.1)	10.2 (9.6; 11.1)	10.2 (9.6; 11.1)	10.2 (9.5; 11.1)	0.183
• Glucose 3 h	7.8 (6.6; 8.8)	7.9 (6.8; 8.8)	7.9 (6.6; 8.8)	7.5 (6.1; 8.7)	0.002
Number of abnormal glucose values	2 (2; 3)	2 (2; 3)	2 (2; 3)	2 (2; 3)	0.594
Autoimmunity against beta cells (%)	9.2	9.0	9.4	9.6	0.904
Gestational age at delivery (weeks)	39 (38;40)	39 (38;40)	39 (38;40)	39 (38;40)	<0.001
Length of follow-up (weeks)	7 (3; 11)	7 (4; 11)	7 (4;10)	6 (3;10)	0.032
Weight gain (kg)	10.2 (7.7; 13.0)	8.2 (5.7; 10.0)	12.2 (9.5; 13.9)	16.0 (13.0; 18.2)	<0.001

IOM: Institute of Medicine; BMI: body mass index; * Variables different from weight gain with a p value < 0.100 after bivariate multinomial regression analysis are displayed in bold characters and used in the multivariate multinomial logistic regression analysis.

Table 2. Independent variables for insufficient or excessive gestational weight gain according to IOM 2009 (multinomial multivariate logistic regression analysis).

	Insufficient Weight Gain				Excessive Weight Gain		
	OR	p	95% CI	Overall p	OR	p	95% CI
Non-Caucasian ethnicity (yes)	1.182	0.500	0.727–1.922		3.283	**<0.001**	**1.984–5.433**
Height (cm)	0.979	**0.008**	**0.963–0.994**	0.001	1.020	0.062	0.999–1.041
Prepregnancy BMI category				<0.001			
• Underweight	0.659	0.137	0.381–1.142		0.487	0.191	0.165–1.433
• Normal weight (reference category)	1				1		
• Overweight	0.301	**<0.001**	**0.235–0.387**		3.190	**<0.001**	**2.403–4.234**
• Obesity	0.603	**0.005**	**0.425–0.857**		5.060	**<0.001**	**3.472–7.375**
Unfavorable obstetric history (yes)	0.520	**<0.001**	**0.387–0.700**	<0.001	0.865	0.399	0.618–1.211
Smoking habit				<0.001			
• Non-smoker (reference category)	1				1		
• Quitter during pregnancy (yes)	0.668	**0.011**	**0.490–0.910**		1.614	**0.010**	**1.121–2.325**
• Active smoker during pregnancy (yes)	0.727	**0.007**	**0.576–0.918**		1.382	**0.030**	**1.031–1.852**
Gestational age at delivery (weeks)	0.855	**<0.001**	**0.806–0.907**	<0.001	1.026	0.527	0.947–1.113
Length of follow-up (weeks)	1.035	**<0.001**	**1.018–1.052**	<0.001	0.980	0.066	0.958–1.001

OR: odds ratio; CI: confidence interval; p value < 0.05 are considered significant; ORs significantly different from the reference category are marked in bold.

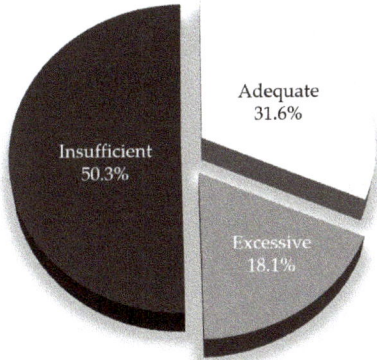

Figure 2. Distribution of gestational weight gain according to Institute of Medicine 2009.

Pregnancy outcomes according to IOM 2009 are presented in Table 3, with significant associations with three maternal (PIH, preeclampsia, cesarean delivery) and eight fetal outcomes (preterm birth, arterial pH < 7.1, LGA, macrosomia, SGA, jaundice requiring treatment, respiratory distress requiring treatment and neonatal hypocalcemia).

Table 3. Pregnancy outcomes of women with gestational diabetes mellitus according to gestational weight gain category.

Outcome	Prevalence (%) in Each GWG Category				Overall p
	Overall	iGWG	aGWG	eGWG	
Pregnancy-induced hypertension	5.3	3.4	5.5	10.1	<0.001
Preeclampsia	2.9	1.3	1.7	6.5	0.031
Insulin treatment	46.8	45.4	46.5	51.4	0.068
Cesarean delivery	24.1	19.9	23.4	36.8	<0.001
Fetal scalp blood pH < 7.25	3.8	3.1	4.0	5.3	0.077
Preterm birth	9.8	13.3	6.9	4.8	<0.001
Apgar at 5 min < 7	0.5	0.6	0.3	0.4	0.735
Arterial pH < 7.1	3.8	3.5	3.1	6.0	0.035
Obstetric trauma	2.3	2.1	2.6	2.4	0.697
LGA newborn	11.2	6.4	10.7	26.1	<0.001
Macrosomia ($\geq$ 4000 g)	5.7	2.4	5.7	14.9	<0.001
SGA newborn	9.9	11.7	9.3	5.9	0.001
Neonatal hypoglycemia	2.5	2.4	2.5	2.7	0.932
Jaundice requiring treatment	5.1	6.1	4.0	4.1	0.040
Respiratory distress requiring treatment	3.3	4.7	1.9	2.0	<0.001
Neonatal hypocalcemia	1.6	2.5	1.0	0.0	0.009
Neonatal polycythemia	1.4	1.3	1.4	1.8	0.662
Perinatal mortality	0.5	0.6	0.5	0.2	0.603

GWG (gestational weight gain), iGWG (insufficient gestational weight gain), aGWG (adequate gestational weight gain), eGWG (excessive gestational weight gain), LGA (large-for-gestational age), SGA (small-for-gestational age). A Chi-square test was used for statistical analyses.

Unadjusted and adjusted OR resulting from logistic regression are presented in Table 4. In the adjusted analysis, GWG according to IOM was significantly associated with PIH, preeclampsia, cesarean delivery, LGA, macrosomia and SGA. With the exception of SGA, eGWG was associated with higher risks and iGWG with lower risks even when for some variables (PIH, preeclampsia and SGA), significance was present for GWG according to IOM but not for individual categories of iGWG and eGWG. Additionally, iGWG was associated with neonatal hypocalcemia (aOR 4.557, 95% CI 1.037–20.003) even when the global association of GWG did not reach significance (overall p 0.133).

Table 4. Risk of different pregnancy outcomes in women with gestational diabetes mellitus according to gestational weight gain.

Outcome	Unadjusted OR Unadjusted CI 95%				Adjusted OR * Adjusted CI 95%			
	iGWG	aGWG	eGWG	Overall p	iGWG	aGWG	eGWG	Overall p
Pregnancy-induced hypertension	**0.604** **0.397–0.920**	1	**1.949** **1.282–2.963**	<0.001	0.655 0.396–1.085	1	1.357 0.818–2.253	0.028
Preeclampsia	0.785 0.109–5.658	1	4.095 0.832–20.161	0.054	1.008 0.077–13.163	1	6.519 0.746–56.939	<0.050
Insulin treatment	0.955 0.805–1.134	1	1.219 0.976–1.523	0.068	—	1	—	ns
Cesarean delivery	**0.812** **0.660–0.999**	1	**1.898** **1.488–2.419**	<0.001	**0.715** **0.556–0.920**	1	**1.641** **1.225–2.197**	<0.001
Fetal scalp blood pH <7.25	0.777 0.492–1.225	1	1.367 0.810–2.306	0.081	—	1	—	ns
Preterm birth	2.029 1.546–2.832	1	0.689 0.424–1.121	<0.001	—	1	—	ns
Apgar at 5 min <7	1.647 0.436–6.226	1	1.182 0.197–7.097	0.739	—	1	—	ns
Arterial pH <7.1	1.138 0.672–1.927	1	2.000 1.113–3.595	0.038	—	1	—	ns
Obstetric trauma	0.793 0.453–1.389	1	0.949 0.466–1.936	0.698	—	1	—	ns
LGA newborn	**0.575** **0.425–0.777**	1	**2.952** **2.200–3.962**	<0.001	**0.569** **0.400–0.810**	1	**2.003** **1.397–2.871**	<0.001
Macrosomia (≥4000g)	**0.412** **0.265–0.640**	1	**2.893** **1.983–4.220**	<0.001	**0.461** **0.282–0.752**	1	**1.822** **1.152–2.881**	<0.001
SGA newborn	1.289 0.947–1.706	1	**0.608** **0.392–0.943**	0.001	1.228 0.893–1.689	1	**0.515** **0.310–0.855**	0.002
Neonatal hypoglycemia	0.951 0.547–1.656	1	1.076 0.534–2.168	0.932	—	1	—	ns
Jaundice requiring treatment	**1.579** **1.052–2.369**	1	1.024 0.583–1.800	0.041	—	1	—	ns
Respiratory distress requiring treatment	**2.558** **1.472–4.447**	1	1.086 0.489–2.413	0.001	—	1	—	ns
Neonatal hypocalcemia	2.529 0.952–6.720	1	odd coefficient 1.310	0.177	**4.557** **1.037–20.003**	1	odd coefficient	0.133
Neonatal polycythemia	0.904 0.433–1.886	1	1.310 0.548–3.132	0.665	—	1	—	ns
Perinatal mortality	1.213 0.364–4.039	1	0.437 0.049–3.917	0.624	—	1	—	ns

OR (odds ratio), CI (confidence interval), iGWG (insufficient gestational weight gain), aGWG (adequate gestational weight gain), eGWG (excessive gestational weight gain), LGA (large-for-gestational age), SGA (small-for-gestational age). Logistic regression analysis was used to calculate ORs. * See methods for variables used for adjustment. ORs significantly different from the reference category are marked in bold, —is indicated when IOM is not included in the last step and OR not available.

In addition to weight gain itself, women in the different categories of gestational weight gain according to IOM differed in 13 out of 20 characteristics.

4. Discussion

The present study in a large cohort of women with GDM and satisfactory overall pregnancy outcomes has shown that GWG was very frequently outside IOM recommendations and GWG, in turn, was associated with PIH, preeclampsia, cesarean delivery, LGA, macrosomia and SGA with eGWG essentially linked with higher risks and iGWG with lower ones.

4.1. Prevalence and of Inadequate GWG

The distribution of GWG according to IOM in this cohort (50.3% insufficient, 31.6% adequate, 18.1% excessive) is far away from IOM recommendations. The rate of eGWG is similar to that in the study of Barquiel et al., also in Spain (14.7%) [19]—iGWG was not reported in this article [19]. In a meta-analysis of more than 80,000 patients with GDM, rates of inadequate GWG were also very high (30% insufficient, 34% adequate and 37% excessive) [13] and this was also the case in a recent article on this subject [31]. However, the GWG distribution in this study is clearly shifted towards iGWG whereas in other publications on this subject, the percentage of insufficient and excessive GWG is more balanced. We partially attribute this difference to the fact that, in the center, the glycemic control goals (90 mg/dL basal/preprandial, <120 mg/dL 1 h postprandial) are tighter than usual (95 mg/dL basal/preprandial, <140 mg/dL 1 h postprandial). This may facilitate that in order to avoid or delay insulin treatment, there is a larger caloric restriction and/or increased exercise. However, we think that the fundamental factor is that in the population herein reported, the percentage of prepregnancy overweight/obesity is much lower than in the aforementioned meta-analysis (34.2% vs. 68%) and we have also seen that this is associated to less eGWG.

4.2. Variables Independently Associated with Inadequate GWG

The study has identified seven independent variables for inadequate GWG, namely non-Caucasian ethnicity, unfavorable obstetric history, maternal height, prepregnancy BMI category, smoking habit, gestational age at delivery and length of follow-up for GDM.

For iGWG, independent variables were unfavorable obstetric history, height, prepregnancy overweight/obesity, active smoking/quitting smoking during pregnancy, gestational age at delivery and length of follow-up, all of them negatively associated with the exception of length of follow-up. For eGWG, independent variables were non-Caucasian ethnicity, prepregnancy overweight/obesity, active smoking/quitting smoking during pregnancy; maternal height and length of follow-up displayed borderline significance.

4.2.1. Ethnicity

The association of ethnicity with eGWG herein described is in line with information in the literature of inadequate GWG being different according to ethnicity both in the general obstetric population [32,33] and in women with GDM [31].

4.2.2. Maternal Anthropometry

The observation that height is associated with GWG is in line with the report of Straube et al., describing that for a given maternal BMI, weight gain during pregnancy increased with maternal height [34], and also with the more recent report of Khanolkar et al., describing that maternal height increases with the category of GWG (insufficient < adequate < excessive) [35].

Our observation of a negative association between prepregnancy overweight/obesity and iGWG and a positive one with eGWG is broadly in line with current information both in the general pregnant population and in women with GDM. In the general pregnant population, Lindberg et al. described that underweight was associated with a higher risk of iGWG, and overweight, and obesity class I and II with eGWG [36]. In women with GDM, Wong et al. also have described that, in relation to women gaining within recommendations, those with eGWG had a higher prepregnancy BMI (28.4 vs. 25.0 kg/m^2), whereas those gaining less than recommended displayed no differences [31].

4.2.3. Unfavorable Obstetric History

We attribute the lower odds of insufficient GWG (OR 0.520, CI 95% 0.387–0.700) with unfavorable obstetric history to the fact that the latter was usually due to a macrosomic baby in a prior pregnancy and eGWG is a well-known risk factor for this condition [35]. We speculate that women with a prior macrosomic baby had eGWG in a prior pregnancy and repeated the pattern of GWG in current pregnancy.

4.2.4. Smoking

It is well-known that nicotine increases energy expenditure, and may reduce appetite, so that smokers tend to have lower body weight and at the same time smoking cessation is commonly followed by weight gain both outside [37] and during pregnancy [36,38]. In the same line, in the current study women beginning pregnancy as smokers and quitting during pregnancy had a higher odds of eGWG (OR 1.614, 1.121–2.325) and a lower odds of iGWG (OR 0.668, 0.490–0.910). However, the observation that women who continued smoking during pregnancy also had a similar pattern of GWG can seem counterintuitive at first glance. Our interpretation is that women who continue to smoke during pregnancy reduce the consumption of cigarettes to a similar or higher extent than those who quit. In the last 10 years, where specific information on number of cigarettes consumed has been collected (N = 234), women who continued to smoke during pregnancy reduced the number of cigarettes in the same range than those who stopped (from 16.9 to 5.9 vs. 8 to 0, data not shown). Thus, the reduction in cigarettes per day would be similar in women who continued smoking during pregnancy and those who quitted, and similar patterns of GWG could be expected. Other studies in the general obstetric population have associated active smoking either with insufficient GWG [36] or smoking (unclear definition) with a twofold risk of excessive GWG [9].

4.2.5. Gestational Age at Delivery and Length of Follow-up

We observed that earlier gestational age at delivery and longer follow-up was associated with a higher frequency of iGWG. The interpretation of higher odds of iGWG with shorter duration of pregnancy is straightforward. As to length follow-up, although we do not have specific information on weight gain before and after initiation of specific follow-up for GDM, we attribute overall results of GWG according to IOM to the impact of the intervention for GDM. The diet initially prescribed is normocaloric but it is modified afterwards (by healthcare providers and by pregnant women themselves) to achieve the metabolic goals [39]. This is in line with the observations of Berglund et al., where women with GDM had a lower total GWG versus women with normal glucose tolerance at the expense of a lower GWG after diagnosis [18], and with those of Hillier et al., who recently reported that obese women with GDM had less eGWG when diagnosed after early screening than at 24–28 weeks (35 vs. 59%) [40]. The current report establishes this fact in a much larger population.

As to independent predictors of GWG, only length of specific follow-up for GDM can be considered as modifiable during pregnancy, in contrast with smoking habit and gestational age at delivery. Follow-up for GDM is required for the treatment of the condition. In addition, taking into account the essentially satisfactory pregnancy outcomes with iGWG, poorer outcomes with eGWG and the association of length of follow-up with both (borderline with eGWG), we conclude that follow-up for GDM likely has an impact on outcomes through GWG.

4.3. Inadequate GWG and Pregnancy Outcomes

4.3.1. PIH and Preeclampsia

With regard to pregnancy outcomes, in the adjusted analysis, hypertensive disorders (both PIH and preeclampsia) were associated with GWG categories even when, individually, iGWG and eGWG were not significantly different from aGWG. The direction of the association was towards a higher risk with eGWG and a lower risk with iGWG. The magnitude of the association was nominally larger for preeclampsia than for PIH (i.e., the aOR and 95%CI for eGWG was 6.519, 0.746–56.939 for preeclampsia vs. 1.357, 0.818–2.253 for PIH).

These observations are in line with data from previous investigations. In the general obstetric population Fortner et al. reported that women with eGWG had a ≃3-fold increased risk for hypertension and a ≃4-fold increased risk for preeclampsia, compared with aGWG [41]. On the other side, there is a reduced risk of hypertensive disorders in association with iGWG [42]. Among women with GDM, the abovementioned meta-analysis also observed a significant association with eGWG with hypertensive disorders of pregnancy (OR 1.65) but no association with iGWG [13]. Interestingly, GWG is positively associated with concurrent blood pressure in all gestational periods [41] and some authors have only observed an association in the third trimester (i.e., Gaillard for preeclampsia [9] or Gonzalez et al. for PIH [43]). Thus, GWG from the diagnosis of GDM onwards could play a relevant a role in the risk of PIH and preeclampsia and we have shown that the length of specific follow-up for GDM is negatively associated with GWG supporting a beneficial role of GDM care.

4.3.2. Cesarean Delivery

We also have observed an association of GWG with cesarean delivery: the risk was higher in women with eGWG (aOR 1.641, 95 % CI 1.225–2.197) and lower in those with iGWG (0.715, 0.556–0.920). This is in agreement with information in the general obstetric population [44] and partially with data in women with GDM where the negative association of iGWG with cesarean delivery did not reach significance [13]. Since GWG in second [45] and third trimesters [46] has been related with cesarean delivery, we consider that the relationships described in this study are partially attributable to GWG taking place after GDM diagnosis and affected by its management.

4.3.3. LGA, Macrosomia and SGA

In this series, eGWG was associated with a higher odds of LGA (aOR 2.003, 95% CI 1.397–2.871) and macrosomia (aOR 1.822, 95% CI 1.152–2.881), results that are perfectly in line with those observed in meta-analyses both in the general obstetric population (respective ORs of 1.85 and 1.95) [47] and in women with GDM (respective RRs of 2.08 and 1.87) [13]. As to SGA newborns, eGWG was associated with less risk (aOR 0.515, 95% CI 0.310–0.855), and iGWG was not significantly different from the reference category (aOR 1.228, 95% CI 0.893–1.689). This is also in line with meta-analysis results in women with GDM where summary figures for individual categories of iGWG (RR 1.40) and eGWG (RR 0.57) were not significantly different from aGWG [13]. However, in the general obstetric population, individual IOM categories display similar risks in terms of SGA and are significantly different from reference (OR 1.53 for iGWG and 0.66 for eGWG) [47]. Thus, the lack of significance in women with GDM is likely attributable to insufficient statistical power. The relationship between GWG and birth-weight-related outcomes is present throughout pregnancy [9,48], so we also consider that observed associations of GWG with these outcomes are partly attributable to weight gain after GDM diagnosis.

We have not observed significant associations of GWG with the additional 12 outcomes addressed in the current investigation. Viecelli et al. did not show an association between GWG with either drug treatment or preterm birth. They did not address the other 10 variables [13]. Overall, GWG was not associated with neonatal hypocalcemia, but the category of iGWG displayed a positive association (OR 4.557, 95% CI 1.037–20.003). The association could be mediated through reduced birthweight [49] and requires confirmation.

4.4. Is iGWG Satisfactory in Women with GDM?

In relation to pregnancy outcomes, eGWG is associated with higher risks, and iGWG with a more favorable pattern. In fact, different authors have suggested that definition of adequate GWG should use more stringent limits in women with GDM [31,50], with approaches such as subtracting 2 kg to the limits indicated by IOM [31] or deriving specific limits using ROC curves [51].

iGWG during pregnancy also raises the issue of ketogenesis, known to be associated with neurocognitive outcomes in the offspring [52]. It is usually recommended to monitor ketones in women with GDM displaying overt hyperglycemia and/or weight loss during follow-up even when this has not been formally tested to improve fetal outcomes [53]. In fact, it has been our practice for decades [54] to recommend urinary ketone monitoring in women with GDM and not only before breakfast [55] in order to identify its presence and introduce modifications for its prevention. Thus, we consider that women in this series, have not displayed significant amounts of urinary ketones during follow-up for GDM or at least, not for long periods.

The observed GWG distribution can be viewed as a good outcome according to the observed association with pregnancy outcomes. However, a recent study in a general obstetric population in Hong Kong has reported that inadequate GWG is associated with adiposity, hypertension and insulin resistance in offspring at 7 years of age, independently of factors such as gestational hyperglycemia or birthweight [56]. The association is present both for excessive and insufficient GWG but more marked for eGWG and especially for extreme values. The relationship of iGWG with long-term adiposity and insulin resistance would be akin to situations such as maternal treatment with metformin [57,58] or prevention of GDM through lifestyle intervention [59]. Should these observations be confirmed in women with GDM, the distribution of GWG herein described should be viewed as less satisfactory.

The results herein presented confirm data in the literature and also include novel observations among predictors of GWG (maternal height, active smoking and length of follow-up) and also among its association with pregnancy outcomes (iGWG associated with a lower rate of cesarean delivery).

The strength of our retrospective study is the large sample size of the cohort. We provide data on more than two thousand women with GDM and have performed a comprehensive analysis of the predictors of inadequate GWG according to IOM 2009 and its association with pregnancy outcomes. The study has several limitations. This is an observational, retrospective, single-center study, hence selection and information bias cannot be ruled out. A second limitation is that only information on total GWG is available and we have not been able to address weight gain after initiation of specific follow-up for GDM. Another limitation is that information on preeclampsia is only available in a reduced subset of women.

5. Conclusions

In summary, in this cohort of women with GDM, inadequate GWG was very common at the expense of iGWG; length of clinical follow-up for GDM was the only independent variable that is modifiable during pregnancy, after GDM diagnosis. The associations of GWG with pregnancy outcomes were essentially favorable for iGWG and unfavorable for eGWG.

Author Contributions: Conceptualization, X.X., J.L. and R.C.; formal analysis, X.X., J.L. and R.C.; investigation, X.X., J.L., I.P., A.L., M.J.M., A.G.-P., J.M.A., G.G., and R.C.; data curation, X.X., J.L., I.P., A.L., M.J.M., A.G.-P., J.M.A., G.G., and R.C.; writing—original draft preparation, X.X., J.L. and R.C.; writing—review and editing, X.X., J.L., I.P., A.L., M.J.M., A.G.-P., J.M.A., G.G., and R.C.; supervision, R.C. All authors have read and agreed to the published version of the manuscript.

Funding: This research received no external funding.

Conflicts of Interest: The authors declare no conflict of interest.

Appendix A

Table A1. Recommendations of GWG according to IOM 2009 [60]:

Pre-Pregnancy BMI Category (kg/m^2)	Recommended Range of GWG During Pregnancy (kg)	
	Singleton Pregnancy	Multiple Pregnancy
Underweight (BMI < 18.5)	12.5–18.0	
Normal weight (BMI = 18.5–24.9)	11.5–16.0	16.8–24.5
Overweight (BMI = 25.0–29.9)	7.0–11.5	14.1–22.7
Obesity (BMI ≥ 30)	5.0–9.0	11.3–19.1

GWG: gestational weight gain, IOM: Institute of Medicine, BMI: body mass index.

Appendix B

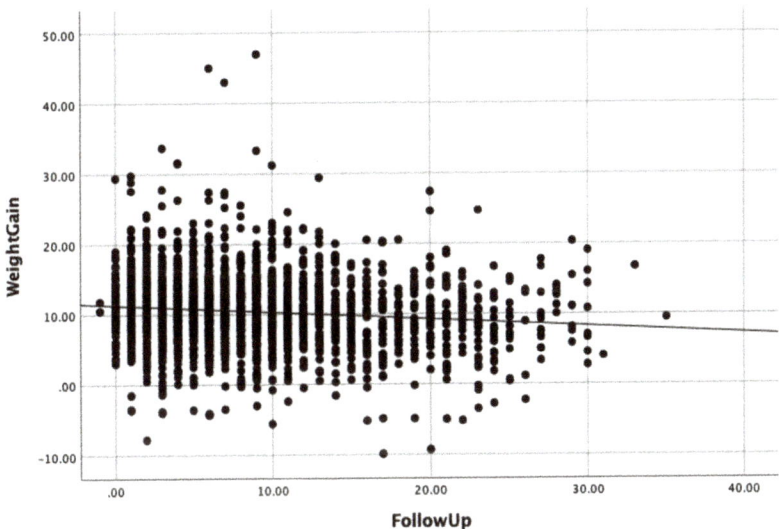

Figure A1. Scatterplot of gestational weight gain (in kg) vs. length of follow-up (in weeks).

References

1. ADA. 2. Classification and Diagnosis of Diabetes: Standards of Medical Care in Diabetes 2020. *Diabetes Care* **2020**, *43*, 14–31. [CrossRef] [PubMed]
2. Albareda, M.; Caballero, A.; Badell, G.; Piquer, S.; Ortiz, A.; De Leiva, A.; Corcoy, R. Diabetes and abnormal glucose tolerance in women with previous gestational diabetes. *Diabetes Care* **2003**, *26*, 1199–1205. [CrossRef]
3. Wendland, E.M.; Torloni, M.R.; Falavigna, M.; Trujillo, J.; Dode, M.A.; Campos, M.A.; Duncan, B.B.; Schmidt, M.I. Gestational diabetes and pregnancy outcomes—A systematic review of the World Health Organization (WHO) and the International Association of Diabetes in Pregnancy Study Groups (IADPSG) diagnostic criteria. *BMC Pregnancy Childbirth* **2012**, *12*, 23. [CrossRef] [PubMed]
4. Bellamy, L.; Casas, J.; Hingorani, A.D.; Williams, D. Type 2 diabetes mellitus after gestational diabetes: A systematic review and meta-analysis. *Lancet* **2009**, *373*, 1773–1779. [CrossRef]
5. Sendag, F.; Terek, M.C.; Itil, I.M.; Oztekin, K.; Bilgin, O. Maternal and perinatal outcomes in women with gestational diabetes mellitus as compared to nondiabetic controls. *J. Reprod. Med.* **2001**, *46*, 1057–1062.
6. Abenhaim, H.A.; Kinch, R.A.; Morin, L.; Benjamin, A.; Usher, R. Effect of prepregnancy body mass index categories on obstetrical and neonatal outcomes. *Arch. Gynecol. Obstet.* **2007**, *275*, 39–43. [CrossRef]

7. Catalano, P.M.; McIntyre, H.D.; Cruickshank, J.K.; McCance, D.R.; Dyer, A.R.; Metzger, B.E.; Lowe, L.P.; Trimble, E.R.; Coustan, D.R.; Hadden, D.R.; et al. The hyperglycemia and adverse pregnancy outcome study: Associations of GDM and obesity with pregnancy outcomes. *Diabetes Care* **2012**, *35*, 780–786. [CrossRef] [PubMed]
8. Ricart, W.; López, J.; Mozas, J.; Pericot, A.; Sancho, M.A.; González, N.; Balsells, M.; Luna, R.; Cortázar, A.; Navarro, P.; et al. Body mass index has a greater impact on pregnancy outcomes than gestational hyperglycaemia. *Diabetologia* **2005**, *48*, 1736–1742. [CrossRef] [PubMed]
9. Gaillard, R.; Durmuş, B.; Hofman, A.; MacKenbach, J.P.; Steegers, E.A.P.; Jaddoe, V.W.V. Risk factors and outcomes of maternal obesity and excessive weight gain during pregnancy. *Obesity* **2013**, *21*, 1046–1055. [CrossRef]
10. Haugen, M.; Brantsæter, A.L.; Winkvist, A.; Lissner, L.; Alexander, J.; Oftedal, B. Associations of pre-pregnancy body mass index and gestational weight gain with pregnancy outcome and postpartum weight retention: A prospective observational cohort study. *BMC Pregnancy Childbirth* **2014**, 201. [CrossRef]
11. Viswanathan, M.; Siega-Riz, A.M.; Moos, M.K.; Deierlein, A.; Mumford, S.; Knaack, J.; Thieda, P.; Lux, L.J.; Lohr, K.N. Outcomes of maternal weight gain. *Evid Rep. Technol. Assess. Full. Rep.* **2008**, 1–223.
12. Siega-Riz, A.M.; Viswanathan, M.; Moos, M.K.; Deierlein, A.; Mumford, S.; Knaack, J.; Thieda, P.; Lux, L.J.; Lohr, K.N. A systematic review of outcomes of maternal weight gain according to the Institute of Medicine recommendations: Birthweight, fetal growth, and postpartum weight retention. *Am. J. Obstet. Gynecol.* **2009**, *201*, 339.e1–339.e14. [CrossRef] [PubMed]
13. Viecceli, C.; Remonti, L.R.; Hirakata, V.N.; Mastella, L.S.; Gnielka, V.; Oppermann, M.L.R.; Silveiro, S.P.; Reichelt, A.J. Weight gain adequacy and pregnancy outcomes in gestational diabetes: A meta-analysis. *Obes. Rev.* **2017**, *18*, 567–580. [CrossRef] [PubMed]
14. American College of Obstetricians and Gynecologists. Weight gain during pregnancy. *Obstet. Gynecol.* **2013**, *121*, 171–173.
15. Stewart, Z.A.; Wallace, E.M.; Allan, C. A Patterns of weight gain in pregnant women with and without gestational diabetes mellitus: An observational study. *Aust. N. Z. J. Obstet. Gynaecol.* **2012**. [CrossRef]
16. Egan, A.M.; Dennedy, M.C.; Al-Ramli, W.; Heerey, A.; Avalos, G.; Dunne, F. ATLANTIC-DIP: Excessive gestational weight gain and pregnancy outcomes in women with gestational or pregestational diabetes mellitus. *J. Clin. Endocrinol. Metab.* **2014**, *99*, 212–219. [CrossRef] [PubMed]
17. Barquiel, B.; Herranz, L.; Meneses, D.; Moreno, Ó.; Hillman, N.; Burgos, M.Á.; Bartha, J.L. Optimal Gestational Weight Gain for Women with Gestational Diabetes and Morbid Obesity. *Matern. Child. Health J.* **2018**, *22*, 1297–1305. [CrossRef]
18. Berglund, S.K.; García-Valdés, L.; Torres-Espinola, F.J.; Segura, M.T.; Martínez-Zaldívar, C.; Aguilar, M.J.; Agil, A.; Lorente, J.A.; Florido, J.; Padilla, C.; et al. Maternal, fetal and perinatal alterations associated with obesity, overweight and gestational diabetes: An observational cohort study (PREOBE). *BMC Public Health* **2016**, *16*, 207. [CrossRef] [PubMed]
19. Barquiel, B.; Herranz, L.; Hillman, N.; Burgos, M.Á.; Grande, C.; Tukia, K.M.; Bartha, J.L.; Pallardo, L.F. HbA1c and gestational weight gain are factors that influence neonatal outcome in mothers with gestational diabetes. *J. Women's Health* **2016**, *25*, 579–585. [CrossRef]
20. Ricart, W.; López, J.; Mozas, J.; Pericot, A.; Sancho, M.A.; González, N.; Balsells, M.; Luna, R.; Cortázar, A.; Navarro, P.; et al. Potential impact of American Diabetes Association (2000) criteria for diagnosis of gestational diabetes mellitus in Spain. *Diabetologia* **2005**, *48*, 1135–1141. [CrossRef] [PubMed]
21. Acosta, D.; Balsells, M.; Ballesteros, M.; Bandres, M.O.; Bartha, J.L.; Bellart, J.; Chico, A.I.; Codina, M.; Corcoy, R.; Cortázar, A.; et al. Asistencia a la gestante con diabetes. Guía de práctica clínica actualizada en 2014. *Av. Diabetol.* **2015**, *31*, 45–59. [CrossRef]
22. National Institute for Health and Care Excellence. NICE Intrapartum Care: Care of Healthy Women and Their Babies During Childbirth Guidance and Guidelines. 2014. Available online: www.nice.org.uk/guidance/cg190 (accessed on 15 December 2014).
23. American College of Obstetricians and Gynecologists. ACOG Committee Opinion No. 644: The Apgar Score. *Obstet. Gynecol.* **2015**, *126*, e52–e55. [CrossRef] [PubMed]
24. Yeh, P.; Emary, K.; Impey, L. The relationship between umbilical cord arterial pH and serious adverse neonatal outcome: Analysis of 51 519 consecutive validated samples. *BJOG Int. J. Obstet. Gynaecol.* **2012**, *119*, 824–831. [CrossRef] [PubMed]

25. Santamaria Lozano, R.; Verdú Martín, L.; Martín Caballero, C.; García López, G. *Tablas Españolas de Pesos Neonatales Según Edad Gestacional*; Ed. Artes Gráficas Beatulo: Badalona, Spain, 1998; Available online: https//www.menarini.es/aviso-legal/509-salud/areas-terapeuticas/ginecologia/3073-tablas-espanolas-de-pesos-neonatales.html (accessed on 15 June 2018).
26. Cornblath, M.; Schwartz, R. Hypoglycemia in the neonate. *J. Pediatr. Endocrinol.* **1993**, *6*, 113–129. [CrossRef]
27. Maisels, M.J. Bilirubin: On understanding and influencing its metabolism in the newborn infant. *Pediatr. Clin. N. Am.* **1972**, *19*, 447–501. [CrossRef]
28. Edwards, M.O.; Kotecha, S.J.; Kotecha, S. Respiratory Distress of the Term Newborn Infant. *Paediatr. Respir. Rev.* **2013**, *14*, 29–37. [CrossRef] [PubMed]
29. Loughead, J.L.; Mimouni, F.; Tsang, R.C. Serum Ionized Calcium Concentrations in Normal Neonates. *Am. J. Dis. Child.* **1988**, *142*, 516–518. [CrossRef]
30. Kates, E.H.; Kates, J.S. Anemia and polycythemia in the newborn. *Pediatr. Rev.* **2007**, *28*, 33–34. [CrossRef]
31. Wong, T.; Barnes, R.A.; Ross, G.P.; Cheung, N.W.; Flack, J.R. Are the Institute of Medicine weight gain targets applicable in women with gestational diabetes mellitus? *Diabetologia* **2017**, *60*, 416–423. [CrossRef]
32. Headen, I.E.; Davis, E.M.; Mujahid, M.S.; Abrams, B. Racial-Ethnic Differences in Pregnancy-Related Weight. *Adv. Nutr.* **2012**, *3*, 83–94. [CrossRef]
33. Cheng, H.R.; Walker, L.O.; Brown, A.; Lee, J.Y. Gestational Weight Gain and Perinatal Outcomes of Subgroups of Asian-American Women, Texas, 2009. *Women's Health Issues* **2015**, *25*, 303–311. [CrossRef]
34. Straube, S.; Voigt, M.; Briese, V.; Schneider, K.T.M.; Voigt, M. Weight gain in pregnancy according to maternal height and weight. *J. Perinat. Med.* **2008**, *36*, 405–412. [CrossRef] [PubMed]
35. Khanolkar, A.R.; Hanley, G.E.; Koupil, I.; Janssen, P.A. 2009 IOM guidelines for gestational weight gain: How well do they predict outcomes across ethnic groups? *Ethn. Health* **2017**, *25*, 1–16. [CrossRef]
36. Lindberg, S.; Anderson, C.; Pillai, P.; Tandias, A.; Arndt, B.; Hanrahan, L. Prevalence and predictors of unhealthy weight gain in pregnancy. *Wis. Med. J.* **2016**, *115*, 233–237.
37. Chiolero, A.; Faeh, D.; Paccaud, F.; Cornuz, J. Consequences of smoking for body weight, body fat distribution, and insulin resistance. *Am. J. Clin. Nutr.* **2008**, *87*, 801–809. [CrossRef]
38. Hulman, A.; Lutsiv, O.; Park, C.K.; Krebs, L.; Beyene, J.; McDonald, S.D. Are women who quit smoking at high risk of excess weight gain throughout pregnancy? *BMC Pregnancy Childbirth* **2016**, *16*, 263. [CrossRef] [PubMed]
39. Hagiwara, Y.; Kasai, J.; Nakanishi, S.; Saigusa, Y.; Miyagi, E.; Aoki, S. Should the IADPSG criteria be applied when diagnosing early-onset gestational diabetes? *Diabetes Res. Clin. Pract.* **2018**, *140*, 154–161. [CrossRef] [PubMed]
40. Hillier, T.A.; Ogasawara, K.K.; Pedula, K.L.; Vesco, K.K.; Oshiro, C.E.S.; Van Marter, J.L. Timing of Gestational Diabetes Diagnosis by Maternal Obesity Status: Impact on Gestational Weight Gain in a Diverse Population. *J. Women's Health* **2020**, *29*, 1–9. [CrossRef]
41. Fortner, R.T.; Pekow, P.; Solomon, C.G.; Markenson, G.; Chasan-Taber, L. Prepregnancy body mass index, gestational weight gain, and risk of hypertensive pregnancy among Latina women. *Am. J. Obstet. Gynecol.* **2009**, *200*, 167.e1–167.e7. [CrossRef]
42. Macdonald-Wallis, C.; Tilling, K.; Fraser, A.; Nelson, S.M.; Lawlor, D.A. Gestational weight gain as a risk factor for hypertensive disorders of pregnancy. *Am. J. Obstet. Gynecol.* **2013**, *209*, 327.e1–327.e17. [CrossRef]
43. Gonzalez-Ballano, I.; Saviron-Cornudella, R.; Esteban, L.M.; Sanz, G.; Castán, S. Pregestational body mass index, trimester-specific weight gain and total gestational weight gain: How do they influence perinatal outcomes? *J. Matern. Neonatal Med.* **2019**, 1–8. [CrossRef] [PubMed]
44. Xiong, C.; Zhou, A.; Cao, Z.; Zhang, Y.; Qiu, L.; Yao, C.; Wang, Y.; Zhang, B. Association of pre-pregnancy body mass index, gestational weight gain with cesarean section in term deliveries of China. *Sci. Rep.* **2016**, *6*, 37168. [CrossRef] [PubMed]
45. Drehmer, M.; Duncan, B.B.; Kac, G.; Schmidt, M.I. Association of Second and Third Trimester Weight Gain in Pregnancy with Maternal and Fetal Outcomes. *PLoS ONE* **2013**, *8*. [CrossRef]
46. Harvey, M.W.; Braun, B.; Ertel, K.A.; Pekow, P.S.; Markenson, G.; Chasan-Taber, L. Prepregnancy Body Mass Index, Gestational Weight Gain, and Odds of Cesarean Delivery in Hispanic Women. *Obesity* **2018**, *26*, 185–192. [CrossRef] [PubMed]

47. Goldstein, R.F.; Abell, S.K.; Ranasinha, S.; Misso, M.; Boyle, J.A.; Black, M.H.; Li, N.; Hu, G.; Corrado, F.; Rode, L.; et al. Association of gestational weight gain with maternal and infant outcomes: A systematic review and meta-analysis. *JAMA J. Am. Med. Assoc.* **2017**, *317*, 2207–2225. [CrossRef]
48. Kramer, C.K.; Campbell, S.; Retnakaran, R. Gestational diabetes and the risk of cardiovascular disease in women: A systematic review and meta-analysis. *Diabetologia* **2019**, *62*, 905–914. [CrossRef]
49. Vuralli, D. Clinical Approach to Hypocalcemia in Newborn Period and Infancy: Who Should Be Treated? *Int. J. Pediatr.* **2019**, *2019*, 1–7. [CrossRef] [PubMed]
50. Gou, B.; Guan, H.; Bi, Y.; Ding, B. Gestational diabetes: Weight gain during pregnancy and its relationship to pregnancy outcomes. *Chin. Med. J. (Engl.)* **2019**, 6–11. [CrossRef]
51. Jiang-nan, W.; Wei-rong, G.; Xi-rong, X.; Yi, Z.; Xiao-tian, L.; Chuan-Min, Y. Gestational weight gain targets during the second and third trimesters of pregnancy for women with gestational diabetes mellitus in China. *Eur. J. Clin. Nutr.* **2018**. [CrossRef]
52. Rizzo, T.; Metzger, B.; Burns, W.; Burns, K. Correlations between antepartum maternal metabolism and intelligence of offspring. *N. Engl. J. Med.* **1991**, *325*, 911–916. [CrossRef]
53. Metzger, B.E.; Buchanan, T.A.; Coustan, D.R.; De Leiva, A.; Dunger, D.B.; Hadden, D.R.; Hod, M.; Kitzmiller, J.L.; Kjos, S.L.; Oats, J.N.; et al. Summary and recommendations of the Fifth International Workshop-Conference on Gestational Diabetes Mellitus. *Diabetes Care* **2007**, *30*. [CrossRef] [PubMed]
54. Corcoy, R.; Codina, M.; Cerqueira, M.J.; Rectoret, G.; Cervera, T.; Cabero, L.; de Leiva, A. Intensive treatment of pregnancy diabetes: Clinical course in 100 patients. *Rev. Clin. Esp.* **1988**, *183*, 344–348. [PubMed]
55. Montaner, P.; Ripollés, J.; Pamies, C.; Corcoy, R. Measurement of fasting ketonuria and capillary blood glucose after main meals in women with gestational diabetes mellitus: How well is the metabolic picture captured? *J. Obstet. Gynaecol. Res.* **2011**, *37*, 722–728. [CrossRef]
56. Tam, C.H.T.; Ma, R.C.W.; Yuen, L.Y.; Ozaki, R.; Li, A.M.; Hou, Y.; Chan, M.H.M.; Ho, C.S.; Yang, X.; Chan, J.C.N.; et al. The impact of maternal gestational weight gain on cardiometabolic risk factors in children. *Diabetologia* **2018**, *61*, 2539–2548. [CrossRef]
57. Jane, L.T.; Aiken, C.E.; Ozanne, S.E. Neonatal, infant, and childhood growth following metformin versus insulin treatment for gestational diabetes: A systematic review and meta-analysis. *PLoS Med.* **2019**, *16*, e1002848.
58. Salomaki, H.; Vahatalo, L.H.; Kirsti, L.; Norma, T.J.; Penttinen, A.-M.; Ailanen, L.; Ilyasizadeh, J.; Pesonen, U.; Koulu, M. Prenatal Metformin Exposure in Mice Programs the Metabolic Phenotype of the Offspring during a High Fat Diet at Adulthood. *PLoS ONE* **2013**, *8*, e56594. [CrossRef]
59. Grotenfelt, N.E.; Wasenius, N.; Eriksson, J.G.; Huvinen, E.; Stach-lempinen, B.; Koivusalo, S.B.; Rönö, K. Effect of maternal lifestyle intervention on metabolic health and adiposity of offspring: Findings from the Finnish Gestational Diabetes Prevention Study (RADIEL). *Diabetes Metab.* **2019**, *46*, 46–53. [CrossRef]
60. Rasmussen, K.; Yaktine, A. Institute of Medicine (US) and National Research Council (US) Committee to Reexamine IOM Pregnancy Weight Guidelines. *Weight Gain Pregnancy Reexamining Guidel.* **2009**. [CrossRef]

Publisher's Note: MDPI stays neutral with regard to jurisdictional claims in published maps and institutional affiliations.

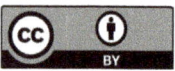

© 2020 by the authors. Licensee MDPI, Basel, Switzerland. This article is an open access article distributed under the terms and conditions of the Creative Commons Attribution (CC BY) license (http://creativecommons.org/licenses/by/4.0/).

Article

Main Fetal Predictors of Adverse Neonatal Outcomes in Pregnancies with Gestational Diabetes Mellitus

Maria-Christina Antoniou [1,*], Leah Gilbert [2], Justine Gross [2,3], Jean-Benoît Rossel [2], Céline Julie Fischer Fumeaux [4], Yvan Vial [2] and Jardena Jacqueline Puder [2]

1. Pediatric Service, Department Woman Mother Child, University Hospital of Lausanne, 1011 Lausanne, Switzerland
2. Obstetric Service, Department Woman Mother Child, University Hospital of Lausanne, 1011 Lausanne, Switzerland; leah.gilbert@chuv.ch (L.G.); justine.gross@chuv.ch (J.G.); jean-benoit.rossel@unisante.ch (J.-B.R.); yvan.vial@chuv.ch (Y.V.); jardena.puder@chuv.ch (J.J.P.)
3. Service of Endocrinology, Diabetes and Metabolism, University Hospital of Lausanne, 1011 Lausanne, Switzerland
4. Clinic of Neonatology, Department Woman Mother Child, University Hospital of Lausanne, 1011 Lausanne, Switzerland; Celine-Julie.Fischer@chuv.ch
* Correspondence: maria-christina.antoniou@chuv.ch; Tel.: +41-79-55-61-663 or +41-21-314-48-773

Received: 11 June 2020; Accepted: 14 July 2020; Published: 28 July 2020

Abstract: The objectives of this study were to (a) assess the utility of fetal anthropometric variables to predict the most relevant adverse neonatal outcomes in a treated population with gestational diabetes mellitus (GDM) beyond the known impact of maternal anthropometric and metabolic parameters and (b) to identify the most important fetal predictors. A total of 189 patients with GDM were included. The fetal predictors included sonographically assessed fetal weight centile (FWC), FWC > 90% and <10%, and fetal abdominal circumference centile (FACC), FACC > 90% and < 10%, at 29 0/7 to 35 6/7 weeks. Neonatal outcomes comprising neonatal weight centile (NWC), large and small for gestational age (LGA, SGA), hypoglycemia, prematurity, hospitalization for neonatal complication, and (emergency) cesarean section were evaluated. Regression analyses were conducted. Fetal variables predicted anthropometric neonatal outcomes, prematurity, cesarean section and emergency cesarean section. These associations were independent of maternal anthropometric and metabolic predictors, with the exception of cesarean section. FWC was the most significant predictor for NWC, LGA and SGA, while FACC was the most significant predictor for prematurity and FACC > 90% for emergency cesarean section. In women with GDM, third-trimester fetal anthropometric parameters have an important role in predicting adverse neonatal outcomes beyond the impact of maternal predictors.

Keywords: gestational diabetes; fetal ultrasound; fetal anthropometry; pregnancy outcomes; neonatal complications

1. Introduction

Gestational diabetes mellitus (GDM) carries an increased risk for short and long-term adverse outcomes, both for the mothers and their offspring [1,2]. In women with GDM, maternal anthropometric and metabolic parameters including prepregnancy BMI, gestational weight gain (GWG), maternal medical treatment requirement (metformin and/or insulin) and HbA1c at the end of pregnancy have been shown to influence and predict neonatal complications, such as small and large for gestational age (SGA, LGA), prematurity, hypoglycemia and cesarean section [3–5].

Third-trimester fetal ultrasound (US) is a helpful tool to predict neonatal outcomes. In the healthy pregnant population, estimated fetal weight (FW) was found to predict birth weight [6], whereas lower

FW and fetal abdominal circumference (FAC) were associated with preterm birth [7,8]. There is a need for studies investigating the association between third-trimester fetal parameters and diverse adverse neonatal outcomes in the context of a population with GDM. Fetal abdominal circumference centile (FACC) cut-offs in association with maternal capillary glycemic values have been used for medical treatment guidance in women with GDM, leading to a reduction in neonatal complications, but these studies were limited to experienced centres and obstetricians [9–11].

To our knowledge, it is not known whether fetal anthropometric parameters have an added value in predicting diverse neonatal outcomes beyond the known impact of different maternal anthropometric and metabolic variables.

When analysing fetal US parameters to guide decisions for monitoring during pregnancy, the utility of each parameter can be assessed. Comparable efficiency between estimated FW and FACC has been shown to predict both SGA and LGA in a mixed population with diabetes [12]. To date, no study has compared the effectiveness of the fetal anthropometric parameters, including fetal weight centile (FWC), FACC and their lower and higher cut-offs, in predicting the most relevant neonatal outcomes in women with GDM.

To answer these questions, the objectives of this study were: (1) to assess the utility of fetal anthropometric parameters to predict the most relevant adverse neonatal outcomes beyond maternal anthropometric and metabolic parameters in a population of women with GDM and (2) to identify the most important fetal predictors for these outcomes.

2. Experimental Section

This is a prospective observational study, which included a consecutive cohort of pregnant women with GDM followed in the Diabetes and Pregnancy Unit in the Centre Hospitalier Universitaire Vaudois (CHUV), Lausanne, Switzerland, between April 2012 and October 2017. Detailed information on the material and methods have been described in a previous study [3]. Briefly, we included all women with GDM who had signed an informed consent. Exclusion criteria were: multiple gestation, pregestational diabetes or diabetes diagnosed before 13 weeks of gestation, missing newborn sex and/or birth weight and missing fetal ultrasound data between 29 0/7 and 35 6/7 gestational weeks. Patients with concomitant pathologies or pregnancy complications were not excluded from the study.

GDM was diagnosed according to the International Association of the Diabetes and Pregnancy Study Groups criteria [13], including a 75-g oral glucose tolerance test at 24–28 weeks GA. The treatment was based on the current guidelines of the American Diabetes Association [14] and of the Endocrine Society [15]. At their first clinical appointment, patients were seen by a diabetes educator specialized in GDM or a medical doctor, received information on GDM, and were taught how to perform the capillary blood glucose test. A dietician saw these women one week later and provided them with advice to optimal glycaemic control, while providing all the nutrients required and to promote optimal weight gain during pregnancy. Women were encouraged to increase physical activity and had the possibility to receive physical activity counselling by a physiotherapist, as well as to participate in GDM physical activity groups. According to international and local guidelines (Vaud Cantonal Diabetes Program [16,17]), women were asked to check their capillary glucose values 4x/day. If, despite lifestyle changes, glucose values remained above targets, metformin or insulin treatment was introduced [13,14,16,17].

2.1. Maternal and Fetal Predictors and Neonatal Outcome Measures

Maternal anthropometric and metabolic predictors included prepregnancy body mass index (BMI), GWG, fasting, 1-h and 2-h blood glucose values during the 75g oGTT at 24–28 weeks of GA, HbA1c at the last visit at the GDM clinic, and maternal glucose lowering medical treatment requirement (metformin and/or insulin). Prepregnancy BMI was calculated based on pre-pregnancy weight that was retrieved from medical charts or self-reported, and on height measured at the first visit at the GDM clinic, using the formula weight(kg)/(height(m))^2. Height at the first GDM visit was measured to the nearest 0.1 cm with a regularly calibrated Seca® height scale. GWG was determined as the difference between the last weight measured before delivery and pre-pregnancy weight. Weight was measured to the nearest 0.1 kg in women wearing light clothes and no shoes with an electronic scale (Seca®). HbA1c at the last visit at the GDM clinic (last visit before delivery) was performed after March 2015, and was measured using a chemical photometric method (conjugation with boronate; Afinion®). Maternal treatment was obtained from medical charts and classified into 2 categories (no treatment, treatment with metformin and/or insulin). The latter category was not subdivided, as only 14 women were treated with metformin alone.

Fetal predictors consisted of FWC (ranging from 0–100%), FWC > 90%, FWC < 10%, FACC (ranging from 0–100%), FACC > 90% and FACC < 10%. All fetal ultrasounds were performed at the CHUV by trained obstetricians. Estimated FW using the Hadlock formula [18] and FAC were obtained during the antenatal ultrasound performed between 29 0/7 and 35 6/7 weeks of gestation. Fetal centiles were calculated using the Intergrowth 21st fetal size application tool [19].

Neonatal outcomes included neonatal weight centile (NWC), large-for-gestational-age (LGA), small-for-gestational-age (SGA), hypoglycemia, prematurity, hospitalization in the neonatal unit for a neonatal complication, 5-min Apgar score < 7, cesarean section (emergency and scheduled together) and emergency cesarean section by itself. All neonatal outcomes, with the exception of NWC, were binary. Neonatal weight (g) was documented at birth as an absolute value; NWCs were calculated using the Intergrowth 21st newborn size application tool [20]. LGA was defined as newborn weight centile > 90% for sex and gestational age. SGA was defined as newborn weight centile < 10% for sex and gestational age. Prematurity was defined as gestational age < 37 weeks. Gestational age was calculated according to the date of the last menstruations, or as assessed by the fetal ultrasound in the cases where gestational age was corrected during the first trimester ultrasound evaluation. According to the centre protocol based on national Swiss guidelines [21], all neonates from mothers with GDM received feeding in the first 2 h of life and were fed every 2–3 h during the first 48 h in order to prevent neonatal hypoglycemia. Systemic blood glucose monitoring was conducted in all newborns [21], and the frequency of the controls depended on whether the mother was treated or not with insulin during her pregnancy (at least 3 controls, and at least 8 controls over 48 h in case of maternal treatment). Neonatal glycemia was also measured if symptoms suggested hypoglycemia. Neonatal hypoglycemia was defined as capillary or venous glucose value ≤ 2.5 mmol/L. The blood glucose value (capillary or venous) was also verified at the CHUV central laboratory, if capillary glycemia measured by the glucometer was ≤ 2.5 mmol/L. Neonates were hospitalized for intravenous glucose infusion when they presented a symptomatic hypoglycemia, or a glycemia ≤ 2.0 mmol/L, or more than one hypoglycemia ≤ 2.5 mmol/L despite administration of dextromaltan and/or formula milk. Any hospitalization in the neonatal unit was documented. Cesarean section occurrence was documented (emergency and total including also scheduled cesarean sections). Emergency cesarean section included all non-scheduled cesarean sections for either a fetal or maternal indication. The exact indication of the emergency cesarean section was not specified. In cases of scheduled cesarean section, the decision for the cesarean section indication was taken by the mother's obstetrician as well the mother. Fetal and neonatal data were obtained from the center patient electronic medical chart for all newborns born in the CHUV.

2.2. Statistical Analysis

All data were analysed using Stata/SE 16.0 (StataCorp LLC, TX, USA). The normality of continuous variables was assessed, and normally distributed continuous variables were described as means and standard deviations (SDs). Binary outcomes were described as N (percentages) (Table 1). Linear and logistic regression analyses with adverse neonatal outcomes as the dependent variable, adjusting for gestational age at birth and neonatal sex where appropriate, and including the fetal and maternal variables as the predictor variables (see above), were initially conducted (Tables A1 and A2 of the Appendix A). In the specific case of emergency cesarean, comparisons were made with scheduled cesarean section. In order to evaluate the role of fetal anthropometric parameters beyond maternal anthropometric and metabolic parameters, the analyses of significant fetal predictors were additionally adjusted for significant maternal predictors (Table 2). Finally, in order to identify the most important fetal predictors for neonatal outcomes, we used stepwise procedures (backward elimination), in order to select the most important variables among those which are highly correlated. (Table 3). This latter analysis was also adjusted for significant maternal predictors in univariate analyses, as well as for gestational age at birth and neonatal sex as indicated before. For all analyses, beta-coefficients (for continuous outcomes such as neonatal centiles) and adjusted odds ratios (aORs-for binary outcomes, e.g., all other neonatal outcomes) are reported along with their 95% confidence intervals (CIs). The significance was set at $p < 0.05$. Due to the small number of some neonatal complications, analysis was only performed for adverse outcomes present in more than 10 cases [22]. Therefore, 5-min Apgar score < 7 was removed from the regression analyses.

Table 1. Descriptive maternal, fetal and neonatal characteristics.

Number of Patients	189
Maternal characteristics	
Age (years)	32.9 ± 5.4
Prepregnancy BMI (kg/m^2)	26.6 ± 5.4
Gestational weight gain (kg)	13.3 ± 7.2
Gestational weight gain until the 1st visit at the GDM clinic (kg)	10.5 ± 6.1
Fasting oGTT glucose value (mmol/L)	5.3 ± 0.7
1-h oGTT glucose value (mmol/L)	10.0 ± 2.1
2-h oGTT glucose value (mmol/L)	7.9 ± 2.0
Gestational age at the 1st visit at the GDM clinic (weeks)	28.2 ± 3.0
Gestational age at the last visit at the GDM clinic * (weeks)	36.1 ± 1.4
HbA1c at the last visit at the GDM clinic * (%)	5.7 ± 0.5
Maternal medical treatment requirement N(%)	104 (58.8)
Fetal characteristics	
Gestational age (weeks)	32.8 ± 1.5
Fetal weight centile * (%)	67.8 ± 21.4
Fetal weight centile > 90% * N(%)	33 (17.5)
Fetal weight centile < 10% * N(%)	0
Fetal abdominal circumference centile * (%)	65.9 ± 29.9
Fetal abdominal circumference centile > 90% * N(%)	54 (28.6)
Fetal abdominal circumference centile < 10% * N(%)	12 (6.4)
Neonatal characteristics	
Male N(%)	96 (50.8)
Gestational age at birth (weeks)	38.8 ± 1.5
Neonatal weight (g)	3252 ± 591
Neonatal weight centile [†] (%)	55.3 ± 31.7
LGA [‡] N(%)	41 (21.7)
SGA [§] N(%)	22 (11.6)
Neonatal Hypoglycemia ** N(%)	25 (13.9)
Prematurity [††] N(%)	16 (8.5)
Hospitalization for neonatal complication N(%)	25 (13.8)
5-min Apgar score < 7 N(%)	6 (3.2)
Cesarean section [‡‡] N(%)	88 (48.1)
Emergency cesarean section N(%)	41 (22.4)

Abbreviations: BMI body mass index, GDM gestational diabetes mellitus, oGTT oral glucose tolerance test, HbA1c glycated hemoglobin, LGA Large for gestational age, SGA Small for gestational age. * for gestational age using the Intergrowth 21st fetal size application tool [19] [†] for sex and gestational age using the Intergrowth 21st newborn size application tool [20]. [‡] LGA: birth weight >90th centile for sex and gestational age using the Intergrowth 21st newborn size application tool [20]. [§] SGA: birth weight < 10th centile for sex and gestational age using the Intergrowth 21st newborn size application tool [20]. ** capillary or venous glucose value ≤ 2.5 mmol/L. [††] gestational age <37 weeks. [‡‡] cesarean section includes scheduled and emergency cesarean sections.

Table 2. Fetal predictors of adverse neonatal outcomes after adjustment for maternal predictors.

Neonatal Outcomes	Fetal Predictors	OR/ Beta-Coefficient	Standard Error	95% CI		p Value
Neonatal Weight Centile (%) *	Fetal weight centile (%) †	0.94 ††	0.09	0.76	1.13	<0.001
	Fetal weight centile >90 (%) †	37.77 ††	5.62	22.66	44.88	<0.001
	Fetal abdominal circumference centile (%) †	0.55 ††	0.07	0.40	0.69	<0.001
	Fetal abdominal circumference centile >90 (%) †	30.27 ††	4.78	20.83	39.71	<0.001
LGA ‡	Fetal weight centile (%) †	1.09	0.03	1.04	1.14	<0.001
	Fetal weight centile >90 (%) †	10.90	7.10	3.04	39.09	<0.001
	Fetal abdominal circumference centile (%) †	1.09	0.03	1.03	1.14	0.001
	Fetal abdominal circumference centile >90 (%) †	9.46	5.54	3.00	29.83	<0.001
SGA §	Fetal weight centile (%) †	0.95	0.01	0.92	0.97	<0.001
	Fetal abdominal circumference centile (%) †	0.97	0.01	0.96	0.99	<0.001
	Fetal abdominal circumference centile >90 (%) †	0.13	0.13	0.02	0.99	0.049
Prematurity ¶	Fetal weight centile (%) †	0.98	0.01	0.95	1.00	0.038
	Fetal abdominal circumference centile (%) †	0.98	0.01	0.97	1.00	0.029
Cesarean section **	Fetal abdominal circumference centile < 10 (%) †	0.38	0.35	0.07	2.27	0.291
Emergency cesarean section **	Fetal weight centile > 90 (%) †	3.08	1.75	1.01	9.38	0.047
	Fetal abdominal circumference centile > 90 (%) †	3.17	1.58	1.20	8.41	0.020

Abbreviations: OR odds ratio BMI body mass index, GDM gestational diabetes mellitus, oGTT oral glucose tolerance test, HbA1c glycated hemoglobin, LGA Large for gestational age, SGA Small for gestational age. * for sex and gestational age using the Intergrowth 21st newborn size application tool [20]. † for gestational age using the Intergrowth 21st fetal size application tool [19]. ‡ LGA: birth weight >90th centile for sex and gestational age using the Intergrowth 21st newborn size application tool [20]. § SGA: birth weight <10th centile for sex and gestational age using the Intergrowth 21st newborn size application tool [20]. ¶ gestational age < 37 weeks. ** cesarean section includes scheduled and emergency cesarean sections. Emergency cesarean sections were compared to scheduled cesarean sections. †† this value corresponds to a beta-coefficient. Linear and logistic regression analyses, adjusted for neonatal sex, gestational age and significant maternal variables presented in Table A1.

Table 3 shows the main fetal predictors of neonatal outcomes using multiple logistic regression analyses. FWC was the most relevant fetal predictor for NWC, LGA, and SGA (inverse association; all $p < 0.001$). FACC was the most relevant predictor for prematurity (inverse association) and FACC > 90% for emergency cesarean section (both $p \leq 0.029$).

Table 3. Main fetal predictors of adverse neonatal and maternal outcomes.

Neonatal Outcomes	Fetal Predictors	OR/ Beta-Coefficient	Standard Error	95% CI		p Value
Neonatal Weight centile (%) *	Fetal weight centile (%) †	0.94 ††	0.09	0.76	1.13	<0.001
	Fetal weight centile > 90(%) †					0.306
	Fetal abdominal circumference centile (%) †					0.616
	Fetal abdominal circumference centile > 90 (%) †					0.887
LGA ‡	Fetal weight centile (%) †	1.09	0.260	1.04	1.14	<0.001
	Fetal weight centile > 90 (%) †					0.569
	Fetal abdominal circumference centile (%) †					0.287
	Fetal abdominal circumference centile > 90 (%) †					0.937
SGA §	Fetal weight centile (%) †	0.950	0.1200	0.920	0.970	<0.001
	Fetal abdominal circumference centile (%) †					0.750
	Fetal abdominal circumference centile > 90 (%) †					0.829
Prematurity ¶	Fetal weight centile (%) †					0.634
	Fetal abdominal circumference centile (%) †	0.98	0.01	0.97	1.00	0.029
Emergency cesarean section **	Fetal weight centile >90 (%) †					0.756
	Fetal abdominal circumference centile >90 (%) †	1.15	0.50	0.18	2.13	0.020

Abbreviations: OR odds ratio BMI body mass index, GDM gestational diabetes mellitus, oGTT oral glucose tolerance test, HbA1c glycated hemoglobin, LGA Large for gestational age, SGA Small for gestational age. * for sex and gestational age using the Intergrowth 21st newborn size application tool [20]. † for gestational age using the Intergrowth 21st fetal size application tool [19]. ‡ LGA: birth weight >90th centile for sex and gestational age using the Intergrowth 21st newborn size application tool [20]. § SGA: birth weight <10th centile for sex and gestational age using the Intergrowth 21st newborn size application tool [20]. ¶ gestational age < 37 weeks. ** emergency cesarean section was compared to scheduled cesarean section. †† this value corresponds to a beta-coefficient. Manual stepwise multiple logistic regression analyses with all significant fetal variables presented in Table A2, adjusted for neonatal sex and gestational age, as well as significant maternal variables presented in Table A1. The outcomes are only shown if at least one predictor remains significative.

2.3. Ethics

Signed informed consent was obtained from all participating women. The study was conducted in accordance with the guidelines of the declaration of Helsinki, and good clinical practice. The Human Research Ethics Committee of the Canton de Vaud approved the study protocol (326/15).

3. Results

Out of a population of 826 adult women with gestational diabetes, 111 women were excluded due to missing informed consent, 9 because they participated in an intervention clinical trial, 128 due to multiple gestation, missing newborn sex and/or birth weight and 389 because of missing fetal ultrasound data between 29 0/7 and 35 6/7 gestational weeks. Overall, 189 women were included in the final analysis.

3.1. Maternal, Fetal and Neonatal Characteristics

Detailed information about the maternal, fetal and neonatal characteristics are shown in Table 1. In summary, women were 32.9 ± 5.4 years old and had a mean prepregnancy BMI of 26.6 ± 5.4 kg/m2. The mean fetal and neonatal weight centiles were $67.8 \pm 21.4\%$, and $55.3 \pm 31.7\%$, respectively.

3.2. Associations Between Maternal and Fetal Predictors and Neonatal Outcomes

Prepregnancy maternal BMI, GWG, fasting, 1h and 2h glucose values at oGTT and need for maternal glucose lowering medical treatment (metformin and/or insulin) showed a significant association with one or more adverse neonatal outcomes such as NWC, LGA, SGA, hypoglycemia, and cesarean section (all $p \leq 0.046$, see Table A1 of the Appendix A). HbA1c at the last GDM visit did not show any association with neonatal outcomes. The maternal medical treatment requirement was the only maternal predictor for neonatal hypoglycemia ($p = 0.02$), whereas none of the maternal parameters were correlated with prematurity, hospitalization for neonatal complications or emergency cesarean section.

One or more of the fetal parameters were correlated with all adverse neonatal outcomes except for hypoglycemia and hospitalization for neonatal complications (all $p \leq 0.047$, see Table A2 of the Appendix A). The significance of fetal predictors did not change after adjusting for significant maternal predictors, with the exception of cesarean section; therefore, the FACC < 10% did not remain significant after adjustment for maternal glycemic values at the oGTT (Table A2 of the Appendix A and Table 2). Thus, after adjustment for maternal predictors, FWC was positively associated with NWC, LGA, and inversely with SGA and prematurity (all $p \leq 0.038$), while FWC > 90% showed a positive correlation with neonatal birth weight, LGA, and emergency cesarean section (all $p \leq 0.047$). Similarly, FACC was positively associated with neonatal birth weight, LGA, and inversely with SGA and prematurity (all $p \leq 0.029$). FACC > 90% showed a positive association with neonatal birth weight, LGA and emergency cesarean section, and an inverse association with SGA (all $p \leq 0.049$).

4. Discussion

The novel finding in this study of 189 clinically followed women with GDM was that third-trimester fetal anthropometric parameters can predict diverse relevant neonatal outcomes, such as anthropometry, prematurity, and emergency cesarean section, independently and beyond the impact of significant maternal anthropometric and metabolic predictors. However, none of the maternal or fetal parameters could predict hospitalization for neonatal complications. Maternal glucose lowering medical treatment requirement was the only predictor for neonatal hypoglycemia. FWC was found to be the most powerful predictor for NWC, LGA, and SGA, whereas FACC was the most powerful predictor for prematurity, and FACC > 90% for emergency cesarean section. Based on our findings, fetal ultrasound is a useful tool in the management of women with GDM, helping to independently predict adverse neonatal outcomes.

More specifically, FWC was an independent predictor for NWC, LGA, SGA and prematurity, while FWC > 90% was an independent predictor for neonatal birth weight, LGA, and emergency cesarean section. The association between FW and neonatal complications in the context of a population with GDM in a clinical setting still remains poorly studied, even in healthy pregnancies, studies mainly focused on anthropometric neonatal outcomes or a single adverse outcome. A previous study in a healthy population showed that estimated FW was a reliable predictor of actual birth weight; sonography appeared marginally more accurate in predicting SGA than macrosomia [6]. Alsulyman et al. compared discrepancies between intrapartum sonographically estimated FW and actual birth weight, and found a similar accuracy between women with (mixed GDM and pre-existent diabetes) and without diabetes [23]. Estimated FW assessed by ultrasound between 36 0/7 and 38 6/7 weeks of gestation predicted emergency cesarean section in a recent retrospective study including a predominantly healthy population (18% GDM) [24]. To our knowledge, this is the first study proving the utility of third-trimester sonographically estimated FW in the prediction of a series of neonatal outcomes, in the context of a population with GDM.

Moreover, FACC (%) independently predicted neonatal birth weight, LGA, SGA and prematurity, while FACC > 90% predicted neonatal birth weight, LGA, SGA and emergency cesarean section. Our study is in accordance with a study by Hawkings et al., which showed that in a healthy population, FACC < 10% was associated with a higher incidence of preterm delivery. Previous studies have used different sonographically assessed FACC cut-offs (>70% or 75% centile) and maternal capillary glycemic values in order to guide the medical treatment in populations with GDM [9–11]. GDM management based on FACC cut-offs, combined with less stringent glycemic criteria, resulted in similar rates of cesarean section, LGA, SGA, neonatal hypoglycemia, and neonatal admission compared to management based on strict glycemic criteria alone in a study by Schaefer-Graf et al. [10] and in lower rates of LGA, macrosomia and SGA in a study by Bonomo et al. [11]. A third-trimester FACC cut-off could be used for treatment guidance in women with GDM, aiming to reduce adverse neonatal outcomes.

We also evaluated the respective importance of FWC and FACCs, and their higher and lower cut-offs in predicting neonatal outcomes. FWC was found to be the most powerful fetal predictor for NWC, LGA, and SGA, while FACC was superior for the prediction of prematurity, and FACC >90% was a stronger predictor for emergency cesarean section. To our knowledge, this is the first study comparing the role of different fetal anthropometric parameters in the prediction of a series of neonatal outcomes in the context of a population with GDM. A previous study by Holcomb et al. demonstrated equal efficiency between sonographically estimated FW and FAC (without using centiles or cut-offs) in the prediction LGA, in a mixed population with diabetes [12]. In our study, FWC was more relevant for the prediction of neonatal anthropometric parameters at birth, whereas FACC was more relevant for the prediction of other outcomes, such as prematurity and emergency cesarean section. Thus, both parameters are useful and non-interchangeable in the follow-up of patients with GDM. In terms of clinical relevance, these parameters may be implemented in clinical practice for maternal treatment guidance, enabling a personalized treatment based on maternal metabolic control and fetal anthropometry.

HbA1c at the last visit at the GDM clinic was not associated with neonatal outcomes, which may be related to a smaller sample size due to missing data.

The strengths of our study included its originality and prospective nature, which ensured the presence of complete detailed information on maternal, fetal and neonatal characteristics. However, some limitations may also be noted. The emergency cesarean section indication was not specified, and the premature population was included as a whole. Dividing the population into emergency cesarean section subgroups (i.e., for maternal or fetal reason), as well as the subclassification of prematurity according to gestational age at delivery, could be interesting, but would lead to smaller sizes and limited statistical power. Moreover, as the exact indication for emergency cesarean was not specified, some of these may have been due to pregnancy complications not directly connected with gestational diabetes. The presence of an instrumentally assisted vaginal birth was also not investigated, due to insufficiently documented data. Lastly, we did not include fetal anthropometric data obtained during the second trimester of pregnancy, due to the limited number of patients followed at our tertiary hospital before the diagnosis of GDM. This was the authors' decision in order to ensure that all ultrasound measurements were performed with the same methodology and by an equally experienced team, in order to ensure data quality.

5. Conclusions

FWC and FACCs assessed in the third trimester predicted diverse relevant adverse neonatal outcomes at birth independently and beyond the impact of maternal anthropometric and metabolic parameters. FWC was found to be the most relevant predictor for neonatal anthropometric parameters (weight centile, LGA, SGA), and FACC and FACC > 90% were the most relevant predictors for prematurity and emergency cesarean section, respectively. Fetal anthropometry is thus a useful tool for risk stratification in pregnancies with GDM. Along with maternal anthropometric and metabolic parameters such as weight (changes) and glycemic control, it could be used for maternal treatment guidance, allowing for a personalized follow-up and eventually a decrease in adverse neonatal outcomes.

6. Patents

Not applicable.

Author Contributions: M.-C.A. participated in the conceptual design of the study, the data collection, analysis and interpretation and wrote the original draft. L.G. participated in the data collection and revised the final draft. J.G. participated in the data collection and revised the final draft. J.-B.R. participated in the statistical analysis and revised the final draft. C.J.F.F. contributed to the design and conceptualization of the study and revised the final draft. Y.V. contributed to the design and conceptualization of the study and revised the final draft. J.J.P. was the coordinator of the study, participated in the conceptual design of the study, the data analysis and interpretation and corrected all drafts. All the authors critically reviewed the article for important intellectual content and approved the final version submitted for publication. All authors have read and agreed to the published version of the manuscript.

Funding: This study was sponsored by an unrestricted educational grant from Novo Nordisk. The funding body did not take part in the design of the study, the collection, analysis, interpretation of data or in the writing of the manuscript. This study is a pilot of a project grant by the Swiss National Science Foundation (SNF 32003B_176119).

Conflicts of Interest: The authors declare no conflict of interest. The funders had no role in the design of the study; in the collection, analyses, or interpretation of data; in the writing of the manuscript, or in the decision to publish the results.

Appendix A

Table A1. Maternal predictors of adverse neonatal outcomes.

Neonatal Outcomes	Maternal Predictors	OR/beta-Coefficient	Standard Error	95% CI		p Value
Neonatal Weight Centile (%) *	Prepregnancy BMI (kg/m^2)	0.9 ‡‡	0.42	0.07	1.74	0.034
	Gestational weight gain (kg)	0.96 ‡‡	0.33	0.30	1.61	0.005
	Fasting oGTT glucose (mmol/L)	5.29 ‡‡	3.55	−1.70	12.29	0.138
	1-h oGTT glucose (mmol/L)	2.29 ‡‡	1.23	−0.14	4.73	0.065
	2-h oGTT glucose (mmol/L)	1.07 ‡‡	1.32	−1.54	3.68	0.419
	HbA1c at the last visit at the GDM clinic (%) †	1.59 ‡‡	9.12	−16.71	19.89	0.862
	Maternal medical treatment requirement	14.6 ‡‡	4.68	5.37	23.84	0.002
LGA ‡	Prepregnancy BMI (kg/m^2)	1.06	0.03	1.00	1.13	0.052
	Gestational weight gain (kg)	1.11	0.03	1.05	1.18	0.001
	Fasting oGTT glucose (mmol/L)	1.87	0.49	1.11	3.13	0.018
	1-h oGTT glucose (mmol/L)	1.22	0.12	1.01	1.48	0.040
	2-h oGTT glucose (mmol/L)	1.16	0.12	0.95	1.41	0.139
	HbA1c at the last visit at the GDM clinic (%) †	2.12	1.44	0.56	8.01	0.267

Table A1. Cont.

Neonatal Outcomes	Maternal Predictors	OR/beta-Coefficient	Standard Error	95% CI		p Value
SGA [§]	Maternal medical treatment requirement	6.61	3.36	2.44	17.89	<0.001
	Prepregnancy BMI (kg/m^2)	0.96	0.04	0.87	1.05	0.333
	Gestational weight gain (kg)	0.98	0.03	0.92	1.05	0.596
	Fasting oGTT glucose (mmol/L)	1.01	0.35	0.51	1.99	0.975
	1-h oGTT glucose (mmol/L)	1.04	0.14	0.81	1.35	0.743
	2-h oGTT glucose (mmol/L)	1.09	0.13	0.86	1.39	0.466
	HbA1c at the last visit at the GDM clinic (%) [†]	0.46	0.61	0.04	6.06	0.559
Neonatal Hypoglycemia [¶]	Maternal medical treatment requirement	0.37	0.18	0.14	0.98	0.046
	Prepregnancy BMI (kg/m^2)	1.03	0.04	0.95	1.11	0.483
	Gestational weight gain (kg)	1.03	0.03	0.97	1.10	0.310
	Fasting oGTT glucose (mmol/L)	0.93	0.31	0.49	1.78	0.831
	1-h oGTT glucose (mmol/L)	1.02	0.12	0.81	1.28	0.868
	2-h oGTT glucose (mmol/L)	1.08	0.13	0.85	1.38	0.534
	HbA1c at the last visit at the GDM clinic (%) [†]	0.34	0.33	0.05	2.31	0.267
Prematurity [**]	Maternal medical treatment requirement	3.83	2.21	1.23	11.88	0.020
	Prepregnancy BMI (kg/m^2)	0.95	0.05	0.86	1.06	0.375
	Gestational weight gain (kg)	0.98	0.04	0.91	1.06	0.609
	Fasting oGTT glucose (mmol/L)	1.35	0.47	0.68	2.68	0.384
	1-h oGTT glucose (mmol/L)	1.21	0.16	0.94	1.56	0.146
	2-h oGTT glucose (mmol/L)	1.23	0.15	0.96	1.56	0.098
	HbA1c at the last visit at the GDM clinic (%) [†]	13.37	18.98	0.82	215.73	0.068
Hospitalization for Neonatal Complication	Maternal medical treatment requirement	0.87	0.55	0.25	2.98	0.823
	Prepregnancy BMI (kg/m^2)	1.04	0.04	0.96	1.14	0.308
	Gestational weight gain (kg)	0.99	0.04	0.92	1.06	0.753
	Fasting oGTT glucose (mmol/L)	1.12	0.34	0.62	2.02	0.701
	1-h oGTT glucose (mmol/L)	1.11	0.12	0.90	1.39	0.329
	2-h oGTT glucose (mmol/L)	1.07	0.13	0.85	1.35	0.567
	HbA1c at the last visit at the GDM clinic (%) [†]	0.63	0.67	0.08	5.07	0.662
Cesarean Section [††]	Maternal medical treatment requirement	1.26	0.65	0.46	3.47	0.651
	Prepregnancy BMI (kg/m^2)	1.06	0.03	1.00	1.12	0.064
	Gestational weight gain (kg)	1.00	0.02	0.96	1.05	0.908
	Fasting oGTT glucose (mmol/L)	1.46	0.39	0.86	2.47	0.161
	1-h oGTT glucose (mmol/L)	1.22	0.12	1.01	1.47	0.038
	2-h oGTT glucose (mmol/L)	1.22	0.12	1.00	1.49	0.045
	HbA1c at the last visit at the GDM clinic (%) [†]	0.33	0.25	0.07	1.48	0.148
Emergency cesarean section	Maternal medical treatment requirement	1.28	0.42	0.68	2.42	0.440
	Prepregnancy BMI (kg/m^2)	0.97	0.04	0.90	1.04	0.370
	Gestational weight gain (kg)	1.01	0.03	0.95	1.07	0.852
	Fasting oGTT glucose (mmol/L)	1.13	0.31	0.66	1.93	0.656
	1-h oGTT glucose (mmol/L)	1.15	0.14	0.90	1.46	0.267
	2-h oGTT glucose (mmol/L)	1.06	0.13	0.84	1.34	0.630
	HbA1c at the last visit at the GDM clinic (%) [†]	3.88	4.16	0.48	31.73	0.206
	Maternal medical treatment requirement	0.93	0.44	0.37	2.35	0.881

Abbreviations: OR odds ratio BMI body mass index, GDM gestational diabetes mellitus, oGTT oral glucose tolerance test, HbA1c glycated hemoglobin, LGA Large for gestational age, SGA Small for gestational age. * for sex and gestational age using the Intergrowth 21st newborn size application tool [20]. [†] this corresponds to the last visit at the GDM clinic. [‡] LGA: birth weight >90th percentile for sex and gestational age using the Intergrowth 21st newborn size application tool [20]. [§] SGA: birth weight < 10th percentile for sex and gestational age using the Intergrowth 21st newborn size application tool [20]. [¶] capillary or venous glucose value ≤ 2.5 mmol/L; [**] gestational age < 37 weeks. [††] cesarean section includes scheduled and emergency cesarean sections. Emergency cesarean sections were compared to scheduled cesarean sections. [‡‡] this value corresponds to a beta-coefficient. Linear and logistic regression analyses, adjusted for neonatal sex and gestational age.

Table A2. Fetal predictors of adverse neonatal outcomes.

Neonatal Outcomes	Fetal Predictors	OR/beta-Coefficient	Standard Error	95% CI		p Value
Neonatal Weight centile (%) *	Fetal weight centile (%) †	0.96 §§	0.08	0.80	1.13	<0.001
	Fetal weight centile > 90 (%) †	37.73 §§	5.42	27.03	48.43	<0.001
	Fetal abdominal circumference centile (%) †	0.59 §§	0.06	0.46	0.71	<0.001
	Fetal abdominal circumference centile > 90(%) †	34.99 §§	4.43	26.26	43.72	<0.001
	Fetal abdominal circumference centile < 10(%) †	−14.63 §§	9.41	−33.19	3.94	0.122
LGA ‡	Fetal weight centile (%) †	1.10	0.18	1.06	1.14	<0.001
	Fetal weight centile > 90 (%) †	9.89	4.22	4.29	22.82	<0.001
	Fetal abdominal circumference centile (%) †	1.09	0.02	1.06	1.13	<0.001
	Fetal abdominal circumference centile > 90(%) †	11.89	4.84	5.35	26.42	<0.001
	Fetal abdominal circumference centile < 10(%) †	− §	− §	− §	− §	− §
SGA ¶	Fetal weight centile (%) †	0.95	0.01	0.93	0.97	<0.001
	Fetal weight centile > 90 (%) †	− §	− §	− §	− §	− §
	Fetal abdominal circumference centile (%) †	0.97	0.01	0.96	0.98	<0.001
	Fetal abdominal circumference centile > 90(%) †	0.10	0.11	0.01	0.78	0.028
	Fetal abdominal circumference centile < 10(%) †	2.77	0.20	0.69	11.14	0.151
Neonatal Hypoglycemia **	Fetal weight centile (%) †	1.00	0.01	0.98	1.02	0.855
	Fetal weight centile > 90 (%) †	0.78	0.46	0.24	2.49	0.674
	Fetal abdominal circumference centile (%) †	1.01	0.01	0.99	1.02	0.322
	Fetal abdominal circumference centile > 90(%) †	1.44	0.65	0.59	3.51	0.428
	Fetal abdominal circumference centile < 10(%) †	0.59	0.65	0.07	5.18	0.634
Prematurity ††	Fetal weight centile (%) †	0.98	0.01	0.95	1.00	0.038
	Fetal weight centile > 90 (%) †	0.67	0.52	0.14	3.11	0.608
	Fetal abdominal circumference centile (%) †	0.98	0.01	0.97	1.00	0.029
	Fetal abdominal circumference centile > 90(%) †	0.55	0.37	0.15	2.03	0.371
	Fetal abdominal circumference centile < 10(%) †	4.10	3.00	0.98	17.20	0.054
Hospitalization for Neonatal Complication	Fetal weight centile (%) †	1.00	0.01	0.98	1.02	0.780
	Fetal weight centile > 90 (%) †	0.94	0.55	0.30	2.98	0.922
	Fetal abdominal circumference centile (%) †	1.00	0.01	0.99	1.02	0.982
	Fetal abdominal circumference centile > 90(%) †	1.55	0.76	0.59	4.07	0.377
	Fetal abdominal circumference centile < 10(%) †	0.53	0.56	0.07	4.22	0.547
Cesarean Section ‡‡	Fetal weight centile (%) †	1.01	0.01	1.00	1.03	0.159
	Fetal weight centile > 90 (%) †	2.22	0.93	0.98	5.04	0.057
	Fetal abdominal circumference centile (%) †	1.01	0.01	1.00	1.02	0.129
	Fetal abdominal circumference centile > 90(%) †	1.45	0.49	0.75	2.80	0.275
	Fetal abdominal circumference centile < 10(%) †	0.21	0.16	0.05	0.92	0.038
Emergency cesarean section	Fetal weight centile (%) †	1.01	0.01	0.99	1.04	0.163
	Fetal weight centile > 90 (%) †	3.08	1.75	1.01	9.38	0.047
	Fetal abdominal circumference centile (%) †	1.01	0.01	0.99	1.03	0.252
	Fetal abdominal circumference centile > 90(%) †	3.17	1.58	1.20	8.41	0.020
	Fetal abdominal circumference centile < 10(%) †	0.23	0.30	0.02	3.02	0.265

Abbreviations: OR odds ratio BMI body mass index, GDM gestational diabetes mellitus, oGTT oral glucose tolerance test, HbA1c glycated hemoglobin, LGA Large for gestational age, SGA Small for gestational age. * for sex and gestational age using the Intergrowth 21st newborn size application tool [20]. † for gestational age using the Intergrowth 21st fetal size application tool [19]. ‡ LGA: birth weight >90th percentile for sex and gestational age using the Intergrowth 21st newborn size application tool [20]. § statistical analysis not possible due to the small number of outcomes. ¶ SGA: birth weight <10th percentile for sex and gestational age using the Intergrowth 21st newborn size application tool [20]. ** capillary or venous glucose value ≤ 2.5 mmol/L. †† gestational age < 37 weeks. ‡‡ cesarean section includes scheduled and emergency cesarean sections. Emergency cesarean sections were compared to scheduled cesarean sections. §§ this value corresponds to a beta-coefficient. Linear and logistic regression analyses, adjusted for neonatal sex and gestational age.

References

1. Ryser Ruetschi, J.; Jornayvaz, F.R.; Rivest, R.; Huhn, E.A.; Irion, O.; Boulvain, M. Fasting glycaemia to simplify screening for gestational diabetes. *BJOG* **2016**, *123*, 2219–2222. [CrossRef] [PubMed]
2. Mitanchez, D.; Yzydorczyk, C.; Siddeek, B.; Boubred, F.; Benahmed, M.; Simeoni, U. The offspring of the diabetic mother–short- and long-term implications. *Best Pract. Res. Clin. Obstet. Gynaecol.* **2015**, *29*, 256–269. [CrossRef] [PubMed]
3. Antoniou, M.C.; Gilbert, L.; Gross, J.; Rossel, J.B.; Fischer Fumeaux, C.J.; Vial, Y.; Puder, J.J. Potentially modifiable predictors of adverse neonatal and maternal outcomes in pregnancies with gestational diabetes mellitus: Can they help for future risk stratification and risk-adapted patient care? *BMC Pregnancy Childbirth* **2019**, *19*, 469. [CrossRef] [PubMed]
4. Li, N.; Liu, E.; Guo, J.; Pan, L.; Li, B.; Wang, P.; Liu, J.; Wang, Y.; Liu, G.; Baccarelli, A.A. Maternal prepregnancy body mass index and gestational weight gain on pregnancy outcomes. *PLoS ONE* **2013**, *8*, e82310. [CrossRef]

5. Barquiel, B.; Herranz, L.; Hillman, N.; Burgos, M.A.; Grande, C.; Tukia, K.M.; Bartha, J.L.; Pallardo, L.F. HbA1c and Gestational Weight Gain Are Factors that Influence Neonatal Outcome in Mothers with Gestational Diabetes. *J. Womens Health (Larchmt)* **2016**. [CrossRef]
6. Eze, C.; Ohagwu, C.; Abonyi, L.; Irurhe, N.; Ibitoye, Z. Reliability of sonographic estimation of fetal weight: A study of three tertiary hospitals in Nigeria. *Saudi J. Med. Med. Sci.* **2017**, *5*, 38–44. [CrossRef]
7. Boghossian, N.S.; Geraci, M.; Edwards, E.M.; Horbar, J.D. Neonatal and fetal growth charts to identify preterm infants <30 weeks gestation at risk of adverse outcomes. *Am. J. Obstet. Gynecol.* **2018**, *219*, 195.e1–195.e14. [CrossRef]
8. Hawkins, L.K.; Schnettler, W.T.; Modest, A.M.; Hacker, M.R.; Rodriguez, D. Association of third-trimester abdominal circumference with provider-initiated preterm delivery. *J. Matern. Fetal Neonatal Med.* **2014**, *27*, 1228–1231. [CrossRef]
9. Kjos, S.L.; Schaefer-Graf, U.; Sardesi, S.; Peters, R.K.; Buley, A.; Xiang, A.H.; Bryne, J.D.; Sutherland, C.; Montoro, M.N.; Buchanan, T.A. A randomized controlled trial using glycemic plus fetal ultrasound parameters versus glycemic parameters to determine insulin therapy in gestational diabetes with fasting hyperglycemia. *Diabetes Care* **2001**, *24*, 1904–1910. [CrossRef]
10. Schaefer-Graf, U.M.; Kjos, S.L.; Fauzan, O.H.; Buhling, K.J.; Siebert, G.; Buhrer, C.; Ladendorf, B.; Dudenhausen, J.W.; Vetter, K. A randomized trial evaluating a predominantly fetal growth-based strategy to guide management of gestational diabetes in Caucasian women. *Diabetes Care* **2004**, *27*, 297–302. [CrossRef]
11. Bonomo, M.; Cetin, I.; Pisoni, M.P.; Faden, D.; Mion, E.; Taricco, E.; Nobile de Santis, M.; Radaelli, T.; Motta, G.; Costa, M. Flexible treatment of gestational diabetes modulated on ultrasound evaluation of intrauterine growth: A controlled randomized clinical trial. *Diabetes Metab.* **2004**, *30*, 237–244. [CrossRef]
12. Holcomb, W.L.; Mostello, D.J.; Gray, D.L. Abdominal circumference vs. estimated weight to predict large for gestational age birth weight in diabetic pregnancy. *Clin. Imaging* **2000**, *24*, 1–7. [CrossRef]
13. International Association of Diabetes and Pregnancy Study Groups Consensus Panel. International Association of Diabetes and Pregnancy Study Groups Recommendations on the Diagnosis and Classification of Hyperglycemia in Pregnancy. *Diabetes Care* **2010**, *33*, 676–682. [CrossRef]
14. Management of Diabetes in Pregnancy: Standards of Medical Care in Diabetes—2020. *Diabetes Care* **2020**, *43* (Suppl. 1), S183–S192. [CrossRef]
15. Blumer, I.; Hadar, E.; Hadden, D.R.; Jovanovič, L.; Mestman, J.H.; Murad, M.H.; Yogev, Y. Diabetes and Pregnancy: An Endocrine Society Clinical Practice Guideline. *J. Clin. Endocrinol. Metab.* **2013**, *98*, 4227–4249. [CrossRef]
16. Diabète programme Cantonal, V. *Recommendations Pour la Pratique Clinique*; Programme Cantonal Diabète: Canton de Vaud, Switzerland, 2017.
17. Arditi, C.; Burnand, B.; Puder, J. Recommendations Pour la Pratique Clinique. 2017. [cited 19 September 2018]. Available online: http://recodiab.ch/RPC22_diabete_gestationnel_20171102.pdf (accessed on 17 February 2020).
18. Hadlock, F.P.; Harrist, R.B.; Sharman, R.S.; Deter, R.L.; Park, S.K. Estimation of fetal weight with the use of head, body, and femur measurements—A prospective study. *Am. J. Obstet. Gynecol.* **1985**, *151*, 333–337. [CrossRef]
19. Papageorghiou, A.T.; Ohuma, E.O.; Altman, D.G.; Todros, T.; Cheikh Ismail, L.; Lambert, A.; Jaffer, Y.A.; Bertino, E.; Gravett, M.G.; Purwar, M.; et al. International standards for fetal growth based on serial ultrasound measurements: The Fetal Growth Longitudinal Study of the INTERGROWTH-21st Project. *Lancet* **2014**, *384*, 869–879. [CrossRef]
20. Villar, J.; Cheikh Ismail, L.; Victora, C.G.; Ohuma, E.O.; Bertino, E.; Altman, D.G.; Lambert, A.; Papageorghiou, A.T.; Carvalho, M.; Jaffer, Y.A.; et al. International standards for newborn weight, length, and head circumference by gestational age and sex: The Newborn Cross-Sectional Study of the INTERGROWTH-21st Project. *Lancet* **2014**, *384*, 857–868. [CrossRef]
21. Tolsa, J.-F.; Truttmann, A.; Giannoni, E.; Muehlethaler, V.; Fischer, C.; Roth-Kleiner, M. *Vademecum de Neonatologie*, 12 December 2013 ed.; CHUV: Lausanne, Switzerland, 2013.
22. Peduzzi, P.; Concato, J.; Kemper, E.; Holford, T.R.; Feinstein, A.R. A simulation study of the number of events per variable in logistic regression analysis. *J. Clin. Epidemiol.* **1996**, *49*, 1373–1379. [CrossRef]

23. Alsulyman, O.M.; Ouzounian, J.G.; Kjos, S.L. The accuracy of intrapartum ultrasonographic fetal weight estimation in diabetic pregnancies. *Am. J. Obstet. Gynecol.* **1997**, *177*, 503–506. [CrossRef]
24. Yang, J.M.; Hyett, J.A.; Mcgeechan, K.; Phipps, H.; de Vries, B.S. Is ultrasound measured fetal biometry predictive of intrapartum caesarean section for failure to progress? *Aust. N. Z. J. Obstet. Gynaecol.* **2018**, *58*, 620–628. [CrossRef] [PubMed]

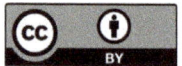

© 2020 by the authors. Licensee MDPI, Basel, Switzerland. This article is an open access article distributed under the terms and conditions of the Creative Commons Attribution (CC BY) license (http://creativecommons.org/licenses/by/4.0/).

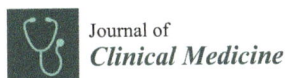

Article

Multidisciplinary Group Education for Gestational Diabetes Mellitus: A Prospective Observational Cohort Study

Caro Minschart [1,*], **Kelly Amuli** [2], **Anouk Delameillieure** [3], **Peggy Calewaert** [1], **Chantal Mathieu** [1] **and Katrien Benhalima** [1]

1. Department of Endocrinology, University Hospital Gasthuisberg, Catholic University Leuven, Leuven 3000, Belgium; peggy.calewaert@uzleuven.be (P.C.); chantal.mathieu@uzleuven.be (C.M.); katrien.benhalima@uzleuven.be (K.B.)
2. Nursing and Midwifery Research Group, Brussel Health Campus, University Hospital Brussel, Brussels 1000, Belgium; KellyAmuli@hotmail.com
3. Department of Chronic Diseases, Metabolism and Ageing, Laboratory of Respiratory Diseases, Catholic University Leuven, Leuven 3000, Belgium; anouk.delameillieure@kuleuven.be
* Correspondence: caro.minschart@kuleuven.be

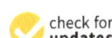

Received: 16 January 2020; Accepted: 11 February 2020; Published: 13 February 2020

Abstract: The value of diabetes education, focusing on lifestyle measures, in women with gestational diabetes mellitus (GDM) is acknowledged, but requires intensive education and input of resources if done on an individual basis. Group education could be a valuable alternative to individual education. This study aims to investigate the impact of multidisciplinary group education on women's knowledge about GDM, education, treatment satisfaction, and emotional status. Two hundred women with GDM were enrolled in a prospective observational study. Dutch speaking women were offered group education at their first visit after GDM diagnosis. Non-Dutch speaking women or women for whom group education was not possible received individual education. Individual follow-up with a dietitian was planned within two weeks for all women. Women receiving individual education ($n = 100$) were more often from an ethnic minority background compared to women in group education ($n = 100$) (32.0% ($n = 31$) vs. 15.3% ($n = 15$), $p = 0.01$). Knowledge about GDM significantly improved after education, with few differences between the two education settings. Both patients in group and individual education were equally satisfied with the content and duration of the initial and follow-up education. Of all group participants, 91.8% ($n = 90$) were satisfied with group size (on average three participants) and 76.5% ($n = 75$) found that group education fulfilled their expectations. In conclusion, women diagnosed with GDM were overall satisfied with the education session's content leading to a better understanding of their condition, independent of the education setting. Group education is a valuable alternative to better manage the increasing workload and is perceived as an added value by GDM patients.

Keywords: gestational diabetes mellitus; treatment; education; group education

1. Introduction

Gestational diabetes mellitus (GDM) is one of the most frequent medical conditions during pregnancy and is defined as diabetes diagnosed in the second or third trimester of pregnancy, provided that overt diabetes early in pregnancy has been excluded [1]. GDM is associated with an increased risk for fetal and maternal complications such as preeclampsia and macrosomia [2,3]. In the long term, women with GDM have a seven-fold increased risk of developing type 2 diabetes mellitus (T2DM). The offspring is also at increased risk of developing obesity, metabolic syndrome, and T2DM [4–8].

The 'International Association of Diabetes and Pregnancy Study Groups' (IADPSG) and the World Health Organization (WHO) currently both recommend a universal one-step strategy with a 75 g oral glucose tolerance test (OGTT) for the screening of GDM [9,10]. As these diagnostic cut-off values are more stringent and one abnormal glucose value is sufficient for the diagnosis of GDM, adoption of the new IADPSG criteria leads to an important increase in the prevalence of GDM, creating an important increase in workload and associated costs [11].

Treatment of women with GDM results in a lesser degree of perinatal complications and can potentially improve the health-related quality of life [2,3,12,13]. Initial treatment of GDM involves non-pharmacological approaches such as medical nutrition therapy, weight management, physical activity, and glucose monitoring [1]. If lifestyle measures are insufficient to reach and maintain glycemic targets, pharmacological therapy should be added [1]. Treatment of GDM should always start with education about medical nutrition therapy, physical activity, weight management, and self-monitoring of blood glucose (SMBG). The concept of self-management is thereby crucial to achieve good maternal and neonatal outcomes [14]. Therefore, diabetes educational programs for women with GDM should be organized in order to help them cope with their condition during pregnancy. However, the management of GDM is a labor-intensive discipline in which the rapidly rising prevalence of GDM poses challenges to maintain high-quality care [11].

Group education is a well-documented alternative to individual education in the organization of diabetes care in general, serving as a method to meet the educational needs of diabetes patients while at the same time providing peer support and motivation [15,16]. However, few studies have investigated the effectiveness of group education for the treatment of GDM. A study investigating multidisciplinary group education in women with GDM found that group sessions were associated with a reduction in carbohydrate consumption, an increase in physical activity level, and a combined clinical time saving of 8–28 h per week [17]. Another observational study in the United States demonstrated that women with GDM in group prenatal care required less insulin treatment, attended post-partum follow-ups more often, and underwent more often postpartum glucose screening compared to women who received conventional obstetrical care [18]. Factors associated with group education such as learning from the experience of peers, a greater connection with health care providers and a motivating group dynamic may partially explain these beneficial results [18]. A recent study demonstrated the benefits of group education sessions delivered by a specialized diabetes midwife and a dietitian on women's knowledge of GDM, but made no comparison with individual education sessions [19]. Additional high-quality studies in this research area are necessary to evaluate the feasibility and impact of group education compared with conventional individual education sessions in the management of GDM. This study aimed therefore to determine the impact of a multidisciplinary group education program for the management of GDM on women's knowledge about GDM, their satisfaction about the education and treatment, and their emotional status.

2. Materials and Methods

This study was performed in compliance with the principles of the Declaration of Helsinki (2008) and received approval from the local Ethics Committee of UZ Leuven (B322201525589). Prior to the first inclusion, the study was registered in Clinicaltrials.gov (NCT02528162). Participants provided written informed consent before inclusion in the study.

2.1. Study Design

This monocentric prospective observational cohort study was conducted at the University Hospital UZ Leuven in Belgium from October 2015 to September 2018. Since October 2015, the endocrinology department of UZ Leuven replaced the initial individual education session for the management of GDM as much as possible by structured group education sessions. Screening for GDM was based on a universal two-step screening strategy with a 50 g glucose challenge test (GCT) and a 75 g oral glucose tolerance test (OGTT) using the IADPSG/2013 WHO criteria. After diagnosis of GDM, Dutch speaking women were invited to attend a multidisciplinary group education session of maximum 1.5 h with a maximum of six participants. The session was organized on a weekly basis and was provided by a certified diabetes educator and a specialized diabetes dietitian. For non-Dutch speaking women or if group education was not possible, the first education session was delivered individually. A structured PowerPoint presentation was used both in the group and individual education sessions to educate about the pathophysiology, consequences and treatment of GDM—including dietary intake, physical activity and SMBG. The structure and content of this presentation was evaluated on a regular basis and adapted if necessary to the most recent guidelines and recommendations. For non-Dutch speaking patients, the presentation was translated to French and English. At the end of the education session, women received the handouts of the presentation, a brochure with information on physical activity, a glucose monitoring diary, a seven-day diet journal, a brochure on specific dietary guidelines with adapted recipes and material for SMBG.

Regardless of the initial education setting, all women were offered an individual follow-up session of 30 min with a dietitian within two weeks after the initial education session. During this session, women received further advice regarding their gestational weight gain and dietary habits based on their seven-day diet journal together with the SMBG results. The glycemic targets of the American Diabetes Association (ADA) were followed (fasting plasma glucose < 95 mg/dL (5.3 mmol/L) and two hours after meals < 120 mg/dL (6.6 mmol/L)) [1]. Further follow-up of glycemic values occurred every two weeks through email, phone or by attending the diabetes outpatient clinic as needed. In case of persistent inadequate glycemic control, treatment with insulin was started in consultation with an endocrinologist and women were followed-up at the outpatient diabetes clinic every two weeks until delivery. As part of normal routine, women with GDM were offered a 75 g OGTT three months after delivery to screen for glucose intolerance according to the ADA criteria [1]. Treatment and follow-up of women participating in the study were in line with normal routine for the management of GDM. There were no additional medical interventions, extra visits or additional blood tests compared to the treatment of women who did not participate in the study.

2.2. Study Participants

Women diagnosed with GDM could participate if at least 18 years old. Women were excluded if they had a history of bariatric surgery, were diagnosed with pregestational diabetes or if they could not speak fluently Dutch, French or English. All other women attending a group or individual education session were invited to participate in the study.

2.3. Study Assessments

Data were collected from the electronic medical records and through questionnaires. Outcome data from women who received the initial education session in group were compared to those from women who received the initial education session individually.

2.3.1. Self-Administered Questionnaires

All participants—both in group and individual education—were asked to complete several questionnaires at three different time points during the multidisciplinary education program: prior to the initial education session, immediately after the initial education session and after the individual follow-up session with the dietitian. The questionnaires aimed to evaluate the education of GDM, the knowledge on GDM and the emotional status. For this purpose, the questionnaires measured sociodemographic characteristics of the subjects, knowledge of GDM, feelings of depression and anxiety associated with the diagnosis of GDM, and the satisfaction with the education and the treatment. It took about 10 to 15 min at each point in time to fill in the questionnaires. All questionnaires were translated into French and English for non-Dutch speaking participants. An overview of the questionnaires administered at each time point is given in Table 1.

Table 1. Overview of the different self-administered questionnaires at the different visits.

	Prior to the Initial Session	after the Initial Session	after the Follow-Up Session
I: questionnaire on sociodemographic characteristics	x		
II: questionnaire on knowledge about GDM	x	x	x
IIIa: questionnaire on satisfaction with the initial session		x	
IIIb: questionnaire on satisfaction with the follow-up session			x
IV: CES-D questionnaire on depression	x	x	x
V: STAI-6 questionnaire on anxiety	x	x	x
VI: DTSQs questionnaire on treatment satisfaction			x

GDM: gestational diabetes mellitus; CES-D: Center for Epidemiologic Studies Depression; STAI: Spielberger State-Trait Anxiety Inventory; DTSQs: Diabetes Treatment Satisfaction Questionnaire—status version.

Questionnaire I on sociodemographic characteristics: A self-designed sociodemographic questionnaire—including data on education level, ethnicity, financial and marital status—was administered at the start of the initial education session. This questionnaire was based on a questionnaire that has previously been used in the Belgian Diabetes in Pregnancy Study [20].

Questionnaire II on knowledge of GDM: Knowledge of GDM was assessed before and after the initial session and after the follow-up session to measure knowledge gains, using a self-designed questionnaire containing 14 multiple-choice questions on risk factors for and consequences of GDM, diagnosis of GDM, treatment of GDM and follow-up after delivery. Proportions of correct responses on the knowledge questionnaire of the total cohort prior to the initial education session were compared to those after the follow-up session in order to evaluate knowledge improvement after education. In order to compare the knowledge about GDM between participants in group education and those in individual education, response rates on the knowledge questionnaire after the initial education session were compared between both groups.

Questionnaire IIIa and IIIb on satisfaction with the education sessions: Two self-designed questionnaires were created to evaluate satisfaction with the education program and whether treatment goals could be achieved. The first education satisfaction questionnaire (IIIa) was administered after the initial education session and evaluated the participant's degree of agreement with the clarity and relevance of the explanation on twelve items that were discussed during the presentation, using a five-point Likert scale. This questionnaire also contained an extra section with multiple choice questions for women attending the group education to evaluate perceptions on the duration of the group session, the advantages and disadvantages of group education and the size of the group. At the end of the questionnaire, an open question was included to share comments about the education session. The second education satisfaction questionnaire (IIIb) was completed after the follow-up session with the dietitian and again assessed participant's satisfaction with the twelve discussed items during the session. An additional set of questions on a five-point Likert scale was included regarding patient satisfaction on accomplishing lifestyle modifications in the week following the initial education session. At the end of this questionnaire, women were given the opportunity to share their opinions about the education session in an open question.

Questionnaire IV on depression: To measure possible feelings of depression, the 'Center for Epidemiologic Studies Depression' (CES-D) questionnaire was completed at all three time points. The CES-D questionnaire is a validated tool to use in pregnancy and consists of 20 items with each item being scored between 0 and 3 on a four-point Likert scale, from respectively 'rarely or none' to 'almost all the time'. Total score on the CES-D questionnaire can range from 0 to 60, with a score of $\geq$ 16 being suggestive for clinical depression [21].

Questionnaire V on anxiety: The validated six-item short-form of the Spielberger State-Trait Anxiety Inventory (STAI-6) questionnaire was administered at each point in time to measure state anxiety level. The six items are scored from 'very much' to 'not at all' with a four-point Likert scale and a total score ranging from 6 to 24, with a higher score referring to a greater level of anxiety [22,23].

Questionnaire VI on treatment satisfaction: The Diabetes Treatment Satisfaction Questionnaire—status version (DTSQs) is a validated tool for measuring satisfaction with diabetes treatment regimens and was administered after the follow-up session. This is an eight-item questionnaire in which each item is scored on a seven-point Likert scale from 0 to 6 [24]. The DTSQs scale score is calculated by summing the six satisfaction item scores. Total scores can range between 0 and 36, with higher scores indicating better treatment satisfaction. Item 2 and 3 are related to perceived frequency of hyperglycemia and hypoglycemia and are analyzed separately. They are reported on a seven-point Likert scale, with lower scores indicating fewer episodes of hyperglycemia or hypoglycemia [25].

2.3.2. Data from the Electronic Medical Records

Data from the participant's electronic medical record (EMR) were collected during pregnancy, at delivery and at three months postpartum. Maternal characteristics recorded were age, ethnicity, height, body weight, body mass index (BMI) at first prenatal visit and at delivery, overweight (BMI $\geq$ 25 kg/m^2), obesity (BMI $\geq$ 30 kg/m^2), gestational weight gain (difference in weight between delivery and first prenatal visit), parity, family history of diabetes, smoking, alcohol intake during pregnancy and history of GDM. Excessive gestational weight gain was defined according to the most recent Institute of Medicine (IOM) guidelines [26].

Data recorded about the diagnosis and treatment of GDM were timing and result of the GCT and OGTT, gestational age at the diagnosis of GDM, HbA1c at the time of the OGTT during pregnancy, time between diagnosis and start of the treatment, whether women received treatment with corticoids during pregnancy, need of insulin, type of insulin and gestational age at the start of insulin, timing and result of the postpartum OGTT.

The following maternal pregnancy outcomes were recorded: gestational hypertension (blood pressure $\geq$ 140/90 mmHg), preeclampsia (hypertension with proteinuria or in combination with reduced fetal growth or the 'Hemolysis Elevated Liver enzymes and Low Platelets' (HELPP)-syndrome), preterm delivery (<37 weeks of gestation) and cesarean section (planned and emergency sections combined). Neonatal pregnancy outcomes recorded were: gender, birth weight, macrosomia (birth weight > 4 kg), large-for-gestational age infants (LGA, birth weight > 90 percentile adjusted for sex and parity according to the Flemish birth charts), small-for-gestational age infants (SGA, birth weight < 10 percentile adjusted for sex and parity according to the Flemish birth charts), shoulder dystocia, Apgar score at five minutes and admission at the neonatal intensive care unit (NICU) [27].

2.4. Statistical Analyses

Statistical analyses were performed using SPSS software for Windows (IBM SPSS Statistics version 25.0, Armonk, NY, USA). Continuous data were expressed as mean and standard deviation (SD) if normally distributed, otherwise, variables were displayed as median and interquartile range (IQR). Categorical data were presented as frequencies and percentages. To compare variables between two groups, independent sample t-tests were used for normally distributed continuous variables, Mann-Whitney U-tests for non-normal variables and Chi-square tests for categorical variables. To evaluate the effect of the education, the Wilcoxon Signed Rank test was used for non-normal variables and McNemar test for categorical variables. Multivariable models were used to correct for significant differences in general patient characteristics between both groups. Linear regression was used for continuous outcomes and logistic regression for binary outcomes. A p-value of <0.05 (two-tailed) was considered significant.

3. Results

A total of 200 pregnant women with a recent diagnosis of GDM were enrolled. The prevalence of GDM over this period was 6.6% (n = 392). Women with GDM who did not participate in the study despite meeting the inclusion criteria (n = 145), were mostly women who received the initial education during hospitalization, were unable to participate due to practical reasons such as arriving too late for the education session, or women who declined to participate. Of all participants, 100 attended the initial education session in group and 100 received the initial education session individually. As this was an observational study, the equal division of participants over the two groups occurred by chance. The average number of women seen in each group education session was three. Results did not differ when excluding non-Dutch speaking women. The supplementary (Tables S1–S8), gives an overview of the general characteristics and comparisons between the individual and group education groups excluding non-Dutch-speaking women from the analyzes.

3.1. General Characteristics

The mean age of the participants was 32.3 ± 5.0 years, 11.2% (n = 13 of 116 women with more than one pregnancy) had a previous history of GDM, 23.7% (n = 47) had an ethnic minority (EM) background. The most frequent EM background was Asian in 10.6% (n = 21), Black-African in 4.0% (n = 8), Northern-African in 4.0% (n = 8), Middle-Eastern in 2.0% (n = 4) and Turkish in 1.5% (n = 3). Women receiving individual education were more often from an EM background than women in group education (32.0% (n = 32) versus 15.3% (n = 15), p = 0.01). There were no other significant differences in characteristics between women in each setting (Table 2). Of all women with GDM, 85.0% (n = 170) attended the postpartum OGTT of which 40.4% (n = 67) had glucose intolerance (Table 2).

Table 2. Baseline characteristics.

	General Cohort n = 200	Group Education n = 100	Individual Education n = 100	p-Value
age (mean ± SD)	32.3 ± 5.0	32.1 ± 5.3	23.6 ± 4.7	0.455
BMI at first prenatal visit (mean ± SD)	26.7 ± 5.4	26.5 ± 5.4	26.8 ± 5.4	0.695
overweight at first prenatal visit	30.6 (60)	29.3 (29)	32.0 (31)	0.917
obese at first prenatal visit % (n)	27.0 (53)	27.3 (27)	26.8 (26)	0.917
EM background % (n)	23.7 (47)	15.3 (15)	32.0 (32)	**0.010**
primigravida % (n)	39.9 (79)	44.0 (44)	35.7 (35)	0.410
first degree relative with T2DM % (n)	20.2 (40)	17.0 (17)	23.5 (23)	0.526
history of GDM (n = 116) % (n)	11.2 (13)	13.0 (7)	9.7 (6)	0.913
high secondary diploma % (n)	84.8 (168)	84.8 (84)	84.8 (84)	0.166
higher degree diploma % (n)	71.5 (138)	69.8 (67)	73.2 (71)	0.716
paid job % (n)	81.0 (158)	83.7 (82)	78.4 (76)	0.409
single % (n)	7.1 (14)	7.1 (7)	7.1 (7)	1.000
week at OGTT (median (IQR))	26 (24–28)	26 (25–27)	26 (24–28)	0.617
Hba1c % at OGTT (mean ± SD)	5.2 ± 0.4	5.2 ± 0.4	5.2 ± 0.4	0.768
insulin treatment % (n)	17.2 (33)	16.3 (16)	18.1 (17)	0.895
present at postpartum OGTT % (n)	85.0 (170)	88.0 (88)	82.0 (82)	0.990 *
weeks after delivery (median (IQR))	14 (10–18)	15 (12–18)	14 (9–19)	0.398 *
abnormal postpartum OGTT % (n)	40.4 (67)	35.6 (31)	45.6 (36)	0.284 *

GDM: gestational diabetes mellitus; BMI = body mass index; OGTT: oral glucose tolerance test; EM: ethnic minority; T2DM: type 2 diabetes mellitus; Statistically significant p-values are in bold; *p-values based on multiple linear and logistic regression adjusting for difference in EM background.

3.2. Pregnancy Outcomes

Of all woman, 21.9% (n = 41) had excessive gestational weight gain, 8.2% (n = 16) had preeclampsia and 30.3% (n = 59) had a cesarean section. Of all babies, 9.3% (n = 18) was LGA, 9.9% (n = 19) SGA and 5.2% (n = 10) had macrosomia. There were no significant differences in pregnancy outcomes between the different education groups (Table 3).

Table 3. Pregnancy outcomes of women in group versus individual education.

	General Cohort n = 200	Group Education n = 100	Individual Education n = 100	p-Value
Maternal Outcomes				
total weeks of gestation (median)	39 (38–40)	39 (37–41)	39 (38–40)	0.803 *
excessive weight gain % (n)	21.9 (42)	18.2 (18)	25.8 (24)	0.847 *
gestational hypertension % (n)	13.8 (27)	16.0 (16)	11.6 (11)	0.401 *
preeclampsia % (n)	8.2 (16)	12.0 (12)	4.2 (4)	0.075 *
preterm delivery % (n)	9.7 (19)	12.0 (12)	7.4 (7)	0.407 *
cesarean section % (n)	30.3 (59)	31.0 (31)	29.5 (28)	0.415 *

Table 3. Cont.

	General Cohort $n = 200$	Group Education $n = 100$	Individual Education $n = 100$	p-Value
Neonatal Outcomes				
macrosomia % (n)	5.2 (10)	5.0 (5)	5.3 (5)	1.000
LGA % (n)	9.3 (18)	6.1 (6)	12.8 (12)	0.069 *
SGA % (n)	9.9 (19)	9.1 (9)	10.8 (10)	0.764 *
shoulder dystocia % (n)	2.1 (4)	2.0 (2)	2.1 (2)	1.000
NICU transfer % (n)	6.2 (12)	7.0 (7)	5.4 (5)	0.774 *
Apgar score < 7 after 5 minutes % (n)	3.2 (6)	1.0 (1)	5.6 (5)	0.104

LGA: large for gestational age; SGA: small for gestational age; NICU: neonatal intensive care unit; Statistically significant p-values are in bold; * p-values based on multiple linear and logistic regression adjusting for difference in EM background.

3.3. Knowledge about GDM

Of all participants, 159 (79.5%) completed the knowledge questionnaire prior to the initial session and after the follow-up session. Women generally had good knowledge about GDM before the initial education session, which improved significantly for almost all items after the follow-up session (Table 4).

Table 4. Comparison of the correct responses on the knowledge questionnaire prior to the initial education session and after the follow-up session.

	Prior to the Initial Session $n = 159$ % (n)	after the Follow-Up Session $n = 159$ % (n)	p-Value
When is GDM diagnosed?			
24–28 weeks	95.6 (152)	98.7 (157)	0.180
How is GDM diagnosed?			
Based on a fasting blood collection in combination with drinking a sugar solution	82.4 (131)	87.4 (139)	0.201
It's more likely to develop gestational diabetes if you:			
Are overweight before pregnancy	78.0 (124)	87.4 (139)	**0.007**
Gain too much weight during the pregnancy	35.2 (56)	53.5 (85)	**<0.0001**
Have had GDM during a previous pregnancy	71.1 (113)	79.9 (127)	**0.011**
Have a first degree relative with diabetes	75.5 (120)	80.5 (128)	0.152
Your age is > 30 years	49.7 (79)	63.5 (101)	**0.002**
What are the consequences for the baby if the treatment of GDM is insufficient?			
Too high birth weight of the baby	85.5 (136)	97.5 155)	**<0.0001**
Increased risk of diabetes for the baby later on	60.4 (96)	74.2 (118)	**0.006**
Increased risk of overweight for the baby later on	50.9 (81)	69.8 (111)	**<0.0001**
What are the risks for you if the treatment of GDM is insufficient?			
An increased risk for a difficult delivery	77.7 (122)	91.7 (144)	**<0.0001**
An increased risk for preeclampsia	22.2 (35)	75.9 (120)	**<0.0001**
An increased risk for a cesarean section	66.5 (105)	89.9 (142)	**<0.0001**
How GDM is initially treated after diagnosis?			
Dietary change and increasing physical activity	59.1 (94)	79.2 (126)	**<0.0001**
Insulin is only started if dietary change and physical activity is insufficient	53.5 (85)	63.5 (101)	**0.049**
Which food products do you have to restrict if you have GDM?			
Pie	88.1 (140)	95.6 (152)	**0.008**
Fruits	19.5 (31)	54.1 (86)	**<0.0001**
Sugared soda	94.3 (150)	98.1 (156)	**0.031**
Fruit juice	74.8 (119)	93.1 (148)	**<0.0001**
Which fasting blood sugar level is normal in the morning?			
< 95 mg/dl	39.0 (62)	98.1 (156)	**<0.0001**

Table 4. Cont.

	Prior to the Initial Session $n = 159$ % (n)	after the Follow-Up Session $n = 159$ % (n)	p-Value
Which blood sugar level is normal 2 hours after eating?			
< 120 mg/dl	25.8 (41)	96.2 (153)	**<0.0001**
How can best be checked if your blood sugar levels are sufficiently under control?			
Based on a finger prick with a glucometer	79.0 (124)	98.7 (155)	**<0.0001**
What do you think about the treatment with insulin for GDM?			
This can lower the risk of an overweight baby	45.9 (72)	73.2 (115)	**<0.0001**
What do you think about breastfeeding after a pregnancy with GDM?			
This is good for the general health of the baby	58.5 (93)	89.9 (143)	**<0.0001**
This can lower the risk of diabetes and overweight in the baby later on	25.2 (40)	37.7 (60)	**0.002**
What do you think that happens with your GDM after your delivery?			
GDM disappears completely but I have a strongly increased risk of 50% to develop T2DM within 10 years	39.0 (62)	83.0 (132)	**<0.0001**

GDM: gestational diabetes mellitus; T2DM: type 2 diabetes mellitus; Statistically significant p-values are in bold.

Women showed an overall good knowledge of most topics after the initial education session, with almost no significant differences between the group and individual education groups (Table 5).

Table 5. Comparison of correct responses on the knowledge questionnaire between group and individual education after the first education session.

	Group Education $n = 98$ % (n)	Individual Education $n = 99$ % (n)	p-Value
When is GDM diagnosed?			
24–28 weeks	99.0 (97)	98.0 (97)	1.000
How is GDM diagnosed?			
Based on a fasting blood collection in combination with drinking a sugar solution	87.8 (86)	88.9 (88)	0.979
It's more likely to develop gestational diabetes if you:			
Are overweight before pregnancy	91.8 (90)	77.8 (77)	**0.011**
Gain too much weight during the pregnancy	38.8 (38)	40.4 (40)	0.930
Have had GDM during a previous pregnancy	77.6 (76)	65.7 (65)	0.091
Have a first degree relative with diabetes	89.8 (88)	75.8 (75)	**0.016**
Your age is > 30 years	62.2 (61)	52.5 (52)	0.217
What are the consequences for the baby if the treatment of GDM is insufficient?			
Too high birth weight of the baby	95.9 (94)	94.9 (94)	1.000
Increased risk of diabetes for the baby later on	80.6 (79)	75.8 (75)	0.514
Increased risk of overweight for the baby later on	73.5 (72)	70.7 (70)	0.785
What are the risks for you if the treatment of GDM is insufficient?			
An increased risk for a difficult delivery	91.8 (90)	90.9 (90)	1.000
An increased risk for preeclampsia	92.9 (91)	93.8 (83)	0.080
An increased risk for a cesarean section	90.8 (89)	90.9 (90)	1.000
How is GDM initially treated after diagnosis?			
Dietary change and increasing physical activity	81.6 (80)	79.8 (79)	0.884
Insulin is only started if dietary change and physical activity is insufficient	74.5 (73)	60.6 (60)	0.054

Table 5. Cont.

	Group Education $n = 98$ % (n)	Individual Education $n = 99$ % (n)	p-Value
Which food products do you have to restrict if you have GDM?			
Pie	96.9 (96)	91.9 (91)	0.221
Fruits	63.6 (62)	51.5 (51)	0.128
Sugared soda	95.9 (94)	94.9 (94)	1.000
Fruit juice	98.0 (96)	94.9 (94)	0.445
Which fasting blood sugar level is normal in the morning?			
< 95 mg/dl	98.0 (96)	92.9 (92)	0.170
Which blood sugar level is normal 2 hours after eating?			
< 120 mg/dl	96.9 (96)	91.9 (91)	0.221
How can best be checked if your blood sugar levels are sufficiently under control?			
Based on a finger prick with a glucometer	94.9 (93)	94.9 (94)	1.000
What do you think about the treatment with insulin for GDM?			
This can lower the risk of an overweight baby	77.6 (76)	71.7 (71)	0.437
What do you think about breastfeeding after a pregnancy with GDM?			
This is good for the general health of the baby	85.7 (84)	93.9 (92)	0.099
This can lower the risk of diabetes and overweight in the baby later on	32.7 (32)	34.7 (34)	0.880
What do you think that happens with your GDM after your delivery?			
GDM disappears completely but I have a strongly increased risk of 50% to develop T2DM within 10 years	85.7 (84)	86.9 (86)	0.977

GDM: gestational diabetes mellitus; T2DM: type 2 diabetes mellitus; Statistically significant p-values are in bold.

3.4. Satisfaction with the Education and Treatment

3.4.1. Satisfaction with the Education Sessions

Patients were overall satisfied with the content and duration of both the initial and follow-up education sessions (Table 6). The majority of all women were satisfied with the explanation that was given on the subject of pathophysiology, risks, treatment, and follow-up of GDM. There were no significant differences in satisfaction rates after the initial education session between women receiving group education and those receiving individual education (Table 6).

Table 6. Satisfaction rates with the given explanation on 12 items after the initial education session for women in group education compared to women in individual education.

	Strongly Disagree		Disagree		Neutral		Agree		Strongly Agree		I Don't Know		p-Value
	G % (n)	I % (n)	G % (n)	I % (n)	G % (n)	I % (n)	G % (n)	I % (n)	G % (n)	I % (n)	G % (n)	I % (n)	
Q1: What is GDM	0.0 (0)	1.0 (1)	0.0 (0)	0.0 (0)	2.0 (2)	0.0 (0)	21.4 (21)	18.4 (18)	75.5 (74)	80.6 (79)	1.0 (1)	0.0 (0)	0.568
Q2: Importance of treatment	0.0 (0)	1.0 (1)	0.0 (0)	0.0 (0)	3.1 (3)	0.0 (0)	16.3 (16)	14.3 (14)	80.6 (79)	84.7 (83)	0.0 (0)	0.0 (0)	0.426
Q3: Risks for myself	0.0 (0)	1.0 (1)	1.0 (1)	0.0 (0)	4.1 (4)	1.0 (1)	20.4 (20)	15.5 (15)	73.5 (72)	82.5 (80)	1.0 (1)	0.0 (0)	0.212
Q4: Risks for my baby	0.0 (0)	1.0 (1)	0.0 (0)	0.0 (0)	2.0 (2)	0.0 (0)	21.4 (21)	19.4 (19)	75.5 (74)	79.6 (78)	1.0 (1)	0.0 (0)	0.688
Q5: Treatment with diet	0.0 (0)	1.0 (1)	0.0 (0)	0.0 (0)	4.1 (4)	2.0 (2)	32.7 (32)	23.5 (23)	63.3 (62)	73.5 (72)	0.0 (0)	0.0 (0)	0.131
Q6: Treatment with physical activity	0.0 (0)	1.0 (1)	1.0 (1)	0.0 (0)	3.1 (3)	2.0 (2)	28.6 (28)	27.6 (27)	66.3 (65)	69.4 (68)	1.0 (1)	0.0 (0)	0.817
Q7: Weight gain	0.0 (0)	2.1 (2)	2.0 (2)	0.0 (0)	12.2 (12)	3.1 (3)	29.6 (29)	37.1 (36)	55.1 (54)	57.7 (56)	1.0 (1)	0.0 (0)	0.534
Q8: Measuring blood sugar levels	0.0 (0)	1.0 (1)	1.0 (1)	0.0 (0)	1.0 (1)	0.0 (0)	17.3 (17)	18.8 (18)	79.6 (78)	80.2 (77)	1.0 (1)	0.0 (0)	0.857
Q9: Treatment with insulin	0.0 (0)	1.0 (1)	3.1 (3)	4.2 (4)	23.7 (23)	11.5 (11)	34.0 (33)	35.4 (34)	37.1 (36)	44.8 (43)	2.1 (2)	3.1 (3)	0.129
Q10: Follow-up after delivery	0.0 (0)	1.0 (1)	1.0 (1)	0.0 (0)	2.0 (2)	2.0 (2)	31.6 (31)	28.6 (28)	64.3 (63)	68.4 (67)	1.0 (1)	0.0 (0)	0.741
Q11: Risk of diabetes after delivery	0.0 (0)	1.0 (1)	1.0 (1)	0.0 (0)	4.1 (4)	0.0 (0)	25.5 (25)	26.5 (26)	68.4 (67)	71.4 (70)	1.0 (1)	1.0 (1)	0.539
Q12: Breastfeeding	0.0 (0)	2.1 (2)	3.1 (3)	1.0 (1)	3.1 (3)	2.1 (2)	27.6 (27)	23.7 (23)	66.3 (65)	71.1 (69)	0.0 (0)	0.0 (0)	0.481

Q = question; G: group education; I: individual education; GDM: gestational diabetes mellitus.

Of all women who completed the additional questions about group education ($n = 98$), 91.8% ($n = 90$) were pleased with the size of the group. A large majority of 76.5% ($n = 75$) indicated that group education fulfilled their expectations, although 22% ($n = 22$) indicated that they would prefer supplementary individual education after group education. Only four women (4.1%) preferred individual education alone. The most frequently reported advantages of group education were 'learning from the questions of others' (74.5%, $n = 73$) and 'learning from the experience of others' (50.0%, $n = 49$), followed by 'feeling supported by the group' (26.5%, $n = 26$) and 'helping you to stick to the advice' (14.3%, $n = 14$). However, 10 women (10.2%) reported no advantages of group education and four women (4.1%) indicated that they felt inhibited by the group.

3.4.2. Satisfaction with the Treatment Regimen

Of all responders ($n = 152$), a large majority agreed that is was possible to follow the advice about diet, physical activity, weight gain, and glycemic measurements. Almost all participants agreed or strongly agreed with the statement that they were confident in the given advice (96.7%, $n = 147$). However, 23.0% ($n = 35$) perceived the advice to be too strict and indicated that they felt starved. There were no significant differences in agreement with the feasibility of the advice between women who received group education and those who received individual education (Table 7).

Mean total score of the DTSQs was 27.3 (± 0.5) and this was not significantly different for women in group or individual education (27.1 $\pm$ 5.4 versus 27.5 $\pm$ 5.6, $p = 0.692$). Mean total score for the two items on perceived hyper- or hypoglycemia was 3.1 (± 2.1) and this was not significantly different between both education groups (2.9 $\pm$ 1.8 versus 3.3 $\pm$ 2.4, $p = 0.240$).

3.5. Emotional Status

Of all responders ($n = 148$), 25.0% ($n = 37$) had a total score ≥ 16 at the CES-D questionnaire prior to the initial education session and were therefore considered at risk for clinical depression. This percentage declined to 18.9% ($n = 28$) after the follow-up session ($p = 0.137$). The median total score on the STAI-6 questionnaire decreased significantly from 12 (10–14) at the start of the initial education session to 11 (8–13) at the end of the follow-up session ($p < 0.0001$).

No significant differences in clinical depression rates (25.6% versus 24.2%, $p = 0.967$) or median anxiety scores (11.0 versus 10.5, $p = 0.294$) were observed between both education groups after the initial education session.

3.6. Comments on the Education Sessions

In general, most women indicated that the explanation was sufficient and felt that all of their questions had been addressed during the education sessions. However, topics such as postpartum follow-up and future risks should have been addressed in more detail according to a few women. Another recurring comment was the demand for specific recipes and nutritional instructions. Women often indicated that they were well aware of what they should not eat, but struggled with deciding what they were allowed to eat instead.

Table 7. Agreement with the feasibility of the advice for the management of GDM.

	Strongly Disagree		Disagree		Neutral		Agree		Strongly Agree		I Don't Know		p-Value
	G % (n)	I % (n)	G % (n)	I % (n)	G % (n)	I % (n)	G % (n)	I % (n)	G % (n)	I % (n)	G % (n)	I % (n)	
Advice about diet	0.0 (0)	0.0 (0)	0.0 (0)	1.2 (1)	8.5 (6)	4.9 (4)	36.6 (26)	42.0 (34)	54.9 (39)	51.9 (42)	0.0 (0)	0.0 (0)	0.821
Advice about physical activity	0.0 (0)	0.0 (0)	5.6 (4)	6.3 (5)	11.1 (8)	8.9 (7)	43.1 (31)	41.8 (33)	40.3 (29)	43.0 (34)	0.0 (0)	0.0 (0)	0.733
Advice about treatment with insulin *	20.0 (1)	0.0 (0)	0.0 (0)	0.0 (0)	0.0 (0)	12.5 (1)	60.0 (3)	37.5 (3)	0.0 (0)	12.5 (1)	20.0 (1)	37.5 (3)	0.435
Advice about weight gain	0.0 (0)	0.0 (0)	1.4 (1)	0.0 (0)	5.8 (4)	11.3 (9)	43.5 (30)	40.0 (32)	49.3 (34)	46.3 (37)	0.0 (0)	2.5 (2)	0.896
Advice about SMBG	0.0 (0)	0.0 (0)	0.0 (0)	0.0 (0)	1.4 (1)	1.3 (1)	36.1 (26)	31.3 (25)	62.5 (45)	67.5 (54)	0.0 (0)	0.0 (0)	0.523
The advice was too strict and I felt starved	22.5 (16)	13.6 (11)	38.0 (27)	43.2 (35)	18.3 (13)	16.0 (13)	14.1 (10)	11.1 (9)	5.6 (4)	14.8 (12)	1.4 (1)	1.2 (1)	0.212
I am confident in the given advice	1.4 (1)	0.0 (0)	0.0 (0)	0.0 (0)	4.2 (3)	1.2 (1)	35.2 (25)	42.0 (34)	59.2 (42)	56.8 (46)	0.0 (0)	0.0 (0)	0.959

* Only those who were treated with insulin and filled in the questionnaire (n = 13); I: individual education; G: group education; GDM: gestational diabetes mellitus; SMBG: self-monitoring of blood glucose.

4. Discussion

Due to the worldwide obesity epidemic and the adoption of the 2013 WHO diagnostic criteria, the prevalence of GDM will continue to increase. This contributes to a number of practical challenges in the management of GDM, such as an increased workload for health care providers and a growing demand for additional resources [11,28]. In order to cope with this increasing burden, it may be useful to reconsider the way in which health care services are currently provided for women with newly diagnosed GDM. Group education is a commonly used approach in the treatment of diabetes, but little is known about the effectiveness of group education in women with GDM in particular. However, gaining sufficient insight into the perceptions of GDM patients with regard to their treatment is crucial to better organize educational programs that are adapted to their needs.

Improved knowledge about GDM in newly diagnosed women might result in better adoption of a healthy lifestyle, better treatment adherence and better self-management. A Malaysian study among 175 women with GDM demonstrated that better knowledge about GDM is related to better glycemic control [29]. Our study showed that a multidisciplinary education program for the management of GDM can effectively improve the knowledge on GDM with almost no difference whether women received group education or individual education. This finding is consistent with a recent Irish study investigating the effectiveness of group education on knowledge of women with newly diagnosed GDM [19]. However, no comparison was made with individual education in the Irish study. A Canadian study further investigated the impact of small-group versus individual nutritional counseling on knowledge improvement of women with GDM and showed that women with GDM can be effectively and cost-efficiently counselled on nutrition in small-group settings. [30].

Patient satisfaction is an important consideration in the organization of medical care, since improved satisfaction rates appear to be associated with a more effective engagement in health care programs [31]. In this prospective study, participants were overall satisfied with the content and duration of both the initial and follow-up education sessions, independent of whether they received group or individual education. The majority agreed with the clarity and relevance of the explanation given about the different aspects of GDM. Furthermore, almost all participants were confident in the given advice. However, a considerable group of women (23.0%) perceived the advice to be too strict and indicated that they felt starved. The same observations were made in the Italian DAWN (Diabetes Attitudes, Wishes, and Needs) Pregnancy Study, which was promoted by the International Diabetes Federation to evaluate the quality of life, wishes and needs in women diagnosed with GDM [32]. In this study, women indicated that they experienced difficulties in following the treatment regimen and that the dietary advice was one of their biggest concerns. This study also showed that the issue of eating habits among immigrant women with GDM is often more difficult compared to indigenous women. To address these concerns, we have developed leaflets in cooperation with specialized diabetes dietitians on specific dietary guidelines and with adapted recipes for Flemish, Asian, and North-African cuisine.

The results of the DTSQs revealed that the participants were generally very satisfied with their treatment, whether they received group or individual education. A Malaysian study in women with GDM showed that higher treatment satisfaction is associated with better glycemic control [25]. Other studies in the field of diabetes research have demonstrated that treatment satisfaction can have a significant impact on clinical outcomes as well as on treatment adherence [33,34]. Determining patient treatment satisfaction levels could therefore be a useful tool in improving healthcare delivery in patients with GDM.

More than 90% of all group participants were satisfied with the group size and almost 80% indicated that group education met their expectations. Only a small minority reported that they felt inhibited by the group and preferred individual education. This is in contrast to the findings of a study from New Zealand, establishing that only a minority of the people surveyed would consider participating in a group session, fearing that less attention would be paid to the individual needs of each patient [35]. In our study, the most important advantages reported with group education were learning from others' questions and experiences. This is in line with another observational study on GDM, showing that the beneficial effects of their prenatal group care program were associated with factors as learning from the experience of peers, a greater connection with health care providers, and a motivating group dynamic [18].

Depression is a common condition in women with GDM, with studies reporting depression rates between 15% and 20% in this population [36,37]. In our cohort, 25% of all women were considered at risk for clinical depression prior to the initial education session, which declined to 18.9% after the follow-up session, although this was not statistically significant. Depression can lead to poor management of GDM, thus increasing the risk of adverse pregnancy outcomes such as macrosomia and neonatal hypoglycemia [38]. Health care providers should therefore be aware of the risk of antenatal depression when treating women with GDM and should regularly screen for depression in order to timely provide appropriate care. GDM can also cause maternal anxiety and stress related to the perception of a high-risk pregnancy, fear of maternal and neonatal complications and the feeling of losing control during the process of dietary management [39]. However, feelings of anxiety tend to decrease throughout pregnancy, which could be related to the understanding that GDM is a self-limiting condition and which might suggest that education and reassurance by health care providers is successful in dissipating anxiety in women diagnosed with GDM [40]. This is in line with the findings in our study, as feelings of anxiety were apparent prior to the initial education but declined significantly after education was given. To our knowledge, no studies have been conducted to compare feelings of depression and anxiety between women with GDM in group versus individual education. We show that there were no significant differences in terms of feelings of depression and anxiety between patients receiving group education and those receiving individual education.

We present the first prospective study on the impact of group education on patient's knowledge about GDM, their satisfaction with the education and treatment, and emotional status. Our study demonstrates that group education is at least as good an alternative to individual education with regard to these outcomes. Moreover, our results did not differ when non-Dutch speaking women were excluded from the analyzes.

Our study has several strengths. We provide prospective data of a large cohort of women with GDM, allowing the evaluation of the impact of group education compared to individual education. In addition, we used several validated questionnaires to evaluate treatment satisfaction and emotional status of women with GDM. When validated questionnaires were not available, we used self-designed questionnaires based on our experience and previous research in women with GDM. We included French and English speaking women in our cohort, ensuring that our results are representative of a multi-ethnic population. However, we could not evaluate group education for non-Dutch-speaking, since group education was only offered to Dutch-speaking women in line with routine care in our hospital.

A limitation of our study is the observational design. Women following individual education were more often from an EM background than women in group education, but we corrected for this difference through multiple regression analysis. In addition, some participation bias is likely since not all eligible patients participated in the study and we have no data available on their characteristics.

5. Conclusions

The results of this study show that women with newly diagnosed GDM are overall satisfied with their education and treatment, and have a better understanding of their condition after education, independent of the education setting. We show that group education is a valuable alternative to better organize education in view of the increasing GDM prevalence and is perceived as an added value by GDM patients.

Supplementary Materials: The following are available online at http://www.mdpi.com/2077-0383/9/2/509/s1, Table S1: Baseline characteristics, Table S2: Pregnancy outcomes of women in group versus individual education, Table S3: Comparison of the correct responses on the knowledge questionnaire prior to the initial education session and after the follow-up session, Table S4: Comparison of correct responses on the knowledge questionnaire between group and individual education after the first education session, Table S5: Satisfaction rates with the given explanation on 12 items after the initial education session for women in group education compared to women in individual education, Table S6: Agreement with the feasibility of the advice for the management of GDM for women in group education compared to women in individual education, Table S7: Emotional status before the initial education session versus after the follow-up session for the complete Dutch cohort, Table S8: Emotional status in group versus individual education at the end of the initial education session.

Author Contributions: Conceptualization, P.C. and K.B.; Data curation, C.M. (Caro Minschart), K.A. and A.D.; Formal analysis, C.M. (Caro Minschart); Investigation, C.M. (Caro Minschart), K.A. and A.D.; Project administration, C.M. (Caro Minschart), K.A., A.D. and P.C.; Visualization, C.M. (Caro Minschart); Writing—original draft, C.M. (Caro Minschart) and K.B.; Writing—review & editing, C.M. (Caro Minschart), K.A., A.D., P.C., C.M. (Chantal Mathieu) and K.B. All authors have read and agreed to the published version of the manuscript.

Funding: This research received no external funding.

Acknowledgments: C.M. has a PhD Fellowship Strategic Basic Research of the Research Foundation– Flanders (FWO). K.B. is the recipient of a 'Fundamenteel Klinisch Navorserschap FWO Vlaanderen'.

Conflicts of Interest: The authors declare no conflict of interest.

References

1. American Diabetes Association. *Standards of Medical Care in Diabetes-2017*. Diabetes Care; American Diabetes Association: Arlington, VA, USA, 2017; Volume 40.
2. Crowther, C.A.; Hiller, J.E.; Moss, J.R.; McPhee, A.J.; Jeffries, W.S.; Robinson, J.S. Effect of Treatment of Gestational Diabetes Mellitus on Pregnancy Outcomes. *N. Engl. J. Med.* **2005**, *352*, 2477–2486. [CrossRef] [PubMed]
3. Landon, M.B.; Spong, C.Y.; Thom, E.; Carpenter, M.W.; Ramin, S.M.; Casey, B.; Wapner, R.J.; Varner, M.W.; Rouse, D.J.; Thorp, J.M., Jr.; et al. A Multicenter, Randomized Trial of Treatment for Mild Gestational Diabetes. *N. Engl. J. Med.* **2009**, *361*, 1339–1348. [CrossRef] [PubMed]
4. Bellamy, L.; Casas, J.P.; Hingorani, A.D.; Williams, D. Type 2 diabetes mellitus after gestational diabetes: A systematic review and meta-analysis. *Lancet* **2009**, *373*, 1773–1779. [CrossRef]
5. Damm, P.; Houshmand-Oeregaard, A.; Kelstrup, L.; Lauenborg, J.; Mathiesen, E.R.; Clausen, T.D. Gestational diabetes mellitus and long-term consequences for mother and offspring: A view from Denmark. *Diabetologia* **2016**, *59*, 1396–1399. [CrossRef]
6. Zhao, P.; Liu, E.; Qiao, Y.; Katzmarzyk, P.T.; Chaput, J.-P.; Fogelholm, M.; Johnson, W.D.; Kuriyan, R.; Kurpad, A.; Lambert, E.V.; et al. Maternal gestational diabetes and childhood obesity at age 9–11: Results of a multinational study. *Diabetologia* **2016**, *59*, 2339–2348. [CrossRef] [PubMed]
7. Clausen, T.D.; Mathiesen, E.R.; Hansen, T.; Pedersen, O.; Jensen, D.M.; Lauenborg, J.; Schmidt, L.; Damm, P. Overweight and the Metabolic Syndrome in Adult Offspring of Women with Diet-Treated Gestational Diabetes Mellitus or Type 1 Diabetes. *J. Clin. Endocrinol. Metab.* **2009**, *94*, 2464–2470. [CrossRef]
8. Clausen, T.D.; Mathiesen, E.R.; Hansen, T.; Pedersen, O.; Jensen, D.M.; Lauenborg, J.; Damm, P. High Prevalence of Type 2 Diabetes and Pre-Diabetes in Adult Offspring of Women with Gestational Diabetes Mellitus or Type 1 Diabetes The role of intrauterine hyperglycemia. *Diabetes Care* **2008**, *31*, 340–346. [CrossRef]
9. International Association of Diabetes and Pregnancy Study Groups Consensus Panel. International Association of Diabetes and Pregnancy Study Groups Recommendations on the Diagnosis and Classification of Hyperglycemia in Pregnancy. *Diabetes Care* **2010**, *33*, 676–682. [CrossRef] [PubMed]
10. Agarwal, M.; Boulvain, M.; Coetzee, E.; Colagiuri, S. Diagnostic criteria and classification of hyperglycaemia first detected in pregnancy: A World Health Organization Guideline. *Diabetes Res. Clin. Pract.* **2014**, *103*, 341–363.
11. Flack, J.R.; Ross, G.P.; Ho, S.; McElduff, A. Recommended changes to diagnostic criteria for gestational diabetes: Impact on workload. *Aust. N. Z. J. Obstet. Gynaecol.* **2010**, *50*, 439–443. [CrossRef] [PubMed]
12. Hartling, L.; Dryden, D.M.; Guthrie, A.; Muise, M.; Vandermeer, B.; Donovan, L. Benefits and Harms of Treating Gestational Diabetes Mellitus: A Systematic Review and Meta-analysis for the U.S. Preventive Services Task Force and the National Institutes of Health Office of Medical Applications of Research. *Ann. Intern Med.* **2013**, *159*, 123–129. [CrossRef] [PubMed]

13. Brown, J.; Alwan, N.A.; West, J.; Brown, S.; McKindlay, C.J.; Farrar, D.; Crowther, C.A. Lifestyle interventions for the treatment of women with gestational diabetes. *Cochrane Database Syst. Rev.* **2017**. [CrossRef] [PubMed]
14. Carolan, M.; Steele, C.; Margetts, H. Attitudes towards gestational diabetes among a multiethnic cohort in Australia. *J. Clin. Nurs.* **2010**, *19*, 2446–2453. [CrossRef] [PubMed]
15. Mensing, C.R.; Norris, S.L. Group Education in Diabetes: Effectiveness and Implementation. *Diabetes Spectr.* **2003**, *16*, 96–103. [CrossRef]
16. Ridge, T. Shared Medical Appointments in Diabetes Care: A Literature Review. *Diabetes Spectr.* **2012**, *25*, 72–75. [CrossRef]
17. Tadesse, W.G.; Dunlevy, F.; Nazir, S.F.; Doherty, H.; Turner, M.J.; Kinsley, B.; Daly, S. Multidisciplinary group education for the treatment of gestational diabetes mellitus. *Am. J. Obstet. Gynecol.* **2016**, *214*, S92–S93. [CrossRef]
18. Mazzoni, S.E.; Hill, P.K.; Webster, K.W.; Heinrichs, G.A.; Hoffman, M.C. Group prenatal care for women with gestational diabetes. *J. Matern. Neonatal Med.* **2016**, *29*, 2852–2856. [CrossRef]
19. Alayoub, H.; Curran, S.; Coffey, M.; Hatunic, M.; Higgins, M. Assessment of the effectiveness of group education on knowledge for women with newly diagnosed gestational diabetes. *Ir. J. Med. Sci.* **2018**, *187*, 65–68. [CrossRef]
20. Benhalima, K.; Van Crombrugge, P.; Verhaeghe, J.; Vandeginste, S.; Verlaenen, H.; Vercammen, C.; Dufraimont, E.; De Block, C.; Jacquemyn, Y.; Mekahli, F.; et al. The Belgian Diabetes in Pregnancy Study (BEDIP-N), a multi-centric prospective cohort study on screening for diabetes in pregnancy and gestational diabetes: Methodology and design. *BMC Pregnancy Childbirth* **2014**, *14*, 226. [CrossRef]
21. Dalfrà, M.G.; Nicolucci, A.; Bisson, T.; Bonsembiante, B.; Lapolla, A. Quality of life in pregnancy and post-partum: A study in diabetic patients. *Qual. Life Res.* **2012**, *21*, 291–298. [CrossRef]
22. Marteau, T.M.; Bekker, H. The development of a six-item short-form of the state scale of the Spielberger State—Trait Anxiety Inventory (STAI). *Br. J. Clin. Psychol.* **1992**, *31*, 301–306. [CrossRef] [PubMed]
23. van der Bij, A.K.; de Weerd, S.; Cikot, R.J.L.M.; Steegers, E.A.P.; Braspenning, J.C.C. Validation of the Dutch Short Form of the State Scale of the Spielberger State-Trait Anxiety Inventory: Considerations for Usage in Screening Outcomes. *Community Genet.* **2003**, *6*, 84–87. [CrossRef]
24. Bradley, C.; Speight, J. Patient perceptions of diabetes and diabetes therapy: Assessing quality of life. *Diabetes Metab. Res. Rev.* **2002**, *18*, 64–69. [CrossRef] [PubMed]
25. Hussain, Z.; Yusoff, Z.M.; Syed Sulaiman, S.A. A study exploring the association of attitude and treatment satisfaction with glycaemic level among gestational diabetes mellitus patients. *Prim. Care Diabetes* **2015**, *9*, 275–282. [CrossRef] [PubMed]
26. IOM (Institute of Medicine); NRC (National Research Council). *Weight Gain during Pregnancy: Reexamining the Guidelines*; The National Academies Press: Washington, DC, USA, 2009.
27. Devlieger, H.; Martens, G.; Bekaert, A.; Eeckels, R. Standaarden van geboortegewicht-voor-zwangerschapsduur voor de Vlaamse boreling. *Tijdschr. Geneeskd.* **2000**, *56*, 1–14. [CrossRef]
28. Benhalima, K.; Damm, P.; Van Assche, A.; Mathieu, C.; Devlieger, R.; Mahmood, T.; Dunne, F. Screening for gestational diabetes in Europe: Where do we stand and how to move forward?: A scientific paper commissioned by the European Board & College of Obstetrics and Gynaecology (EBCOG). *Eur. J. Obstet. Gynecol.* **2016**, *201*, 192–196.
29. Hussain, Z.; Yusoff, Z.M.; Syed Sulaiman, S.A. Evaluation of knowledge regarding gestational diabetes mellitus and its association with glycaemic level: A Malaysian study. *Prim. Care Diabetes* **2015**, *9*, 184–190. [CrossRef]
30. Murphy, A.; Guilar, A.; Donat, D. Nutrition Education for Women with Newly Diagnosed Gestational Diabetes Mellitus: Small-group vs. Individual Counselling. *Can. J. Diabetes* **2004**, *28*, 1–5.
31. Schauffler, H.H.; Rodriguez, T. Availability and Utilization of Health Promotion Programs and Satisfaction with Health Plan. *Med. Care* **1994**, *32*, 1182–1196. [CrossRef]
32. Lapolla, A.; Di Cianni, G.; Di Benedetto, A.; Franzetti, I.; Napoli, A.; Sciacca, L.; Torlone, E.; Tonutti, L.; Vitacolonna, E.; Mannino, D. Quality of Life, Wishes, and Needs in Women with Gestational Diabetes: Italian DAWN Pregnancy Study. *Int. J. Endocrinol.* **2012**, *2012*. [CrossRef]
33. Biderman, A.; Noff, E.; Harris, S.B.; Friedman, N.; Levy, A. Treatment satisfaction of diabetic patients: What are the contributing factors? *Fam. Pract.* **2009**, *26*, 102–108. [CrossRef] [PubMed]

34. Alazri, M.H.; Neal, R.D. The association between satisfaction with services provided in primary care and outcomes in Type 2 diabetes mellitus. *Diabet. Med.* **2003**, *20*, 486–490. [CrossRef] [PubMed]
35. Kapur, S.R. Service evaluation of patient satisfaction for antenatal diabetes education in Christchurch Women's Hospital, New Zealand. *N. Z. Med. Stud. J.* **2015**, *20*, 10–14.
36. Ross, G.P.; Falhammar, H.; Chen, R.; Barraclough, H.; Kleivenes, O.; Gallen, I. Relationship between depression and diabetes in pregnancy: A systematic review. *World J. Diabetes* **2016**, *7*, 554–571. [CrossRef]
37. Byrn, M.; Penckofer, S. The Relationship between Gestational Diabetes and Antenatal Depression. *J. Obstet. Gynecol. Neonatal Nurs.* **2015**, *44*, 246–255. [CrossRef] [PubMed]
38. Byrn, M.; Penckofer, S. Antenatal Depression and Gestational Diabetes: A Review of Maternaland Fetal Outcomes. *Nurs. Womens Health* **2013**, *17*, 22–33. [CrossRef] [PubMed]
39. Nicklas, J.M.; Miller, L.J.; Zera, C.A.; Davis, R.B.; Levkoff, S.E.; Seely, E.W. Factors Associated with Depressive Symptoms in the Early Postpartum Period among Women with Recent Gestational Diabetes Mellitus. *Matern. Child Health J.* **2013**, *17*, 1665–1672. [CrossRef]
40. Daniells, S.; Grenyer, B.F.S.; Davis, W.S.; Coleman, K.J.; Burgess, J.-A.P.; Moses, R.G. Gestational Diabetes Mellitus: Is a diagnosis associated with an increase in maternal anxiety and stress in the short and intermediate term? *Diabetes Care* **2003**, *26*, 385–389. [CrossRef]

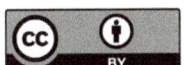

© 2020 by the authors. Licensee MDPI, Basel, Switzerland. This article is an open access article distributed under the terms and conditions of the Creative Commons Attribution (CC BY) license (http://creativecommons.org/licenses/by/4.0/).

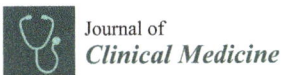

Review

The Oral Glucose Tolerance Test—Is It Time for a Change?—A Literature Review with an Emphasis on Pregnancy

Delia Bogdanet [1,2,*], Paula O'Shea [1,3], Claire Lyons [3], Amir Shafat [1] and Fidelma Dunne [1,2]

1. Department of Medicine, School of Medicine, National University of Ireland Galway, H91TK33 Galway, Ireland; PaulaM.OShea@hse.ie (P.O.); amir.shafat@nuigalway.ie (A.S.); fidelma.dunne@nuigalway.ie (F.D.)
2. Department of Diabetes and Endocrinology, Saolta University Health Care Group (SUHCG), University Hospital Galway, H91YR71 Galway, Ireland
3. Department of Clinical Biochemistry, SUHCG, University Hospital Galway, H91YR71 Galway, Ireland; Claire.lyons11@gmail.com
* Correspondence: deliabogdanet@gmail.com; Tel.: +00-353-8310-27771

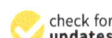

Received: 1 September 2020; Accepted: 22 October 2020; Published: 27 October 2020

Abstract: Globally, gestational diabetes (GDM) is increasing at an alarming rate. This increase is linked to the rise in obesity rates among women of reproductive age. GDM poses a major global health problem due to the related micro- and macro-vascular complications of subsequent Type 2 diabetes and the impact on the future health of generations through the long-term impact of GDM on both mothers and their infants. Therefore, correctly identifying subjects as having GDM is of utmost importance. The oral glucose tolerance test (OGTT) has been the mainstay for diagnosing gestational diabetes for decades. However, this test is deeply flawed. In this review, we explore a history of the OGTT, its reproducibility and the many factors that can impact its results with an emphasis on pregnancy.

Keywords: oral glucose tolerance test; reproducibility; diabetes; gestational diabetes

---

1. Introduction

1.1. Diabetes and Gestational Diabetes—Historical Aspects

Diabetes mellitus has been recognised since 1500 BC [1]. Diabetes with onset during pregnancy was first described in 1824 in Germany [2]. Lambie in 1926 determined that the first manifestation of diabetes in pregnancy occurs in the 5th or 6th month of pregnancy. He advocated the use of the 50 g oral glucose challenge test (OGCT) to calculate ketogenic-anti-ketogenic balance [3]. Based on Hoet's study [4], in 1957, Wilkerson [5] developed a protocol proposing a 3 h oral glucose tolerance test (OGTT) for patients at high risk for developing diabetes. Additionally, for women with no risk factors, he recommended a 2-step approach: 1 h blood glucose measurement after a 50 g glucose load which, if abnormal, was followed by a 3 h OGTT.

The clinical equipoise regarding the best approach to screen and diagnose gestational diabetes (GDM) was the impetus for Norbet Freinkel to organise the First International Workshop on GDM in 1979 [6]. A core outcome of this event was the emergence of a model for GDM screening and the suggestion that screening should be carried out between 24 and 28 weeks' gestation. This model was updated in 1984 at the Second International Workshop on GDM [7], which concluded that all pregnant women should be screened for glucose intolerance with a 50 g OGCT, irrespective of the time of the last meal or time of day, and for diagnostic purposes the 100 g OGTT was to be employed. In 1990, at the Third International Workshop on GDM [8], screening and diagnostic criteria were confirmed. This panel agreed that the 75 g 2 h OGTT should be used to screen women at high risk of developing GDM [8].

The seminal Hyperglycaemia and Adverse Pregnancy Outcome (HAPO) Study in 2008 [9] addressed the importance of having all three glucose values (fasting, 1-h and 2-h post glucose load) in the OGTT since none of the glucose values were significantly correlated, and no single value was better in predicting a GDM diagnosis.

1.2. OGTT

The OGTT has been used in clinical medicine for over 100 years [10] and was first described by Conn [11]. His findings were based on the work of Jacobsen in 1913, who demonstrated that carbohydrate ingestion leads to glucose fluctuations [10]. Since then, the OGTT has been contested [12]. The main concerns raised by Unger in 1957 were the diagnostic values at each time point, the timing of samples, diet (at that time 300 g of carbohydrates for 3 consecutive days prior to the test was recommended), exercise, age, gastrointestinal factors (e.g., gastric emptying time or gastrointestinal absorption rates) and stress prior to the test that may influence the values of the test. In 1964, Nadon et al. [13] completed a comparative analysis between OGTT and the intravenous glucose tolerance test (IVGTT) and found considerable disagreement between both in the identification of diabetes. They concluded that, in the future, diabetes "may be diagnosed without reliance on glucose tolerance tests alone" [13].

1.3. Reproducibility

In 1965, McDonald et al. examined the reproducibility of the OGTT [14]. In this work, 400 male volunteers free of diabetes underwent a series of six separate OGTTs and demonstrated that blood glucose levels for individuals varied considerably. A decade later, these findings were corroborated by Olefsky et al. [15].

In 1991, Harlass et al. [16] found OGTT reproducibility of only 78% in women with an elevated glucose concentration 1 h post a glucose load when repeated within 2 weeks. Catalano [17] reported poor reproducibility for the OGTT in diagnosing GDM in 24% (9 of 38) of pregnant women tested. The authors hypothesised that this was likely due to a norepinephrine-mediated process where maternal stress leads to increased concentrations of glucose and insulin. This theory was supported by Ko et al. [18], who found the overall reproducibility of the OGTT to be 65.5% with subjects showing an improvement in glycaemic status on repeat testing. More recently, Munang et al. [19] showed the reproducibility of the OGTT for GDM in a sub-Saharan African population to be 74.2%. In this study, 70 women underwent the OGTT at 24–28 weeks of gestation and again one week later. However, the generalisability of the results of this study to other populations is questionable due to the small cohort, the short time interval between repeat testing and the fact that glucose was measured on capillary blood samples and not plasma as is more usual.

Despite scientists raising concerns about the reproducibility of the OGTT for over 50 years, it remains the only available test and the current "gold standard" for diagnosing Type 2 Diabetes Mellitus (T2DM) and GDM. In this review, the myriad of variables that affect the reproducibility and accuracy of the OGTT are discussed in terms of the Total Testing Process: pre-analytical, analytical and post-analytical phases (Figure 1).

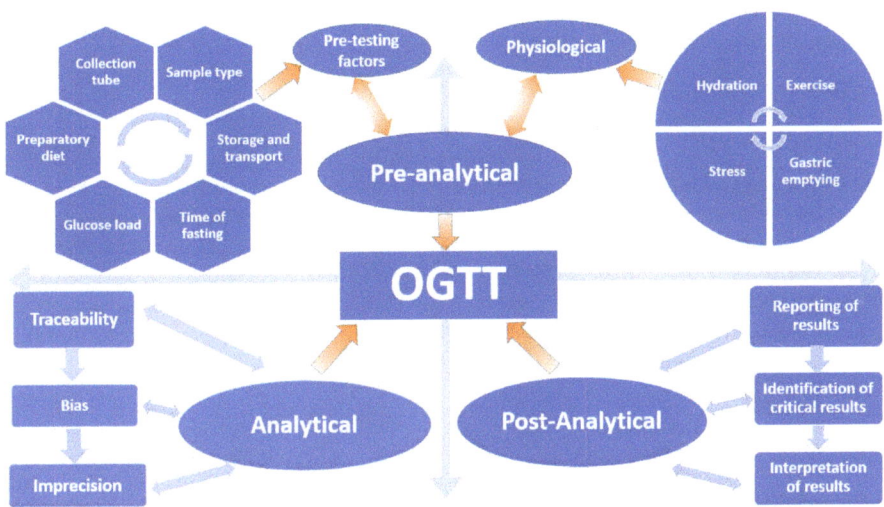

Figure 1. Variables that influence the oral glucose tolerance test (OGTT).

1.4. Screening

Diagnosing GDM is important not only for the short-term adverse outcomes related to pregnancy and delivery, but also for the long-term consequences affecting both the mother and the child such as development of T2DM, obesity, metabolic, cardiovascular, neurological and psychiatric problems [20]. The main purpose of GDM screening is the identification of GDM cases, thus facilitating early lifestyle interventions and treatment. Randomised clinical trials (RCTs) have shown that treatment of GDM through lifestyle changes and pharmacological interventions leads to a reduction in adverse perinatal outcomes (large/small for gestational age, macrosomia, prematurity, neonatal hypoglycaemia and caesarean section delivery) [21,22].

Debate continues on the optimum screening strategy to diagnose GDM [23]. Universal screening is an approach where all pregnant women are screened. Critics of this approach highlight the fact that, if adopted, universal screening would mean that many women without GDM would be subjected to unnecessary invasive testing and that the cost implications for healthcare systems would be significant [24]. The alternative approach is selective screening based on the presence of risk factors. Selective screening is less costly as fewer women are tested. However, unscreened women may develop GDM and remain undiagnosed with the potential for increased adverse outcomes. Risk factors for GDM include age ≥30 years, family history of diabetes, increased body mass index (BMI), previous GDM, miscarriage, polycystic ovarian syndrome (PCOS) and a previous large for gestational age (LGA) or macrosomic baby [25]. The Atlantic Diabetes in Pregnancy (Atlantic DIP) study group evaluated the difference in GDM prevalence using three distinct guidelines for selective screening in a cohort of universally screened pregnant women [26]. This research found that by using 2008 National Institute for Health and Care Excellence (NICE) [27], 2010 Irish [28] and 2013 American Diabetes Association (ADA) guidelines [29], 20%, 16% and 5% of women, respectively, would have been misdiagnosed as not having GDM. In an Italian study, Pintaudi et al. [30] found that when universal screening was applied, 11.1% of pregnant women were identified as having GDM, but when selective screening was applied to the same cohort, 23% of GDM cases would have been missed.

In an effort to provide universal screening such that no case of pregnancy dysglycaemia is missed, researchers are intensifying the quest to identify an alternative biomarker/test that would easily, accurately, reproducibly and economically detect this at-risk maternal population. Identifying a minimally invasive biomarker that could be used as a single test in the non-fasting state would have clear advantages over the current fasting OGTT.

2. The Total Testing Process

2.1. Pre-Analytical Phase

The importance of the pre-analytical phase of the total testing process is often underappreciated and accounts for 46–68% of all laboratory errors [31]. An inaccurate glucose measurement due to sampling without standard timepoints can lead to a missed diagnosis of GDM or mismanagement of a patient with GDM with the potential for increased adverse outcomes and healthcare costs. This is particularly relevant when using the International Association of the Diabetes and Pregnancy Study Groups (IADPSG) criteria, as only one of three values is required to be met or exceeded to make the diagnosis.

2.2. Physiological Factors

2.2.1. Exercise

The benefits of exercise on physical and mental health have been widely documented from improvement of cardiovascular fitness and outcomes to significant reduction in depression and anxiety [32,33]. Many researchers have looked at the impact of exercise on blood glucose levels to build evidence on the importance of exercise in the management and prevention of glucose intolerance and diabetes.

In 2007, Andersen et al. [34] showed that an exercise session carried out 14 h before having a high carbohydrate meal significantly reduced post prandial levels of glucose compared to controls ($p \leq 0.05$). Slentz et al. [35] studied the effects of different intensities of exercise on the OGTT in individuals with prediabetes. These authors found significant reductions in fasting glucose levels only when low amount of moderate exercise and diet was combined. Higher levels of exercise were associated with improved glucose concentrations at 30 min post OGTT but was less effective when compared to the combination of diet and exercise. When overall improvement in glucose tolerance was assessed, low amounts of moderate exercise alone was determined to be half as effective as diet and exercise combined but twice as effective as high amounts of high intensity exercise. These findings are supported by Houmard et al. [36], who found that exercise sessions of low and moderate intensity have a positive effect on improving insulin sensitivity and fasting plasma glucose. These results contradict previous studies [37,38] that found no improvement in the OGTT results after moderate intensity training but noticed a 30% decrease in glucose levels on the OGTT after sustained vigorous exercise sessions.

Castleberry et al. [39] examined the impact of various workout patterns (no exercise, a single exercise session, alternative days of exercise or consecutive days of exercise) on glycaemic control on the OGTT 12–14 h post the exercise session and found that the type of exercise pattern made no difference to the glucose results.

Despite contradictory data in the literature on the length and intensity of the exercise session, physical activity influences the way our body processes nutrients. Most of the studies on this topic have been carried out on healthy subjects or individuals with diabetes and there are no studies evaluating the impact of exercise on the antepartum OGTT results. Hence, further research is required to determine whether a single exercise session prior to the antepartum OGTT lowers/improves glucose results. Such evidence is also necessary to ensure that patient preparation for the OGTT is standardised with respect to the amount of exercise, if any, pregnant women should do in the days prior to testing.

2.2.2. Gastric Emptying

Absorption of glucose is negligible from the mouth and the stomach, so the ingested glucose dose cannot enter the blood compartment until it is emptied from the stomach, digested to monosaccharides and transported across the intestinal epithelia. The ability of the small and large bowel for transport far exceeds the rate of delivery of the 75 g glucose challenge, and so a major rate limiting step for the absorption of glucose is gastric emptying rate. Gastric emptying in one of the main factors influencing the glucose response in the first hour after the OGTT or after a meal and is responsible for 30–35% of the variability in post-prandial glycaemia in healthy controls [40,41] and diabetic patients [42]. This supports the hypothesis that an augmentation in the volume or reduction in the osmolality of a meal may result in an intensification in the speed of gastric emptying with a consequent rise in glucose [43]. Studies have shown that the faster the gastric emptying post glucose load, the higher the postprandial glucose levels will be [40,44]. Horowitz et al. [40] found that the 2 h glucose level post OGTT was inversely related to the gastric emptying rate—the slower the gastric emptying, the higher the 2 h blood glucose level. Their hypothesis for this finding was that high blood glucose levels may influence gastric motility, slowing it down in order to reduce further glucose absorption.

We cannot control (but should always consider) the individual variability of the rate of gastric emptying. Guidelines recommend the glucose load should be drank slowly over a period of 5 min. However, this is difficult to achieve and control for in clinical practice with individual wide variations in the glucose load drinking time.

2.2.3. Hydration

Research into the impact of hydration status on glycemic levels is limited. In 2015, Murry [45] explored the effects of mild hypohydration on glucose tolerance within individuals diagnosed with T2DM by evaluating blood glucose levels over two 120-min time periods in euhydrated and hypo-hydrated states, respectively. He found that reduced water consumption resulted in increased glucose concentration before and during the OGTT. Johnson et al. [46] found similar findings, concluding that 3 days of decreased total water intake in people with T2DM acutely modifies blood glucose levels during an OGTT with higher glucose measurements in the hypohydrated group. In 2016, Caroll et al. [47] piloted a study ($n = 5$) in which ~12 h hypo-hydration (sauna plus fluid restriction) induced a higher glycaemic response to a glucose load compared with sauna plus rehydration. The same group [48] however, 3 years later, found contradictory evidence indicating that acute hypohydration did not modify the glycaemic response, suggesting that when OGTTs are done in healthy subjects, hydration status may not necessarily influence the glycemic response during the OGTT. In 2019, Jansen et al. [49] conducted a crossover trial looking at the acute effect of osmotically stimulated arginine vasopressin (AVP) on glucose response in 60 healthy adults and found that acute osmotic stimulation increased glucose levels during the OGTT.

Additional findings that might reflect the importance of hydration status come from studies assessing the impact of seasonal variation on the OGTT and GDM prevalence. Numerous studies [50–53] have had consistent findings of higher GDM prevalence during the summer months with higher 1 h and 2 h values on the OGTT and no impact on fasting glucose levels. While these results can be attributed to other seasonal factors such as nutrition quality, exercise level, light-sensitive hormones or increased blood flow due to increased temperature, hydration status may be more likely to explain these higher glucose values observed. The rationale being that where increased temperature is not accompanied by adequate fluid intake, this could lead to hypohydration, hypovolemia and increased glucose concentration.

Even though there are no studies examining the impact of hydration status on the OGTT in pregnancy, we can extrapolate on previous findings and consider that the effects of hypo-hydration or hyper-hydration are not negligible and have the potential to lead to a misdiagnosis. Currently, there are no guidelines on water intake in the days prior to the OGTT.

2.2.4. Stress and Sleep

In 1991, Spirito et al. [54] explored the impact of stress and coping mechanisms on glucose levels in 72 pregnant women without diabetes (mean age 27.8 years) and 125 women (mean age 27.7 years) with GDM. While levels of emotional distress and methods of coping did not show any significant difference between groups, disconnection and detachment significantly influenced daily blood glucose variability. In 2011, Hosler et al. [55] found that having any number of stressors one year prior to delivery was significantly associated with pregnant women failing their glucose test. One of the possible explanations for this is that psychological stress alters the hypothalamic-pituitary adrenocortical system and stimulates the release of cortisol thus increasing glucose levels. Importantly, both GDM studies were retrospective cohort studies, therefore the knowledge of one's GDM diagnosis could potentially influence the woman's disease awareness creating a recall bias for stressors.

Experiencing acute psychological stress is associated with hyperglycemia and increased risk of T2DM and glucose intolerance [56]. In 2016, Horsch et al. [57] found that intense stress (major life events) and psychological stress responses (depression, anxiety and sleep length) led to increased glucose levels during pregnancy even prior to women being tested for GDM. The variables that were associated most with increased levels of fasting blood glucose were increased distress and short sleep duration. The association between sleep duration and quality and glucose homeostasis has been highlighted by additional studies [58,59] that found that shorter sleep duration is associated with higher glucose levels, particularly the fasting and 2 h glucose level on the OGTT. Retrukatul et al. [60] found that pregnant women with reduced sleep duration (less than 7 h per night) have an increased risk of developing GDM; in fact, each hour of reduced sleep leads to a 4% increase in blood glucose levels. These results are supported by Myoga et al. [61], who also found that pregnant women who sleep less than 5 h per night had higher random blood glucose levels.

Stress can impact glycaemic status not only through hormonal responses but also through the development of unhealthy lifestyle behaviours such as overeating, smoking, increased alcohol intake [62,63]. Given the glucose response to stress and to decreased sleep duration/quality, it would seem possible that pregnant women could be erroneously diagnosed as having GDM using the OGTT.

2.3. Pre-Testing Patient Preparation Factors

2.3.1. Length of Time Spent in the Fasting State

A regular meal can significantly influence glucose levels [64]. Similarly, fasting also influences the levels of glucose. Salehi et al. [65] noticed a significant decrease in glucose after a complete period of fasting during Ramadan of 13 h in young healthy males, while Saada et al. [66] found that glucose levels increased significantly after 10–12 h fast in women with T2DM.

The OGTT is performed after an overnight fast. However, the period of fasting is not standardised and varies between 8 h and 16 h. Despite a low level of evidence (grade B), the ADA guidelines recommend that the glucose sample should be taken in the morning, after a period of fasting of at least 8 h, with no constraints on the amount of water allowed to be consumed by the patient during this time [67,68].

Variation in the period of fasting prior to testing may influence OGTT results. In 2011, Moebus et al. [69] challenged the necessity for fasting >8 h and found that a fasting length of 3 h was adequate for a reliable glucose measurement. In the British Regional Heart Study [70], a cross-sectional study of men aged between 60–79 years, there was no difference in plasma glucose levels in those fasting for 6 h or ≥6 h.

Patient adherence to instructions for fasting prior to the OGTT must also be considered. In 2013, Kackov et al. [71] explored how well patients were informed regarding the fasting protocol for laboratory blood testing and whether patients arrived for phlebotomy appropriately prepared for testing. These authors found that 46% of the participants believed that the precise time of their last meal prior to fasting was unimportant, as long as the last meal was on the day prior to the blood test.

Notwithstanding, only 60% of participants arrived for blood testing having adhered to instructions for fasting. Furthermore, 52% of study participants had not been informed about the pre-testing preparation requirements for blood testing.

Therefore, while there is no clear evidence regarding impact of the duration of time spent fasting prior to the OGTT, it is critical to standardise the duration spent fasting prior to laboratory OGTT and to give clear, consistent instructions to our patients to prevent inaccurate results.

2.3.2. Preparatory Diet

Many centers recommend that the OGTT is preceded by a 3-day diet of 150 g carbohydrate per day. The concept of this is based on the original work of Conn [11]. The length of the diet preceding the OGTT and the quantity of carbohydrate recommended have been randomly selected. Conn's 3-day diet contained in fact 300 g carbohydrate per day. Conn showed that by keeping a low-carbohydrate diet prior to the glucose test the number of false-positive cases of diabetes would increase. However, this study was small and only 3 of the 9 study participants were women.

The Fourth International Workshop-Conference on GDM [72] recommended the 3-day diet with a minimum of 150 g carbohydrate per day prior to the OGTT in order to prevent patients being misdiagnosed as having diabetes.

However, other studies [73–75] found that the carbohydrate ratio of the diet prior to the OGTT did not impact upon the test results indicating that a specific diet prior to the OGTT is not mandatory for women with normal dietary habits.

There is not enough evidence to recommend a pre-set diet/carbohydrate intake prior to the OGTT. Perhaps maintaining one's normal, regular diet prior to undergoing the OGTT would best reflect the individual's capacity to metabolise glucose. However, in order to maintain a standardised approach to OGTT, adherence to current guidelines should be recommend for now.

2.3.3. Glucose Load

In 1998, Sievenpiper et al. [76] investigated the post-prandial glycaemic response (PGR) after the ingestion of 25 g glucose, sucrose or fructose dissolved in either 200 mL or 600 mL of water. They established that PGR was not only influenced by carbohydrate type but also by the volume dose. By increasing the meal volume from 200 mL to 600 mL, PGR areas were significantly increased for all three sugars. Building on these results, Sievenpiper investigated the effects of a 2- and 3-fold increase in the volume of a 300 mL 75-g OGTT on glycaemic concentrations [77]. He found that there was a significant statistical difference between the means of the area under the curve (AUC) for the 300 mL, 600 mL and 900 mL OGTTs ($p = 0.006$). While post prandial glucose levels were not affected by the increase in volume from 300 mL to 600 mL, glucose levels were significantly increased when the volume was increased to 900 mL.

Fifty years ago, in an effort to reframe and strengthen this analysis, the Committee of the Statistics of the American Diabetes Association (ADA) suggested that the glucose load used during the OGTT should be based on an estimation of the individual body surface area (BSA) [78]; However, despite this recommendation, in 1980 the World Health Organization (WHO) endorsed the use of the 75 g glucose load for the OGTT irrespective of the individual BSA [79,80]. Subsequently, the glucose dose was set at 1.75 g/kg body weight with a maximum of 75 g [72,81]. Practically, this means that all patients over 43 kg are tested using the maximal dose of 75 g glucose. Furthermore, a number of studies have shown an association between a person's height and their 2 h glucose values on the OGTT [82,83], which supports the ADA's findings. In 2019, Palmu et al. [84] showed that the BSA has a considerable impact on the blood glucose levels from a standardised 75 g OGTT, with smaller individuals more likely to be diagnosed with diabetes or glucose intolerance compared to individuals with a larger BSA.

Therefore, emerging research has made a strong case for glucose loading to be individualised according to BSA. Additionally, research is steering practitioners to reexamine if 75 g glucose load is an appropriate dose regardless of the patient's physical characteristics. Indicators are showing that the glucose values following a 75 g glucose load is expected to differ according to variable factors such as pancreatic beta cell function, gut hormones and neural responses to carbohydrate ingestion. The problem becomes clear when individuals with a small BSA are diagnosed with diabetes or glucose intolerance, despite their daily glucose values not exceeding the diabetes threshold. Moreover, individuals with an increased BSA might not reveal an abnormal glucose response, even though their daily glucose values meet the diabetes diagnostic criteria because the 75 g glucose dose is inadequate to increase the glucose level to ≥11.1 mmol/L compared to their normal daily caloric intake required to maintain their BMI. Consequently, the parameters for loading dose of glucose in the tolerance test should ideally be individualised according to BSA, activity level, or necessary caloric intake calculated for the individuals basal metabolic rate in order to increase its usefulness in the identification of glucose intolerance.

There are several options regarding the preparation and delivery of the standard 75 g glucose load. One of the most popular options has been the use of Lucozade (Energy Original), which contained 70 kcal and 17 g of carbohydrates per 100 mL. To obtain 75 g of glucose required the consumption of 410 mL. The current reformulated product has a ~50% reduction in calories (available April 2017), contains 37 kcal and 8.7 g of carbohydrate per 100 mL, and to deliver a 75 g glucose load requires the consumption of a large volume, 860 mL. This change in formulation of Lucozade makes it unsuitable for use in the OGTT. To overcome this issue, an alternative form of 75 g anhydrous glucose (glucose monohydrate 82.5 g) comes in powder form in a ready-to-use sachet. It requires dissolving in 250 mL of water (to give final volume of 300 mL). Polycal® (Nutricia) (Nutricia Ltd., White Horse Business Park, Newmarket Avenue, Trowbridge, Wiltshire, UK)comes in liquid form and necessitates having access to a sufficiently accurate measuring vessel to accurately measure out 113 mL (equivalent to 75 g glucose) to which water is then added and mixed to give a final total volume of 250–300 mL. Rapilose® OGTT Solution (Penlan Healthcare Ltd., Abbey House, Wellington Way, Weybridge, UK) comes in liquid form and is available in a ready-to-use 300 mL pouch containing 75 g anhydrous glucose. Rapilose® has be customised for patients with a body weight ≥43 kg where they should consume the entire contents of one pouch but patients who weigh under 43 kg should have the volume adjusted accordingly.

2.4. Pre-Analysis Sample Handling

2.4.1. Sampling Site

In order to improve the interpretation of glucose results, it is imperative to understand the difference in results between samples collected from different sites (capillary plasma, capillary whole blood, venous plasma and venous whole blood). For example, the glucose levels in plasma are 11% higher than the levels in whole blood despite the fact that in clinical practice the words "plasma" and "blood" are used interchangeably [85].

Under normal physiological conditions, the post-prandial, capillary glucose levels are higher than the venous glucose levels as determined by the rate at which glucose is extracted from blood by tissues. Exploring this anomaly, Kuwa et al. [86] examined the difference in glucose levels between capillary and venous samples during the OGTT in 75 healthy individuals. They found that venous and capillary glucose levels were comparable in the fasting state, but the post-load capillary sample had significantly higher glucose levels compared to the venous one.

Stahl et al. [87] investigated whether capillary whole blood glucose levels used for analysis can be expressed as plasma results (as recommended by the ADA and WHO). Results from this study confirm that translation from capillary to plasma values may be acceptable for mean values but should not be used for individual glucose levels. These findings were confirmed by Colagiuri et al. [88], assessing the correlation between glucose levels in capillary and venous samples in fasting state, 2 h after oral glucose load and random glucose levels. These authors established that both fasting and random capillary samples gave lower glucose values than venous samples but the 2 h post glucose load capillary sample gave higher glucose values than the venous sample.

Adding to these research conclusions, D'Orazio et al. [89] maintain that due to the difference in glucose concentrations observed between whole blood and plasma, the glucose levels are not interchangeable. They also recommend that the reporting of glucose measurements should be in plasma only as the concentration of glucose in plasma is independent of hematocrit.

Preferably, the best model is one where blood glucose levels are reported from plasma samples where glycolysis has been delayed or inhibited. Alternatively, glucose level measurement reports should have clear information on the sample type being used and if any conversion factors had been applied in the reporting process.

2.4.2. Specimen Collection Tube

A prominent source of pre-analytical error in determining plasma glucose levels in vitro is glycolysis. It is reported that glycolysis leads to 5–7% decrease in glucose levels per hour at room temperature [68]. There are two main approaches to inhibit glycolysis. The first requires immediate separation of plasma/serum (within 30 min of sampling) from blood cells prior to analysis. The second approach involves collecting venous whole blood into specimen tubes containing a glycolytic inhibitor.

Sodium fluoride is one such glycolytic inhibitor and acts to inhibit enolase activity [90] stabilising the glucose levels in the long term. However, enolase is late in the glycolytic pathway such that glycolysis continues during the first hours after the sample has been collected. The rate of glucose loss is similar during the first 90 min regardless of the presence of sodium fluoride [68,91]. Furthermore, using sodium fluoride as a glycolytic inhibitor leads to an error in glucose levels that ranges between 0.28 and 0.39 mmol/L (5–7 mg/dL), and can be as high as 1.1 mmol/L (20 mg/dL) if plasma is left unseparated for more than 3 h post collection [92]. These findings are supported by Chen et al. [93] who confirmed the failure of sodium fluoride to inhibit glycolysis one hour after sample collection and recommending that the best way to reduce glycolysis and improve glucose integrity in samples in vitro was through immediate separation of plasma from blood cells.

Therefore, using sodium fluoride alone as a glycolytic inhibitor is considered insufficient. To circumvent this issue, Uchida et al. [94] showed that acidification quickly inhibits glycolysis through the inhibition of hexokinase and phosphofructokinase. In 2013, Garcia del Pino et al. [95] determined that citric acid immediately inhibits glycolysis. These authors showed that the glucose levels in samples taken in sodium fluoride tubes was significantly lower when compared to the glucose levels taken in temporally paired citrate tubes. Comparable results were reported by Norman et al. [96] evaluating paired fasting plasma glucose samples collected into sodium fluoride and citrate tubes and found higher glucose levels in the samples collected into the citrate tubes. This was reaffirmed in 2019 by Jamieson et al. [97], seeking to compare plasma glucose stability over time in 501 samples taken at the time of the OGTT after 24 weeks of gestation and found that the samples containing citrate as a glycolytic inhibitor offered the best short and long-term stability for glucose levels even compared with fluoride samples placed immediately on ice. They suggested that the use of sample tubes containing citrate would not require services to make any changes in the sample collection protocols (such as the addition of ice or immediate plasma separation). However, the authors advised that the diagnostic criteria for glucose intolerance may need revision as glucose values were, on average, 0.2 mmol/L higher when using fluoride-citrate sample tubes compared to those obtained by research methodology. In support of these findings, Lyons et al., 2018, assessed the stability of glucose in citrate-fluoride-oxalate buffered plasma (FC-Mix tubes) stored at 4 °C and 18–22 °C for 8.5 days and found that glucose results were maintained within 0.20 mmol/L of those determined using WHO specifications [98].

In clinical practice, where delays of sample transport and processing are regularly encountered, the use of citrate tubes delivers the best option in inhibiting glycolysis and preserving the integrity of blood glucose levels ex vivo. The use of citrate buffered specimen tubes is recommended by the ADA especially if the sample processing is likely to be more than 30 min post-collection [68].

2.4.3. Sample Storage and Transport

In 1985, the WHO recommended "rapid plasma separation from samples collected in fluoride tubes" in order to prevent or delay glycolysis [99]. The AACC and ADA guideline [68] recommends that samples "be immediately immersed in an ice-slurry and analyzed within 30 min of collection or rapid centrifugation after collection". However, compliance with these guidelines is particularly challenging in the case of the OGTT due to that fact that fasting and post glucose samples are usually held at the point of patient care until the test is completed, invariably over 2 h.

Consequently, diabetes prevalence will be underestimated in research studies in which sample handling and analysis is delayed as indicated by Potter et al. [100], who compared OGTT results (sodium fluoride tubes) between early centrifugation (within 10 min) and delayed centrifugation (at the end of the OGTT test) in over 12,000 women. They found the mean glucose levels for fasting, 1 h, and 2 h OGTT samples were higher using early centrifugation ($p < 0.0001$ for all) compared to delayed processing, increasing the GDM prevalence from 11.6% ($n = 869/7509$) to 20.6% ($n = 1007/4887$). In the commentary accompanying this study, Price et al. [101] highlight that "without strict pre-analytical OGTT sample handling in routine clinical practice, our ability to accurately diagnose GDM and report GDM prevalence data will be flawed".

The pre-analytical blood sampling protocol for pregnancy OGTT requires revision and standardisation [102]. Consideration of the difficulties that rapid centrifugation (within 30 min of sampling) or placement of samples on ice in busy clinics illustrates that value and pragmatism of the use of citrate blood tubes for sample collection. However, the use of citrate tubes has the potential to give a positive bias of 0.2 mmol/L, falsely increasing the rate of GDM diagnosis, such that a correction factor or revision of the diagnostic thresholds may be required [96,103,104]. An alternative approach could be to measure glucose in lithium heparin plasma analysed on the critical care analyser at the point of care (POC). In 2018, Lyons et al., recruited 12 volunteers to undergo the OGTT measuring blood glucose at each time point on the critical care analyser (ABL90FLEX®/Glucose oxidase), (Manor Court, Manor Royal, Crawley, West Sussex, England) and concomitantly in whole blood collected into fluoride-oxalate tubes immersed immediately in ice-slurry and analysed within 30 min using the central laboratory (Roche Cobas® 8000 modular analyzer series/Hexokinase) (Roche Diagnostics GmbH, Sandhoferstrasse 116, Mannheim, Germany) [105]. These authors demonstrated good agreement of glucose results with the WHO recommended method with results within the total allowable error analytical goal for plasma glucose of < 5.5%.

While clear recommendations exist regarding glucose sample transport and storage, the challenge is the practicality and applicability of these guidelines to the routine clinical practice settings that are not resourced for immediate sample handling and processing. Outside of research specific laboratories, worldwide, very few centers are likely equipped to adhere to such strict glucose processing methodology. Citrate buffered specimen tubes offer the best practical solution and their use is recommended by the ADA.

2.5. Analytical Phase

2.5.1. Traceability and Methodology

Central Laboratory

Global standardisation of clinical assay's aims to produce accurate and reproducible test results across space and time (traceability) through a reduction in method variability. To minimise assay bias, methods for measuring glucose should be calibrated (traceable) to reference methods. Currently, there are two reference methods for blood glucose measurement recommended by the Joint Committee for Traceability in Laboratory Medicine: isotope dilution mass spectrometry (ID-MS) [106], and enzymatic (Hexokinase-Glucose-6-Phosphate Dehydrogenase) [107]. The maximum allowable deviation for the alignment of the central laboratory method with a reference method is 4%. In the routine clinical central laboratory setting, glucose is invariably measured using one of three common enzymatic methods: hexokinase, glucose 1-dehydrogenase and glucose oxidase in reactions that either are coupled to a chromophore or generate an electric current.

2.5.2. Point of Care (POC)

Blood Glucose Meters (BGM)

Glucose is measured using capillary blood glucose concentrations. All POC meters use enzymes to measure glucose. These enzymes are oxidoreductases, can be classified in several categories each with its specific characteristics but, ultimately, have as a primary role to oxidise glucose [108]. Electron transfer to an electrode is then measured (third generation sensors). Of note, none are completely specific for glucose.

In 2020, O'Malley and colleagues [109] studied the use of POC glucose measurements in diagnosing GDM in women undergoing an antepartum OGTT. These authors found the diagnostic accuracy of POC glucose for GDM to be 83.0% (95% confidence interval (CI), 74.2–89.8) and concluded that there is no justification for the use of POC in centers that have adequate sample handling facilities. However, they noted that POC might be acceptable in low- and medium-resource settings, where processes to inhibit glycolysis are not available.

Critical Care Analysers (Blood Gas Analysers)

Whole blood (venous/arterial) is collected into balanced sodium heparinised (plasma) syringes and glucose is measured by a fixed enzyme electrode or via a reagent cassette. Glucose oxidase is the enzyme most commonly used [110].

2.6. Analytical Quality

2.6.1. Central Laboratory

Generally, laboratory testing quality should not be one of the variables influencing GDM prevalence and should not cause any glucose variability though the measurement process. The total laboratory analytical error has two main components: (1) precision, which is the capacity of the test to reproduce replicate measurements and it is expressed as the coefficient of variation (CV); and (2) bias, which is the difference between the laboratory result and the true value of the test. A good laboratory test should have minimal imprecision and bias and should conform with the specified analytical regulatory criteria. Laboratories compare their test result and the performance of their measurements against objective quality requirements such as the National Academy of Clinical Biochemistry (NACB) guidelines for total maximum allowable error (TEa). For glucose, the recommended targets are imprecision < 2.9%, bias < 2.2% and TEa < 6.9% [68]. The analytical imprecision for central laboratories is of the order of 1–2%.

However, glucose measurements, even within permissible limits, can influence GDM incidence and prevalence significantly. The true value of a laboratory test ranges within a 95% confidence interval of the reported value. In 2015, Agarwal et al. [111] examined the impact the analytical quality of a laboratory can have on GDM prevalence by comparing the total analytical error in one laboratory with the TEa as recommended by the NACB. This was a prospective study with over 2000 study participants. The research team found that, irrespective of criteria used to diagnose GDM (IADPSG, ADA, CDA), the analytical variation in glucose measurement had both a statistically significant impact on the GDM prevalence and also a significant impact on pregnant women that would be incorrectly reassured as not having GDM. These authors suggest that laboratories with decreased quality performance that report glucose measurements outside the 95% CI will ultimately lead to an increased reported GDM prevalence and an increase in false positive GDM cases. Based on total analytical variation of glucose for glucose in the laboratory performing the analyses, in their cohort, the prevalence of GDM ranged from 27% to 71% with an absolute prevalence of 45.3% (independent of the diagnostic criteria used). The authors concluded that the reported GDM prevalence has the potential to vary from 0.5–2.0-fold even if the laboratory meets the NACB recommendation of TEa < 6.9%, and urge laboratories to strive to improve their analytical performance even beyond the NACB recommendation in order to avoid misclassifying patients. Supporting these findings, Nielsen et al. [112] found that at 0% bias, an increase in imprecision from 2.7% to 3.7% increased the prevalence of diabetes by 90%.

Clinicians should always seek to use accredited laboratories but must be aware that TEa does not take into account pre-analytical factors that may influence glucose results. For example, a delay of more than 4 h in processing (centrifugation and separation of plasma from blood cells) the fasting sample of the OGTT would exceed the TEa for glucose.

2.6.2. POC—BGM

The analytical variation for BGM is commonly of the order of 5%. POC guidelines recommend that 95% of glucose results from BGM should be within ± 12.5% of the central laboratory glucose results ≥ 5.55 mmol/L (100 mg/dL) and within 0.67 mmol/L (12 mg/dL) for values < 5.55 mmol/L (100 mg/dL); furthermore, that 98% of BGM glucose results should be within ± 20% of the central laboratory glucose values ≥ 4.2 mmol/L (75 mg/dL) and within ± 0.83 mmol/L (15 mg/dL) for glucose values < 4.2 mmol/L (75 mg/dL) [113].

2.6.3. POC—Critical Care Analysers (Blood Gas Analysers)

The analytical imprecision for critical care analysers is of the order of 1–2% and similar to that of the central laboratory [114,115].

2.7. Post-Analytical Phase

The next phase of the total testing process is the post-analytical phase, which includes the following steps:

Processing of results into a report format (paper or electronic).
Identification of critical results and communication to the requesting clinician.
Interpretation of the results and if deemed necessary provision of advice for further tests.
Transmission of final report to the requesting clinician.

In the context of the OGTT, the diagnostic criteria are not uniform and are the subject of much debate.

In 1964, O'Sullivan et al. [116] proposed that "screening, diagnosis and treatment of hyperglycaemia in women who are not known to have diabetes improves outcomes". The diagnostic criteria proposed were based on the 3 h–100 g glucose OGTT, which were subsequently validated for the development of future maternal T2DM [116]. The values proposed for GDM diagnosis were: fasting, 6.1 mmol/L (110 mg/dL); 1 h, 9.4 mmol/L (170 mg/dL); 2 h, 6.7 mmol/L (120 mg/dL) and 3 h, 6.1 mmol/L (110 mg/dL). Women with at least two abnormal values were diagnosed with GDM.

In 2008, the HAPO study showed that mild hyperglycemia was associated with adverse neonatal outcomes even below the previous GDM diagnostic criteria [9]. Based on these findings, in 2010 the IADPSG recommended a one-step 75 g OGTT and modified the GDM diagnostic cut-off points: fasting glucose: 5.1 mmol/L, 1 h glucose: 10.0 mmol/L and 2 h glucose: 8.5 mmol/L (fasting glucose: 92 mg/dL, 1 h glucose: 180 mg/dL and 2 h glucose: 153 mg/L) [81]. A single abnormal value confirms a diagnosis of GDM. Some critics of the new IADPSG diagnostic criteria indicate that the HAPO study did not take into account all pre-specified adverse outcomes and factors such as the rates of cesarean section or neonatal hypoglycemia in the determination of diagnostic cut-off points. Another criticism was that the single abnormal value required for diagnosis and the low glucose threshold of the new criteria to identify women as having GDM meant that such women would be in a very low risk category [117].

The IADPSG criteria were embraced by many international organisations including the ADA [118], WHO [119], the International Federation of Gynaecology and Obstetrics (FIGO) [120] and European

Board and College of Obstetrics and Gynaecology (EBCOG) (2015). At the same time, some international bodies have not incorporated the IADPSG criteria: American College of Obstetricians and Gynecologists (ACOG) Practice Bulletin [121], the National Institutes of Health (NIH) consensus statement [122] and Society of Obstetricians and Gynaecologists of Canada (SOGC) [123]. The reasons given for not adopting the IADPSG criteria were (1) the benefit of treating women with mild GDM is not well established; (2) the increased prevalence of GDM will lead to additional healthcare costs; (3) caesarean section delivery and neonatal intensive care unit (NICU) admission rates will increase; and (4) patients identified as having GDM will develop additional psychosocial burdens which will decrease their Quality of Life (QoL).

Inconsistencies in GDM diagnostic criteria worldwide have led to challenges in making meaningful comparisons between study results (through systematic reviews and metanalysis). Cost analysis studies should always include clinical adverse outcome prevention through diagnosis and treatment in their analysis. A very well designed study by Duran et al. [124] found that the use of the IADPSG criteria was associated with an improvement in the prevalence of maternal and neonatal adverse outcomes (pregnancy induced hypertension, prematurity, caesarean sections, NICU admissions, LGA and SGA) that was cost-effective despite a 3.5-fold rise in GDM prevalence.

2.7.1. COVID-19: Implications for GDM Testing

In the context of the coronavirus 2019 (COVID-19) pandemic, travel restrictions, the time (up to 3 h) spent in a potentially infectious environment while the OGTT is carried out and the requisite glucose samples collected, together with the additional number of clinical visits consequent to a positive GDM diagnosis, have combined to reduce the use of the OGTT. In fact, McIntyre et al. [125], have highlighted that international bodies have already moved to using one or more of the following alternative approaches to GDM diagnosis: fasting venous plasma glucose [126], random venous plasma glucose and/or HbA$_{1c}$ [127]. Unfortunately, both approaches, while safer in the context of the SARS-CoV-2 pandemic, will lead to many women with GDM not being diagnosed. Gemert et al. [128] have shown that by only using a fasting plasma glucose ≤ 4.6 mmol/L for the diagnosis of GDM, 29% of women would have been missed. Similarly, van-de- l'Isle et al. [129] found that by using the Royal College of Obstetrics and Gynecologists recommendations for the diagnosis of GDM (fasting glucose ≥ 5.3 mmol/L or HbA$_{1c}$ ≥ 39 mmol/mol or random plasma glucose ≥ 9 mmol/L), 57% of women would have been wrongly diagnosed as not having GDM. The likely consequence of this will be an increase in GDM-related complications as these women will not have received the appropriate treatment for GDM. In their commentary, Mcintyre et al. [130] emphasise the need for validation and regulatory approval of alternative, less cumbersome strategies for the diagnosis and classification of GDM by using new non-fasting biomarkers such as plasma glycated CD59, a complement regulatory protein, which is showing promise. The need for change to the way in which the diagnosis of GDM is made has been recognised for many decades now. The current global COVID-19 pandemic has reignited the urgent quest for the rapid identification of a new, reliable and feasible biomarker to diagnose GDM.

2.7.2. Emerging Biomarkers

The current COVID-19 pandemic has highlighted what the scientific community has known for years [13]—that it is time to identify new tests that can accurately and robustly diagnose GDM, tests that require less preparatory and sampling time and that are less affected, if at all, by the pre-analytical factors mentioned in this article. There are now several biomarkers showing great potential to meet this clinical need. They include amino acids, peptides, proteins, lipids, enzymes, saccharides, microRNA, etc. The following biomarkers are a cross-section of the emerging data in this field.

Adiponectin is a protein hormone and adipokine involved in glucose metabolism. Many researchers have shown that adiponectin levels can diagnose GDM and can also predict GDM when analysed in early pregnancy. In 2008, Lain et al. [131] showed that women with a low first trimester level of adiponectin were 10 times more likely to be diagnosed with GDM later in pregnancy. In 2013,

Rasanen et al. [132] supported this work showing that first trimester adiponectin levels were associated with the development of GDM. Additionally, an Irish study [133] found that high first trimester adiponectin levels were associated with a reduced risk of developing GDM validating the work of Rasanen et al. Furthermore, there is evidence to suggest that adiponectin may also be used in predicting the development of post-partum glucose intolerance in women with a history of GDM [134]. However, despite these promising results, in 2016 a study by Iliodromiti et al. [135] found the sensitivity and specificity of adiponectin in predicting GDM diagnosis to be 60.3% and 81.3%, respectively. Prospective studies to confirm the adiponectin role as a GDM diagnostic biomarker are warranted.

Emerging research on GDM has shown that CD59, a glycoprotein biomarker, has the potential to diagnose GDM. Gosh et al. [136] determined that glycated CD59 (gCD59) accurately predicted the development of GDM with a sensitivity of 85% and a specificity of 92%. These authors found that GDM patients had 10-fold higher levels of gCD59 compared to controls. These findings are supported in work by Ma et al. [137], showing that gCD59 levels in pregnant women before 20 weeks of pregnancy accurately predict the results of the OGTT. In addition, gCD59 levels were also associated with higher risk of delivering a baby large for gestational age (LGA). Prospective studies are ongoing to assess the potential of gCD59 to identify GDM early in pregnancy and improve prediction of adverse pregnancy outcomes [138].

Extracellular vesicles (EV) have also shown diagnostic potential as indicated in a study by Salomon et al. [139], who found a 2-fold higher concentration of exosomes (small EV) in GDM pregnancies compared to normal pregnancies. These findings have been further supported by several recent studies [140,141] which found higher concentrations of EV in women who developed GDM compared to controls.(add references) Jayabala et al. [142] examined the differences in protein content in EVs between women with GDM and women with normal glucose tolerance. They found a total of 78 proteins that were significantly differentially expressed in GDM women compared to women with normal glucose tolerance. Despite this, there are no studies comparing the levels of EV concentrations between different types of pregnancy complications (gestational hypertension/preeclampsia, foetal growth abnormalities, foetal malformations, etc). There are no studies assessing the trimester-specific EV levels in normal and GDM pregnancies or studies assessing the robustness of the test by comparing different analysis method, different methods for purifying and separating exosomes or different types of blood sample used, nor also studies investigating concentrations of EV released from placenta vs. non-placental sources. EV are an emerging biomarker with great potential; however, further studies are required to establish the exact role of EV in GDM diagnosis.

Nesfatin-1 is a polypeptide involved in food regulation and water intake and has a glucose-dependent insulinotropic action. In 2012, Aslan et al. [143] found lower nesfatin-1 levels in GDM women compared to controls. These findings are supported by Kucukler et al. [144], who similarly found lower levels of nesfatin-1 in women who developed GDM compared to women without GDM but also found a positive correlation between nesfatin-1 and insulin levels. In a recent prospective study, Mierzynski et al. [145] also observed that women with GDM had significantly lower levels of nesfatin-1 compared to women with normal glucose tolerance but also found a strong correlation between nesfatin-1 levels and pre-pregnancy BMI. However, a study by Zang et al. [146] found opposite results with nesfatin-1 levels higher in GDM patients compared to controls with a positive correlation between nesfatin-1 levels and BMI, while Deniz et al. [147] showed a negative correlation between nesfatin-1 levels and BMI. The discrepancy of these results might arise from the different study participants' characteristics or the timing of the sample collection. While it is clear that nesfatin-1 plays a role in GDM pathophysiology, further studies are required to define its potential as a diagnostic biomarker.

Several biomarkers show potential advantages over the historical OGTT. The breadth of this emerging trend shows the activity within the research community to identify an appropriate new test for GDM diagnosis. Those mentioned above provide a mere snapshot of the evolving evidence, and an in-depth analysis is beyond the scope of this paper. This review has explored the fallacy of the OGTT, the current "gold standard" for GDM, a test that is easily affected by many variables, potentially leading to false results and has drawn attention to promising emerging alternative biomarkers. Through ongoing collaboration, researchers in this field can make a critical breakthrough on a new test for GDM diagnosis.

3. Conclusions

The OGTT is subject to several factors spanning the total testing process that have the potential to influence its results and negatively impact patient care. Clear guidance is needed to ensure a universal standardised approach to performing and interpreting the OGTT for the diagnosis of GDM. This will permit global harmonisation of the detection of GDM, improve the accuracy and reproducibility of the OGTT and provide for better outcomes for mothers and their offspring. Alongside this, the search for better biomarkers to diagnose GDM and ultimately replace the OGTT is gaining pace with several biomarkers currently under evaluation. However, the diagnostic accuracy and clinical usefulness of many of these novel biomarkers remain to be fully validated.

Author Contributions: D.B., P.O. and F.D. contributed to the study concept and researched the data. D.B. wrote first draft of the manuscript. All authors, D.B., P.O., C.L., A.S. and F.D. reviewed, critically revised and approved the final version of the manuscript. All authors have read and agreed to the published version of the manuscript.

Funding: This research received no external funding.

Conflicts of Interest: The authors have no conflict of interest to declare.

References

1. Ghalioungui. *PTEPANET, Commentaries and Glossaries*; Academy of Scientific Research and Technology: Cairo, Egypt, 1987.
2. Bennewitz, H.G. *De Diabete Mellito Graviditatis Symptomate*; Typis Ioannis Friderici Starckii: Berlin, Germany, 1824.
3. Lambie, C.G. Diabetes and Pregnancy. *Trans. Edinb. Obstet. Soc.* **1927**, *47*, 43–59. [CrossRef] [PubMed]
4. Hoet, J.P.; Lukens, F.D.W. Carbohydrate Metabolism during Pregnancy. *Diabetes* **1954**, *3*, 1–12. [CrossRef] [PubMed]
5. Wilkerson, H.L.C.; Remein, Q.R. Studies of Abnormal Carbohydrate Metabolism in Pregnancy: The Significance of Impaired Glucose Tolerance. *Diabetes* **1957**, *6*, 324–329. [CrossRef]
6. Freinkel, N. Gestational Diabetes 1979: Philosophical and Practical Aspects of a Major Public Health Problem. *Diabetes Care* **1980**, *3*, 399–401. [CrossRef]
7. Freinkel, N. *Proceedings of the Second International Workshop-Conference on Gestational Diabetes Mellitus*; American Diabetes Association: Alexandria, VA, USA, 1985; Volume 34, pp. 123–126.
8. Metzger, B.E. Summary and Recommendations of the Third International Workshop-Conference on Gestational Diabetes Mellitus. *Diabetes* **1991**, *40*, 197–201. [CrossRef]
9. Metzger, B.E.; Lowe, L.P.; Dyer, A.R.; Trimble, E.R.; Chaovarindr, U.; Coustan, D.R.; Hadden, D.R.; McCance, D.R.; Hod, M.; McIntyre, H.D.; et al. Hyperglycemia and adverse pregnancy outcomes. *N. Engl. J. Med.* **2008**, *358*, 1991–2002. [PubMed]
10. Jacobsen, A. Untersuchungen über den Einfluss verschiedener Nahrungsmittel auf den Blutzucker bei normalen, zuckerkranken und graviden Personen. *Biochem. Z.* **1913**, *56*, 471–494.
11. Conn, J. Interpretation of the glucose tolerance test. The necessity of a standard preparatory diet. *Am. J. Med. Sci.* **1940**, *199*, 555–564. [CrossRef]
12. Unger, R.H. The standard two-hour oral glucose tolerance test in the diagnosis of diabetes mellitus in subjects without fasting hyperglycemia. *Ann. Intern. Med.* **1957**, *47*, 1138–1153. [CrossRef]
13. Nadon, G.W.; Little, J.A.; Hall, W.E.; O'Sullivan, M.O. A Comparison of the Oral and Intravenous Glucose Tolerance Tests in Non-Diabetic, Possible Diabetic and Diabetic Subjects. *Can. Med. Assoc. J.* **1964**, *91*, 1350–1353. [PubMed]
14. McDonald, G.W.; Fisher, G.F.; Burnham, C. Reproducibility of the Oral Glucose Tolerance Test. *Diabetes* **1965**, *14*, 473–480. [CrossRef] [PubMed]
15. Olefsky, J.M.; Reaven, G.M. Insulin and glucose responses to identical oral glucose tolerance tests performed forty-eight hours apart. *Diabetes* **1974**, *23*, 449–453. [CrossRef] [PubMed]

16. Harlass, F.E.; Brady, K.; Read, J.A. Reproducibility of the oral glucose tolerance test in pregnancy. *Am. J. Obstet. Gynecol.* **1991**, *164*, 564–568. [CrossRef]
17. Catalano, P.M.; Avallone, D.A.; Drago, N.M.; Amini, S.B. Reproducibility of the oral glucose tolerance test in pregnant women. *Am. J. Obstet. Gynecol.* **1993**, *169*, 874–881. [CrossRef]
18. Ko, G.T.; Chan, J.C.; Woo, J.; Lau, E.; Yeung, V.T.; Chow, C.C.; Cockram, C. S The reproducibility and usefulness of the oral glucose tolerance test in screening for diabetes and other cardiovascular risk factors. *Ann. Clin. Biochem.* **1998**, *35*, 62–67. [CrossRef]
19. Munang, Y.N.; Noubiap, J.J.; Danwang, C.; Sama, J.D.; Azabji-Kenfack, M.; Mbanya, J.C.; Sobngwi, E. Reproducibility of the 75 g oral glucose tolerance test for the diagnosis of gestational diabetes mellitus in a sub-Saharan African population. *BMC Res. Notes* **2017**, *10*, 622. [CrossRef] [PubMed]
20. Metzger, B.E. Long-term outcomes in mothers diagnosed with gestational diabetes mellitus and their offspring. *Clin. Obstet. Gynecol.* **2007**, *50*, 972–979. [CrossRef]
21. Landon, M.B.; Spong, C.Y.; Thom, E.; Carpenter, M.W.; Ramin, S.M.; Casey, B.; Wapner, R.J.; Varner, M.W.; Rouse, D.J.; Thorp, J.M., Jr.; et al. A multicenter, randomized trial of treatment for mild gestational diabetes. *N. Engl. J. Med.* **2009**, *361*, 1339–1348. [CrossRef]
22. Crowther, C.A.; Hiller, J.E.; Moss, J.R.; McPhee, A.J.; Jeffries, W.S.; Robinson, J.S. Australian Carbohydrate Intolerance Study in Pregnant Women (ACHOIS) Trial Group Effect of treatment of gestational diabetes mellitus on pregnancy outcomes. *N. Engl. J. Med.* **2005**, *352*, 2477–2486. [CrossRef]
23. McIntyre, H.D.; Colagiuri, S.; Roglic, G.; Hod, M. Diagnosis of GDM: A suggested consensus. *Best Pract. Res. Clin. Obstet. Gynaecol.* **2015**, *29*, 194–205. [CrossRef]
24. Gillespie, P.; O'Neill, C.; Avalos, G.; O'Reilly, M.; Dunne, F.; Collaborators, A.D. The cost of universal screening for gestational diabetes mellitus in Ireland. *Diabetes Med.* **2011**, *28*, 912–918. [CrossRef]
25. Egan, A.M.; Vellinga, A.; Harreiter, J.; Simmons, D.; Desoye, G.; Corcoy, R.; Adelantado, J.M.; Devlieger, R.; Van Assche, A.; Galjaard, S.; et al. Epidemiology of gestational diabetes mellitus according to IADPSG/WHO 2013 criteria among obese pregnant women in Europe. *Diabetologia* **2017**, *60*, 1913–1921. [CrossRef]
26. Avalos, G.E.; Owens, L.A.; Dunne, F. Applying Current Screening Tools for Gestational Diabetes Mellitus to a European Population: Is It Time for Change? *Diabetes Care* **2013**, *36*, 3040–3044. [CrossRef]
27. Guideline Development Group. Management of diabetes from preconception to the postnatal period: Summary of NICE guidance. *BMJ* **2008**, *336*, 714–717. [CrossRef] [PubMed]
28. Health Service Executive. *Guidelines for the Management of Pre-Gestational and Gestational Diabetes Mellitus from Pre-Conception to the Postnatal Period*; Health Service Executive: Dublin, Ireland, 2010. Available online: https://www.hse.ie/eng/services/list/2/primarycare/east-coast-diabetes-service/management-of-type-2-diabetes/diabetes-and-pregnancy/guidelines-for-the-management-of-pre-gestational-and-gestational-diabetes-mellitus-from-pre-conception-to-the-postnatal-period.pdf. (accessed on 1 September 2020).
29. Association, A.D. Standards of medical care in diabetes—2013. *Diabetes Care* **2013**, *36*, S11–S66. [CrossRef]
30. Pintaudi, B.; Di Vieste, G.; Corrado, F.; Lucisano, G.; Pellegrini, F.; Giunta, L.; Nicolucci, A.; D'Anna, R.; Di Benedetto, A. Improvement of selective screening strategy for gestational diabetes through a more accurate definition of high-risk groups. *Eur. J. Endocrinol.* **2014**, *170*, 87–93. [CrossRef]
31. Plebani, M. The detection and prevention of errors in laboratory medicine. *Ann. Clin. Biochem.* **2010**, *47*, 101–110. [CrossRef] [PubMed]
32. Hansen, D.; De Strijcker, D.; Calders, P. Impact of Endurance Exercise Training in the Fasted State on Muscle Biochemistry and Metabolism in Healthy Subjects: Can These Effects be of Particular Clinical Benefit to Type 2 Diabetes Mellitus and Insulin-Resistant Patients? *Sports Med.* **2017**, *47*, 415–428. [CrossRef] [PubMed]
33. Stubbs, B.; Vancampfort, D.; Rosenbaum, S.; Firth, J.; Cosco, T.; Veronese, N.; Salum, G.A.; Schuch, F.B. An examination of the anxiolytic effects of exercise for people with anxiety and stress-related disorders: A meta-analysis. *Psychiatry Res.* **2017**, *249*, 102–108. [CrossRef]
34. Andersen, E.; Høstmark, A.T. Effect of a single bout of resistance exercise on postprandial glucose and insulin response the next day in healthy, strength-trained men. *J. Strength Cond. Res.* **2007**, *21*, 487–491.
35. Slentz, C.A.; Bateman, L.A.; Willis, L.H.; Granville, E.O.; Piner, L.W.; Samsa, G.P.; Setji, T.L.; Muehlbauer, M.J.; Huffman, K.M.; Bales, C.W.; et al. Effects of exercise training alone vs a combined exercise and nutritional lifestyle intervention on glucose homeostasis in prediabetic individuals: A randomised controlled trial. *Diabetologia* **2016**, *59*, 2088–2098. [CrossRef] [PubMed]

36. Houmard, J.A.; Tanner, C.J.; Slentz, C.A.; Duscha, B.D.; McCartney, J.S.; Kraus, W.E. Effect of the volume and intensity of exercise training on insulin sensitivity. *J. Appl. Physiol.* **2004**, *96*, 101–106. [CrossRef] [PubMed]
37. Kang, J.; Robertson, R.J.; Hagberg, J.M.; Kelley, D.E.; Goss, F.L.; DaSilva, S.G.; Suminski, R.R.; Utter, A.C. Effect of exercise intensity on glucose and insulin metabolism in obese individuals and obese NIDDM patients. *Diabetes Care* **1996**, *19*, 341–349. [CrossRef] [PubMed]
38. Seals, D.R.; Hagberg, J.M.; Hurley, B.F.; Ehsani, A.A.; Holloszy, J.O. Effects of endurance training on glucose tolerance and plasma lipid levels in older men and women. *JAMA* **1984**, *252*, 645–649. [CrossRef] [PubMed]
39. Castleberry, T.; Irvine, C.; Deemer, S.E.; Brisebois, M.F.; Gordon, R.; Oldham, M.D.; Duplanty, A.A.; Ben-Erza, V. Consecutive days of exercise decrease insulin response more than a single exercise session in healthy, inactive men. *Eur. J. Appl. Physiol.* **2019**, *119*, 1591–1598. [CrossRef]
40. Horowitz, M.; Edelbroek, M.A.; Wishart, J.M.; Straathof, J.W. Relationship between oral glucose tolerance and gastric emptying in normal healthy subjects. *Diabetologia* **1993**, *36*, 857–862. [CrossRef]
41. Horowitz, M.; Cunningham, K.M.; Wishart, J.M.; Jones, K.L.; Read, N.W. The effect of short-term dietary supplementation with glucose on gastric emptying of glucose and fructose and oral glucose tolerance in normal subjects. *Diabetologia* **1996**, *39*, 481–486. [CrossRef]
42. Jones, K.L.; Horowitz, M.; Wishart, M.J.; Maddox, A.F.; Harding, P.E.; Chatterton, B.E. Relationships between gastric emptying, intragastric meal distribution and blood glucose concentrations in diabetes mellitus. *J. Nucl. Med.* **1995**, *36*, 2220–2228.
43. Hunt, J.N.; Smith, J.L.; Jiang, C.L. Effect of meal volume and energy density on the gastric emptying of carbohydrates. *Gastroenterology* **1985**, *89*, 1326–1330. [CrossRef]
44. Thompson, D.G.; Wingate, D.L.; Thomas, M.; Harrison, D. Gastric emptying as a determinant of the oral glucose tolerance test. *Gastroenterology* **1982**, *82*, 51–55. [CrossRef]
45. Murry, W. Hypohydration and Glucose Regulation in Adult Males with Type II Diabetes Mellitus. Bachelor's Thesis, University of Arkansas, Fayetteville, NC, USA, 2015. Available online: http://scholarworks.uark.edu/biscuht/6 (accessed on 1 September 2020).
46. Johnson, E.C.; Bardis, C.N.; Jansen, L.T.; Adams, J.D.; Kirkland, T.W.; Kavouras, S.A. Reduced water intake deteriorates glucose regulation in patients with type 2 diabetes. *Nutr. Res.* **2017**, *43*, 25–32. [CrossRef] [PubMed]
47. Carroll, H.A.; Johnson, L.; Betts, J. Effect of hydration status on glycemic control: A pilot study. *Med. Sci. Sports Exerc.* **2016**, *48*, 745. [CrossRef]
48. Carroll, H.A.; Templeman, I.; Chen, Y.C.; Edinburgh, R.M.; Burch, E.K.; Jewitt, J.T.; Povey, G.; Robinson, T.D.; Dooley, W.L.; Jones, R.; et al. Effect of acute hypohydration on glycemic regulation in healthy adults: A randomized crossover trial. *J. Appl. Physiol.* **2019**, *126*, 422–430. [CrossRef] [PubMed]
49. Jansen, L.T.; Suh, H.; Adams, J.D.; Sprong, C.A.; Seal, A.D.; Scott, D.M.; Butts, C.L.; Melander, O.; Kirkland, T.W.; Vanhaecke, T.; et al. Osmotic stimulation of vasopressin acutely impairs glucose regulation: A counterbalanced, crossover trial. *Am. J. Clin. Nutr.* **2019**, *110*, 1344–1352. [CrossRef]
50. Moses, R.G.; Wong, V.C.; Lambert, K.; Morris, G.J.; Gil, F.S. Seasonal Changes in the Prevalence of Gestational Diabetes Mellitus. *Diabetes Care* **2016**, *39*, 1218–1221. [CrossRef] [PubMed]
51. Katsarou, A.; Claesson, R.; Ignell, C.; Shaat, N.; Berntorp, K. Seasonal Pattern in the Diagnosis of Gestational Diabetes Mellitus in Southern Sweden. *J. Diabetes Res.* **2016**, *2016*, 1–6. [CrossRef] [PubMed]
52. Molina-Vega, M.; Gutiérrez-Repiso, C.; Muñoz-Garach, A.; Lima-Rubio, F.; Morcillo, S.; Tinahones, F.J.; Picón-César, M.J. Relationship between environmental temperature and the diagnosis and treatment of gestational diabetes mellitus: An observational retrospective study. *Sci. Total Environ.* **2020**, *744*, 140994. [CrossRef]
53. Vasileiou, V.; Kyratzoglou, E.; Paschou, S.A.; Kyprianou, M.; Anastasiou, E. The impact of environmental temperature on the diagnosis of gestational diabetes mellitus. *Eur. J. Endocrinol.* **2018**, *178*, 209–214. [CrossRef]
54. Spirito, A.; Russo, D.C.; Masek, B.J. Behavioral interventions and stress management training for hospitalized adolescents and young adults with cystic fibrosis. *Gen. Hosp. Psychiatry* **1984**, *6*, 211–218. [CrossRef]
55. Hosler, A.S.; Nayak, S.G.; Radigan, A.M. Stressful events, smoking exposure and other maternal risk factors associated with gestational diabetes mellitus. *Paediatr. Périnat. Epidemiol.* **2011**, *25*, 566–574. [CrossRef]
56. Faulenbach, M.; Uthoff, H.; Schwegler, K.; Spinas, G.A.; Schmid, C.; Wiesli, P. Effect of psychological stress on glucose control in patients with Type 2 diabetes. *Diabetes Med.* **2012**, *29*, 128–131. [CrossRef] [PubMed]

57. Horsch, A.; Kang, J.S.; Vial, Y.; Ehlert, U.; Borghini, A.; Marques-Vidal, P.; Jacobs, I.; Puder, J.J. Stress exposure and psychological stress responses are related to glucose concentrations during pregnancy. *Br. J. Health Psychol.* **2016**, *21*, 712–729. [CrossRef] [PubMed]
58. Ford, E.S.; Wheaton, A.G.; Chapman, D.P.; Li, C.; Perry, G.S.; Croft, J.B. Associations between self-reported sleep duration and sleeping disorder with concentrations of fasting and 2-h glucose, insulin, and glycosylated hemoglobin among adults without diagnosed diabetes. *J. Diabetes* **2014**, *6*, 338–350. [CrossRef]
59. Byberg, S.; Hansen, A.-L.S.; Christensen, D.L.; Vistisen, D.; Aadahl, M.; Linneberg, A.; Witte, D.R. Sleep duration and sleep quality are associated differently with alterations of glucose homeostasis. *Diabetes Med.* **2012**, *29*, e354–e360. [CrossRef] [PubMed]
60. Reutrakul, S.; Zaidi, N.; Wroblewski, K.; Kay, H.H.; Ismail, M.; Ehrmann, D.A.; Van Cauter, E. Sleep Disturbances and Their Relationship to Glucose Tolerance in Pregnancy. *Diabetes Care* **2011**, *34*, 2454–2457. [CrossRef]
61. Myoga, M.; Tsuji, M.; Tanaka, R.; Shibata, E.; Askew, D.J.; Aiko, Y.; Senju, A.; Kawamoto, T.; Hachisuga, T.; Araki, S.; et al. Impact of sleep duration during pregnancy on the risk of gestational diabetes in the Japan environmental and Children's study (JECS). *BMC Pregnancy Childbirth* **2019**, *19*, 1–7. [CrossRef]
62. Williams, E.D.; Magliano, D.J.; Tapp, R.J.; Oldenburg, B.; Shaw, J.E. Psychosocial Stress Predicts Abnormal Glucose Metabolism: The Australian Diabetes, Obesity and Lifestyle (AusDiab) Study. *Ann. Behav. Med.* **2013**, *46*, 62–72. [CrossRef]
63. Lloyd, C.; Smith, J.; Weinger, K. Stress and Diabetes: A review of the links. *Diabetes Spectr.* **2005**, *18*, 121–127. [CrossRef]
64. Lima-Oliveira, G.; Salvagno, G.L.; Lippi, G.; Gelati, M.; Montagnana, M.; Danese, E.; Picheth, G.; Guidi, G.C. Influence of a Regular, Standardized Meal on Clinical Chemistry Analytes. *Ann. Lab. Med.* **2012**, *32*, 250–256. [CrossRef]
65. Salehi, M.; Neghab, M. Effects of Fasting and a Medium Calorie Balanced Diet During the Holy Month Ramadan on Weight, BMI and Some Blood Parameters of Overweight Males. *Pak. J. Biol. Sci.* **2007**, *10*, 968–971. [CrossRef]
66. Saada, A.; Sa, G.; Belkacemi, L.; Ait chabane, O.; Italhi, M.; Bekada, A.M.; Kati, D. Effect of Ramadan fasting on glucose, glycosylated haemoglobin, insulin, lipids and proteinous concentrations in women with non-insulin dependent diabetes mellitus. *Afr. J. Biotech.* **2010**, *9*, 87–94.
67. Mellitus, D. The Expert Committee on the Diagnosis and Classification of Diabetes Mellitus Report of the Expert Committee on the Diagnosis and Classification of Diabetes Mellitus. *Diabetes Care* **1997**, *20*, 1183–1197.
68. Sacks, D.B.; Arnold, M.; Bakris, G.L.; Bruns, D.E.; Horvath, A.R.; Kirkman, M.S.; Lernmark, A.; Metger, B.E.; Nathan, D.M. Guidelines and recommendations for laboratory analysis in the diagnosis and management of diabetes mellitus. *Clin. Chem.* **2011**, *57*, e1–e47. [CrossRef]
69. Moebus, S.; Göres, L.; Lösch, C.; Jöckel, K.H. Impact of time since last caloric intake on blood glucose levels. *Eur. J. Epidemiol.* **2011**, *26*, 719–728. [CrossRef] [PubMed]
70. Emberson, J.R.; Whincup, P.H.; Walker, M.; Thomas, M.; Alberti, K.G. Biochemical measures in a population-based study: Effect of fasting duration and time of day. *Ann. Clin. Biochem.* **2002**, *39*, 493–501. [CrossRef]
71. Kackov, S.; Simundic, A.M.; Gatti-Drnic, A. Are patients well informed about the fasting requirements for laboratory blood testing? *Biochem. Med. (Zagreb)* **2013**, *23*, 326–331. [CrossRef]
72. Metzger, B.E.; Coustan, D.R. Summary and recommendations of the Fourth International Workshop-Conference on Gestational Diabetes Mellitus. The Organizing Committee. *Diabetes Care* **1998**, *21* (Suppl. 2), B161–B167. [PubMed]
73. Entrekin, K.; Work, B.; Owen, J. Does a high carbohydrate preparatory diet affect the 3-h oral glucose tolerance test in pregnancy? *J. Matern. Fetal. Med.* **1998**, *7*, 68–71. [PubMed]
74. Crowe, S.M.; Mastrobattista, J.M.; Monga, M. Oral glucose tolerance test and the preparatory diet. *Am. J. Obs. Gynecol.* **2000**, *182*, 1052–1054. [CrossRef] [PubMed]
75. Buhling, K.J.; Elsner, E.; Wolf, C.; Harder, T.; Engel, B.; Wascher, C.; Siebert, G.; Dudenhausen, J.W. No influence of high- and low-carbohydrate diet on the oral glucose tolerance test in pregnancy. *Clin. Biochem.* **2004**, *37*, 323–327. [CrossRef]

76. Sievenpiper, J.L.; Vuksan, V.; Wong, E.Y.; Mendelson, R.A.; Bruce-Thompson, C. Effect of meal dilution on the postprandial glycemic response: Implications for glycemic testing. *Diabetes Care* **1998**, *21*, 711–716. [CrossRef]
77. Sievenpiper, J.L.; Jenkins, D.J.; Josse, R.G.; Vuksan, V. Dilution of the 75-g oral glucose tolerance test increases postprandial glycemia: Implications for diagnostic criteria. *CMAJ* **2000**, *162*, 993–996. [PubMed]
78. American Diabetes Association. Standardization of the oral glucose tolerance test. Report of the Committee on Statistics of the American Diabetes Association June 14, 1968. *Diabetes* **1969**, *18*, 299–307. [CrossRef]
79. Keen, H.; Jarrett, R.J.; Alberti, K.G.M.M. Diabetes mellitus: A new look at diagnostic criteria. *Diabetol.* **1980**, *18*, 81. [CrossRef]
80. WHO Expert Committee. WHO Expert Committee on Diabetes Mellitus: Second report. *World Health Organ. Tech. Rep. Ser.* **1980**, *646*, 1–80.
81. Metzger, B.E.; Gabbe, S.G.; Persson, B.; Buchanan, T.A.; Catalano, P.A.; Damm, P.; Dyer, A.R.; Leiva, A.D.; Hod, M.; Kitzmiler, J.L.; et al. International association of diabetes and pregnancy study groups recommendations on the diagnosis and classification of hyperglycemia in pregnancy. *Diabetes Care* **2010**, *33*, 676–682. [CrossRef]
82. Sicree, R.A.; Zimmet, P.Z.; Dunstan, D.W.; Cameron, A.J.; Welborn, T.A.; Shaw, J.E. Differences in height explain gender differences in the response to the oral glucose tolerance test- the AusDiab study. *Diabet Med.* **2008**, *25*, 296–302. [CrossRef]
83. Rehunen, S.K.J.; Kautiainen, H.; Eriksson, J.G.; Korhonen, P.E. Adult height and glucose tolerance: A re-appraisal of the importance of body mass index. *Diabetes Med.* **2017**, *34*, 1129–1135. [CrossRef] [PubMed]
84. Palmu, S.; Rehunen, S.; Kautiainen, H.; Eriksson, J.G.; Korhonen, P.E. Body surface area and glucose tolerance—The smaller the person, the greater the 2-h plasma glucose. *Diabetes Res. Clin. Pract.* **2019**, *157*, 107877. [CrossRef]
85. Burrin, J.M.; Alberti, K.G. What is blood glucose: Can it be measured? *Diabetes Med.* **1990**, *7*, 199–206. [CrossRef] [PubMed]
86. Kuwa, K.; Nakayama, T.; Hoshino, T.; Tominaga, M. Relationships of glucose concentrations in capillary whole blood, venous whole blood and venous plasma. *Clin. Chim. Acta* **2001**, *307*, 187–192. [CrossRef]
87. Stahl, M.; Brandslund, I.; Jørgensen, L.G.M.; Petersen, P.H.; Borch-Johnsen, K.; Olivarius, N.D.F. Can capillary whole blood glucose and venous plasma glucose measurements be used interchangeably in diagnosis of diabetes mellitus? *Scand. J. Clin. Lab. Investig.* **2002**, *62*, 159–166. [CrossRef] [PubMed]
88. Colagiuri, S.; Sandbaek, A.; Carstensen, B.; Christensen, J.; Glümer, C.; Lauritzen, T.; Borch-Johnsen, K.; Sandbæk, A. Comparability of venous and capillary glucose measurements in blood. *Diabetes Med.* **2003**, *20*, 953–956. [CrossRef] [PubMed]
89. D'Orazio, P.; Burnett, R.W.; Fogh-Andersen, N.; Jacobs, E.; Kuwa, K.; Külpmann, W.R.; Larsson, L.; Lewenstam, A.; Maas, A.H.; Mager, G.; et al. Approved IFCC Recommendation on Reporting Results for Blood Glucose (Abbreviated). *Clin. Chem.* **2005**, *51*, 1573–1576. [CrossRef] [PubMed]
90. Qin, J.; Chai, G.; Brewer, J.M.; Lovelace, L.L.; Lebioda, L. Fluoride inhibition of enolase: Crystal structure and thermodynamics. *Biochemistry* **2006**, *45*, 793–800. [CrossRef]
91. Alberti, K.G.; Zimmet, P.Z. Definition, diagnosis and classification of diabetes mellitus and its complications. Part 1: Diagnosis and classification of diabetes mellitus provisional report of a WHO consultation. *Diabetes Med.* **1998**, *15*, 539–553. [CrossRef]
92. Gambino, R. Sodium fluoride: An ineffective inhibitor of glycolysis. *Ann. Clin. Biochem.* **2013**, *50*, 3–5. [CrossRef]
93. Chan, H.; Lunt, H.; Thompson, H.; Heenan, H.F.; Frampton, C.M.; Florkowski, C.M. Plasma glucose measurement in diabetes: Impact and implications of variations in sample collection procedures with a focus on the first hour after sample collection. *Clin. Chem. Lab. Med.* **2014**, *52*, 1061–1068. [CrossRef]
94. Uchida, K.; Matuse, R.; Toyoda, E.; Okuda, S.; Tomita, S. A new method of inhibiting glycolysis in blood samples. *Clin. Chim. Acta* **1988**, *172*, 101–108. [CrossRef]
95. del Pino, I.G.; Constanso, I.; Mourín, L.V.; Safont, C.B.; Vázquez, P.R. Citric/citrate buffer: An effective antiglycolytic agent. *Clin. Chem. Lab. Med.* **2013**, *51*, 1943–1949. [CrossRef]
96. Norman, M.; Jones, I. The shift from fluoride/oxalate to acid citrate/fluoride blood collection tubes for glucose testing—The impact upon patient results. *Clin. Biochem.* **2014**, *47*, 683–685. [CrossRef] [PubMed]

97. Jamieson, E.L.; Spry, E.P.; Kirke, A.B.; Atkinson, D.N.; Marley, J.V. Real-World Gestational Diabetes Screening: Problems with the Oral Glucose Tolerance Test in Rural and Remote Australia. *Int. J. Environ. Res. Public Health* **2019**, *16*, 4488. [CrossRef] [PubMed]
98. Lyons, C.; Griffin, T.P.; Islam, M.N.; Hamon, S.M.; Mellet, T.; O'Shea, P.M. Maintaining glucose integrity ex-vivo: Comparison of Citrate- Fluoride-Oxalate with Fluoride-Oxalate additives to stabilize plasma glucose. *IRISH J. Med. Sci.* **2018**, *187*, s212.
99. Diabetes mellitus. Report of a WHO Study Group. *World Health Organ Tech. Rep. Ser.* **1985**, *727*, 1–113.
100. Potter, J.M.; Hickman, P.E.; Oakman, C.; Woods, C.; Nolan, C.J. Strict Preanalytical Oral Glucose Tolerance Test Blood Sample Handling Is Essential for Diagnosing Gestational Diabetes Mellitus. *Diabetes Care* **2020**, *43*, 1438–1441. [CrossRef]
101. Price, S.A.; Moses, R.G. Gestational Diabetes Mellitus and Glucose Sample Handling. *Diabetes Care* **2020**, *43*, 1371–1372. [CrossRef]
102. Bruns, D.E.; Metzger, B.E.; Sacks, D.B. Diagnosis of Gestational Diabetes Mellitus Will Be Flawed until We Can Measure Glucose. *Clin. Chem.* **2020**, *66*, 265–267. [CrossRef]
103. van den Berg, S.A.; Thelen, M.H.; Salden, L.P.; van Thiel, S.W.; Boonen, K.J. It takes acid, rather than ice, to freeze glucose. *Sci. Rep.* **2015**, *5*, 8875. [CrossRef]
104. Carey, R.; Lunt, H.; Heenan, H.F.; Frampton, C.M.; Florkowski, C.M. Collection tubes containing citrate stabiliser over-estimate plasma glucose, when compared to other samples undergoing immediate plasma separation. *Clin. Biochem.* **2016**, *49*, 1406–1411. [CrossRef]
105. Lyons, C.; Mustafa, M.; Khattak, A.; Griffin, T.P.; Bogdanet, D.; Dunne, F.; O'Shea, P. Glucose measurement using point of care (POC) testing compared to central laboratory testing during the Oral Glucose Tolerance Test (OGTT). *IRISH J. Med. Sci.* **2018**, *187*, s211–s212.
106. Zhang, T.; Zhang, C.; Zhao, H.; Zeng, J.; Zhang, J.; Zhou, W.; Yan, Y.; Wang, Y.; Wang, M.; Chen, W. Determination of serum glucose by isotope dilution liquid chromatography-tandem mass spectrometry: A candidate reference measurement procedure. *Anal. Bioanal. Chem.* **2016**, *408*, 7403–7411. [CrossRef] [PubMed]
107. Armbruster, D.; Miller, R.R. The Joint Committee for Traceability in Laboratory Medicine (JCTLM): A global approach to promote the standardisation of clinical laboratory test results. *Clin. Biochem. Rev.* **2007**, *28*, 105–113. [PubMed]
108. Ferri, S.; Kojima, K.; Sode, K. Review of glucose oxidases and glucose dehydrogenases: A bird's eye view of glucose sensing enzymes. *J. Diabetes Sci. Technol.* **2011**, *5*, 1068–1076. [CrossRef] [PubMed]
109. O'Malley, E.G.; Reynolds, C.M.E.; O'Kelly, R.; Killalea, A.; Sheehan, S.R.; Turner, M.J. A Prospective Evaluation of Point-of-Care Measurements of Maternal Glucose for the Diagnosis of Gestational Diabetes Mellitus. *Clin. Chem.* **2020**, *66*, 316–323. [CrossRef]
110. Le, H.T.; Harris, N.S.; Estilong, A.J.; Olson, A.; Rice, M.J. Blood glucose measurement in the intensive care unit: What is the best method? *J. Diabetes Sci. Technol.* **2013**, *7*, 489–499. [CrossRef]
111. Agarwal, M.M.; Dhatt, G.S.; Othman, Y. Gestational diabetes mellitus prevalence: Effect of the laboratory analytical variation. *Diabetes Res. Clin. Pract.* **2015**, *109*, 493–499. [CrossRef]
112. Nielsen, A.A.; Petersen, P.H.; Green, A.; Christensen, C.; Christensen, H.; Brandslund, I. Changing from glucose to HbA1c for diabetes diagnosis: Predictive values of one test and importance of analytical bias and imprecision. *Clin. Chem. Lab. Med.* **2014**, *52*, 1069–1077. [CrossRef]
113. Cunningham, S.; Slingerland, R.; Mesotten, D.; Karon, B.S.; Nichols, J. How Should Glucose Meters Be Evaluated For Critical Care 2017. Available online: https://www.ifcc.org/media/477215/ifcc_wg-gmecc_terms_1-2.pdf (accessed on 2 October 2020).
114. LaCara, R.T.; Domagtoy, R.C.; Lickliter, R.D.; Quattrocchi, R.K.; Snipes, R.L.; Kuszaj, R.J.; Prasnikar, R.M. Comparison of Point-of-Care and Laboratory Glucose Analysis in Critically Ill Patients. *Am. J. Crit. Care* **2007**, *16*, 336–346. [CrossRef]
115. Kapoor, D.; Singh, P.; Srivastava, M. Point of care blood gases with electrolytes and lactates in adult emergencies. *Int. J. Crit. Illn. Inj. Sci.* **2014**, *4*, 216–222. [CrossRef]
116. O'Sullivan, J.B.; Mahan, C.M. CRITERIA FOR THE ORAL GLUCOSE TOLERANCE TEST IN PREGNANCY. *Diabetes* **1964**, *13*, 278–285.
117. d'Emden, M.C. Reassessment of the new diagnostic thresholds for gestational diabetes mellitus: An opportunity for improvement. *Med. J. Aust.* **2015**, *202*, 133. [CrossRef] [PubMed]

118. American Diabetes Association. Standards of Medical Care in Diabetes—2014. *Diabetes Care* **2014**, *37*, S14–S80. [CrossRef] [PubMed]
119. Agarwal, M.M.; Boulvain, M.; Coetzee, E.; Colagiuri, S.; Falavigna, M.; Hod, M.; Meltzer, S.; Metzger, B.; Omori, Y.; Rasa, I.; et al. Diagnostic criteria and classification of hyperglycaemia first detected in pregnancy: A World Health Organization Guideline. *Diabetes Res. Clin. Pract.* **2014**, *103*, 341–363.
120. Hod, M.; Kapur, A.; Sacks, D.A.; Hadar, E.; Agarwal, M.; Di Renzo, G.C.; Roura, L.C.; McIntyre, H.D.; Morris, J.L.; Divakar, H. The International Federation of Gynecology and Obstetrics (FIGO) Initiative on gestational diabetes mellitus: A pragmatic guide for diagnosis, management, and care. *Int. J. Gynaecol. Obstet.* **2015**, *131*, S173–S211. [CrossRef]
121. Committee on Practice Bulletins. Practice Bulletin No. 180: Gestational Diabetes Mellitus. *Obstet Gynecol.* **2017**, *130*, e17–e37. [CrossRef] [PubMed]
122. National Institutes of Health. Consensus Development Conference Statement: Diagnosing gestational diabetes mellitus, March 4–6, 2013. *Obstet. Gynecol.* **2013**, *122*, 358–369. [CrossRef]
123. Berger, H.; Gagnon, R.; Sermer, M.; Basso, M.; Bos, H.; Brown, R.N.; Bujold, E.; Cooper, S.L.; Gagnon, R.; Gouin, K.; et al. Diabetes in Pregnancy. *J. Obstet. Gynaecol. Can.* **2016**, *38*, 667–679.e1. [CrossRef]
124. Duran, A.; Sáenz, S.; Torrejón, M.J.; Bordiú, E.; Del Valle, L.; Galindo, M.; Perez, N.; Herraiz, M.A.; Izquierdo, N.; Rubio, M.A.; et al. Introduction of IADPSG Criteria for the Screening and Diagnosis of Gestational Diabetes Mellitus Results in Improved Pregnancy Outcomes at a Lower Cost in a Large Cohort of Pregnant Women: The St. Carlos Gestational Diabetes Study. *Diabetes Care* **2014**, *37*, 2442–2450. [CrossRef]
125. McIntyre, H.D.; Gibbons, K.S.; Ma, R.C.; Tam, W.H.; Sacks, D.A.; Lowe, J.; Madsen, L.R.; Catalano, P.M. Testing for gestational diabetes during the COVID-19 pandemic. An evaluation of proposed protocols for the United Kingdom, Canada and Australia. *Diabetes Res. Clin. Pract.* **2020**, *167*, 108353. [CrossRef]
126. Torlone, E.; Festa, C.; Formoso, G.; Scavini, M.; Sculli, M.A.; Succurro, E.; Sciacca, L.; Di Bartolo, P.; Purrello, F.; Lapolla, A. Italian recommendations for the diagnosis of gestational diabetes during COVID-19 pandemic: Position statement of the Italian Association of Clinical Diabetologists (AMD) and the Italian Diabetes Society (SID), diabetes, and pregnancy study group. *Nutr. Metab. Cardiovasc. Dis.* **2020**, *30*, 1418–1422. [CrossRef]
127. Thangaratinam, S.; Cooray, S.D.; Sukumar, N.; Huda, M.S.B.; Devlieger, R.; Benhalima, K.; McAuliffe, F.; Saravanan, P.; Teede, H.J. ENDOCRINOLOGY IN THE TIME OF COVID-19: Diagnosis and management of gestational diabetes mellitus. *Eur. J. Endocrinol.* **2020**, *183*, G49–G56. [CrossRef] [PubMed]
128. Van Gemert, T.E.; Moses, R.G.; Pape, A.V.; Morris, G.J. Gestational diabetes mellitus testing in the COVID-19 pandemic: The problems with simplifying the diagnostic process. *Aust. New Zealand J. Obstet. Gynaecol.* **2020**, *60*, 671–674. [CrossRef] [PubMed]
129. Van De L'Isle, Y.; Steer, P.J.; Coote, I.W.; Cauldwell, M. Impact of changes to national UK Guidance on testing for gestational diabetes screening during a pandemic: A single-centre observational study. *BJOG Int. J. Obstet. Gynaecol.* **2020**. [CrossRef]
130. McIntyre, H.D.; Moses, R.G. The Diagnosis and Management of Gestational Diabetes Mellitus in the Context of the COVID-19 Pandemic. *Diabetes Care* **2020**, *43*, 1433–1434. [CrossRef] [PubMed]
131. Lain, K.Y.; Daftary, A.R.; Ness, R.B.; Roberts, J.M. First trimester adipocytokine concentrations and risk of developing gestational diabetes later in pregnancy. *Clin. Endocrinol.* **2008**, *69*, 407–411. [CrossRef] [PubMed]
132. Rasanen, J.P.; Snyder, C.K.; Rao, P.V.; Mihalache, R.; Heinonen, S.; Gravett, M.G.; Roberts, C.T.; Nagalla, S.R. Glycosylated Fibronectin as a First-Trimester Biomarker for Prediction of Gestational Diabetes. *Obstet. Gynecol.* **2013**. [CrossRef] [PubMed]
133. Corcoran, S.; Achamallah, N.; Loughlin, J.O.; Stafford, P.; Dicker, P.; Malone, F.D.; Breathnach, F. First trimester serum biomarkers to predict gestational diabetes in a high-risk cohort: Striving for clinically useful thresholds. *Eur. J. Obstet. Gynecol. Reprod. Biol.* **2018**, *222*, 7–12. [CrossRef]
134. Ryan, A.S. Inflammatory Markers in Older Women with a History of Gestational Diabetes and the Effects of Weight Loss. *J. Diabetes Res.* **2018**, *2018*, 5172091. [CrossRef] [PubMed]
135. Iliodromiti, S.; Sassarini, J.; Kelsey, T.W.; Lindsay, R.S.; Sattar, N.; Nelson, S.M. Accuracy of circulating adiponectin for predicting gestational diabetes: A systematic review and meta-analysis. *Diabetologia* **2016**, *59*, 692–699. [CrossRef]
136. Ghosh, P.; Luque-Fernandez, M.-A.; Vaidya, A.; Ma, N.; Sahoo, R.; Chorev, M.; Zera, C.; McElrath, T.F.; Williams, M.A.; Seely, E.W.; et al. Plasma Glycated {CD59}, a Novel Biomarker for Detection of Pregnancy-Induced Glucose Intolerance. *Diabetes Care* **2017**, *40*, 981–984. [CrossRef]

137. Ma, D.; Luque-Fernez, M.A.; Bogdanet, D.; Desoye, G.; Dunne, F.; Halperin, J.A. Plasma Glycated CD59 Predicts Early Gestational Diabetes and Large for Gestational Age Newborns. *J. Clin. Endocrinol. Metab.* **2020**, *105*, e1033–e1040. [CrossRef] [PubMed]
138. Bogdanet, D.; O'Shea, P.M.; Halperin, J.; Dunne, F. Plasma glycated CD59 (gCD59), a novel biomarker for the diagnosis, management and follow up of women with Gestational Diabetes (GDM)—Protocol for prospective cohort study. *BMC Pregnancy Childbirth* **2020**, *20*, 412. [CrossRef] [PubMed]
139. Salomon, C.; Scholz-Romero, K.; Sarker, S.; Sweeney, E.; Kobayashi, M.; Correa, P.; Longo, S.; Duncombe, G.; Mitchell, M.D.; Rice, G.E.; et al. Gestational Diabetes Mellitus Is Associated With Changes in the Concentration and Bioactivity of Placenta-Derived Exosomes in Maternal Circulation Across Gestation. *Diabetes* **2016**, *65*, 598–609. [CrossRef] [PubMed]
140. Arias, M.; Monteiro, L.J.; Acuña-Gallardo, S.; Varas-Godoy, M.; Rice, G.E.; Monckeberg, M.; Díaz, P.; Illanes, S.E. Vesículas extracelulares como predictores tempranos de diabetes gestacional [Extracellular vesicle concentration in maternal plasma as an early marker of gestational diabetes]. *Rev. Med. Chil.* **2019**, *147*, 1503–1509. (In Spanish) [CrossRef] [PubMed]
141. Monteiro, L.J.; Varas-Godoy, M.; Monckeberg, M.; Realini, O.; Hernández, M.; Rice, G.; Romero, R.; Saavedra, J.F.; Illanes, S.E.; Chaparro, A. Oral extracellular vesicles in early pregnancy can identify patients at risk of developing gestational diabetes mellitus. *PLoS ONE* **2019**, *14*, e0218616. [CrossRef] [PubMed]
142. Jayabalan, N.; Lai, A.; Nair, S.; Guanzon, D.; Scholz-Romero, K.; Palma, C.; McIntyre, H.D.; Lappas, M.; Salomon, C. Quantitative Proteomics by SWATH-MS Suggest an Association Between Circulating Exosomes and Maternal Metabolic Changes in Gestational Diabetes Mellitus. *Proteomics* **2019**, *19*, e1800164. [CrossRef] [PubMed]
143. Aslan, M.; Celik, O.; Celik, N.; Turkcuoglu, I.; Yilmaz, E.; Karaer, A.; Simsek, Y.; Celik, E.; Aydin, S. Cord blood nesfatin-1 and apelin-36 levels in gestational diabetes mellitus. *Endocrine* **2012**, *41*, 424–429. [CrossRef] [PubMed]
144. Kucukler, F.K.; Gorkem, U.; Simsek, Y.; Kocabas, R.; Gulen, S.; Guler, S. Low level of Nesfatin-1 is associated with gestational diabetes mellitus. *Gynecol. Endocrinol.* **2016**, *32*, 759–761. [CrossRef] [PubMed]
145. Mierzyński, R.; Poniedziałek-Czajkowska, E.; Dłuski, D.; Patro-Małysza, J.; Kimber-Trojnar, Ż.; Majsterek, M.; Leszczyńska-Gorzelak, B. Nesfatin-1 and Vaspin as Potential Novel Biomarkers for the Prediction and Early Diagnosis of Gestational Diabetes Mellitus. *Int. J. Mol. Sci.* **2019**, *20*, 159. [CrossRef] [PubMed]
146. Zhang, Y.; Lu, J.H.; Zheng, S.Y.; Yan, J.H.; Chen, L.; Liu, X.; Wu, W.Z.; Wang, F. Serum levels of nesfatin-1 are increased in gestational diabetes mellitus. *Gynecol. Endocrinol.* **2017**, *33*, 621–624. [CrossRef] [PubMed]
147. Deniz, R.; Gurates, B.; Aydin, S.; Celik, H.; Sahin, I.; Baykus, Y.; Catak, Z.; Aksoy, A.; Citil, C.; Gungor, S. Nesfatin-1 and other hormone alterations in polycystic ovary syndrome. *Endocrine* **2012**, *42*, 694–699. [CrossRef] [PubMed]

Publisher's Note: MDPI stays neutral with regard to jurisdictional claims in published maps and institutional affiliations.

© 2020 by the authors. Licensee MDPI, Basel, Switzerland. This article is an open access article distributed under the terms and conditions of the Creative Commons Attribution (CC BY) license (http://creativecommons.org/licenses/by/4.0/).

Review

Emerging Protein Biomarkers for the Diagnosis or Prediction of Gestational Diabetes—A Scoping Review

Delia Bogdanet [1,2,*], Catriona Reddin [2], Dearbhla Murphy [2], Helen C. Doheny [2], Jose A. Halperin [3], Fidelma Dunne [1,2] and Paula M. O'Shea [2]

1. College of Medicine Nursing and Health Sciences, National University of Ireland Galway, H91TK33 Galway, Ireland; fidelma.dunne@nuigalway.ie
2. Centre for Diabetes Endocrinology and Metabolism, Galway University Hospital, Newcastle Road, H91YR71 Galway, Ireland; reddin.catriona@gmail.com (C.R.); dearbhlaa.murphy@hse.ie (D.M.); helen.doheny@hse.ie (H.C.D.); paulaM.OShea@hse.ie (P.M.O.)
3. Divisions of Haematology, Brigham & Women's Hospital, Boston, MA 02115, USA; jhalperin@bwh.harvard.edu
* Correspondence: deliabogdanet@gmail.com; Tel.: +35-38-3102-7771

Abstract: Introduction: Gestational diabetes (GDM), defined as hyperglycemia with onset or initial recognition during pregnancy, has a rising prevalence paralleling the rise in type 2 diabetes (T2DM) and obesity. GDM is associated with short-term and long-term consequences for both mother and child. Therefore, it is crucial we efficiently identify all cases and initiate early treatment, reducing fetal exposure to hyperglycemia and reducing GDM-related adverse pregnancy outcomes. For this reason, GDM screening is recommended as part of routine pregnancy care. The current screening method, the oral glucose tolerance test (OGTT), is a lengthy, cumbersome and inconvenient test with poor reproducibility. Newer biomarkers that do not necessitate a fasting sample are needed for the prompt diagnosis of GDM. The aim of this scoping review is to highlight and describe emerging protein biomarkers that fulfill these requirements for the diagnosis of GDM. **Materials and Methods:** This scoping review was conducted according to preferred reporting items for systematic reviews and meta-analyses (PRISMA) guidelines for scoping reviews using Cochrane Central Register of Controlled Trials (CENTRAL), the Cumulative Index to Nursing & Allied Health Literature (CINAHL), PubMed, Embase and Web of Science with a double screening and extraction process. The search included all articles published in the literature to July 2020. **Results:** Of the 3519 original database citations identified, 385 were eligible for full-text review. Of these, 332 (86.2%) were included in the scoping review providing a total of 589 biomarkers studied in relation to GDM diagnosis. Given the high number of biomarkers identified, three post hoc criteria were introduced to reduce the items set for discussion: we chose only protein biomarkers with at least five citations in the articles identified by our search and published in the years 2017–2020. When applied, these criteria identified a total of 15 biomarkers, which went forward for review and discussion. **Conclusions:** This review details protein biomarkers that have been studied to find a suitable test for GDM diagnosis with the potential to replace the OGTT used in current GDM screening protocols. Ongoing research efforts will continue to identify more accurate and practical biomarkers to take GDM screening and diagnosis into the 21st century.

Keywords: gestational diabetes; biomarker; protein biomarker

1. Introduction

Gestational diabetes (GDM) is defined as hyperglycemia with onset or initial recognition during pregnancy [1]. GDM is a common complication of pregnancy, with a prevalence of 5.8–12.9% globally, the prevalence varying by region, and diagnostic criteria [2]. GDM is associated with substantial short and long-term adverse outcomes for both mother and child. Short-term complications include preeclampsia and pregnancy-induced hypertension, increased risk of delivery by cesarean section, macrosomia, and neonatal hypoglycemia [3,4]. Long-term complications include increased risk of type 2 diabetes mellitus (T2DM), obesity and cardiovascular complications for both mother and offspring [5,6]. Studies have established that effective treatment of GDM reduces the rate of short-term perinatal complications and improves the quality of life of the mother [7,8]. Given this evidence, it is of utmost importance that we identify those at risk and accurately diagnose GDM [9]. Current diagnostic strategies use the oral glucose tolerance test (OGTT) performed between 24 and 28 weeks of gestation, with universal screening advised in populations with a high prevalence of T2DM [10].

As with any screening program, we must continue to re-evaluate the test suitability, accuracy, and reproducibility. The OGTT was first described in 1957 [11] and has been the gold standard for the diagnosis of GDM for decades [12]. The OGTT is onerous, lengthy and requires a fasting state [13]. A recent review by our research group [14] has detailed the numerous factors contributing to its poor reproducibility [15].

In view of the cumbersome nature and poor reproducibility of the OGTT, it is necessary to look for and identify a more robust, convenient, and accurate biomarker for the diagnosis of GDM. Over recent years, substantial progress has been made in this field of biomarkers. There is an unmet clinical need to identify an easily measurable biomarker, which is superior to the traditional OGTT. In addition, a more convenient biomarker could be used to diagnose GDM in early pregnancy, reducing the period of intra-uterine hyperglycemic exposure. This scoping review aims to synthesize the literature on emerging biomarkers for GDM diagnosis.

2. Materials and Methods

2.1. Scoping Review Question

What are the emerging biomarkers reported in the literature for the diagnosis of gestational diabetes?

2.2. Aim

The aim of this scoping review was to systematically identify the evidence available on emerging biomarkers with the potential to diagnose GDM (beyond glucose, fructosamine and HbA1c).

2.3. Methods

This review was conducted based on the framework for scoping reviews recommended by Arksey and O'Malley [16] and the later improvements to this method [17,18]. By contrast to systematic reviews, this approach was found to be more appropriate for a comprehensive search reflecting the vast number of biomarkers with a potential to diagnose GDM at the same time, enabling us to provide an in-depth analysis of selected key biomarkers [19]. Scoping reviews are a method for recording evidence from a particular research area by presenting existing research results and highlighting gaps in the evidence at the same time.

Preferred reporting items for systematic reviews and meta-analyses (PRISMA) guidelines were followed using the PRISMA extension for scoping reviews checklist [20].

No review protocol for this study has been published.

2.4. Data Sources and Search Strategy

Using a broad-based search strategy, the following databases were searched for relevant studies from database inception through July 2020: Cochrane Central Register of Controlled Trials (CENTRAL), the Cumulative Index to Nursing and Allied Health Literature (CINAHL), PubMed, Embase and Web of Science. Search terms used included "gestational diabetes", "GDM", "emerging/novel/new", "biomarkers", "tests", and "diagnoses" combined as appropriate using the Boolean operators "AND" and "OR" (Supplemental Material).

Results were inputted into the reference manager, Rayyan web application [21], and duplicates were identified and removed. Two reviewers (DB and CR) screened the titles and the abstracts. The reference lists of included studies were also reviewed. Full texts of the remaining articles were independently assessed by two reviewers (DB and CR) for eligibility based on predefined criteria. Disagreements were resolved by consensus. Where a resolution was not reached by discussion, two other reviewers were consulted (FD, POS). The electronic search strategy can be found in (Supplemental Material)

2.5. Eligibility Criteria

Studies were eligible for inclusion if study participants were pregnant women, and the study reported on a biomarker for GDM diagnosis. All study designs were eligible for inclusion. We did not apply a language restriction. However, if translation to English was not possible, the study was excluded. There was no time restriction on the date of publication of the studies. Only full-text articles were included in this review. When the full text was unavailable, the corresponding authors were contacted.

2.6. Data extraction and Synthesis

Data were extracted independently by two authors (DB and CR) using a standardized predetermined data collection form. For each study, we extracted the title, year of publication, journal, and biomarker (which was identified on review of the methods and results section of each paper).

Extracted data were compared for inconsistencies and merged into a final database. Disagreement was resolved through discussion and, where necessary, consultation with two further reviewers (FD, POS).

The biomarkers identified were grouped alphabetically together with all the papers citing the specific biomarker for easier identification.

It was decided that if the number of potential biomarkers identified was considerable, rendering the analysis and discussion impractical, post hoc criteria would be implemented. This would help focus the discussion on the most recent, most cited protein biomarkers.

2.7. Post Hoc Inclusion Criteria

Once all the biomarkers were identified, we selected for analysis and discussion biomarkers that fulfilled 3 criteria:
1. Protein biomarkers;
2. Biomarkers that had at least 5 citations in our search results;
3. Study publication year: 2017–2020.

The resulting biomarkers were grouped into categories and brought forward for discussion.

3. Results

A total of 3519 articles were identified after the database search (Figure 1). Following title screening and deletion of duplicates, 843 abstracts were selected. A total of 458 articles were further excluded after abstract screening by two researchers, thereby reducing the articles eligible for full-paper screening to 385. A total of 53 articles were excluded (articles not in English n = 5, the test assessed was not used for GDM diagnosis n = 13, no biomarker was discussed n = 4, duplicates n = 8 and conference proceeding/abstract publication only n = 23). Finally, 332 articles were selected for data extraction. Following data extraction, a total of 589 biomarkers were identified (Supplemental Table S1).

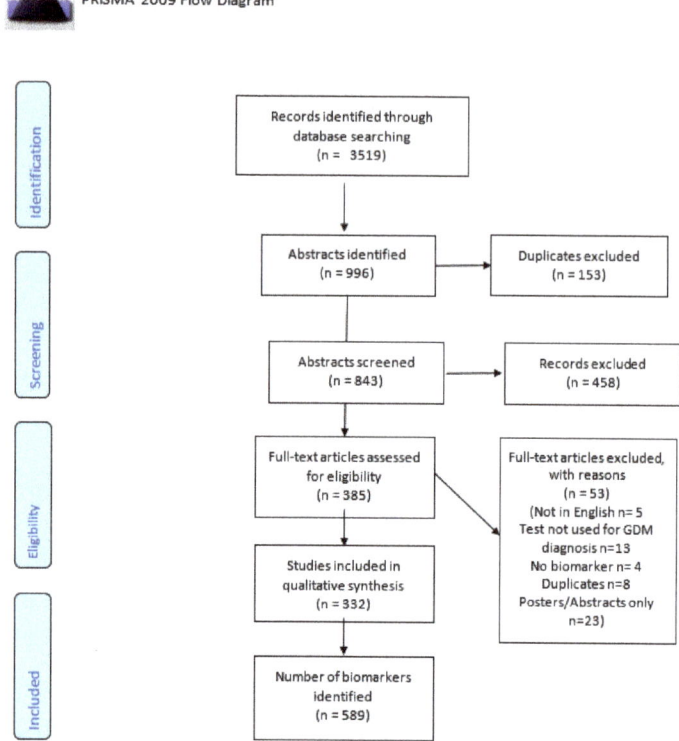

Figure 1. Prisma diagram.

After the application of the post hoc criteria, 15 biomarkers were identified, reviewed, and discussed. These biomarkers were grouped into 3 categories: cytokines, glycoproteins, and other proteins (Table 1). The biomarkers' testing performance at the time of GDM and as a predictive indicator of GDM are shown in Tables 2 and 3, and Supplemental Material Figures S1 and S2.

Table 1. Protein biomarkers (n = 15) identified post-application of post hoc criteria.

Biomarker	Function	Molecular Characteristics
	Cytokines	
* Adiponectin	Regulation of glucose and lipid metabolism. Role in cell apoptosis, inflammation and angiogenesis	Molecular mass 30 kDa; consists of 244 aa in multimeric circulating forms: a 90-kDa low molecular weight trimer, a middle molecular weight hexamer of 180 kDa and a high molecular weight multimer of ~360 kDa
* Chemerin	Adipogenesis regulation and adipocyte metabolism; role in glucose and lipid metabolism; pro/anti-inflammatory modulator	Molecular mass of 18 kDa; chemerin is translated as a 163 aa preproprotein that is secreted as a 143 aa (18 kDa) proprotein following proteolytic cleavage of a signal peptide
* Fetuin	Transport of fatty acids in the circulation with a role in insulin resistance; inhibits vascular calcification; role in inflammatory responses	Molecular mass of 64 kDa; comprises a two-chain form whose N-terminal heavy chain (321 amino acid residues) is disulfide bonded to the C-terminal light chain (27 aa)
* Leptin	Regulation of food intake and energy balance	Molecular mass of 16 kDa; consists of 146 aa structured in four antiparallel α-helices

Table 1. Cont.

Biomarker	Function	Molecular Characteristics
* Omentin	Role in glucose and lipid metabolism and adipocyte mediated inflammation	Molecular mass of 34 kDa; consists of 313 aa; contains a secretory signal sequence and a fibrinogen-related domain and appears as a glycolyzed trimer of 120 kDa molecular weight in its negative form
IL-6	Role in immunity as a mediator of the acute phase response. Acts as both a proinflammatory cytokine and an anti-inflammatory myokine. Additional role in adipocyte-mediated inflammation and glucose metabolism	Molecular mass of 21 kDa; single, non-glycosylated polypeptide chain with a four–α-helix structure containing 185 aa
TNF	Role in the regulation of immune cells, growth regulation, inflammation, viral replication, tumorigenesis, and autoimmune diseases	Molecular mass of 17.3 kDa; homotrimer composed of 233 aa
Glycoproteins		
Afamin	Vitamin E transport. Possible role in glucose and lipid metabolism	Molecular mass of 87 kDa with 55% aa sequence similarity to albumin; composed of a 21-aa leader peptide, followed by 578aa of the mature protein and consists of 2 structural domains
hCG	Maintains the production of progesterone from the corpus luteum during pregnancy; role in glucose and insulin metabolism; role in adipocyte-mediated inflammation	Molecular mass of 36.7 kDa, (~14.5 αhCG and 22.2 kDa βhCG), composed of 237 aa; it is heterodimeric, with an α subunit identical to that of luteinizing, follicle-stimulating and thyroid-stimulating hormone and an β subunit that is unique to hCG
CD59	Inhibits the complement membrane attack complex action	Molecular mass of 14.2 kDa; consists of 128 aa
SHBG	Binding protein for testosterone and estradiol; regulates sex steroid effects in target cells by direct action; role in lipid and glucose metabolism	Molecular mass of 43.7 kDa; homodimer, each monomer consists of 402 aa
Other Proteins		
CRP	Activation of the complement system, promoting phagocytosis by macrophages Role in the innate immune system	Molecular mass of 120 kDa, belonging to the family of pentraxins; consists of five identical subunits that contain each 206 aa
Nefatin-1	Regulation of food intake and glucose homeostasis	Molecular mass of 9.7 kDa containing 82 aa residues
PAPP-A	Cleavage of insulin-like growth factor-binding proteins promoting somatic growth	Molecular mass of 400 kDa composed of two 200-kDa disulfide-bound subunits, each subunit consists of 1547 aa: belonging to the pappalysin protein family
RBP4	Transporter protein for retinol; role in insulin resistance and tumor growth	Molecular mass of 21 kDa consisting of 184 aa; the entire molecule consists of an N-terminal loop, a β-barrel structure, an alpha helix and a C-terminal loop

* adipokines; IL-6—interleukin 6; TNF—tumor necrosis factor; hCG—human chorionic gonadotropin; SHBG—sex hormone-binding globulin; CRP—C-reactive protein; PAPP-A—placental associated plasma protein A; RBP4—retinol-binding protein 4; aa—amino acids.

Table 2. Summary of test performance at the time of gestational diabetes (GDM) diagnosis *.

Biomarker	First Author (Ref.)	Analytical Method	Diagnostic Sensitivity %	Diagnostic Specificity %	AUC	Cutoff Value
Cytokines						
Adiponectin	Bozkurt et al. [22]	RIA	NS	ns	0.62	ns
	Weerakiet et al. [23]	ELISA	91.7	30.8	0.63	10 µg/mL
Chemerin	Wang et al. [24]	ELISA	73.3	76	0.82	6.78 µg/L
Leptin	Bozkurt et al. [22]	RIA	ns	ns	0.61	ns
	Boyadzhieva et al. [25]	ELISA	81.2	64.2	0.82	28.7 ng/mL
Glycoproteins						
CD59	Ghosh et al. [26]	ELISA	85	92	0.92	ns
	Ma et al. [27]	ELISA	54	93	0.86	ns
SHBG	Tawfeek et al. [28]	ELISA	96	95	0.91	50 nmol/L

Table 2. Cont.

Biomarker	First Author (Ref.)	Analytical Method	Diagnostic Sensitivity %	Diagnostic Specificity %	AUC	Cutoff Value
		Other Proteins				
RBP4	Du et al. [29]	ELISA	79.4	79.1	0.87	34.84 µg/mL

* no information on test performance at the time of GDM diagnosis was found for the following biomarkers: fetuin, omentin, IL-6, TNF, afamin, hCG, CRP, nesfatin-1, PAPP-A. AUC—area under the curve; IL-6—interleukin 6; TNF—tumor necrosis factor; hCG—human chorionic gonadotropin; SHBG—sex hormone-binding protein; CRP—C-reactive protein; PAPP-A—pregnancy-associated plasma protein A; RBP4—retinol-binding protein 4; RIA—radioimmunoassay; ELISA—enzyme-linked immunosorbent assay; ns—not stated.

Table 3. Summary of test performance as a predictive indicator of GDM *.

Biomarker	First Author, Year (Ref.)	Analytical Method	Diagnostic Sensitivity %	Diagnostic Specificity %	AUC	Cutoff Value
		Cytokines				
Adiponectin	Georgiou et al. [30]	ELISA	85 [1]	85.7 [1]	0.86	3.5 µg/mL
	Ferreira et al. [31]	ELISA	ns	ns	0.85 [2]	ns
	Madhu et al. [32]	ELISA	100	95.6	ns	9.1 µg/mL
Fetuin	Iliodromiti et al. [33] **	ns	64.7	77.8	0.78	ns
	Kansu-Celik et al. [34]	ELISA	58.6	76.2	0.33	166 ng/mL
	Jin et al. [35]	ELISA	64.4	58.5	0.61	305.9 pg/mL
Leptin	Bawah et al. [36]	ELISA	95.7	68.6	0.81	18.9 ng/mL
TNF	Syngelaki et al. [37]	ELISA	ns	ns	0.82	ns
		Glycoproteins				
Afamin	Tramontana et al. [38]	ELISA	ns	ns	0.66 [3]	ns
	Koninger et al. [39] **	ELISA	79.3	79.4	0.78	88.6 mg/L
	Ravnsborg et al. [40] **	nanoLC-MS	ns	ns	0.67	ns
SHBG	Caglar et al. [41]	RIA	46.7	84.1	0.87	97.47 nmol/L
	Maged et al. [42]	ELISA	85.2	37	0.69	211.5 nmol/L
	Veltman-Verhulst et al. [43] **	ECL	81	82.8	0.86	58.5 nmol/L
	Badon et al. [44] **	ELISA	ns	ns	0.71 [2]	44.2 nmol/L
		Other Proteins				
CRP	Kansu-Celik et al. [34]	Nephelometry	86.2	50.8	0.70	ns
	Lovati et al. [45]	DELFIA	81.4 [2]	50.5 [2]	0.70 [2]	ns
	Ramezani et al. [46]	ELISA	73.3	57.3	0.61	1896 mU/L
	Ramezani et al. [46]	ELISA	34.4	83.2	0.62	0.3 mU/L
PAPP-A	Ren et al. [47]	TRFIA	72.5	82.3	0.86	16.34 ng/mL
	Snyder et al. [48]	DELFIA	75.7 [2]	55.5 [2]	0.71 [2]	ns
	Xiao et al. [49]	DELFIA	ns	ns	0.53; 0.68 [2]	ns
	Syngelaki et al. [50]	DELFIA	ns	ns	0.84 [2]	ns
RBP4	Yuan et al. [51]	EIA	63.6	75	0.72	30.45 µg/mL

* no information on test performance as a predictive indicator of GDM was found for the following biomarkers: chemerin, omentin, IL-6, CD59, hCG, nesfatin-1. AUC—area under the curve; IL-6—interleukin 6; TNF—tumor necrosis factor; hCG—human chorionic gonadotropin; SHBG—sex hormone-binding protein; CRP—C-reactive protein; PAPP-A—pregnancy-associated plasma protein A; RBP4—retinol-binding protein 4; RIA—radioimmunoassay; ELISA—enzyme-linked immunosorbent assay; nanoLC-MS—nano-flow liquid chromatography-tandem mass spectrometry; ECL—electrochemiluminescence; DELFIA—dissociation-enhanced lanthanide fluorescent immunoassay, TRFIA—time-resolved fluorescence immunoassay analyzer; EIA—enzyme immunoassay; ns—not stated; [1] combined model with insulin levels; [2] combined model with risk factors; [3] combined model with BMI; ** prior to pregnancy.

4. Cytokines

Cytokines are cell-signaling proteins, peptides or glycoproteins that are secreted by specific cells of the immune system. They regulate and modulate both the innate and adaptive immune response to inflammation and infection.

4.1. Adipokines

The adipokines are cytokines secreted by the adipose tissue and comprise a group of over 600 molecules that have paracrine and endocrine functions [52]. Inflammation and dysfunction of the adipose tissue lead to a pattern of adipokines secretion, which reflects a proinflammatory, dysmetabolic and diabetogenic model [52,53].

4.1.1. Adiponectin

Adiponectin is a protein secreted primarily by the fat tissue but also by the brain, the skeletal muscle, and the placenta [54–56], comprising 244 amino acids. Adiponectin has a role in insulin sensitivity [57,58], reduces liver gluconeogenesis [59] and enhances skeletal muscle fatty acid oxidation [60]. Low adiponectin levels are associated with an increased incidence of T2DM [61,62], and furthermore, low adiponectin levels were found in women with GDM [63,64]. This raised the question of adiponectin can be used to diagnose GDM.

Hedderson et al. [65] looked at the relationship of prepregnancy adiponectin levels and the risk of subsequent development of GDM in a case–control study within a cohort of 4098 women (GDM women n = 256, 100 g 3 h OGTT, American College of Obstetricians and Gynecologists criteria [66] controls n = 497). The team found that low adiponectin levels measured as far as six years prior to pregnancy were associated with an increased risk of developing GDM independent of age, BMI, family history or ethnicity. This finding suggests that adiponectin could have the potential to identify women at high risk of developing GDM, who otherwise would not be classified as high risk. This study, however, does not capture the changes in lifestyle, diet, and exercise between the baseline adiponectin measurement and the GDM diagnosis, and it also does not provide any information on body composition, such as percentage of fat or anthropomorphic measurements. One study has found that the first-trimester of pregnancy adiponectin is significantly lower in GDM cases compared to controls and has the potential to determine the risk of developing GDM [30] with an AUC of 0.86, thus showing promise despite the small sample size of their cohorts (n = 28). Similar results come from Williams et al. [67] and Ferreira et al. [31], who found that adiponectin levels taken at 13 weeks of gestation were lower in women, who developed GDM compared to controls. Choosing a cutoff point of 9.1 µg/mL for the first-trimester adiponectin levels, Madhu et al. [32] found the test to have a sensitivity of 100% and a specificity of 95.6% in predicting GDM.

In 2018 Bozkurt et al. [22] investigated the relationship between adiponectin levels and the development of GDM. The study included 223 participants, who were assessed for their glycemic status (75 g 2 h OGTT, IADPSG criteria) and adiponectin level at the first visit (<21 weeks of gestation) and at the second visit (24–28 weeks of gestation). The team found that adiponectin levels were significantly lower in women that developed GDM, and the association between adiponectin levels and GDM was even stronger in study participants that developed early GDM (<21 weeks), with a calculated predictive value for GDM of 0.67 (95% CI 0.57 to 0.77). Adiponectin taken during the OGTT at 24–28 weeks of gestation could predict GDM with an AUC of 0.65 (95% CI 0.57–0.74). These findings were independent of the prepregnancy maternal BMI; this is consistent with previous studies [68,69] that found adiponectin levels to be similar between individuals with a normal BMI and obese individuals that are classified as being metabolically healthy (based on lipid levels, glycemic status and blood pressure readings) compared to obese individuals classified as metabolically unhealthy. Therefore, in pregnancy, low adiponectin levels may indicate a prepregnancy predisposition for metabolic complications, such as diabetes, hypertension, or dyslipidemia, rather than a reflection on the individual's adipose tissue mass. Weerakiet et al. [23] measured adiponectin levels in 359 women at the same time as the glucose challenge test between 21st and 27th week of gestation and, while the results were consistent with previous findings in that adiponectin level are lower in women that develop GDM independent of age and BMI, in terms of screening. However, the AUC of adiponectin was less than the glucose challenge test (GCT) AUC (0.63 (95% CI 0.53–0.67) Vs. 0.73 (95% CI 0.71–080) and had a sensitivity of 91.7% and a specificity of 30.8%. These calculations, however, were based on an arbitrarily chosen cutoff value for adiponectin at 10 µg/mL.

Xu et al. [70], in their systematic review and meta-analysis, looked at the association between adiponectin and GDM and included 15 studies and 560 GDM patients. They found that adiponectin levels were significantly decreased in women who developed GDM compared to controls, independent of BMI, similar to previous studies. The study, however, had its limitations, including large variability in adiponectin cutoff points and a high degree of heterogeneity. Iliodromiti et al. [33] conducted a systematic review and meta-analysis on the accuracy of adiponectin in predicting GDM and included 11 studies and data on 794 GDM women. They found that pooled sensitivity for adiponectin as a GDM diagnostic biomarker was 64.7% (95% CI 51%, 76.4%), and the pooled specificity was 77.8% (95% CI 66.4%, 86.1% with an AUC of 0.78 (95% CI 0.74, 0.81). While the researchers conclude that adiponectin has a moderate predictive value, there are several limitations to their paper, including the study heterogeneity, the limited access to data (2 studies), the variability of adiponectin levels cutoff points for "low" or "high" levels, the diversity of ethnicities in the populations involved and the various study designs and retrospective nature of the data that may have contributed to the results.

Adiponectin is a very promising biomarker for the diagnosis of GDM and has a significant advantage over the OGTT/GCT of not mandating a fasting state for measurements [71]. While some studies determined less than ideal performance parameters for adiponectin, we need to consider that in the first-trimester, fasting glucose has been shown to have a sensitivity of 47%, a specificity of 77% and AUC of 0.62 [72], improving in the second-trimester [73]; HbA1c has a sensitivity of 32% and a specificity of 94% [74] and fructosamine has a sensitivity of 12.2% and a specificity of 94.7% [75]. More so, there are no studies assessing adiponectin level cutoff points for best prognostic/diagnostic capacity, nor are any studies on adiponectin-trimester-specific interval ranges.

Large prospective studies together with health economic input analyzing best diagnostic cutoff points, natural level variation in GDM and normal glucose tolerance (NGT) cohorts, the impact of confounders, such as ethnicity, percentage of body fat, etc. are required to accurately determine the true value of adiponectin in diagnosing GDM.

4.1.2. Chemerin

Discovered more than 20 years ago [76], chemerin (163 amino acids) is an inflammatory adipokine with a role in adipogenesis, adipocyte metabolism [77] and insulin resistance [78] secreted from the adipose tissue, liver, intestine [79] and placenta [80]. Chemerin plays a role in adipocyte metabolism, inflammation, insulin resistance and metabolic processes [77,78,81], and chemerin levels have been associated with adverse pregnancy outcomes [82–84].

Yang et al. [85] measured chemerin levels in the first-trimester of pregnancy (8–12 weeks' gestation) in 212 women and in 39 women (GDM n = 19, IADPSG criteria) after the 75 g 2 h OGTT. Chemerin levels were significantly lower in the GDM group compared to NGT in the first-trimester but significantly higher in the third-trimester. In both GDM and NGT groups, chemerin significantly rose between the first and third-trimester, paralleling the rise in HOMA-IR.

In 2020 Wang et al. [24] found that the AUC of chemerin (cutoff value 6.78 µg/L) in the diagnosis of GDM (24–28 weeks of gestation) was 0.82 (95% CI 0.74–0.89) with a sensitivity of 73.3% and specificity of 76%.

Pfau et al. [86] measured chemerin levels in 40 GDM women and, while the levels were higher in GDM subjects, there was no significant difference when compared to controls; there was, however, an independent association between chemerin and markers of insulin resistance. Guelfi et al. [87] measured adipokine levels, including chemerin in 123 pregnant women at 14 and 28 weeks of gestation and found no change in chemerin concentration between the two time points and no difference in chemerin levels between women who developed GDM compared to those who did not (unlike adiponectin and leptin that showed significant changes). The cohort in this study included only women with a history of GDM with a different metabolic profile compared to the general population, so the results cannot be extrapolated. Van Poppel et al. [88] found no difference in chemerin levels between GDM (n = 15, IADPSG criteria) and NGT subjects. However, chemerin levels were significantly higher in obese women compared to non-obese women. In their systematic review and meta-analysis (10 studies), Sun et al. [89] did not find any difference in chemerin levels between GDM and NGT women but did find a positive correlation between chemerin and BMI. These results contradict the findings of Zhou et al. [90], who conducted a systematic review and meta-analysis (11 studies) looking specifically at chemerin levels and GDM and found that chemerin levels are significantly raised in the GDM population compared to NGT women. While both systematic reviews and meta-analyses had significant heterogeneity, the discrepancy in results may arise either from the different studies comprising the analysis or either from the type of subanalysis and confounders included.

The main reason for the discordant results is the fact that chemerin is influenced by numerous factors, such as inflammation, insulin resistance, metabolic syndrome, obesity, diabetes, nutrition, activity level and pregnancy [80,82,91–95]. It seems that chemerin may play a better role as a risk-stratifying tool rather than a GDM diagnostic biomarker, identifying women at risk of GDM, but future research might prove otherwise.

4.1.3. Fetuin

Fetuins are a group of adipokines mainly secreted by the liver. Fetuin-A is secreted from the liver and adipose tissue with elevated levels in obesity [96,97], metabolic syndrome [98], fatty liver disease [99], and T2DM [100,101]. Fetuin-B, secreted by hepatocytes, tongue and placenta [102], is increased in hepatic steatosis and is linked to gluconeogenesis through insulin suppression [103,104]. Based on the association with insulin resistance and glucose metabolism, it was hypothesized that fetuins could serve as markers for GDM diagnosis.

Kansu-Celik et al. [34] measured first-trimester fetuin-A as a biomarker for GDM diagnosis in 88 pregnant women (GDM n = 29, GCT/OGTT, Carpenter and Coustan criteria) and found significantly lower levels in GDM women compared with controls. Fetuin-A below 166 ng/mL could predict GDM with a sensitivity of 58.6%, specificity of 76.2% and AUC of 0.337 (95% CI 0.21–0.46). Kalabay et al. [105] measured fetuin-A in 134 pregnant women (GDM n = 30, 75 g 2 h OGTT, 1999 WHO criteria) and 30 non-pregnant women in each-trimester of pregnancy (including at the time of the OGTT) and found significantly higher levels of fetuin-A in GDM women at all time points compared to the NGT and non-pregnant women; fetuin-A was also positively associated with markers of insulin resistance, TNF-α and leptin levels. Iydir et al. [106] also found higher fetuin-A levels (sample collected at the time of the OGTT) in GDM women (n = 26, Carpenter and Coustan criteria [107]) compared to NGT and decreased post-partum. The authors found a positive correlation between fetuin-A and HbA1c levels. Jin et al. [35] measured fetuin-A in 270 women (GDM n = 135, IADPSG criteria) in the first and second-trimester of pregnancy and found significantly higher levels of fetuin-A in GDM women compared to controls at both time points, and it was positively correlated with the changes in the markers of insulin resistance. In this study, a fetuin-A cutoff value of 305.9 pg/mL in the first-trimester would predict GDM with a sensitivity of 64.4%, specificity of 58.5% and AUC of 0.61 (95% CI 0.54 to 0.68).

Farhan et al. [108] measured fetuin-A in 20 women (GDM n = 10) at the time of the 75 g 2 h OGTT (28 weeks of gestation) and 3 months post-partum; they found no difference in fetuin-A levels between GDM and NGT study participants at any time point.

The discrepancy between these study results arises from the different study designs, different population characteristics and sample size, and the different time-point sampling making the results inconsistent and difficult to compare.

It is unclear what the exact role of fetuin-A is in the pathophysiology of GDM. Some hypotheses suggest that its main action is through insulin resistance through the inhibition of the insulin receptor, while others suggest that fetuin-A induces adipose tissue inflammation, which leads to lipid-induced insulin resistance. There is even less information on fetuin-B, as its mode of action, signaling, and even receptor have not been adequately described. However, the minimal studies available show promising results. Prospective studies with a longitudinal sampling of both fetuins while assessing correlations with markers of insulin resistance are required.

4.1.4. Leptin

Leptin (167 amino acids), the first adipokine to be discovered in 1994, [109] is predominantly secreted by adipose cells [110], but also by the stomach [111], placenta [112] and the brain [113]. Leptin has a role in energy homeostasis by inhibiting hunger and mediating food intake [114,115] through its action on the hypothalamus, dopamine system and brain stem [116]. More so, in both animal and human models, leptin administration improved hyperinsulinemia, hyperglycemia, insulin resistance and hyperlipidemia [117–119].

While leptin levels rise in pregnancy compared to the non-pregnant state, peaking between 20 and 30 weeks of gestation most likely secondary to fat accumulation [71,120], even higher leptin levels have been associated with GDM.

Bawah et al. [36] found that first-trimester leptin levels (11–13 weeks of gestation) in 140 women (GDM n = 70, 75 g 2 h OGTT, American Diabetes Association (ADA) criteria [121]) could predict the development of GDM with a sensitivity of 95.7%, specificity of 68.6% and AUC of 0.81.

Kautzky-Willer et al. [122] measured leptin levels at 28 weeks of gestation in GDM women (n = 55, 1999 WHO criteria [1]), women with NGT (n = 25) and women with T1DM (n = 10). These samples were collected in a fasting state and 30 minutes after the glucose load during the OGTT. They found that leptin levels were higher in women with GDM compared to NGT and T1DM and similar between NGT women and T1DM women, all matched for BMI. There were no differences between leptin levels between fasting and post-glucose-load values, indicating that this test could be done in a non-fasting state. Boyadzhieva et al. [25] measured fasting leptin levels during the OGTT in 286 women (GDM n = 127, IADPSG criteria) and found significantly higher levels in the GDM group compared to the controls. They also assessed if leptin could be used as a screening test and, setting the cutoff value at 28.7 ng/mL; the test could exclude GDM with a sensitivity of 81.2%, a specificity of 64.2% and AUC of 0.827. Bozkurt et al. [22] found higher levels of leptin in women with GDM compared to controls, but the predictive value for GDM was 0.66 (95% CI 0.57 to 0.74). Leptin taken during the OGTT at 24–28 weeks of gestation could identify GDM with an AUC of 0.61 (95% CI 0.53–0.69).

Contradictory results come from the work of McLachlan et al. [123], who found higher leptin levels in the control group compared to GDM. However, this was of borderline significance $p = 0.05$. More so, the number of women in this study was small (19 women in each arm) but well-matched, and the measurements for leptin levels were taken during an intravenous glucose tolerance test (IVGTT) in the third-trimester of pregnancy. While the OGTT is preferred over the IVGTT in detecting glucose intolerance [124], we also know from previous studies [71,120] that leptin levels peak up to 30 weeks of gestation and start decreasing thereafter.

In a systematic review and meta-analysis, Xu et al. [70] found that high levels of leptin in early pregnancy may be predictive for developing GDM independent of BMI. In their systematic review (which included 9 prospective studies), Bao et al. [125] found that leptin levels taken in the first or second-trimester of pregnancy were 7.25 ng/mL higher (95% CI 3.27–11.22) in women who were subsequently diagnosed with GDM compared to women with NGT.

The data on leptin is slightly contradictory, and that may be due to the leptin correlation with adipose tissue. Despite that, most studies show great promise. While there is some evidence that stress, sleep deprivation or exercise influence leptin levels [126–128], similar to the OGTT [14], the test can be done in a non-fasting state, which is a clear advantage over the OGTT. Similar to adiponectin, prospective studies are required to determine-trimester-specific reference ranges for the non-diabetic pregnant population,-trimester-specific cutoff points for the GDM population, the impact of confounders (including adiposity markers) on leptin levels and association with pregnancy outcomes.

4.1.5. Omentin

Omentin (313 amino acids) is an adipose-tissue-specific factor selectively expressed in visceral tissue relative to subcutaneous adipose tissue. Omentin has a role in fat distribution, energy expenditure and insulin action modulation [129,130]. In 2007, de Souza Batista et al. [131] found that omentin levels correlated negatively with BMI/obesity, leptin level, and markers of insulin resistance and correlated positively with HDL and adiponectin levels in healthy subjects.

Barker et al. [132] studied the effects of pregnancy on omentin levels, also assessing the impact of BMI and GDM on omentin levels. Blood samples were collected in the first and second-trimester from 83 pregnant women (GDM n = 39, 75 g 2 h OGTT, Australasian Diabetes in Pregnancy Society (ADIPS) [133]). The study found significantly decreased omentin levels in non-obese GDM women compared to controls with no difference in levels between obese GDM and NGT study participants. Omentin was negatively associated with fasting glucose, and maternal BMI and no association was found between omentin and adiponectin or leptin levels. While the subgroup numbers were small and the outcomes most likely underpowered, this research was one of the first to explore the role of omentin in pregnancy and GDM, raising further questions, such as what is the balance between omentin secretion and clearance at each stage of the pregnancy; does the ratio between adipose tissue omentin secretion and placental tissue omentin secretion change during pregnancy?

Abell et al. [134] measured omentin levels in the first-trimester of pregnancy in 103 women (25 of whom later developed GDM) and found lower omentin-1 levels in women with GDM compared to controls and a negative association with 1 h and 2 h glucose levels of the OGTT. They also found that omentin-1 levels less than 38.36 ng/mL were associated with a 4-fold increased risk of GDM and that for 1 ng/mL increase in omentin levels, the risk of GDM was OR 0.97 (95% CI 0.94–0.99). Limitations of the study include that all the participants in this study were at high risk for GDM with all pregnant women being overweight or obese, and the women were initially screened with a GCT followed by the OGTT if deemed necessary with arguably milder GDM cases being missed (thus this is only attributable to the very highest risk group and not suitable for population screening). Regardless, this study also highlights that-trimester 1 omentin may have the potential to predict GDM.

Contradictory data comes from Franz et al. [135], who measured omentin levels in 192 pregnant women (GDM n = 96, German and Austrian Society for Diabetes criteria based on the hyperglycemia and adverse pregnancy outcomes (HAPO) study [136]) at the time of the OGTT, at 32 weeks and from the umbilical cord at the time of the delivery. While omentin levels were lower in the GDM group compared to the NGT group at all timepoints, this was only statistically significant at the delivery timepoint. Omentin levels were also lower in women with a higher BMI and a lower HDL cholesterol.

In a systematic review and meta-analysis, which included 20 studies (GDM n = 1493), Sun et al. [89] found that omentin levels were significantly lower in women with GDM than in healthy controls. The authors also suggested that age and BMI may be important parameters influencing omentin levels in GDM patients. While there was significant heterogeneity in this review and a limited number of studies identified, the authors conclude that omentin has the potential to be a novel biomarker for early GDM diagnosis.

Omentin shows some promise as a GDM diagnostic biomarker, however further studies are required to clarify the actual role in GDM pathophysiology—if it is linked to visceral adiposity, vascular/endothelial dysfunction in either visceral adipose tissue or placenta or insulin mediation. Prospective studies are required to detect specific reference ranges and cut-offs and assess the impact of adiposity and inflammation on omentin levels and consecutively on omentin capacity to diagnose GDM. More so, omentin levels are influenced by fasting state [137,138], which makes it a less attractive biomarker compared to other biomarkers discussed.

4.1.6. Interleukin 6 (IL-6)

IL-6 is an inflammatory cytokine [139] secreted by monocytes/macrophages, but also endothelial cells, myocytes, adipocytes, pancreatic cells and placenta [139,140] with primary roles in immune response regulation, inflammation and hematopoiesis [141], but also roles in obesity, insulin resistance and T2DM [142–144]. Some of the mechanisms proposed for its role in metabolism are the percentage of body fat [145], the degree of visceral fat [146], IL-6 direct effect on hepatocytes [142,147], the immune response induced dyslipidemia, IL6 lipolytic effect [148] or even a central effect of IL-6 on food intake [149,150]. A systematic review and meta-analysis by Liu et al. (Liu 2016) explored the association between IL-6 and T2DM. It comprised 16 studies involving 24,929 subjects and found that IL-6 was a strong predictor of developing T2DM. In pregnancy, the role of IL-6 in GDM prediction has given conflicting results.

Sudharshana Murthy et al. [151] explored the role of IL-6 in GDM. IL-6 levels were taken at the time of the OGTT in 60 pregnant women (GDM n = 30, OGTT) and found significantly raised IL-6 levels at the time of diagnosis. Siddiqui et al. [152], using a very similar study design, measured IL-6 levels in 103 pregnant women (GDM n = 53, OGTT, ADA criteria) at the time of the OGTT and found significantly increased IL-6 levels in the GDM cohort compared to the NGT and a strong association between IL-6 levels and prepregnancy BMI and fasting and post-prandial glucose levels. The participants in both studies were Asian with a median normal/normal-high BMI. A prospective study by Braga et al. [153] involving 176 South American pregnant women (GDM n = 78, 100 g OGTT, Carpenter and Coustan criteria) found no difference in IL-6 levels (taken at the time of the OGTT) between GDM and NGT women. Similar results were found by Simjak et al. [154] in 24 European pregnant women (GDM n = 12, OGTT, IADPSG criteria) with normal BMI, who examined IL-6 levels in the second and third-trimester and post-partum and found no difference between GDM and NGT women.

Driven by the discordance in results, a recent systematic review by Amirian et al. [155] has explored the relationship between Il-6 and GDM in studies published between 2009 and 2020 and included 24 articles. The study highlighted the diversity of ethnicities involved, the different measurement methods, but also the numerous criteria used to diagnose GDM (14 different diagnostic criteria) in the studies selected, making significant research synthesis difficult. The common denominator for all studies, however, was the small sample size with the largest cohort in a study by Abdel Gader et al. [156], who found no difference in IL-6 levels between GDM and NGT women. Out of 24 studies, 16 found a positive association between IL-6 levels and GDM, the authors concluding that IL-6 can be used as a GDM biomarker. However, such a statement requires more scientific evidence. The heterogeneity of the studies to date involved in assessing the relationship between IL-6 and GDM is too high to be able to make any meaningful comparison.

Conceptually, IL-6 could be linked to GDM pathogenesis either through a higher degree of inflammation in GDM pregnancies [157], driven by increased subcutaneous or visceral adipose tissue [158] or increased IL-6 secretion by the placenta in GDM pregnancies [159]. While IL-6 might prove to be a good GDM biomarker in the future, there are too many unanswered questions at present for such a claim. Larger studies with increased homogeneity in GDM diagnostic methods and criteria are required with serial IL-6 measurements in each-trimester of pregnancy for identification of-trimester-specific ranges, measurements of subcutaneous and visceral adipose tissue, which might be the driver for its increase, and associations with adverse pregnancy outcomes.

4.1.7. Tumor Necrosis Factor (TNF)

TNF is an inflammatory cytokine family primarily secreted by monocytes/macrophages [160] with two main components TNF-α (also secreted from the placenta [161]) and TNF-β. The initial role for TNF was thought to be the death of tumor cells [162], but it was soon discovered that TNF plays an important role in inflammatory diseases [163], neurodegenerative disease [164], and depression [165]. Given its pro-inflammatory effects, TNF has been identified as a marker of metabolic syndrome [166,167], obesity [168] and insulin resistance [169,170]. Evidence suggests that TNF stimulates the secretion of IL-6 [171,172], inhibits the secretion of adiponectin [173], induces apoptosis in adipose cells [174,175] and inhibits the insulin receptor, thus promoting insulin resistance [170,176]. A recent study by Alzamil et al. [177] examined the correlation between TNF-α and insulin resistance, T2DM and obesity in 128 Asian subjects (T2DM n = 65). These authors found significantly higher TNF-α in T2DM subjects compared to controls, in obese subjects (T2DM or non-T2DM) compared to non-obese subjects, and TNF-α levels were positively correlated with HbA1c levels and HOMA-IR highlighting the role TNF-α plays in the pathogenesis of insulin resistance and T2DM and the link with both obesity and glucose intolerance.

Guillemette et al. [178] studied TNF-α levels in both the first-trimester of pregnancy and at the time of GDM diagnosis and its relationship to GDM in 756 pregnant women (GDM n = 61, GCT/OGTT, IADPSG criteria). They found a positive association between TNF-α levels and BMI, adiponectin, and insulin levels in the first-trimester and HOMA-IR, BMI, triglycerides, and fasting insulin levels in the third-trimester. The authors also showed that TNF-α levels are strongly positively linked to insulin resistance and that it behaves differently during the OGTT in insulin-sensitive and insulin-resistant women.

Kirwan et al. [179] described longitudinal changes in TNF-α levels and the association with maternal insulin resistance in 15 women (GDM n = 5, euglycemic-hyperinsulinemic clamp, Carpenter and Coustan criteria). They found that TNF-α in normal pregnancy had lower levels in early pregnancy, increasing in late pregnancy paralleling insulin sensitivity changes, with higher levels in GDM women compared to lean NGT women. They also found that TNF-α was positively correlated with insulin sensitivity independent of BMI or glycemic status. Proposed mechanisms for this were either increased TNF-α secretion by the placenta in GDM women and direct inhibition of the insulin receptor. This hypothesis is also supported by Desoye et al. [159]. Syngelaky et al. [37] studied the link between first-trimester TNF-α and the development of GDM in 1000 women (GDM n = 200, random glucose/OGTT, WHO criteria) and found higher TNF-α levels in women with GDM compared to controls. The authors calculated that TNF-α could predict GDM development with an AUC of 0.82, but adding TNF-α levels to a multi-variable prediction model did not improve any of the estimated variables. While this was a large study, the GDM diagnostic method may have omitted milder cases of GDM that could have been included in the NGT group. A recent study by Wang et al. [24] explored TNF-α levels at GDM diagnosis in 110 Chinese pregnant women (GDM n = 60, OGTT, ADA 2017 criteria) and found significantly higher TNF-α levels in GDM women compared to controls.

No correlation between TNF-α levels (samples were taken in both first-trimester and at GDM diagnosis) and GDM development was found by Georgiou et al. [30] in 250 women (GDM n = 14, OGTT, ADIPS criteria).

A systematic review and meta-analysis by Xu et al. [70] on the association between GDM and TNF-α levels comprised 10 studies, and despite the increased heterogeneity of the studies and missing confounders from the analysis, the authors found overall significant high levels of TNF-α in GDM pregnancies compared to controls independent of BMI.

The discrepancy in study results most likely lies in the different sample sizes, ethnicities, diagnostic methods and criteria and concentration limits employed. In addition, fasting, exercise and stress influence TNF-α levels [180–184], and this needs to be taken into account when considering new diagnostic tests. While there is no doubt that TNF-α plays a role in the pathogenesis of GDM and insulin resistance, the actual predictability value of this biomarker is yet to be established.

4.2. Glycoproteins

4.2.1. Afamin

Afamin is a glycoprotein present in plasma, cerebrospinal fluid, ovarian and seminal fluid [185,186], primarily expressed in the liver, but also expressed in the brain and kidneys and its main role to bind and transport vitamin E [185,187] to peripheral tissues and organs.

Studies examining afamin levels in polycystic ovary syndrome (PCOS) cohorts, despite a relatively small sample size, have found an association between afamin and insulin resistance and metabolic syndrome [188,189]. In a large multicenter study (n = 20,136), Kollerits et al. [190] found that afamin was a strong predictor for the development of T2DM and strongly correlated with insulin levels, HOMA-IR and insulin resistance, suggesting that afamin has the potential to be a biomarker for early prediction for future development of T2DM.

In pregnancy, afamin levels raise progressively with each-trimester of pregnancy, decreasing back to baseline post-partum with even higher levels in pregnancies complicated by preeclampsia or hypertension [191]. Based on the previous findings, which linked afamin with the development of insulin resistance and diabetes, it has been hypothesized that afamin may serve as a predictor for GDM. In two studies, Tramontana et al. [38,192] explored the relationship between first-trimester afamin and pregnancy complications in 4948 pregnant women and found significantly higher levels of afamin in women who subsequently developed GDM (n = 207, IADPSG criteria) compared to NGT women. Afamin (cutoff value > 65 mg/L) was shown to be an independent predictor for developing GDM with a risk ratio of 2.07 (95% CI 1.33–3.22) and an AUC of 0.66. Koninger et al. [39] looked at prepregnancy afamin levels in predicting GDM in a PCOS population (n = 63, GDM n = 29) and found higher afamin levels and HOMA-IR in women who developed GDM compared to controls with a strong positive correlation between afamin and HOMA-IR. The team showed that an afamin level of 88.6 mg/L identified GDM patients with a sensitivity of 79.3%, specificity of 79.4% and an AUC of 0.78 (95% CI 0.65–0.90). Ravnsborg et al. [40] studied potential GDM biomarkers in 270 first-trimester samples with shotgun proteomics (GDM n = 135), diagnosed according to the Danish guidelines [193] and found higher afamin levels in GDM women compared with controls and that afamin could predict GDM diagnosis with an AUC of 0.67 (95% CI 0.53–0.81).

Koninger et al. [194] studied the predictive power of afamin in diagnosing GDM in both the first-trimester (n = 110, of which 59 developed GDM) and the second-trimester of pregnancy (n = 105, of which 29 developed GDM). GDM was diagnosed according to the German Diabetes Association (DDG) and the German Association for Gynecology and Obstetrics (DGGG) [195]. They found that both first and second-trimester afamin levels were higher in GDM women compared to NGT. Because this study comprised two different cohorts for first and second-trimester samples, the samples were not taken longitudinally. Therefore, the team was not able to determine-trimester-specific cutoff values for afamin levels. Another limitation of the study is the heterogeneity of the GDM diagnosis method and criteria used as not all women were screened with 75 g 2 h OGTT, and milder cases of GDM might have been missed.

Afamin is a very novel biomarker for GDM. It is not fully clear what is the exact mechanism through which afamin is linked to insulin resistance, metabolic syndrome, and glucose intolerance. In previous studies [186,196], there has been observed no variation in afamin levels between fasting and non-fasting state, no circadian variation, no variation with the menstrual cycle or gender variation, suggesting that afamin is a stable biomarker for longitudinal measurements. There is not enough evidence to clearly state the true potential of afamin in predicting GDM, but the results to date are promising.

4.2.2. CD59

CD59 is an 18–20 kDa glycoprotein, which is also known as membrane attack complex (MAC) inhibitory protein (MAC-IP) [197,198]. Its main role is to restrict MAC formation in the cell membrane, thus preventing cell lysis and cell death. While CD59 is a protein bound to the cell membrane, soluble forms are present in the blood, urine, and saliva [199–201].

The link between diabetes complications and increased MAC deposits has been well documented [202–207]. The first paper linking the increased MAC deposits in diabetes with CD59 inactivation was by Acosta et al. [208]. They showed that in vitro CD59 exposure to glucose reduced its protection role leading to cell lysis. Building on this work,

Qin et al. [207] measured CD59 levels in the red blood cells (RBC) of subjects with and without T2DM and found that there are significantly lower levels of CD59 in diabetic RBC compared to subjects without T2DM.

In 2013, Ghosh et al. [209] hypothesized that glycated CD59 (gCD59) levels might mirror glucose control in human subjects and developed a sandwich ELISA assay to identify plasma gCD59, which they tested initially in 24 participants with and without T2DM (T2DM n = 14 HbA1c > 48 mmol/mol) and then validated it in 190 subjects (T2DM n = 100). gCD59 levels were significantly higher in the 14 individuals with T2DM from the initial testing set compared to controls and were strongly associated with HbA1c levels. gCD59 was able to identify T2DM with a sensitivity of 93%, specificity of 100% and AUC of 0.98. In the follow-up testing set, gCD59 levels were indeed higher in the T2DM group and positively associated with HbA1c levels, with the test generating an AUC of 0.88. Continuing this work, Ghosh et al. [210] explored the link between gCD59 and glycemic variables, such as HbA1c (in 400 subjects (T2DM n = 226) and glucose levels during the OGTT (n = 109). The results supported previous findings, with gCD59 levels higher in diabetic vs. participants without diabetes and independently associated with HbA1c and with the 2 h glucose level on the OGTT. More so, the team also showed an acute response of gCD59 levels to insulin therapy in 21 poorly controlled subjects, with changes in levels in 2 weeks of treatment, while HbA1c and fructosamine took 6–8 weeks to respond. This rapid turnover of values would have particular importance in pregnancy and GDM where time is limited and in utero exposure to hyperglycemia not without consequences.

Ma et al. [27] studied gCD59's capacity to predict GDM earlier in pregnancy (sample collected and OGTT performed <20 week's gestation) and the association with adverse pregnancy outcomes using 770 frozen samples collected as part of the vitamin D and lifestyle intervention (DALI) study (Simmons D 2017). All the participants in the DALI study had a BMI $\geq$ 29 kg/m^2 and underwent 3 OGTT s (<20 weeks GDM n = 207, 24–28 weeks GDM n= 77 and 35 weeks of gestation) and were diagnosed according to the IADPSG criteria. gCD59 levels were higher in GDM women diagnosed <20 weeks of gestation independent of age, BMI or ethnicity and predicted the OGTT results <20 weeks with an adjusted AUC of 0.86 (95% CI, 0.83–0.90). Restricting the analysis to the OGTT performed between 14 and 20 weeks of gestation, the AUC was calculated at 0.90 (95% CI 0.86–0.93). Early gCD59 predicted GDM at 24–28 weeks with an AUC of 0.68 (95% CI 0.64–0.73). The team also found that higher gCD59 levels were associated with the risk of delivering an LGA baby. Some limitations of the study include the retrospective nature of the study, the inclusion of only high-risk women with a BMI $\geq$ of 29 kg/m^2 and low ethnic diversity.

In 2017, Ghosh et al. [26] explored the association between gCD59 and the results of the GCT, the results of the OGTT and the prevalence of large for gestational age (LGA) babies in 1000 pregnant women at 26 weeks of gestation (500 women passed the GCT and were controls and 500 women failed the GCT and underwent a 3 h OGTT). gCD59 was 8.5 times higher in women who failed the GCT compared to those who passed it and 10 times higher in women who were diagnosed with GDM (n = 127) on the 3 h OGTT (Carpenter and Coustan criteria). gCD59 predicted GCT failure with a sensitivity of 90%, specificity of 88% and adjusted AUC of 0.92 (95% CI 0.88–0.93) and predicted the development of GDM compared to controls with a sensitivity of 85%, specificity of 92% and adjusted AUC of 0.92 (95% CI 0.77–0.91), independent of age, BMI, ethnicity of history of diabetes. More so, the team also identified significantly higher gCD59 levels in women who gave birth to an LGA baby. There are some limitations to this study, including its observational nature, the use of GCT (which may not be done in the morning), the 3 h-OGTT and the Carpenter and Coustan criteria for GDM diagnosis arguably missing milder cases of GDM.

gCD59 is a very promising biomarker that has shown much potential in the diagnosis and early diagnosis of GDM and the prediction of LGA-born infants. The rapid turnover of values and the lack of need for fasting certainly is a significant advantage for a pregnancy biomarker. However, there are still unanswered questions, such as: what are the-trimester-specific cutoff values? Are there any discrepancies in cutoff values among different ethnicities? Could early pregnancy gCD59 predict the 24–28 OGTT results in a BMI diverse population? Larger prospective studies are required to answer these questions, and one such study is currently underway [211].

4.2.3. Human Chorionic Gonadotropin (hCG)

HCG is a glycoprotein hormone, mainly secreted by the placenta, whose main role is in embryo implantation and control of embryogenesis [212]. Recently, however, Ma et al. [213] have shown that hCG influences insulin sensitivity and induces adipocyte-mediated inflammation and consequently may contribute to GDM pathogenesis. The beta isoform of hCG (β-hCG) is part of the first-trimester screening for fetal aneuploidy.

Sirikunalai et al. [214] retrospectively studied the link between β-hCG levels and adverse pregnancy outcomes, including GDM in 13,620 pregnant Thai women and found that high first-trimester β-hCG levels were associated with a decreased risk of developing GDM. This finding was not sustained in the second-trimester. While this study had a large sample size, a high number of women had incomplete data, and due to the retrospective nature of the study, adequate adjustments and multivariate analysis could not be done due to the lack of absent confounders. Ong et al. [215] measured β-hCG levels between 10 and 14 weeks of gestation in 5584 pregnant women. Women were diagnosed with GDM with a 2 h OGTT and diagnosed according to the 1980 WHO criteria [216]. The team found significantly lower β-hCG levels in women that developed GDM (n = 49) compared to NGT, suggesting that first-trimester β-hCG could predict second-trimester GDM diagnosis. A limitation of this study and an explanation for the small number of GDM cases detected is the GDM diagnosis criteria used, which would only identify severe cases of GDM, with milder cases not being included in the study. The use of IADPSG criteria in this cohort would have led to a more representative sample of the general population and ease the generalizability of results. Xiong et al. [217] retrospectively analyzed β-hCG levels in 1596 cases, 11 days after single blastocyst transfers (assisted reproduction) with 370 live births and found significantly higher rates of GDM (GDM total n = 61) in women with low levels of β-hCG compared to women with high levels of β-hCG. Beyond the retrospective nature of the study, no information is provided on the GDM diagnosis and criteria used; the number of GDM women in the low-level β-hCG subgroup is quite small (n = 5) and insufficient for a robust comparison. Controversially, Yue et al. [218] measured β-hCG levels between 14 and 20 weeks of gestation in 8333 pregnant Asian women, 1336, of which developed GDM (ADA criteria) and found high β-hCG levels are an independent risk factor for the development of GDM. A possible explanation for this discrepancy may be the more advanced week of gestation when the sample was collected with reactive β-hCG levels secreted by a hypoxic placenta as a response to hyperglycemia; also, the overall BMI of the cohort was very low compared to previous studies.

In a retrospective study, Tul et al. [219] measured first-trimester β-hCG levels in 1136 Caucasian women (GDM n = 27) and found lower yet not statistically significant levels in women who developed GDM. In this cohort, GDM was diagnosed with the 3 h OGTT and given the number diagnosed, and it would equate to a GDM prevalence of 2.37%, which is extremely low compared with the overall European GDM prevalence. It is unclear from the paper whether this low prevalence is due to missing data. However, these results are supported by Savvidou et al. [220], who retrospectively assessed β-hCG levels at 11–13 weeks of gestation in 42,102 pregnant women. GDM (n = 779) was diagnosed with a 2-step approach, the women undergoing an OGTT only if the random plasma glucose at 24–28 weeks of gestation was higher than 6.7 mmol/L. The team found no difference in β-hCG levels between women who developed GDM and NGT. No correlation in first-trimester β-hCG levels and GDM development was also found in Beneventi et al. [221] (GDM n = 228, GCT/ 100 g 3 h OGTT, Carpenter and Coustan criteria) or Sweeting et al. [222] (GDM n=248, OGTT, Australian Diabetes in Pregnancy Society criteria [133]).

There is quite a high degree of heterogeneity in design, populations and GDM diagnosis methods leading to inconsistent results. None of the studies looked at the longitudinal trend of β-hCG levels in the first and second-trimester and GDM diagnosis, which would have clarified the cause of variable levels—low levels in the first-trimester secondary to compromised placentation or reduced placental mass; high levels in the second-trimester of pregnancy secondary to hyperglycemia-induced placental hypoperfusion. It seems, however, that studies, which involved a higher-risk population for the development of GDM (assisted reproduction, GDM diagnosis criteria that identifies more severe cases of GDM, etc.) were more likely to find an association between β-hCG levels and GDM. Perhaps single β-hCG levels could be used to identify a possible at-risk GDM population that should be adequately followed up and screened. However, current evidence does not support this, and future more consistent studies are required.

4.2.4. Sex-Hormone Binding Protein (SHBG)

SHBG is a glycoprotein produced by the liver, brain, uterus, testes and placenta [223], and its main role is to bind and transport biologically active androgens and estrogens [224]. SHBG is linked to adipose tissue with lower levels in obese subjects [225], which increases when weight loss is achieved [226,227]. SHBG also has been linked to insulin resistance [228,229], metabolic syndrome [230–232] and the development of non-alcoholic fatty liver disease (NAFLD) independent of BMI and T2DM [233–235]. Potential mechanisms suggested for this are either a direct effect of insulin on SHBG production [236,237] or fat accumulation in the liver and/or increased hepatic triglycerides levels leading to decreased SHBG gene expression [238–240]. The role of SHBG in GDM diagnosis has been explored in numerous studies at different time points during pregnancy, including prepregnancy, with overall promising results.

Veltman-Verhulst et al. [43], in a prospective study, measured SHBG in 50 women with PCOS prior to pregnancy (median 35 weeks) following fertility treatment. GDM diagnosis was made based on a 3 h OGTT at 24–28 weeks of gestation (GDM n=21). SHBG levels were significantly lower in the GDM group compared to NGT and, with a cutoff level of 58.5 nmol/L, SHBG could predict GDM with a sensitivity of 81.%, specificity of 82.8% and AUC of 0.86 (95% CI 0.75–0.97). Hedderson et al. [241] studied the link between prepregnancy (median 6.2 years) levels of SHBG and the subsequent development of GDM in a case–control study (GDM n = 267, 3 h OGTT, Carpenter and Coustan criteria) and found a significantly lower level of SHBG in women, who developed GDM independent of GDM risk-factors. This study showed that SHBG levels measured years (min. 6 years) prior to pregnancy could predict the development of GDM even in very low-risk women, and this is of high clinical importance. Study limitations include the lack of longitudinal anthropomorphic data, additional SHBG measurements during pregnancy and the lack of markers of visceral adiposity. Badon et al. [44] measured SHBG in a case–control study within a cohort of 4098 pregnant women (GDM n = 267) at a median 7 years prior to pregnancy and similar to previous studies found significantly lower SHBG levels in women who subsequently developed GDM compared to controls with a predictive value of 0.71.

In a longitudinal study, Li et al. [242] measured SHBG levels in 321 women (GDM n = 107) in all 3-trimesters of pregnancy. SHBG levels increased progressively with the-trimester of pregnancy in both GDM and NGT groups, with significantly lower levels in GDM compared to controls in the first-trimester. This significance disappeared in late pregnancy, suggesting that perhaps the best time to measure SHBG is early in pregnancy as lifestyle changes or treatment for GDM in late pregnancy may influence SHBG levels. They also found SHBG levels to be negatively associated with markers of insulin resistance. This study confirmed the results of a previous study by Smirnakis et al. [243], who measured SHBG levels in 145 women (GDM n = 37, GCT, ACOG criteria [244]) at 11 and 17 weeks of gestation and found lower levels in women, who subsequently developed GDM compared to controls, with the stronger association at 11 weeks of gestation. Caglar et al. [41] found that an SHBG cutoff level of 97.47 nmol/L (at 13–16 weeks of gestation) could predict GDM with a sensitivity of 46.7%, specificity 84.1% and AUC 0.67 (95% CI 0.55–0.79), while

Maged et al. [42] using a first-trimester SHBG cutoff value of 211.5 nmol/L calculated a sensitivity of 85.2%, specificity 37% and AUC of 0.69.

Tawfeek et al. [28], in a case control study, measured SHBG levels at the time of the OGTT at 24–28 weeks of gestation (GDM n = 45, 75 g 2 h OGTT, IADPSG criteria) and found significant lower SHBG levels in the GDM group compared to NGT. At a cutoff value of 50 nmol/L, SHBG could identify GDM with a sensitivity of 96%, specificity of 95% and AUC of 0.91 (95% CI 0.82–1.) A similar study in the same population by Siddiqui et al. [245] (GDM n = 53, OGTT, ADA criteria) also found lower levels of SHBG in GDM women compared to controls, but only in nulliparous women with a positive correlation with gestational age. Limitations of both studies include the small sample size with a relatively high BMI and ethnically confined to Asian participants, which tend to have a higher prevalence of metabolic syndrome [246].

McElduff et al. [247], however, found no difference in SHBG levels between GDM and NGT groups in their cross-sectional study, which included 220 pregnant women (GDM n = 642, GCT/OGTT, Carpenter and Coustan criteria). Despite a robust study methodology similar to previous studies, the main reason for these discordant results lies in the difference in population characteristics and diagnostic method.

SHBG is a straightforward, low-cost test that does not require fasting [248] and has no diurnal variation [249]. This test has shown some promise as a predictor of GDM when used prior to or in the first-trimester of pregnancy, and this might be because the difference in insulin resistance markers reduces as the pregnancy progresses. Catalano et al. [250] found higher levels of insulin resistance in the first-trimester of pregnancy in women with NGT in the first-trimester, who eventually developed GDM compared to women with NGT all throughout. In most studies, the link between SHBG and GDM was independent of subcutaneous adiposity, suggesting, perhaps, that liver adiposity would be a better marker for SHBG production [251]. However, further studies are required to measure SHBG levels, markers of insulin resistance, glycemic control and hepatic steatosis for a better understanding of the role of SHBG in GDM. Beyond that, however, we cannot ignore the positive results in studies assessing prepregnancy and first-trimester predictability of GDM development, which would allow for early interventions on the modifiable factors involved in GDM development. Standardization of prepregnancy and-trimester-specific cut-offs, GDM diagnosis cutoff value, exploration of the variability of levels in different populations and standardizations of assays would make SHBG a very promising marker for the early diagnosis of GDM.

4.3. Other Proteins

4.3.1. C-Reactive Protein (CRP)

CRP is an acute-phase protein secreted and released by numerous cells in the context of inflammation [252,253]. Obesity, which is a proinflammatory state, is a known risk factor of GDM. CRP is a nonspecific marker, which may be elevated in settings, such as infection or obesity, in the absence of GDM [254–256]. High levels of CRP have been described in the association with insulin resistance and metabolic syndrome [257–260]. Numerous studies have found an association between obesity and high CRP levels independent of insulin resistance [261–263]. Therefore, it is biologically plausible that inflammatory markers, such as C-reactive protein (CRP), could be a promising biomarker of GDM.

Alamolhoda et al. [264] prospectively studied the relationship between first-trimester CRP levels and the risk of developing GDM in 120 pregnant women (GDM n = 11, OGTT) and found a significant difference between GDM women and controls independent of BMI. The sample size, however, was small, and the cutoff value for fasting glucose at diagnosis was 7 mmol/L (126 mg/dL), which selected only the more severe cases, fasting glucose of 7 mmol/L being the cutoff diagnostic value for T2DM. In a case–control study involving 372 women (GDM n = 124, OGTT, WHO criteria), Savvidou et al. [265] also found higher first-trimester CRP levels in women who subsequently developed GDM compared to controls. While the sample size was larger, similar to the previous study, the fasting glucose cutoff was 7 mmol/L (126 mg/dL). Kansu-Celik et al. [34] investigated first-trimester high-sensitivity CRP (hsCRP) as a biomarker for GDM diagnosis in 88 pregnant women (GDM n = 29, GCT/OGTT, Carpenter and Coustan criteria) and found that hsCRP was significantly higher in women, who subsequently developed GDM independent of BMI with a sensitivity of 86.2%, specificity of 50.8% and AUC of 0.70 (95% CI 0.59–0.81) at a cutoff value for hsCRP of 4.65 ng/mL. Wolf et al. [266] measured first-trimester CRP levels in 131 women (GDM n = 43, GCT/OGTT, ADA criteria) and found that women diagnosed with GDM had higher CRP levels in the first-trimester of pregnancy with a strong positive correlation between CRP levels and 1 h post glucose load levels and systolic blood pressure. The team also found that the addition of BMI in a multivariate model attenuated the correlation between CRP and GDM diagnosis suggesting the influence of adipose tissue on CRP levels. Some of the limitations of this study include the small sample size, the single time point measurement of CRP and the lack of additional adiposity markers beyond BMI (such as waist circumference, visceral fat).

Alyas et al. [267] measured high-sensitivity CRP (hsCRP) levels at 14–18 weeks of gestation and 24–28 weeks of gestation in 158 women (GDM n = 58, OGTT, IADPSG criteria) and found significantly higher CRP levels at both time points in women diagnosed with GDM compared to controls. No analysis on BMI category was done in this study.

Conflicting results are found in a cross-sectional study by Korkmazer et al. [268], who measured hsCRP at GDM screening time point in 116 women, who underwent a GCT followed by an OGTT and were classified in GDM (n = 39, failed GCT and OGTT, Carpenter and Coustan criteria) and glucose intolerant (n = 37, abnormal GCT, normal OGTT) and controls. The team found no differences in hsCRP levels between the three groups. The sample size was small, which may explain these findings, and no analysis was done between the GDM and glucose intolerance groups together and the controls. Corcoran et al. [269] evaluated hsCRP in 225 pregnant women with one or more risk factors for GDM in the first-trimester (46, of which developed GDM, OGTT, IADPSG criteria) and found no difference in hsCRP levels between the GDM and the control group findings also supported by Adam et al. [270]. Retnakaran et al. [255] measured CRP levels at the time of the OGTT in 180 women (GDM n =39, impaired glucose tolerance n = 48, GCT/OGTT, National Diabetes Data Group (NDDG) criteria [271]) and found no association between CRP levels and glycemic pregnancy status, but did describe a strong association between CRP levels and prepregnancy BMI and fasting glucose.

A systematic review by Amirian et al. [272] investigated the association between CRP and GDM diagnosis and included 31 articles. Even though no meta-analysis was done in this study due to the lack of clinical data, the authors found a positive association between high CRP levels and GDM development in 20 studies (CRP n = 8 articles, hsCRP n = 12 articles), while 11 studies (CRP n = 6 articles, hsCRP n = 5 articles) did not identify any correlation. The main reasons for these discrepancies are the variations in diagnostic methods and criteria, the difference in sample size and population characteristics, different methods to quantify CRP levels or the lack of adjustment for BMI and other confounders.

While CRP/hsCRP shows some potential, the literature shows inconsistent and contradictory data, with most studies having small sample size cohorts. This arises from the wide arrays of methodology and study population features. A big disadvantage of using CRP as a diagnostic biomarker is its nonspecificity as a high result will possibly lead to a wide range of investigations, some unnecessary, increasing costs and the pregnant woman's stress levels. Further research is required to clarify the correlation between adiposity (subcutaneous or visceral) and CRP levels and the reflection of this association in glycemic status. CRP may play a more meaningful role as a risk assessment tool for GDM screening rather than GDM diagnosis.

4.3.2. Nesfatin-1

Nesfatin-1, initially described in 2006, is a neuropeptide produced primarily by the hypothalamus and brain stem, and its main role is in food and water intake regulation, control of appetite with anorexigenic properties [273]. Research on animal models [274,275] found that intravenous nesfatin-1 regulated fatty acid metabolism, reduced insulin levels, improved insulin sensitivity and reduced blood glucose levels in mice. Li et al. [276] measured nesfatin-1 levels in healthy adults and adults with T1DM and T2DM and found significantly lower nesfatin-1 levels in individuals with T2DM compared to controls (not valid for T1DM) independent of BMI and no significant change in levels during the OGTT. A systematic review and meta-analysis by Zhai et al. [277] studied the association between T2DM and nesfatin-1 and comprised 7 studies and 627 participants (T2DM n = 328), with 6 out of 7 studies being carried out in China. The authors found significantly higher nesfatin-1 levels in newly diagnosed T2DM compared to controls; however, overall, when all participants were included, there was no significant association between T2DM and nesfatin-1. All the studies included had small size numbers of participants, and there was no subanalysis on the duration of diabetes, BMI subcategory, insulin resistance markers or glycemic control (HbA1c) on or off treatment.

Given the anorexigenic, the antihyperglycemic effect of nesfatin-1 and moderate evidence of the association with T2DM, studies have also assessed a possible implication of nesfatin-1 in GDM. A prospective study by Kucukler et al. [278] measured nesfatin-1 levels at 24–28 weeks of gestation in 79 pregnant women (GDM n = 38, GCT/OGTT, ADA criteria) and found significantly lower nesfatin-1 levels in the GDM group compared to NGT at diagnosis. Nesfatin-1 was negatively associated with BMI, fasting glucose, and HOMA-IR. Measurements at 24–28 weeks of gestation were also taken by Ademoglu et al. [279] in 70 pregnant women (GDM n = 30, GCT/OGTT, Carpenter and Coustan criteria) and similar to previous studies found lower nesfatin-1 levels in women with GDM compared to NGT women independent of age, BMI, fasting glucose and HOMA-IR at diagnosis. No correlation was found between nesfatin-1 and fasting glucose, BMI, or markers of insulin resistance. In a larger study, Mierzynski et al. [280] measured nesfatin-1 levels at 24–28 weeks of gestation in 237 women (GDM n = 153, OGTT, WHO criteria) and found lower nesfatin-1 levels in GDM subjects compared to controls. There was a positive association between nesfatin-1 levels and BMI, glucose levels and gestational age.

Nesfatin-1 is a recent biomarker with only a few small size studies exploring its role in GDM pathogenesis. It is a possibility that nesfatin-1 could act as an antidiabetic agent by enhancing insulin action/ secretion, reducing glucose levels, and reducing food intake, and a decrease in nesfatin-1 levels in pregnant women may lead to insulin resistance and GDM. Another theory is that insulin resistance and hyperinsulinemia may inhibit the secretion of nesfatin-1. There are no studies assessing nesfatin-1 levels dynamically in a normal pregnancy or any studies measuring first-trimester levels in women who will develop GDM. Nesfatin-1 has been shown to be an important component of the glucose dysregulation pathway in both GDM and T2DM, but the exact mechanisms and the exact cutoff values required for accurate interpretation require substantial future studies.

4.3.3. Pregnancy-Associated Plasma Protein A (PAPP-A)

PAPP-A is a zinc-binding matrix metalloproteinase secreted by the trophoblast and can be measured as early as 28 days of pregnancy [281]. PAPP-a has been used as a screening test in the first-trimester of pregnancy for aneuploidy and for identifying certain adverse pregnancy outcomes [282,283]. Through its properties, PAPP-A increases insulin-like growth factor 1 (IGF-1) bioavailability through its cleavage from the IGF binding protein-4, suggesting a possible link between PAPP-A and insulin sensitivity. Pellitero et al. [284] found lower PAPP-A levels in diabetic patients compared to controls with a negative association between PAPP-A levels and HbA1c. In addition, it has been documented that TNF-α (an inflammatory cytokine with a role in insulin resistance) strongly stimulates PAPP-A secretion [285]. Therefore, it has been hypothesized that low PAPP-A levels are linked to insulin resistance in pregnancy through low levels of IGF-1 that led to hyperinsulinemia.

Lovati et al. [45], in a case–control study, explored the association of first-trimester levels of PAPP-A and GDM development in 673 Caucasian pregnant women (GDM n = 307,

100 g 3 h OGTT/ 75 g 2 g OGTT) and found significantly lower levels in women, who were diagnosed with GDM and even lower levels in women that required insulin therapy. PAPP-A (in addition to clinical risk factors) could predict GDM development with a sensitivity of 81.4%, specificity of 50.5% and an AUC of 0.70 (95% CI 0.66–0.73). Similar results are found by Ramezani et al. [46], who prospectively measured first-trimester PAPP-A in 286 Middle Eastern women (GDM n = 45, OGTT, IADPSG criteria) and found significantly lower PAPP-A levels in women who developed GDM. PAPP-A could identify the future development of GDM with a sensitivity of 73.3%, specificity of 57.3% and AUC of 0.61. This study, however, did not record certain variables, and adequate adjustments in the analysis have not been made. A similar design study [47] in a comparative size Asian cohort (GDM n = 45, OGTT, IADPSG criteria) found that PAPP-A could predict GDM with a sensitivity of 72.5%, specificity of 82.3% and AUC of 0.86.

In a large retrospective study, Snyder et al. [48] studied clinical and biomarker models for early GDM diagnosis in 66,687 (GDM n = 4874) in ethnically and racially diverse pregnant women. Samples were collected in both the first and second-trimesters of pregnancy. The team found significantly lower levels of PAPP-A in women who subsequently developed GDM compared to controls with no difference between groups in second-trimester samples. The addition of PAPP-A to the clinical risk prediction model only slightly improved the prediction accuracy of the model. These findings are supported by other studies [49,50], who did not find a significant change to AUC by the addition of PAPP-A to the clinical prediction model. While this was a large study, it only included nulliparous women, there was no information on the GDM diagnostic method or criteria used, and there was no BMI category sub-analysis. These findings suggest that PAPP-A could be useful as the first-trimester of pregnancy predictor for GDM development with limited utility as in GDM diagnosis in the second-trimester of pregnancy.

A systematic review and meta-analysis by Donovan et al. [286] included 13 studies and 83,921 subjects (GDM n = 3786). While the study identified a high degree of heterogeneity mostly due to the analysis method, the GDM diagnostic criteria and the ethnicity of subjects involved, the overall analysis and sub-analysis identified significantly lower first-trimester PAPP-A levels in women who developed GDM compared with controls with even lower levels in GDM women diagnosed prior to 24 weeks of gestation. This correlation was not as strong in women of Asian origin. The correlation between PAPP-A levels and the degree of glucose intolerance in GDM was also highlighted by Wells et al. [287], who found lower levels of PAPP-A in women with early GDM diagnosis compared to late diagnosis and the lowest levels of PAPP-A in women diagnosed with T2DM.

Research to date has not clarified if low levels of PAPP-A promote or are rather the result of impaired glucose metabolism and insulin resistance. The reduced observed levels of PAPP-A in GDM pregnancies may reflect a defect in placentation or placental insufficiency encountered in GDM pathology. The studies, however, have consistent results with overall lower PAPP-A first-trimester levels in GDM pregnancies. Moreover, these findings are also supported by studies exploring exosomes profiles as a biomarker for GDM diagnosis [288]. Despite the variable reported predictive value across the literature, which is mostly due to patients' characteristics, sample size and GDM diagnostic criteria variability, PAPP-A is routinely assessed in first-trimester abnormalities screening, and it may identify women at high risk for early development of GDM. Further prospective studies are required to elucidate the clinical utility of this biomarker on its own or incorporated in risk identification models.

4.3.4. Retinol-Binding Protein 4 (RBP4)

RBP4 is secreted mainly by the liver and adipose tissue. Its main role is to transport retinol (vitamin A) from the liver to the peripheral tissues [289]. RBP4 also has a role in inflammation and adipose tissue dysfunction [290], in increasing hepatic glucose output, in reducing insulin signaling in the muscle and in increasing insulin resistance [291].

Jin et al. [292] measured RBP4 levels in the first and second-trimester of pregnancy in 270 women (GDM n = 135, IADPSG criteria) and found that GDM women had higher first-trimester levels of RBP4 compared to NGT women, that higher levels of RBP4 were associated with a higher risk of developing GDM and that RBP4 levels in both-trimesters were positively independently associated with markers of insulin resistance. Yuan et al. [51] measured a panel of biomarkers with the potential to diagnose GDM in 359 pregnant women (GDM n = 86, IADPSG criteria) at 16–18 weeks of gestation. RBP4 was significantly higher in women that developed GDM compared to NGT. The study also found that RPB4 (cutoff value >30.45 µg/mL) could predict the development of GDM with a sensitivity of 63.6%, specificity of 75% and AUC 0.72 (95% CI 0.64–0.79) and that RPB4/adiponectin ratio (cutoff >0.37) could predict GDM with a sensitivity of 81.8%, specificity of 75.6% and AUC of 0.80 (95% CI 0.73–0.87). A retrospective study by Du et al. [29] found that second-trimester RBP4 levels were significantly higher in the GDM group (n = 194, OGTT, IADPSG criteria) compared to NGT women with a strong association between RBP4 levels, insulin levels and HOMA-IR. The authors found that RBP4 (cutoff levels 34.84 µg/mL) can predict GDM with a sensitivity of 79.4%, specificity of 79.1% and AUC of 0.87 (85% CI 0.83–0.92).

Discordant results are found in a study by Khovidhunkit et al. [293], who measured RBP4 in 532 women (GDM n = 171, GCT/OGTT, Carpenter and Coustan criteria) between 24 and 28 weeks of gestation and found no difference in RBP4 levels between GDM and NGT women and no correlation with insulin levels and HOMA-IR. They did find a positive independent association with fasting triglycerides and weight gain in pregnancy. All the women in this study were of Thai ethnicity with a low/normal BMI, which may account for the discordant result with previous studies along with different diagnosis methods (OGTT/GCT) and different sampling gestational weeks.

Two meta-analyses [294,295] studied the link between RBP4 and GDM. Huang et al. [294] included 14 studies (GDM n = 884) and found that RBP4 levels were significantly higher in women with GDM compared to NGT women, independent of age or BMI. On subgroup analysis, however, this significant difference was only maintained for Asian populations with no difference in levels in non-Asian populations. This study had a low probability of bias but a high degree of heterogeneity; the link between RBP4 levels and GDM varied with GDM diagnostic criteria (WHO criteria—higher levels of RBP4 in GDM patients compared to controls; ADA criteria—no difference in levels between groups) and varied with different assays used for RBP4 determination. These findings are supported by a meta-analysis by Jia et al. [296], who found higher levels of RBP4 in patients of Asian ethnicity compared to controls, but not in patients of European ethnicity compared to controls. A meta-analysis by Hu et al. [295] pooled results from 14 studies (case–control) (GDM n = 647) and found that RBP4 levels taken between 24 and 28 weeks of gestation were associated with the risk of developing GDM. Similar to the previous meta-analysis, there was no difference between groups in studies that used the ADA criteria for GDM diagnosis, suggesting that higher glucose levels on the OGTT are associated with higher RBP4 levels.

There are contradictory findings in the literature, with some studies finding a positive link between RBP4 and GDM [293,297–300] (Asian population), while other studies could not determine an association [301–304] (non-Asian population), and there is scarce evidence on the first-trimester of pregnancy RBP4 and the risk of GDM. If ethnicity plays such an important role in RBP4 levels, this requires further evaluation in much larger studies with multi-ethnic participation.

It is unclear if the free or bound RBP4 (or total) serves as a better predictor for GDM. Some studies [302,305] suggest that, in fact, the RBP4/transthyretin (RBP s binding protein) ratio may be a better marker for insulin resistance and GDM compared to RBP4 alone.

A possible cause for discordant results is the different assays used in the measurement of RBP4. Graham et al. [306] measured RBP4 levels in subjects with insulin resistance and glucose intolerance and insulin-sensitive subjects with NGT using three commercial assays and a quantitative Western blotting assay and found substantial inconsistency among the results with enzyme immunoassays underestimating RBP4 levels concluding that Western blotting is the most reliable method for measuring RBP4.

5. Discussion

This scoping review highlighted the large number of biomarkers described in the literature investigated for their potential to identify GDM and described 15 protein biomarkers selected based on the higher number of citations in very recent publications in our literature search.

5.1. The Current Screening Methods for GDM Pose Several Issues

5.1.1. Universal vs. Selective Screening

Numerous studies [307–310] have shown that universal screening offers a significant advantage over selective screening by identifying all GDM cases, enabling timely lifestyle interventions and treatment, leading to a reduction in GDM associated adverse events. Proponents of selective screening invoke reduced complications associated with milder cases of GDM that would be diagnosed through universal screening as the argument in addition to the increased healthcare costs of screening. It is well known that GDM poses a long-term threat to the health of the mother and child through chronic metabolic diseases in a young population that will considerably increase the lifetime overall healthcare costs. Identifying GDM and intervening to prevent long-term issues has been shown to be cost-effective. A systematic review by Mo et al. [311] included 10 economic evaluations on different GDM screening strategies and found that universal screening is more likely to be cost-effective compared to selective screening. This finding is supported by other studies [312,313].

Beyond the costs, the focus should be on the accurate identification of causes and the prevention of adverse outcomes. In a Malaysian population, Idris et al. [307] found that when universal screening was employed, the OGTT yielded a sensitivity of 83.5% and specificity of 82.6%. When the selective screening was employed, the sensitivity and specificity of the OGTT were lower, 76.1% and 60.9%, respectively, leading to 23.8% of women with GDM being missed. In a European cohort, Miaihle et al. [314] showed that selective screening would have missed one-sixth of GDM cases. Similar results were found by Cosson et al. [315] in a retrospective study, which included 18,775 pregnancies. The authors found that applying selective screening criteria would lead to 34.7% of GDM cases being missed.

It was suggested that low-risk women with GDM would have a good prognosis, and not being diagnosed with GDM would not lead to adverse pregnancy outcomes. The literature has conflicting data, with some studies finding no benefit on adverse pregnancy outcomes when universal screening was applied [314,316], while others have shown significant benefits [317–319].

As selective screening would miss a significant number of women with GDM, and as universal screening has been shown to be cost-effective compared to selective screening, most international bodies now recommend universal screening. One of the barriers to the implementation of universal screening is the logistics of performing OGTT in the entire pregnant population. Accurate biomarkers as an alternative to the OGTT would allow universal screening to become a reality.

5.1.2. Time of Screening

Standard GDM screening occurs between 24 and 28 weeks of gestation. This arguably leaves a very narrow window for intervention. Some studies suggest that women that develop GDM early in pregnancy (<12 weeks of gestation) have outcomes comparable to women with prepregnancy diabetes despite treatment [320,321], while others found that early diagnosis and treatment may lead to a reduction in LGA [322]. Research has focused on the differences in pregnancy outcomes between women with GDM diagnosed in the first and late second-trimester, but we also need to consider the possible long-term impact of the fetal intrauterine exposure to hyperglycemia between onset and diagnosis and, while this may not be obvious at birth, the hyperglycemia-triggered fetal metabolic programming can lead to metabolic syndrome, insulin resistance and obesity in young adults [323]. One of the concerns with early screening is that while some women with more severe forms of GDM will be diagnosed early in pregnancy, others will only develop glucose abnormalities later in pregnancy and will require another test at 24–28. A single non-fasting biomarker would allow repetitive testing through pregnancy to facilitate rapid identification of hyperglycemia.

5.1.3. Diagnostic Criteria

As illustrated, it is difficult to make a meaningful comparison between studies when different criteria are employed to diagnose GDM. Studies that use a two-step approach with higher glucose cutoff thresholds will select a population with more severe forms of GDM, and the results cannot be extrapolated to the general population. Using a common new diagnostic biomarker will lead to harmonization of GDM diagnosis and all data synthesis to be performed

5.1.4. OGTT

Women are currently diagnosed with GDM using an OGTT. This test is unreliable with poor reproducibility and high vulnerability to external and internal factors [14]. More so, the OGTT does not identify the continuous correlation between hyperglycemia in the mother and pregnancy complications and possibly omits milder forms of glucose abnormalities that may identify pregnancy risks. Studies to date evaluating novel biomarkers as diagnostic tests/tools in GDM use the OGTT as the gold standard for comparison. However, how valid are the results if the comparator test is flawed? It may be more accurate to assess the predictive power of the biomarker to identify adverse pregnancy outcomes. Hyperglycemia is not the only contributor to adverse pregnancy outcomes, and other metabolic factors, such as adiposity, dyslipidemia, inflammation, should be considered when considering a test (or panel of tests) with the highest potential to identify pregnant women at risk. Changing the focus from the glucose value to the outcomes we need to prevent—and the factors contributing to them—will bring the research community closer to identifying the next screening test. This would start with a consensus on what are the outcomes we are aiming to prevent (macrosomia, LGA, hypertensive disorders of pregnancy, polyhydramnios, etc.), a reflection on the pathophysiology of the outcome and a reassessment of novel biomarkers not in their capacity to identify an out-of-range glucose value but in their capacity to capture the cumulus of mechanisms that lead to adverse pregnancy outcomes.

The COVID-19 pandemic has highlighted the difficulties in performing the OGTT in such a challenging environment, leading to OGTT screening being terminated and a high number of women being undiagnosed. This further emphasizes the urgent need for a single non-fasting sample biomarker test that could be performed in a family practice setting (GP) rather than a hospital setting.

Identifying a biomarker for the accurate diagnosis of GDM would have numerous practical benefits. A single blood test would reduce the appointment length, would enable a greater number of women to be screened (aiming for universal screening) and would enable the test to be performed in a non-hospital setting. A test that does not require fasting would not only considerably reduce the discomfort a pregnant woman experiences but would also enable appointments for sample collection throughout the day, thus increasing the number of women being screened. A test that does not require glucose loading, reducing adverse experiences, such as nausea, vomiting, pre-syncopal episodes, would considerably increase compliance with testing. Studies assessing the robustness of novel biomarkers to pre-analytical and analytical variables, time-to-result analysis and cost-effectiveness analysis will be required in the future.

Biomarker research has grown exponentially in recent years out of a need for more accurate, more direct measurement of disease and has proven to be a powerful tool in the understanding of physiology and pathophysiology. However, while biomarkers have many advantages, much like other tests, several things need to be considered and assessed when conducting biomarker research: (1) interindividual variability; (2) intraindividual variability; (3) sample collection/transportation/storage; (4) biomarker validity; (5) predictive power; (6) confounding variables; (7) normal ranges and (8) cost [324].

The main limitation of this study lies in the nature of its design. Scoping reviews do not formally evaluate the quality of evidence, and the evidence is collected from studies of different designs and methodology. Therefore, the data collected cannot be presented in a systematic way; but instead, it gives an overall view of the existent literature. The scope of this review was to offer the reader an insight into the vast number of molecules studied in relation to GDM diagnosis and the potential diagnostic value of the selected novel protein biomarkers. This approach, however, led to a certain degree of selection bias. Another limitation of the study is the time lapse between the systematic review search and the publication of the manuscript leading to very recent research not being included in our study.

5.2. Perspectives

Given the limitation mentioned above, several protein biomarkers did not fulfill our inclusion criteria and were not included in the discussion. Therefore, we want to give a short overview of promising protein biomarkers evaluated for GDM prognosis/diagnosis in articles published between January 2020 and March 2021 that should be considered in the future.

Secreted frizzled-related protein 4 (sFRP4) has been shown to play a role in glucose metabolism, reflecting islet inflammation and impaired insulin secretion [325]. Schuitemaker et al. [326] found significantly higher first-trimester levels of sFRP4 in women, who subsequently developed GDM (n = 50, diagnostic criteria fasting glucose ≥ 7.0 mmol/L, 2 h glucose ≥ 7.8 mmol/L) compared to controls and a predictive capacity expressed as AUC of 0.60 (95% CI 0.50–0.70). The correlation between sFRP4 and GDM is supported by other studies [327,328].

Amini et al. [329] studied alfa-fetoprotein (AFP) as a predictor for GDM in the early second-trimester (14–17 weeks of gestation) in 523 pregnant women. The authors found that AFP alone could predict GDM diagnosis with a sensitivity of 70%, specificity of 93% and AUC of 0.58 (95% CI 0.51–0.62) and AFP combined with unconjugated estriol and β-hCG levels can predict GDM with a sensitivity of 95%, specificity of 86% and AUC of 0.91 (95% CI 0.87–0.98).

Wnt1-inducible signaling pathway protein-1 (WISP1) was studied by Liu et al. [330] in 313 pregnant women (GDM n = 61, 2 h 75 g OGTT, IADPSG criteria). The samples were taken at the time of the OGTT. The authors found that WISP1 levels were significantly higher in GDM patients with prepregnancy overweight or obesity compared to normoglycemic and normal-weight subjects, suggesting a possible role of this protein in the mechanisms involved in obesity-induced insulin resistance in GDM. This hypothesis was also suggested by Sahin Esroy et al. [331].

Irisin levels were measured by AL-Ghazali et al. [332] in 90 pregnant women (GDM n = 60, 2 h 75 g OGTT, IADPSG criteria) at the time of the OGTT and found significantly lower levels of irisin in women with GDM compared to controls. Diagnostic capacity (i.e., AUC) was not calculated. These findings are supported by other studies [333,334].

Asprosin levels [335] were found to be significantly higher in women with GDM compared with controls at the time of OGTT, but also as early as 18–20 weeks of gestation, suggesting a potential role as an early biomarker. Similarly, spexin and subfatin levels [336] and fibrinogen-like protein 1 (FGL-1) [337] were found to be higher in women with GDM compared with controls (samples taken at the time of the OGTT).

Finally, coiled-coil domain-containing 80 (CCDC80) levels [338] and complement C1q tumor necrosis factor-related protein 1 (CTRP1) levels [339] taken at the time of the OGTT (2 h 75 g OGTT, IADPSG criteria) were significantly lower in women with GDM compared with controls. Additionally, CCDC80 could identify GDM cases with an AUC of 0.61 (95% CI 0.53–0.68), which increased to 0.74 when additional variables were included in the model (maternal age, gestational age, BMI, blood pressure).

6. Conclusions

This review has identified and described 15 promising biomarkers that could potentially replace the OGTT and be used to both predict and diagnose GDM. Steps required to move the biomarker agenda forward should include large multicenter, multi-ethnic prospective studies using uniform screening and diagnostic criteria for GDM, with longitudinal sampling in all three trimesters and with well-recorded patient characteristics. One such study would answer many questions and help identify the best candidate marker. Recently, the Lames Lindt Alliance (Priority Setting Partnerships) has identified the top 10 research priorities for GDM, one of which is identifying the best test to diagnose GDM [340]. The scientific community agrees that the OGTT is a dated, cumbersome, imperfect test and needs to be replaced, and this review highlights some very promising contenders.

Supplementary Materials: The following are available online at https://www.mdpi.com/article/10.3390/jcm10071533/s1, Supplemental Material: PubMed Search Strategy; Supplemental Table S1: Biomarkers identified through the scoping review in alphabetical order; Figure S1: Reported AUC at the time of GDM diagnosis; Figure S2: Reported AUC for prediction of GDM.

Author Contributions: D.B., P.M.O. and F.D. were responsible for the conception and design of the study. D.B., C.R., D.M. screened, collected, extracted, and analyzed the data. D.B. drafted the manuscript. All authors (D.B., C.R., D.M., H.C.D., J.A.H., P.M.O., F.D.) made substantial contributions to the interpretation of data, critically revised the manuscript for important intellectual content and approved the final version to be published. D.B. is responsible for the integrity of the work as a whole. All authors have read and agreed to the published version of the manuscript.

Funding: This research received no external funding.

Conflicts of Interest: The authors declare no conflict of interest.

References

1. Alberti, K.G.; Zimmet, P.Z. Definition, diagnosis and classification of diabetes mellitus and its complications. Part 1: Diagnosis and classification of diabetes mellitus provisional report of a WHO consultation. *Diabet. Med.* **1998**, *15*, 539–553. [CrossRef]
2. Zhu, Y.; Zhang, C. Prevalence of Gestational Diabetes and Risk of Progression to Type 2 Diabetes: A Global Perspective. *Curr. Diabetes Rep.* **2016**, *16*, 1–11. [CrossRef]
3. Goedegebure, E.A.R.; Koning, S.H.; Hoogenberg, K.; Korteweg, F.J.; Lutgers, H.L.; Diekman, M.J.M.; Stekkinger, E.; Berg, P.P.V.D.; Zwart, J.J. Pregnancy outcomes in women with gestational diabetes mellitus diagnosed according to the WHO-2013 and WHO-1999 diagnostic criteria: A multicentre retrospective cohort study. *BMC Pregnancy Childbirth* **2018**, *18*, 152. [CrossRef]
4. Koivunen, S.; Viljakainen, M.; Männistö, T.; Gissler, M.; Pouta, A.; Kaaja, R.; Eriksson, J.; Laivuori, H.; Kajantie, E.; Vääräsmäki, M. Pregnancy outcomes according to the definition of gestational diabetes. *PLoS ONE* **2020**, *15*, e0229496. [CrossRef]
5. Metzger, B.E. Long-term Outcomes in Mothers Diagnosed With Gestational Diabetes Mellitus and Their Offspring. *Clin. Obstet. Gynecol.* **2007**, *50*, 972–979. [CrossRef]
6. O'Sullivan, E.P.; Avalos, G.; O'Reilly, M.; Dennedy, M.C.; Gaffney, G.; Dunne, F.P. Atlantic DIP: The prevalence and consequences of gestational diabetes in Ireland. *Ir. Med. J.* **2012**, *105*, 13–15. [PubMed]
7. Crowther, C.A.; Hiller, J.E.; Moss, J.R.; McPhee, A.J.; Jeffries, W.S.; Robinson, J.S. Effect of treatment of gestational diabetes mellitus on pregnancy outcomes. *N. Engl. J. Med.* **2005**, *352*, 2477–2486. [CrossRef] [PubMed]
8. Landon, M.B.; Spong, C.Y.; Thom, E.; Carpenter, M.W.; Ramin, S.M.; Casey, B.; Wapner, R.J.; Varner, M.W.; Rouse, D.J.; Thorp, J.M.; et al. A Multicenter, Randomized Trial of Treatment for Mild Gestational Diabetes. *N. Engl. J. Med.* **2009**, *361*, 1339–1348. [CrossRef] [PubMed]
9. Koivusalo, S.B.; Rönö, K.; Klemetti, M.M.; Roine, R.P.; Lindström, J.; Erkkola, M.; Kaaja, R.J.; Pöyhönen-Alho, M.; Tiitinen, A.; Huvinen, E.; et al. Gestational Diabetes Mellitus Can Be Prevented by Lifestyle Intervention: The Finnish Gestational Diabetes Prevention Study (RADIEL): A Randomized Controlled Trial. *Diabetes Care* **2016**, *39*, 24–30. [CrossRef]

10. International Association of Diabetes and Pregnancy Study Groups Consensus Panel. International Association of Diabetes and Pregnancy Study Groups Recommendations on the Diagnosis and Classification of Hyperglycemia in Pregnancy. *Diabetes Care* **2010**, *33*, 676–682. [CrossRef]
11. Wilkerson, H.L.C.; Remein, Q.R. Studies of Abnormal Carbohydrate Metabolism in Pregnancy: The Significance of Impaired Glucose Tolerance. *Diabetes* **1957**, *6*, 324–329. [CrossRef] [PubMed]
12. Metzger, B.E.; Gabbe, S.G.; Persson, B.; Lowe, L.P.; Dyer, A.R.; Oats, J.J.; Buchanan, T.A. International Association of Diabetes and Pregnancy Study Groups Recommendations on the Diagnosis and Classification of Hyperglycemia in Pregnancy: Response to Weinert. *Diabetes Care* **2010**, *33*, e98. [CrossRef]
13. Lachmann, E.H.; Fox, R.A.; Dennison, R.A.; Usher-Smith, J.A.; Meek, C.L.; Aiken, C.E. Barriers to completing oral glucose tolerance testing in women at risk of gestational diabetes. *Diabet. Med.* **2020**, *37*, 1482–1489. [CrossRef]
14. Bogdanet, D.; O'Shea, P.; Lyons, C.; Shafat, A.; Dunne, F. The Oral Glucose Tolerance Test—Is It Time for a Change?—A Literature Review with an Emphasis on Pregnancy. *J. Clin. Med.* **2020**, *9*, 3451. [CrossRef] [PubMed]
15. Catalano, P.M.; Avallone, D.A.; Drago, N.M.; Amini, S.B. Reproducibility of the oral glucose tolerance test in pregnant women. *Am. J. Obstet. Gynecol.* **1993**, *169*, 874–881. [CrossRef]
16. Arksey, H.; O'Malley, L. Scoping studies: Towards a methodological framework. *Int. J. Soc. Res. Methodol.* **2005**, *8*, 19–32. [CrossRef]
17. Levac, D.; Colquhoun, H.; O'Brien, K.K. Scoping studies: Advancing the methodology. *Implement Sci.* **2010**, *5*, 69. [CrossRef] [PubMed]
18. Peters, M.D.; Godfrey, C.M.; Khalil, H.; McInerney, P.; Parker, D.; Soares, C.B. Guidance for conducting systematic scoping reviews. *Int. J. Evid. Based Health* **2015**, *13*, 141–146. [CrossRef]
19. Munn, Z.; Peters, M.D.J.; Stern, C.; Tufanaru, C.; McArthur, A.; Aromataris, E. Systematic review or scoping review? Guidance for authors when choosing between a systematic or scoping review approach. *BMC Med. Res. Methodol.* **2018**, *18*, 1–7. [CrossRef]
20. Tricco, A.C.; Lillie, E.; Zarin, W.; O'Brien, K.K.; Colquhoun, H.; Levac, D.; Moher, D.; Peters, M.D.; Horsley, T.; Weeks, L.; et al. PRISMA Extension for Scoping Reviews (PRISMA-ScR): Checklist and Explanation. *Ann. Intern. Med.* **2018**, *169*, 467–473. [CrossRef] [PubMed]
21. Ouzzani, M.; Hammady, H.; Fedorowicz, Z.; Elmagarmid, A. Rayyan—A web and mobile app for systematic reviews. *Syst. Rev.* **2016**, *5*, 1–10. [CrossRef] [PubMed]
22. Bozkurt, L.; Göbl, C.S.; Baumgartner-Parzer, S.; Luger, A.; Pacini, G.; Kautzky-Willer, A. Adiponectin and Leptin at Early Pregnancy: Association to Actual Glucose Disposal and Risk for GDM—A Prospective Cohort Study. *Int. J. Endocrinol.* **2018**, *2018*, 1–8. [CrossRef] [PubMed]
23. Weerakiet, S.; Lertnarkorn, K.; Panburana, P.; Pitakitronakorn, S.; Vesathada, K.; Wansumrith, S. Can adiponectin predict gestational diabetes? *Gynecol. Endocrinol.* **2006**, *22*, 362–368. [CrossRef] [PubMed]
24. Wang, X.; Liu, J.; Wang, D.; Zhu, H.; Kang, L.; Jiang, J. Expression and correlation of Chemerin and FABP4 in peripheral blood of gestational diabetes mellitus patients. *Exp. Ther. Med.* **2019**, *19*, 710–716. [CrossRef] [PubMed]
25. Boyadzhieva, M.; Atanasova, I.; Zacharieva, S.; Kedikova, S. Adipocytokines during pregnancy and postpartum in women with gestational diabetes and healthy controls. *J. Endocrinol. Investig.* **2013**, *36*, 944–949.
26. Ghosh, P.; Luque-Fernandez, M.A.; Vaidya, A.; Ma, N.; Sahoo, R.; Chorev, M.; Zera, C.; McElrath, T.F.; Williams, M.A.; Seely, E.W.; et al. Plasma Glycated CD59, a Novel Biomarker for Detection of Pregnancy-Induced Glucose Intolerance. *Diabetes Care* **2017**, *40*, 981–984. [CrossRef]
27. Ma, D.; Luque-Fernandez, M.A.; Bogdanet, D.; Desoye, G.; Dunne, F.; Halperin, J.A. Plasma Glycated CD59 Predicts Early Gestational Diabetes and Large for Gestational Age Newborns. *J. Clin. Endocrinol. Metab.* **2020**, *105*, e1033–e1040. [CrossRef]
28. Tawfeek, M.A.; Alfadhli, E.M.; Alayoubi, A.M.; El-Beshbishy, H.A.; Habib, F.A. Sex hormone binding globulin as a valuable biochemical marker in predicting gestational diabetes mellitus. *BMC Women's Health* **2017**, *17*, 1–5. [CrossRef]
29. Du, X.; Dong, Y.; Xiao, L.; Liu, G.-H.; Qin, W.; Yu, H. Association between retinol-binding protein 4 concentrations and gestational diabetes mellitus (A1GDM and A2GDM) in different pregnancy and postpartum periods. *Ann. Transl. Med.* **2019**, *7*, 479. [CrossRef]
30. Georgiou, H.M.; Lappas, M.; Georgiou, G.M.; Marita, A.; Bryant, V.J.; Hiscock, R.; Permezel, M.; Khalil, Z.; Rice, G.E. Screening for biomarkers predictive of gestational diabetes mellitus. *Acta Diabetol.* **2008**, *45*, 157–165. [CrossRef]
31. Ferreira, A.F.A.; Rezende, J.C.; Vaikousi, E.; Akolekar, R.; Nicolaides, K.H. Maternal Serum Visfatin at 11–13 Weeks of Gestation in Gestational Diabetes Mellitus. *Clin. Chem.* **2011**, *57*, 609–613. [CrossRef]
32. Madhu, S.V.; Bhardwaj, S.; Jhamb, R.; Srivastava, H.; Sharma, S.; Raizada, N. Prediction of Gestational Diabetes from First Tri-mester Serum Adiponectin Levels in Indian Women. *Indian J Endocrinol Metab.* **2019**, *23*, 536–539. [CrossRef] [PubMed]
33. Iliodromiti, S.; Sassarini, J.; Kelsey, T.W.; Lindsay, R.S.; Sattar, N.; Nelson, S.M. Accuracy of circulating adiponectin for predicting gestational diabetes: A systematic review and meta-analysis. *Diabetologia* **2016**, *59*, 692–699. [CrossRef]
34. Kansu-Celik, H.; Ozgu-Erdinc, A.S.; Kisa, B.; Findik, R.B.; Yilmaz, C.; Tasci, Y. Prediction of gestational diabetes mellitus in the first trimester: Comparison of maternal fetuin-A, N-terminal proatrial natriuretic peptide, high-sensitivity C-reactive protein, and fasting glucose levels. *Arch. Endocrinol. Metab.* **2019**, *63*, 121–127. [CrossRef] [PubMed]

35. Jin, C.; Lin, L.; Han, N.; Zhao, Z.; Liu, Z.; Luo, S.; Xu, X.; Liu, J.; Wang, H. Effects of dynamic change in fetuin-A levels from the first to the second trimester on insulin resistance and gestational diabetes mellitus: A nested case–control study. *BMJ Open Diabetes Res. Care* **2020**, *8*, e000802. [CrossRef] [PubMed]
36. Bawah, A.T.; Seini, M.M.; Abaka-Yawason, A.; Alidu, H.; Nanga, S. Leptin, resistin and visfatin as useful predictors of gestational diabetes mellitus. *Lipids Health Dis.* **2019**, *18*, 1–8. [CrossRef]
37. Syngelaki, A.; Visser, G.H.; Krithinakis, K.; Wright, A.; Nicolaides, K.H. First trimester screening for gestational diabetes mellitus by maternal factors and markers of inflammation. *Metabolism* **2016**, *65*, 131–137. [CrossRef]
38. Tramontana, A.; Pablik, E.; Stangl, G.; Hartmann, B.; Dieplinger, H.; Hafner, E. Combination of first trimester serum afamin levels and three-dimensional placental bed vascularization as a possible screening method to detect women at-risk for adverse pregnancy complications like pre-eclampsia and gestational diabetes mellitus in low-risk pregnancies. *Placenta* **2018**, *62*, 9–15. [CrossRef]
39. Köninger, A.; Iannaccone, A.; Hajder, E.; Frank, M.; Schmidt, B.; Schleussner, E.; Kimmig, R.; Gellhaus, A.; Dieplinger, H. Afamin predicts gestational diabetes in polycystic ovary syndrome patients preconceptionally. *Endocr. Connect.* **2019**, *8*, 616–624. [CrossRef]
40. Ravnsborg, T.; Svaneklink, S.; Andersen, L.L.T.; Larsen, M.R.; Jensen, D.M.; Overgaard, M. First-trimester proteomic profiling identifies novel predictors of gestational diabetes mellitus. *PLoS ONE* **2019**, *14*, e0214457. [CrossRef]
41. Caglar, G.S.; Ozdemir, E.D.; Cengiz, S.D.; Demirtaş, S. Sex-hormone-binding globulin early in pregnancy for the prediction of severe gestational diabetes mellitus and related complications. *J. Obstet. Gynaecol. Res.* **2012**, *38*, 1286–1293. [CrossRef]
42. Maged, A.M.; Moety, G.A.F.; Mostafa, W.A.; Hamed, D.A. Comparative study between different biomarkers for early prediction of gestational diabetes mellitus. *J. Matern. Neonatal Med.* **2014**, *27*, 1108–1112. [CrossRef] [PubMed]
43. Veltman-Verhulst, S.M.; Van Haeften, T.W.; Eijkemans, M.J.C.; De Valk, H.W.; Fauser, B.C.J.M.; Goverde, A.J. Sex hormone-binding globulin concentrations before conception as a predictor for gestational diabetes in women with polycystic ovary syndrome. *Hum. Reprod.* **2010**, *25*, 3123–3128. [CrossRef]
44. Badon, S.E.; Zhu, Y.; Sridhar, S.B.; Xu, F.; Lee, C.; Ehrlich, S.F.; Quesenberry, C.P.; Hedderson, M.M. A Pre-Pregnancy Biomarker Risk Score Improves Prediction of Future Gestational Diabetes. *J. Endocr. Soc.* **2018**, *2*, 1158–1169. [CrossRef] [PubMed]
45. Lovati, E.; Beneventi, F.; Simonetta, M.; Laneri, M.; Quarleri, L.; Scudeller, L.; Albonico, G.; Locatelli, E.; Cavagnoli, C.; Tinelli, C.; et al. Gestational diabetes mellitus: Including serum pregnancy-associated plasma protein-A testing in the clinical management of primiparous women? A case–control study. *Diabetes Res. Clin. Pr.* **2013**, *100*, 340–347. [CrossRef] [PubMed]
46. Ramezani, S.; Doulabi, M.A.; Saqhafi, H.; Alipoor, M. Prediction of Gestational Diabetes by Measuring the Levels of Pregnancy Associated Plasma Protein-A (PAPP-A) During Gestation Weeks 11-14. *J. Reprod. Infertil.* **2020**, *21*, 130–137.
47. Ren, Z.; Zhe, D.; Li, Z.; Sun, X.-P.; Yang, K.; Lin, L. Study on the correlation and predictive value of serum pregnancy-associated plasma protein A, triglyceride and serum 25-hydroxyvitamin D levels with gestational diabetes mellitus. *World J. Clin. Cases* **2020**, *8*, 864–873. [CrossRef]
48. Snyder, B.M.; Baer, R.J.; Oltman, S.P.; Robinson, J.G.; Breheny, P.J.; Saftlas, A.F.; Bao, W.; Greiner, A.L.; Carter, K.D.; Rand, L.; et al. Early pregnancy prediction of gestational diabetes mellitus risk using prenatal screening biomarkers in nulliparous women. *Diabetes Res. Clin. Pr.* **2020**, *163*, 108139. [CrossRef]
49. Xiao, D.; Chenhong, W.; Yanbin, X.; Lu, Z. Gestational diabetes mellitus and first trimester pregnancy-associated plasma protein A: A case-control study in a Chinese population. *J. Diabetes Investig.* **2018**, *9*, 204–210. [CrossRef]
50. Syngelaki, A.; Kotecha, R.; Pastides, A.; Wright, A.; Nicolaides, K.H. First-trimester biochemical markers of placentation in screening for gestational diabetes mellitus. *Metabolism* **2015**, *64*, 1485–1489. [CrossRef]
51. Yuan, X.; Shi, H.; Wang, H.; Yu, B.; Jiang, J. Ficolin-3/adiponectin ratio for the prediction of gestational diabetes mellitus in pregnant women. *J. Diabetes Investig.* **2017**, *9*, 403–410. [CrossRef] [PubMed]
52. Blüher, M. Adipose Tissue Dysfunction in Obesity. *Exp. Clin. Endocrinol. Diabetes* **2009**, *117*, 241–250. [CrossRef]
53. Blüher, M. Adipokines—Removing road blocks to obesity and diabetes therapy. *Mol. Metab.* **2014**, *3*, 230–240. [CrossRef] [PubMed]
54. Maeda, K.; Okubo, K.; Shimomura, I.; Funahashi, T.; Matsuzawa, Y.; Matsubara, K. cDNA Cloning and Expression of a Novel Adipose Specific Collagen-like Factor, apM1 (AdiposeMost Abundant Gene Transcript 1). *Biochem. Biophys. Res. Commun.* **1996**, *221*, 286–289. [CrossRef] [PubMed]
55. Martinez-Huenchullan, S.F.; Tam, C.S.; Ban, L.A.; Ehrenfeld-Slater, P.; McLennan, S.V.; Twigg, S.M. Skeletal muscle adiponectin induction in obesity and exercise. *Metabolism* **2020**, *102*, 154008. [CrossRef]
56. Chen, J.; Tan, B.; Karteris, E.; Zervou, S.; Digby, J.; Hillhouse, E.W.; Vatish, M.; Randeva, H.S. Secretion of adiponectin by human placenta: Differential modulation of adiponectin and its receptors by cytokines. *Diabetologia* **2006**, *49*, 1292–1302. [CrossRef] [PubMed]
57. Yamauchi, T.; Kamon, J.; Waki, H.; Terauchi, Y.; Kubota, N.; Hara, K.; Mori, Y.; Ide, T.; Murakami, K.; Tsuboyama-Kasaoka, N.; et al. The fat-derived hormone adiponectin reverses insulin resistance associated with both lipoatrophy and obesity. *Nat. Med.* **2001**, *7*, 941–946. [CrossRef]
58. Berg, A.H.; Combs, T.P.; Du, X.; Brownlee, M.; Scherer, P.E. The adipocyte-secreted protein Acrp30 enhances hepatic insulin action. *Nat. Med.* **2001**, *7*, 947–953. [CrossRef]

59. Combs, T.P.; Berg, A.H.; Obici, S.; Scherer, P.E.; Rossetti, L. Endogenous glucose production is inhibited by the adipose-derived protein Acrp30. *J. Clin. Invest.* **2001**, *108*, 1875–1881. [CrossRef]
60. Fruebis, J.; Tsao, T.S.; Javorschi, S.; Ebbets-Reed, D.; Erickson, M.R.; Yen, F.T.; Bihain, B.E.; Lodish, H.F. Proteolytic cleavage product of 30-kDa adipocyte complement-related protein increases fatty acid oxidation in muscle and causes weight loss in mice. *Proc. Natl. Acad. Sci. USA* **2001**, *98*, 2005–2010. [CrossRef]
61. Duncan, B.B.; Schmidt, M.I.; Pankow, J.S.; Bang, H.; Couper, D.; Ballantyne, C.M.; Hoogeveen, R.C.; Heiss, G. Adiponectin and the Development of Type 2 Diabetes: The Atherosclerosis Risk in Communities Study. *Diabetes* **2004**, *53*, 2473–2478. [CrossRef]
62. Wang, Y.; Meng, R.-W.; Kunutsor, S.K.; Chowdhury, R.; Yuan, J.-M.; Koh, W.-P.; Pan, A. Plasma adiponectin levels and type 2 diabetes risk: A nested case-control study in a Chinese population and an updated meta-analysis. *Sci. Rep.* **2018**, *8*, 406. [CrossRef] [PubMed]
63. Mohammadi, T.; Paknahad, Z. Adiponectin Concentration in Gestational Diabetic Women: A Case-Control Study. *Clin. Nutr. Res.* **2017**, *6*, 267–276. [CrossRef] [PubMed]
64. Ranheim, T.; Haugen, F.; Staff, A.C.; Braekke, K.; Harsem, N.K.; Drevon, C.A. Adiponectin is reduced in gestational diabetes mellitus in normal weight women. *Acta Obstet. Gynecol. Scand.* **2004**, *83*, 341–347. [CrossRef]
65. Hedderson, M.M.; Darbinian, J.; Havel, P.J.; Quesenberry, C.P.; Sridhar, S.; Ehrlich, S.; Ferrara, A. Low Prepregnancy Adiponectin Concentrations Are Associated With a Marked Increase in Risk for Development of Gestational Diabetes Mellitus. *Diabetes Care* **2013**, *36*, 3930–3937. [CrossRef] [PubMed]
66. Committee opinion no. 504: Screening and diagnosis of gestational diabetes mellitus. *Obstet Gynecol.* **2011**, *118*, 751–753. [CrossRef]
67. Williams, M.A.; Qiu, C.; Muy-Rivera, M.; Vadachkoria, S.; Song, T.; Luthy, D.A. Plasma Adiponectin Concentrations in Early Pregnancy and Subsequent Risk of Gestational Diabetes Mellitus. *J. Clin. Endocrinol. Metab.* **2004**, *89*, 2306–2311. [CrossRef]
68. Aguilar-Salinas, C.A.; García, E.G.; Robles, L.; Riaño, D.; Ruiz-Gomez, D.G.; García-Ulloa, A.C.; Melgarejo, M.A.; Zamora, M.; Guillen-Pineda, L.E.; Mehta, R.; et al. High Adiponectin Concentrations Are Associated with the Metabolically Healthy Obese Phenotype. *J. Clin. Endocrinol. Metab.* **2008**, *93*, 4075–4079. [CrossRef]
69. Ahl, S.; Guenther, M.; Zhao, S.; James, R.; Marks, J.; Szabo, A.; Kidambi, S. Adiponectin Levels Differentiate Metabolically Healthy vs. Unhealthy among Obese and Nonobese White Individuals. *J. Clin. Endocrinol. Metab.* **2015**, *100*, 4172–4180. [CrossRef] [PubMed]
70. Xu, J.; Zhao, Y.H.; Chen, Y.P.; Yuan, X.L.; Wang, J.; Zhu, H.; Lu, C.M. Maternal Circulating Concentrations of Tumor Necrosis Factor-Alpha, Leptin, and Adiponectin in Gestational Diabetes Mellitus: A Systematic Review and Meta-Analysis. *Sci. World J.* **2014**, *2014*, 1–12. [CrossRef]
71. Sattar, N.; Wannamethee, S.G.; Forouhi, N.G. Novel biochemical risk factors for type 2 diabetes: Pathogenic insights or prediction possibilities? *Diabetologia* **2008**, *51*, 926–940. [CrossRef]
72. Yeral, M.I.; Ozgu-Erdinc, A.S.; Uygur, D.; Seckin, K.D.; Karsli, M.F.; Danisman, A.N. Prediction of gestational diabetes mellitus in the first trimester, comparison of fasting plasma glucose, two-step and one-step methods: A prospective randomized controlled trial. *Endocrine* **2013**, *46*, 512–518. [CrossRef] [PubMed]
73. Trujillo, J.; Vigo, A.; Reichelt, A.; Duncan, B.; Schmidt, M. Fasting plasma glucose to avoid a full OGTT in the diagnosis of gestational diabetes. *Diabetes Res. Clin. Pr.* **2014**, *105*, 322–326. [CrossRef]
74. Thewjitcharoen, Y.; Elizabeth, A.J.; Butadej, S.; Nakasatien, S.; Chotwanvirat, P.; Wanothayaroj, E.; Krittiyawong, S.; Himathongkam, T.; Himathongkam, T. Performance of HbA1c versus oral glucose tolerance test (OGTT) as a screening tool to diagnose dysglycemic status in high-risk Thai patients. *BMC Endocr. Disord.* **2019**, *19*, 1–8. [CrossRef] [PubMed]
75. Aziz, N.L.; Abdelwahab, S.; Moussa, M.; Georgy, M. Maternal fructosamine and glycosylated haemoglobin in the prediction of gestational glucose intolerance. *Clin. Exp. Obstet. Gynecol.* **1992**, *19*, 235–241. [PubMed]
76. Nagpal, S.; Patel, S.; Jacobe, H.; Disepio, D.; Ghosn, C.; Malhotra, M.; Teng, M.; Duvic, M.; Chandraratna, R.A. Tazarotene-induced Gene 2 (TIG2), a Novel Retinoid-Responsive Gene in Skin. *J. Investig. Dermatol.* **1997**, *109*, 91–95. [CrossRef] [PubMed]
77. Goralski, K.B.; McCarthy, T.C.; Hanniman, E.A.; Zabel, B.A.; Butcher, E.C.; Parlee, S.D.; Muruganandan, S.; Sinal, C.J. Chemerin, a Novel Adipokine That Regulates Adipogenesis and Adipocyte Metabolism. *J. Biol. Chem.* **2007**, *282*, 28175–28188. [CrossRef]
78. Sell, H.; Laurencikiene, J.; Taube, A.; Eckardt, K.; Cramer, A.; Horrighs, A.; Arner, P.; Eckel, J. Chemerin Is a Novel Adipocyte-Derived Factor Inducing Insulin Resistance in Primary Human Skeletal Muscle Cells. *Diabetes* **2009**, *58*, 2731–2740. [CrossRef]
79. Huang, J.; Zhang, J.; Lei, T.; Chen, X.; Zhang, Y.; Zhou, L.; Yu, A.; Chen, Z.; Zhou, R.; Yang, Z. Cloning of porcine chemerin, ChemR23 and GPR1 and their involvement in regulation of lipogenesis. *BMB Rep.* **2010**, *43*, 491–498. [CrossRef] [PubMed]
80. Garces, M.; Sanchez, E.; Acosta, B.; Angel, E.; Ruíz, A.; Rubio-Romero, J.; Diéguez, C.; Nogueiras, R.; Caminos, J. Expression and regulation of chemerin during rat pregnancy. *Placenta* **2012**, *33*, 373–378. [CrossRef]
81. Bozaoglu, K.; Bolton, K.; McMillan, J.; Zimmet, P.; Jowett, J.; Collier, G.; Walder, K.; Segal, D. Chemerin Is a Novel Adipokine Associated with Obesity and Metabolic Syndrome. *Endocrinology* **2007**, *148*, 4687–4694. [CrossRef] [PubMed]
82. Stepan, H.; Philipp, A.; Roth, I.; Kralisch, S.; Jank, A.; Schaarschmidt, W.; Lössner, U.; Kratzsch, J.; Blüher, M.; Stumvoll, M.; et al. Serum levels of the adipokine chemerin are increased in preeclampsia during and 6months after pregnancy. *Regul. Pept.* **2011**, *168*, 69–72. [CrossRef] [PubMed]
83. Duan, D.-M.; Niu, J.-M.; Lei, Q.; Lin, X.-H.; Chen, X. Serum levels of the adipokine chemerin in preeclampsia. *J. Périnat. Med.* **2011**, *40*, 121–127. [CrossRef]

84. Xu, Q.-L.; Zhu, M.; Jin, Y.; Wang, N.; Xu, H.-X.; Quan, L.-M.; Wang, S.-S.; Li, S.-S. The predictive value of the first-trimester maternal serum chemerin level for pre-eclampsia. *Peptides* **2014**, *62*, 150–154. [CrossRef]
85. Yang, X.; Quan, X.; Lan, Y.; Ye, J.; Wei, Q.; Yin, X.; Fan, F.; Xing, H. Serum chemerin level during the first trimester of pregnancy and the risk of gestational diabetes mellitus. *Gynecol. Endocrinol.* **2017**, *33*, 770–773. [CrossRef]
86. Pfau, D.; Stepan, H.; Kratzsch, J.; Verlohren, M.; Verlohren, H.-J.; Drynda, K.; Lössner, U.; Blüher, M.; Stumvoll, M.; Fasshauer, M. Circulating Levels of the Adipokine Chemerin in Gestational Diabetes Mellitus. *Horm. Res. Paediatr.* **2010**, *74*, 56–61. [CrossRef]
87. Guelfi, K.J.; Ong, M.J.; Li, S.; Wallman, K.E.; Doherty, D.A.; Fournier, P.A.; Newnham, J.P.; Keelan, J.A. Maternal circulating adipokine profile and insulin resistance in women at high risk of developing gestational diabetes mellitus. *Metabolism* **2017**, *75*, 54–60. [CrossRef]
88. Van Poppel, M.N.; Zeck, W.; Ulrich, D.; Schest, E.C.; Hirschmugl, B.; Lang, U.; Wadsack, C.; Desoye, G. Cord blood chemerin: Differential effects of gestational diabetes mellitus and maternal obesity. *Clin. Endocrinol.* **2014**, *80*, 65–72. [CrossRef] [PubMed]
89. Sun, J.; Ren, J.; Zuo, C.; Deng, D.; Pan, F.; Chen, R.; Zhu, J.; Chen, C.; Ye, S. Circulating apelin, chemerin and omentin levels in patients with gestational diabetes mellitus: A systematic review and meta-analysis. *Lipids Health Dis.* **2020**, *19*, 1–15. [CrossRef]
90. Zhou, Z.; Chen, H.; Ju, H.; Sun, M. Circulating chemerin levels and gestational diabetes mellitus: A systematic review and meta-analysis. *Lipids Health Dis.* **2018**, *17*, 169. [CrossRef]
91. El-Mesallamy, H.O.; El-Derany, M.O.; Hamdy, N.M. Serum omentin-1 and chemerin levels are interrelated in patients with Type 2 diabetes mellitus with or without ischaemic heart disease. *Diabet. Med.* **2011**, *28*, 1194–1200. [CrossRef] [PubMed]
92. Sell, H.; Divoux, A.; Poitou, C.; Basdevant, A.; Bouillot, J.-L.; Bedossa, P.; Tordjman, J.; Eckel, J.; Clément, K. Chemerin Correlates with Markers for Fatty Liver in Morbidly Obese Patients and Strongly Decreases after Weight Loss Induced by Bariatric Surgery. *J. Clin. Endocrinol. Metab.* **2010**, *95*, 2892–2896. [CrossRef] [PubMed]
93. Kukla, M.; Żwirska-Korczala, K.; Hartleb, M.; Waluga, M.; Chwist, A.; Kajor, M.; Ciupińska-Kajor, M.; Berdowska, A.; Wozniak-Grygiel, E.; Buldak, R. Serum chemerin and vaspin in non-alcoholic fatty liver disease. *Scand. J. Gastroenterol.* **2010**, *45*, 235–242. [CrossRef] [PubMed]
94. Chakaroun, R.; Raschpichler, M.; Klöting, N.; Oberbach, A.; Flehmig, G.; Kern, M.; Schön, M.R.; Shang, E.; Lohmann, T.; Dreßler, M.; et al. Effects of weight loss and exercise on chemerin serum concentrations and adipose tissue expression in human obesity. *Metabolism* **2012**, *61*, 706–714. [CrossRef]
95. Weigert, J.; Neumeier, M.; Wanninger, J.; Filarsky, M.; Bauer, S.; Wiest, R.; Farkas, S.; Scherer, M.N.; Schäffler, A.; Aslanidis, C.; et al. Systemic chemerin is related to inflammation rather than obesity in type 2 diabetes. *Clin. Endocrinol.* **2010**, *72*, 342–348. [CrossRef]
96. Brix, J.M.; Stingl, H.; Höllerl, F.; Schernthaner, G.H.; Kopp, H.-P.; Schernthaner, G. Elevated Fetuin-A Concentrations in Morbid Obesity Decrease after Dramatic Weight Loss. *J. Clin. Endocrinol. Metab.* **2010**, *95*, 4877–4881. [CrossRef] [PubMed]
97. Trepanowski, J.F.; Mey, J.; Varady, K.A. Fetuin-A: A novel link between obesity and related complications. *Int. J. Obes.* **2015**, *39*, 734–741. [CrossRef] [PubMed]
98. Ix, J.H.; Shlipak, M.G.; Brandenburg, V.M.; Ali, S.; Ketteler, M.; Whooley, M.A. Association between human fetuin-A and the metabolic syndrome: Data from the Heart and Soul Study. *Circulation* **2006**, *113*, 1760–1767. [CrossRef]
99. Ou, H.-Y.; Yang, Y.-C.; Wu, H.-T.; Wu, J.-S.; Lu, F.-H.; Chang, C.-J. Increased Fetuin-A Concentrations in Impaired Glucose Tolerance with or without Nonalcoholic Fatty Liver Disease, But Not Impaired Fasting Glucose. *J. Clin. Endocrinol. Metab.* **2012**, *97*, 4717–4723. [CrossRef] [PubMed]
100. Jensen, M.K.; Bartz, T.M.; Mukamal, K.J.; Djoussé, L.; Kizer, J.R.; Tracy, R.P.; Zieman, S.J.; Rimm, E.B.; Siscovick, D.S.; Shlipak, M.; et al. Fetuin-A, Type 2 Diabetes, and Risk of Cardiovascular Disease in Older Adults: The Cardiovascular Health Study. *Diabetes Care* **2012**, *36*, 1222–1228. [CrossRef]
101. Ou, H.-Y.; Yang, Y.; Wu, H.-T.; Wu, J.-S.; Lu, F.-H.; Chang, C. Serum fetuin—A concentrations are elevated in subjects with impaired glucose tolerance and newly diagnosed type 2 diabetes. *Clin. Endocrinol.* **2011**, *75*, 450–455. [CrossRef]
102. Denecke, B.; Gräber, S.; Schäfer, C.; Heiss, A.; Wöltje, M.; Jahnen-Dechent, W. Tissue distribution and activity testing suggest a similar but not identical function of fetuin-B and fetuin-A. *Biochem. J.* **2003**, *376*, 135–145. [CrossRef] [PubMed]
103. Meex, R.C.; Hoy, A.J.; Morris, A.; Brown, R.D.; Lo, J.C.; Burke, M.; Goode, R.J.; Kingwell, B.A.; Kraakman, M.J.; Febbraio, M.A.; et al. Fetuin B Is a Secreted Hepatocyte Factor Linking Steatosis to Impaired Glucose Metabolism. *Cell Metab.* **2015**, *22*, 1078–1089. [CrossRef]
104. Peter, A.; Kovarova, M.; Staiger, H.; Machann, J.; Schick, F.; Königsrainer, A.; Königsrainer, I.; Schleicher, E.; Fritsche, A.; Häring, H.-U.; et al. The hepatokines fetuin-A and fetuin-B are upregulated in the state of hepatic steatosis and may differently impact on glucose homeostasis in humans. *Am. J. Physiol. Metab.* **2018**, *314*, E266–E273. [CrossRef] [PubMed]
105. Kalabay, L.; Cseh, K.; Pajor, A.; Baranyi, E.; Csákány, G.M.; Melczer, Z.; Speer, G.; Kovács, M.; Siller, G.; Karádi, I.; et al. Correlation of maternal serum fetuin/alpha2-HS-glycoprotein concentration with maternal insulin resistance and anthropometric parameters of neonates in normal pregnancy and gestational diabetes. *Eur. J. Endocrinol.* **2002**, *147*, 243–248. [CrossRef] [PubMed]
106. Iyidir, O.T.; Degertekin, C.K.; Yilmaz, B.A.; Altinova, A.E.; Toruner, F.B.; Bozkurt, N.; Ayvaz, G.; Akturk, M. Serum levels of fetuin A are increased in women with gestational diabetes mellitus. *Arch. Gynecol. Obstet.* **2014**, *291*, 933–937. [CrossRef] [PubMed]
107. Coustan, D.R.; Carpenter, M.W. The diagnosis of gestational diabetes. *Diabetes Care* **1998**, *21* (Suppl. 2), B5–B8.
108. Farhan, S.; Handisurya, A.; Todoric, J.; Tura, A.; Pacini, G.; Wagner, O.; Klein, K.; Jarai, R.; Huber, K.; Kautzky-Willer, A. Fetuin-A Characteristics during and after Pregnancy: Result from a Case Control Pilot Study. *Int. J. Endocrinol.* **2012**, *2012*, 1–5. [CrossRef]

109. Zhang, Y.; Proenca, R.; Maffei, M.; Barone, M.; Leopold, L.; Friedman, J.M. Positional cloning of the mouse obese gene and its human homologue. *Nature* **1994**, *372*, 425–432. [CrossRef]
110. Considine, R.V.; Sinha, M.K.; Heiman, M.L.; Kriauciunas, A.; Stephens, T.W.; Nyce, M.R.; Ohannesian, J.P.; Marco, C.C.; McKee, L.J.; Bauer, T.L.; et al. Serum Immunoreactive-Leptin Concentrations in Normal-Weight and Obese Humans. *N. Engl. J. Med.* **1996**, *334*, 292–295. [CrossRef]
111. Bado, A.; Levasseur, S.; Attoub, S.; Kermorgant, S.; Laigneau, J.-P.; Bortoluzzi, M.-N.; Moizo, L.; Lehy, T.; Guerre-Millo, M.; Le Marchand-Brustel, Y.; et al. The stomach is a source of leptin. *Nature* **1998**, *394*, 790–793. [CrossRef]
112. Masuzaki, H.; Ogawa, Y.; Sagawa, N.; Hosoda, K.; Matsumoto, T.; Mise, H.; Nishimura, H.; Yoshimasa, Y.; Tanaka, I.; Mori, T.; et al. Nonadipose tissue production of leptin: Leptin as a novel placenta-derived hormone in humans. *Nat. Med.* **1997**, *3*, 1029–1033. [CrossRef] [PubMed]
113. Wilkinson, M.; Morash, B.; Ur, E. The brain is a source of leptin. *Front. Horm. Res.* **1999**, *26*, 106–126. [CrossRef]
114. Considine, R.V. Human Leptin: An Adipocyte Hormone with Weight-Regulatory and Endocrine Functions. *Semin. Vasc. Med.* **2005**, *5*, 15–24. [CrossRef] [PubMed]
115. Brennan, A.M.; Mantzoros, C.S. Drug Insight: The role of leptin in human physiology and pathophysiology—Emerging clinical applications. *Nat. Clin. Pr. Endocrinol. Metab.* **2006**, *2*, 318–327. [CrossRef]
116. Robertson, S.A.; Leinninger, G.M.; Myers, M.G. Molecular and neural mediators of leptin action. *Physiol. Behav.* **2008**, *94*, 637–642. [CrossRef] [PubMed]
117. Harris, R.B.; Zhou, J.; Redmann, S.M.; Smagin, G.N.; Smith, S.R.; Rodgers, E.; Zachwieja, J.J. A leptin dose-response study in obese (ob/ob) and lean (+/?) mice. *Endocrinology* **1998**, *139*, 8–19. [CrossRef] [PubMed]
118. Gavrilova, O.; Marcus-Samuels, B.; Graham, D.; Kim, J.K.; Shulman, G.I.; Castle, A.L.; Vinson, C.; Eckhaus, M.; Reitman, M.L. Surgical implantation of adipose tissue reverses diabetes in lipoatrophic mice. *J. Clin. Investig.* **2000**, *105*, 271–278. [CrossRef]
119. Farooqi, I.S.; Matarese, G.; Lord, G.M.; Keogh, J.M.; Lawrence, E.; Agwu, C.; Sanna, V.; Jebb, S.A.; Perna, F.; Fontana, S.; et al. Beneficial effects of leptin on obesity, T cell hyporesponsiveness, and neuroendocrine/metabolic dysfunction of human congenital leptin deficiency. *J. Clin. Invest.* **2002**, *110*, 1093–1103. [CrossRef]
120. Lewandowski, K.; Horn, R.; O'Callaghan, C.J.; Dunlop, D.; Medley, G.F.; O'Hare, P.; Brabant, G. Free leptin, bound leptin, and soluble leptin receptor in normal and diabetic pregnancies. *J. Clin. Endocrinol. Metab.* **1999**, *84*, 300–306. [CrossRef]
121. Association, A.D. Diagnosis and classification of diabetes mellitus. *Diabetes Care* **2010**, *33* (Suppl. 1), S62–S69. [CrossRef]
122. Kautzky-Willer, A.; Pacini, G.; Tura, A.; Bieglmayer, C.; Schneider, B.; Ludvik, B.; Prager, R.; Waldhäusl, W. Increased plasma leptin in gestational diabetes. *Diabetologia* **2001**, *44*, 164–172. [CrossRef] [PubMed]
123. McLachlan, K.A.; O'Neal, D.; Jenkins, A.; Alford, F.P. Do adiponectin, TNFα, leptin and CRP relate to insulin resistance in pregnancy? Studies in women with and without gestational diabetes, during and after pregnancy. *Diabetes Metab. Res. Rev.* **2006**, *22*, 131–138. [CrossRef] [PubMed]
124. Olefsky, J.M.; Farquhar, J.W.; Reaven, G.M. Do the Oral and Intravenous Glucose Tolerance Tests Provide Similar Diagnostic Information in Patients with Chemical Diabetes Mellitus? *Diabetes* **1973**, *22*, 202–209. [CrossRef]
125. Bao, W.; Baecker, A.; Song, Y.; Kiely, M.; Liu, S.; Zhang, C. Adipokine levels during the first or early second trimester of pregnancy and subsequent risk of gestational diabetes mellitus: A systematic review. *Metabolism* **2015**, *64*, 756–764. [CrossRef] [PubMed]
126. Otsuka, R.; Yatsuya, H.; Tamakoshi, K.; Matsushita, K.; Wada, K.; Toyoshima, H. Perceived Psychological Stress and Serum Leptin Concentrations in Japanese Men. *Obesity* **2006**, *14*, 1832–1838. [CrossRef]
127. Knutson, K.L.; Spiegel, K.; Penev, P.; Van Cauter, E. The metabolic consequences of sleep deprivation. *Sleep Med. Rev.* **2007**, *11*, 163–178. [CrossRef]
128. De Salles, B.F.; Simão, R.; Fleck, S.J.; Dias, I.; Kraemer-Aguiar, L.G.; Bouskela, E. Effects of resistance training on cytokines. *Int. J. Sports Med.* **2010**, *31*, 441–450. [CrossRef] [PubMed]
129. Yang, R.-Z.; Lee, M.-J.; Hu, H.; Pray, J.; Wu, H.-B.; Hansen, B.C.; Shuldiner, A.R.; Fried, S.K.; McLenithan, J.C.; Gong, D.-W. Identification of omentin as a novel depot-specific adipokine in human adipose tissue: Possible role in modulating insulin action. *Am. J. Physiol. Metab.* **2006**, *290*, E1253–E1261. [CrossRef]
130. Schäffler, A.; Neumeier, M.; Herfarth, H.; Fürst, A.; Schölmerich, J.; Büchler, C. Genomic structure of human omentin, a new adipocytokine expressed in omental adipose tissue. *Biochim. Biophys. Acta* **2005**, *1732*, 96–102. [CrossRef]
131. De Souza Batista, C.M.; Yang, R.Z.; Lee, M.J.; Glynn, N.M.; Yu, D.Z.; Pray, J.; Ndubuizu, K.; Patil, S.; Schwartz, A.; Kligman, M. Omentin plasma levels and gene expression are decreased in obesity. *Diabetes* **2007**, *56*, 1655–1661. [CrossRef]
132. Barker, G.; Lim, R.; Georgiou, H.M.; Lappas, M. Omentin-1 Is Decreased in Maternal Plasma, Placenta and Adipose Tissue of Women with Pre-Existing Obesity. *PLoS ONE* **2012**, *7*, e42943. [CrossRef] [PubMed]
133. Hoffman, L.; Nolan, C.; Wilson, J.D.; Oats, J.J.; Simmons, D. Gestational diabetes mellitus–management guidelines. The Australasian Diabetes in Pregnancy Society. *Med. J. Aust.* **1998**, *169*, 93–97. [CrossRef] [PubMed]
134. Abell, S.K.; Shorakae, S.; Harrison, C.L.; Hiam, D.; Moreno-Asso, A.; Stepto, N.K.; De Courten, B.; Teede, H.J. The association between dysregulated adipocytokines in early pregnancy and development of gestational diabetes. *Diabetes Metab. Res. Rev.* **2017**, *33*, e2926. [CrossRef]
135. Franz, M.; Polterauer, M.; Springer, S.; Kuessel, L.; Haslinger, P.; Worda, C.; Worda, K. Maternal and neonatal omentin-1 levels in gestational diabetes. *Arch. Gynecol. Obstet.* **2018**, *297*, 885–889. [CrossRef] [PubMed]

136. Metzger, B.; Lowe, L.; Dyer, A.; Trimble, E.; Chaovarindr, U.; Coustan, D.; Hadden, D.; McCance, D.; Hod, M.; McIntyre, H.; et al. Hyperglycemia and Adverse Pregnancy Outcomes. *Obstet. Anesth. Dig.* **2009**, *29*, 39–40. [CrossRef]
137. Ebrahimi, S.; Gargari, B.P.; Izadi, A.; Imani, B.; Asjodi, F. The effects of Ramadan fasting on serum concentrations of vaspin and omentin-1 in patients with nonalcoholic fatty liver disease. *Eur. J. Integr. Med.* **2018**, *19*, 110–114. [CrossRef]
138. Kiyak Caglayan, E.; Engin-Ustun, Y.; Sari, N.; Gocmen, A.Y.; Polat, M.F. The effects of prolonged fasting on the levels of adiponectin, leptin, apelin, and omentin in pregnant women. *J. Obs. Gynaecol.* **2016**, *36*, 555–558. [CrossRef]
139. Kamimura, D.; Ishihara, K.; Hirano, T. IL-6 signal transduction and its physiological roles: The signal orchestration model. *Rev. Physiol. Biochem. Pharmacol.* **2003**, *149*, 1–38. [CrossRef]
140. Van Snick, J. Interleukin-6: An overview. *Annu. Rev. Immunol.* **1990**, *8*, 253–278. [CrossRef]
141. Jordan, S.C.; Choi, J.; Kim, I.; Wu, G.; Toyoda, M.; Shin, B.; Vo, A. Interleukin-6, A Cytokine Critical to Mediation of Inflammation, Autoimmunity and Allograft Rejection: Therapeutic Implications of IL-6 Receptor Blockade. *Transplantation* **2017**, *101*, 32–44. [CrossRef] [PubMed]
142. Senn, J.J.; Klover, P.J.; Nowak, I.A.; Mooney, R.A. Interleukin-6 Induces Cellular Insulin Resistance in Hepatocytes. *Diabetes* **2002**, *51*, 3391–3399. [CrossRef]
143. Kim, J.H.; Bachmann, R.A.; Chen, J. Interleukin-6 and insulin resistance. *Vitam. Horm.* **2009**, *80*, 613–633.
144. Hoene, M.; Weigert, C. The role of interleukin-6 in insulin resistance, body fat distribution and energy balance. *Obes. Rev.* **2007**, *9*, 20–29. [CrossRef]
145. Carey, A.L.; Bruce, C.R.; Sacchetti, M.; Anderson, M.J.; Olsen, D.B.; Saltin, B.; Hawley, J.A.; Febbraio, M.A. Interleukin-6 and tumor necrosis factor-? Are not increased in patients with Type 2 diabetes: Evidence that plasma interleukin-6 is related to fat mass and not insulin responsiveness. *Diabetologia* **2004**, *47*, 1029–1037. [CrossRef] [PubMed]
146. Dekker, M.J.; Lee, S.; Hudson, R.; Kilpatrick, K.; Graham, T.E.; Ross, R.; Robinson, L.E. An exercise intervention without weight loss decreases circulating interleukin-6 in lean and obese men with and without type 2 diabetes mellitus. *Metabolism* **2007**, *56*, 332–338. [CrossRef]
147. Suzuki, T.; Imai, J.; Yamada, T.; Ishigaki, Y.; Kaneko, K.; Uno, K.; Hasegawa, Y.; Ishihara, H.; Oka, Y.; Katagiri, H. Interleukin-6 enhances glucose-stimulated insulin secretion from pancreatic beta-cells: Potential involvement of the PLC-IP3-dependent pathway. *Diabetes* **2011**, *60*, 537–547. [CrossRef] [PubMed]
148. Trujillo, M.E.; Sullivan, S.; Harten, I.; Schneider, S.H.; Greenberg, A.S.; Fried, S.K. Interleukin-6 regulates human adipose tissue lipid metabolism and leptin production in vitro. *J. Clin. Endocrinol. Metab.* **2004**, *89*, 5577–5582. [CrossRef]
149. Wallenius, K.; Wallenius, V.; Sunter, D.; Dickson, S.L.; Jansson, J.-O. Intracerebroventricular interleukin-6 treatment decreases body fat in rats. *Biochem. Biophys. Res. Commun.* **2002**, *293*, 560–565. [CrossRef]
150. Stenlöf, K.; Wernstedt, I.; Fjällman, T.; Wallenius, V.; Wallenius, K.; Jansson, J.-O. Interleukin-6 Levels in the Central Nervous System Are Negatively Correlated with Fat Mass in Overweight/Obese Subjects. *J. Clin. Endocrinol. Metab.* **2003**, *88*, 4379–4383. [CrossRef]
151. Sudharshana Murthy, K.A.; Bhandiwada, A.; Chandan, S.L.; Gowda, S.L.; Sindhusree, G. Evaluation of Oxidative Stress and Proinflammatory Cytokines in Gestational Diabetes Mellitus and Their Correlation with Pregnancy Outcome. *Indian J. Endocrinol. Metab.* **2018**, *22*, 79–84. [CrossRef] [PubMed]
152. Siddiqui, S.; Waghdhare, S.; Goel, C.; Panda, M.; Soneja, H.; Sundar, J.; Banerjee, M.; Jha, S.; Dubey, S. Augmentation of IL-6 production contributes to development of gestational diabetes mellitus: An Indian study. *Diabetes Metab. Syndr. Clin. Res. Rev.* **2019**, *13*, 895–899. [CrossRef]
153. Braga, F.O.; Negrato, C.A.; Matta, M.D.F.B.D.; Carneiro, J.R.I.; Gomes, M.B. Relationship between inflammatory markers, glycated hemoglobin and placental weight on fetal outcomes in women with gestational diabetes. *Arch. Endocrinol. Metab.* **2019**, *63*, 22–29. [CrossRef]
154. Šimják, P.; Cinkajzlová, A.; Anderlová, K.; Kloučková, J.; Kratochvílová, H.; Lacinová, Z.; Kaválková, P.; KREJČÁ, H.; Mráz, M.; PAŘÁZEK, A.; et al. Changes in plasma concentrations and mRNA expression of hepatokines fetuin A, fetuin B and FGF21 in physiological pregnancy and gestational diabetes mellitus. *Physiol. Res.* **2018**, *67* (Suppl. 3), S531–S542. [CrossRef]
155. Amirian, A.; Mahani, M.B.; Abdi, F. Role of interleukin-6 (IL-6) in predicting gestational diabetes mellitus. *Obstet. Gynecol. Sci.* **2020**, *63*, 407–416. [CrossRef]
156. Abdel Gader, A.G.; Khashoggi, T.Y.; Habib, F.; Awadallah, S.B. Haemostatic and cytokine changes in gestational diabetes mellitus. *Gynecol. Endocrinol.* **2011**, *27*, 356–360. [CrossRef] [PubMed]
157. Wolf, M.; Sauk, J.; Shah, A.; Smirnakis, K.V.; Jimenez-Kimble, R.; Ecker, J.L.; Thadhani, R. Inflammation and Glucose Intolerance: A prospective study of gestational diabetes mellitus. *Diabetes Care* **2003**, *27*, 21–27. [CrossRef]
158. Wedell-Neergaard, A.-S.; Lehrskov, L.L.; Christensen, R.H.; Legaard, G.E.; Dorph, E.; Larsen, M.K.; Launbo, N.; Fagerlind, S.R.; Seide, S.K.; Nymand, S.; et al. Exercise-Induced Changes in Visceral Adipose Tissue Mass are Regulated by IL-6 Signaling: A Randomized Controlled Trial. *SSRN Electron. J.* **2018**, *29*, 844–855. [CrossRef]
159. Desoye, G.; Mouzon, S.H.-D. The Human Placenta in Gestational Diabetes Mellitus: The insulin and cytokine network. *Diabetes Care* **2007**, *30*, S120–S126. [CrossRef]
160. Grivennikov, S.I.; Tumanov, A.V.; Liepinsh, D.J.; Kruglov, A.A.; Marakusha, B.I.; Shakhov, A.N.; Murakami, T.; Drutskaya, L.N.; Förster, I.; Clausen, B.E. Distinct and Nonredundant In Vivo Functions of TNF Produced by T Cells and Macrophages/Neutrophils-Protective and Deleterious Effects. *Immunity* **2005**, *22*, 93–104. [CrossRef]

161. Chen, H.L.; Yang, Y.P.; Hu, X.L.; Yelavarthi, K.K.; Fishback, J.L.; Hunt, J.S. Tumor necrosis factor alpha mRNA and protein are present in human placental and uterine cells at early and late stages of gestation. *Am. J. Pathol.* **1991**, *139*, 327–335.
162. Carswell, E.A.; Old, L.J.; Kassel, R.L.; Green, S.; Fiore, N.; Williamson, B. An endotoxin-induced serum factor that causes necrosis of tumors. *Proc. Natl. Acad. Sci. USA* **1975**, *72*, 3666–3670. [CrossRef] [PubMed]
163. Williams, R.O.; Paleolog, E.; Feldmann, M. Cytokine inhibitors in rheumatoid arthritis and other autoimmune diseases. *Curr. Opin. Pharmacol.* **2007**, *7*, 412–417. [CrossRef] [PubMed]
164. Tweedie, D.; Sambamurti, K.; Greig, N.H. TNF-α Inhibition as a Treatment Strategy for Neurodegenerative Disorders: New Drug Candidates and Targets. *Curr. Alzheimer Res.* **2007**, *4*, 378–385. [CrossRef] [PubMed]
165. Bortolato, B.; Carvalho, A.F.; Soczynska, J.K.; Perini, G.I.; McIntyre, R.S. The Involvement of TNF-α in Cognitive Dysfunction Associated with Major Depressive Disorder: An Opportunity for Domain Specific Treatments. *Curr. Neuropharmacol.* **2015**, *13*, 558–576. [CrossRef]
166. Mohammadi, M.; Gozashti, M.H.; Aghadavood, M.; Mehdizadeh, M.R.; Hayatbakhsh, M.M. Clinical Significance of Serum IL-6 and TNF-α Levels in Patients with Metabolic Syndrome. *Rep. Biochem. Mol. Biol.* **2017**, *6*, 74–79.
167. Emanuela, F.; Grazia, M.; Marco, D.R.; Paola, L.M.; Giorgio, F.; Marco, B. Inflammation as a Link between Obesity and Metabolic Syndrome. *J. Nutr. Metab.* **2012**, *2012*, 1–7. [CrossRef]
168. Bastard, J.-P.; Maachi, M.; Lagathu, C.; Kim, M.J.; Caron, M.; Vidal, H.; Capeau, J.; Feve, B. Recent advances in the relationship between obesity, inflammation, and insulin resistance. *Eur. Cytokine Netw.* **2006**, *17*, 4–12. [PubMed]
169. Lorenzo, M.; Fernández-Veledo, S.; Vila-Bedmar, R.; Garcia-Guerra, L.; De Alvaro, C.; Nieto-Vazquez, I. Insulin resistance induced by tumor necrosis factor-α in myocytes and brown adipocytes. *J. Anim. Sci.* **2008**, *86*, E94–E104. [CrossRef]
170. Nieto-Vazquez, I.; Fernández-Veledo, S.; Krämer, D.K.; Vila-Bedmar, R.; Garcia-Guerra, L.; Lorenzo, M. Insulin resistance associated to obesity: The link TNF-alpha. *Arch. Physiol. Biochem.* **2008**, *114*, 183–194. [CrossRef] [PubMed]
171. Wang, B.; Trayhurn, P. Acute and prolonged effects of TNF-α on the expression and secretion of inflammation-related adipokines by human adipocytes differentiated in culture. *Pflügers Arch.* **2006**, *452*, 418–427. [CrossRef] [PubMed]
172. Patel, A.B.; Tsilioni, I.; Weng, Z.; Theoharides, T.C. TNF stimulates IL-6, CXCL8 and VEGF secretion from human keratinocytes via activation of mTOR, inhibited by tetramethoxyluteolin. *Exp. Dermatol.* **2017**, *27*, 135–143. [CrossRef] [PubMed]
173. Chang, E.; Choi, J.M.; Kim, W.J.; Rhee, E.-J.; Oh, K.W.; Lee, W.-Y.; Park, S.E.; Park, S.W.; Park, C.-Y. Restoration of adiponectin expression via the ERK pathway in TNFα-treated 3T3-L1 adipocytes. *Mol. Med. Rep.* **2014**, *10*, 905–910. [CrossRef] [PubMed]
174. Prins, J.B.; Niesler, C.U.; Winterford, C.M.; Bright, N.A.; Siddle, K.; O'Rahilly, S.; Walker, N.I.; Cameron, D.P. Tumor necrosis factor-alpha induces apoptosis of human adipose cells. *Diabetes* **1997**, *46*, 1939–1944. [CrossRef] [PubMed]
175. Nisoli, E.; Briscini, L.; Giordano, A.; Tonello, C.; Wiesbrock, S.M.; Uysal, K.T.; Cinti, S.; Carruba, M.O.; Hotamisligil, G.S. Tumor necrosis factor alpha mediates apoptosis of brown adipocytes and defective brown adipocyte function in obesity. *Proc. Natl. Acad. Sci. USA* **2000**, *97*, 8033–8038. [CrossRef]
176. Hotamisligil, G.S.; Peraldi, P.; Budavari, A.; Ellis, R.; White, M.F.; Spiegelman, B.M. IRS-1-Mediated Inhibition of Insulin Receptor Tyrosine Kinase Activity in TNF-alpha- and Obesity-Induced Insulin Resistance. *Science* **1996**, *271*, 665–670. [CrossRef] [PubMed]
177. Alzamil, H. Elevated Serum TNF-α Is Related to Obesity in Type 2 Diabetes Mellitus and Is Associated with Glycemic Control and Insulin Resistance. *J. Obes.* **2020**, *2020*, 5076858. [CrossRef]
178. Guillemette, L.; Lacroix, M.; Battista, M.-C.; Doyon, M.; Moreau, J.; Ménard, J.; Ardilouze, J.-L.; Perron, P.; Hivert, M.-F. TNFα Dynamics During the Oral Glucose Tolerance Test Vary According to the Level of Insulin Resistance in Pregnant Women. *J. Clin. Endocrinol. Metab.* **2014**, *99*, 1862–1869. [CrossRef] [PubMed]
179. Kirwan, J.P.; Mouzon, S.H.-D.; Lepercq, J.; Challier, J.-C.; Huston-Presley, L.; Friedman, J.E.; Kalhan, S.C.; Catalano, P.M. TNF-α Is a Predictor of Insulin Resistance in Human Pregnancy. *Diabetes* **2002**, *51*, 2207–2213. [CrossRef]
180. Mushtaq, R.; Akram, A.; Mushtaq, R.; Khwaja, S.; Ahmed, S. The role of inflammatory markers following Ramadan Fasting. *Pak. J. Med. Sci.* **2018**, *35*, 77–81. [CrossRef] [PubMed]
181. Shojaie, M.; Ghanbari, F.; Shojaie, N. Intermittent fasting could ameliorate cognitive function against distress by regulation of inflammatory response pathway. *J. Adv. Res.* **2017**, *8*, 697–701. [CrossRef] [PubMed]
182. Chandrashekara, S.; Jayashree, K.; Veeranna, H.; Vadiraj, H.; Ramesh, M.; Shobha, A.; Sarvanan, Y.; Vikram, Y.K. Effects of anxiety on TNF-α levels during psychological stress. *J. Psychosom. Res.* **2007**, *63*, 65–69. [CrossRef]
183. Stewart, L.K.; Flynn, M.G.; Campbell, W.W.; Craig, B.A.; Robinson, J.P.; Timmerman, K.L.; Mcfarlin, B.K.; Coen, P.M.; Talbert, E. The Influence of Exercise Training on Inflammatory Cytokines and C-Reactive Protein. *Med. Sci. Sports Exerc.* **2007**, *39*, 1714–1719. [CrossRef] [PubMed]
184. Paolucci, E.M.; Loukov, D.; Bowdish, D.M.; Heisz, J.J. Exercise reduces depression and inflammation but intensity matters. *Biol. Psychol.* **2018**, *133*, 79–84. [CrossRef]
185. Jerković, L.; Voegele, A.F.; Chwatal, S.; Kronenberg, F.; Radcliffe, C.M.; Wormald, M.R.; Lobentanz, E.M.; Ezeh, B.; Eller, P.; Dejori, N.; et al. Afamin Is a Novel Human Vitamin E-Binding Glycoprotein Characterization and In Vitro Expression. *J. Proteome Res.* **2005**, *4*, 889–899. [CrossRef]
186. Dieplinger, B.; Egger, M.; Gabriel, C.; Poelz, W.; Morandell, E.; Seeber, B.; Kronenberg, F.; Haltmayer, M.; Mueller, T.; Dieplinger, H. Analytical characterization and clinical evaluation of an enzyme-linked immunosorbent assay for measurement of afamin in human plasma. *Clin. Chim. Acta* **2013**, *425*, 236–241. [CrossRef] [PubMed]

187. Voegele, A.F.; Jerković, L.; Wellenzohn, B.; Eller, P.; Kronenberg, F.; Liedl, K.R.; Dieplinger, H. Characterization of the vitamin E-binding properties of human plasma afamin. *Biochemistry* **2002**, *41*, 14532–14538. [CrossRef] [PubMed]
188. Köninger, A.; Edimiris, P.; Koch, L.; Enekwe, A.; Lamina, C.; Kasimir-Bauer, S.; Kimmig, R.; Dieplinger, H. Serum concentrations of afamin are elevated in patients with polycystic ovary syndrome. *Endocr. Connect.* **2014**, *3*, 120–126. [CrossRef]
189. Seeber, B.; Morandell, E.; Lunger, F.; Wildt, L.; Dieplinger, H. Afamin serum concentrations are associated with insulin resistance and metabolic syndrome in polycystic ovary syndrome. *Reprod. Biol. Endocrinol.* **2014**, *12*, 1–7. [CrossRef]
190. Kollerits, B.; Lamina, C.; Huth, C.; Marques-Vidal, P.; Kiechl, S.; Seppälä, I.; Cooper, J.; Hunt, S.C.; Meisinger, C.; Herder, C.; et al. Plasma Concentrations of Afamin Are Associated With Prevalent and Incident Type 2 Diabetes: A Pooled Analysis in More Than 20,000 Individuals. *Diabetes Care* **2017**, *40*, 1386–1393. [CrossRef] [PubMed]
191. Hubalek, M.; Buchner, H.; Mörtl, M.G.; Schlembach, D.; Huppertz, B.; Firulovic, B.; Köhler, W.; Hafner, E.; Dieplinger, B.; Wildt, L.; et al. The vitamin E-binding protein afamin increases in maternal serum during pregnancy. *Clin. Chim. Acta* **2014**, *434*, 41–47. [CrossRef] [PubMed]
192. Tramontana, A.; Dieplinger, B.; Stangl, G.; Hafner, E.; Dieplinger, H. First trimester serum afamin concentrations are associated with the development of pre-eclampsia and gestational diabetes mellitus in pregnant women. *Clin. Chim. Acta* **2018**, *476*, 160–166. [CrossRef] [PubMed]
193. Jensen, D.M.; Mølsted-Pedersen, L.; Beck-Nielsen, H.; Westergaard, J.G.; Ovesen, P.; Damm, P. Screening for gestational diabetes mellitus by a model based on risk indicators: A prospective study. *Am. J. Obstet. Gynecol.* **2003**, *189*, 1383–1388. [CrossRef]
194. Köninger, A.; Mathan, A.; Mach, P.; Frank, M.; Schmidt, B.; Schleussner, E.; Kimmig, R.; Gellhaus, A.; Dieplinger, H. Is Afamin a novel biomarker for gestational diabetes mellitus? A pilot study. *Reprod. Biol. Endocrinol.* **2018**, *16*, 1–11. [CrossRef] [PubMed]
195. Kleinwechter, H.; Schäfer-Graf, U.; Bührer, C.; Hoesli, I.; Kainer, F.; Kautzky-Willer, A.; Pawlowski, B.; Schunck, K.; Somville, T.; Sorger, M. Gestational diabetes mellitus (GDM) diagnosis, therapy and follow-up care: Practice Guideline of the German Diabetes Association(DDG) and the German Association for Gynaecologyand Obstetrics (DGGG). *Exp. Clin. Endocrinol. Diabetes* **2014**, *122*, 395–405. [PubMed]
196. Dieplinger, H.; Dieplinger, B. Afamin—A pleiotropic glycoprotein involved in various disease states. *Clin. Chim. Acta* **2015**, *446*, 105–110. [CrossRef]
197. Morgan, B.P. Complement regulatory molecules: Application to therapy and transplantation. *Immunol. Today* **1995**, *16*, 257–259. [CrossRef]
198. Maio, M.; Brasoveanu, L.I.; Coral, S.; Sigalotti, L.; Lamaj, E.; Gasparollo, A.; Visintin, A.; Altomonte, M.; Fonsatti, E. Structure, distribution, and functional role of protectin (CD59) in complement-susceptibility and in immunotherapy of human malignancies (Review). *Int. J. Oncol.* **1998**, *13*, 305–323. [CrossRef]
199. Vakeva, A.; Lehto, T.; Takala, A.; Meri, S. Detection of a Soluble Form of the Complement Membrane Attack Complex Inhibitor CD59 in Plasma after Acute Myocardial Infarction. *Scand. J. Immunol.* **2000**, *52*, 411–414. [CrossRef]
200. Lehto, T.; Honkanen, E.; Teppo, A.-M.; Meri, S. Urinary excretion of protectin (CD59), complement SC5b-9 and cytokines in membranous glomerulonephritis. *Kidney Int.* **1995**, *47*, 1403–1411. [CrossRef]
201. Meri, S.; Lehto, T.; Sutton, C.W.; Tyynelä, J.; Baumann, M. Structural composition and functional characterization of soluble CD59: Heterogeneity of the oligosaccharide and glycophosphoinositol (GPI) anchor revealed by laser-desorption mass spectrometric analysis. *Biochem. J.* **1996**, *316*, 923–935. [CrossRef]
202. Gehrs, K.M.; Jackson, J.R.; Brown, E.N.; Allikmets, R.; Hageman, G.S. Complement, age-related macular degeneration and a vision of the future. *Arch. Ophthalmol.* **2010**, *128*, 349–358. [CrossRef] [PubMed]
203. Gerl, V.B.; Bohl, J.; Pitz, S.; Stoffelns, B.; Pfeiffer, N.; Bhakdi, S. Extensive deposits of complement C3d and C5b-9 in the choriocapillaris of eyes of patients with diabetic retinopathy. *Investig. Ophthalmol. Vis. Sci.* **2002**, *43*, 1104–1108.
204. Nevo, Y.; Ben-Zeev, B.; Tabib, A.; Straussberg, R.; Anikster, Y.; Shorer, Z.; Fattal-Valevski, A.; Ta-Shma, A.; Aharoni, S.; Rabie, M.; et al. CD59 deficiency is associated with chronic hemolysis and childhood relapsing immune-mediated polyneuropathy. *Blood* **2013**, *121*, 129–135. [CrossRef] [PubMed]
205. Rosoklija, G.B.; Dwork, A.J.; Younger, D.S.; Karlikaya, G.; Latov, N.; Hays, A.P. Local activation of the complement system in endoneurial microvessels of diabetic neuropathy. *Acta Neuropathol.* **2000**, *99*, 55–62. [CrossRef] [PubMed]
206. Falk, R.J.; Scheinman, J.I.; Mauer, S.M.; Michael, A.F. Polyantigenic Expansion of Basement Membrane Constituents in Diabetic Nephropathy. *Diabetes* **1983**, *32*, 34–39. [CrossRef] [PubMed]
207. Qin, X.; Goldfine, A.; Krumrei, N.; Grubissich, L.; Acosta, J.; Chorev, M.; Hays, A.P.; Halperin, J.A. Glycation Inactivation of the Complement Regulatory Protein CD59: A Possible Role in the Pathogenesis of the Vascular Complications of Human Diabetes. *Diabetes* **2004**, *53*, 2653–2661. [CrossRef]
208. Acosta, J.; Hettinga, J.; Flückiger, R.; Krumrei, N.; Goldfine, A.; Angarita, L.; Halperin, J. Molecular basis for a link between complement and the vascular complications of diabetes. *Proc. Natl. Acad. Sci. USA* **2000**, *97*, 5450–5455. [CrossRef]
209. Ghosh, P.; Sahoo, R.; Vaidya, A.; Cantel, S.; Kavishwar, A.; Goldfine, A.; Herring, N.; Bry, L.; Chorev, M.; Halperin, J.A. A specific and sensitive assay for blood levels of glycated CD59: A novel biomarker for diabetes. *Am. J. Hematol.* **2013**, *88*, 670–676. [CrossRef]
210. Ghosh, P.; Vaidya, A.; Sahoo, R.; Goldfine, A.; Herring, N.; Bry, L.; Chorev, M.; Halperin, J.A. Glycation of the Complement Regulatory Protein CD59 Is a Novel Biomarker for Glucose Handling in Humans. *J. Clin. Endocrinol. Metab.* **2014**, *99*, E999–E1006. [CrossRef]

211. Bogdanet, D.; O'Shea, P.; Halperin, J.; Dunne, F. Plasma glycated CD59 (gCD59), a novel biomarker for the diagnosis, management and follow up of women with Gestational Diabetes (GDM)—protocol for prospective cohort study. *BMC Pregnancy Childbirth* **2020**, *20*, 1–6. [CrossRef]
212. Licht, P.; Lösch, A.; Dittrich, R.; Neuwinger, J.; Siebzehnrübl, E.; Wildt, L. Novel insights into human endometrial paracrinology and embryo-maternal communication by intrauterine microdialysis. *Hum. Reprod. Updat.* **1998**, *4*, 532–538. [CrossRef] [PubMed]
213. Ma, Q.; Fan, J.; Wang, J.; Yang, S.; Cong, Q.; Wang, R.; Lv, Q.; Liu, R.; Ning, G. High levels of chorionic gonadotrophin attenuate insulin sensitivity and promote inflammation in adipocytes. *J. Mol. Endocrinol.* **2015**, *54*, 161–170. [CrossRef] [PubMed]
214. Sirikunalai, P.; Wanapirak, C.; Sirichotiyakul, S.; Tongprasert, F.; Srisupundit, K.; Luewan, S.; Traisrisilp, K.; Tongsong, T. Associations between maternal serum free beta human chorionic gonadotropin (β-hCG) levels and adverse pregnancy outcomes. *J. Obstet. Gynaecol.* **2016**, *36*, 178–182. [CrossRef]
215. Ong, C.Y.T.; Liao, A.W.; Spencer, K.; Munim, S.; Nicolaides, K.H. First trimester maternal serum free β human chorionic gonadotrophin and pregnancy associated plasma protein A as predictors of pregnancy complications. *BJOG* **2000**, *107*, 1265–1270. [CrossRef] [PubMed]
216. WHO Expert Committee on Diabetes Mellitus: Second Report. *World Health Organ Tech Rep Ser.* **1980**, *646*, 1–80.
217. Xiong, F.; Li, G.; Sun, Q.; Chen, P.; Wang, Z.; Wan, C.; Yao, Z.; Zhong, H.; Zeng, Y. Obstetric and perinatal outcomes of pregnancies according to initial maternal serum HCG concentrations after vitrified–warmed single blastocyst transfer. *Reprod. Biomed. Online* **2019**, *38*, 455–464. [CrossRef] [PubMed]
218. Yue, C.-Y.; Zhang, C.-Y.; Ying, C.-M. Serum markers in quadruple screening associated with adverse pregnancy outcomes: A case–control study in China. *Clin. Chim. Acta* **2020**, *511*, 278–281. [CrossRef]
219. Tul, N.; Pusenjak, S.; Osredkar, J.; Spencer, K.; Novak-Antolic, Z. Predicting complications of pregnancy with first-trimester maternal serum free-betahCG, PAPP-A and inhibin-A. *Prenat. Diagn.* **2003**, *23*, 990–996. [CrossRef]
220. Savvidou, M.D.; Syngelaki, A.; Muhaisen, M.; Emelyanenko, E.; Nicolaides, K.H. First trimester maternal serum free β-human chorionic gonadotropin and pregnancy-associated plasma protein A in pregnancies complicated by diabetes mellitus. *BJOG: Int. J. Obstet. Gynaecol.* **2012**, *119*, 410–416. [CrossRef]
221. Beneventi, F.; Simonetta, M.; Lovati, E.; Albonico, G.; Tinelli, C.; Locatelli, E.; Spinillo, A. First trimester pregnancy-associated plasma protein-A in pregnancies complicated by subsequent gestational diabetes. *Prenat. Diagn.* **2011**, *31*, 523–528. [CrossRef] [PubMed]
222. Sweeting, A.N.; Wong, J.; Appelblom, H.; Ross, G.P.; Kouru, H.; Williams, P.F.; Sairanen, M.; Hyett, J.A. A first trimester prediction model for gestational diabetes utilizing aneuploidy and pre-eclampsia screening markers. *J. Matern. Neonatal Med.* **2017**, *31*, 2122–2130. [CrossRef] [PubMed]
223. Hammond, G.L.; Bocchinfuso, W.P. Sex Hormone-Binding Globulin: Gene Organization and Structure/Function Analyses. *Horm. Res.* **1996**, *45*, 197–201. [CrossRef]
224. Hammond, G.L. Diverse Roles for Sex Hormone-Binding Globulin in Reproduction. *Biol. Reprod.* **2011**, *85*, 431–441. [CrossRef] [PubMed]
225. Glass, A.R.; Swerdloff, R.S.; Bray, G.A.; Dahms, W.T.; Atkinson, R.L. Low Serum Testosterone and Sex-Hormone-Binding-Globulin in Massively Obese Men. *J. Clin. Endocrinol. Metab.* **1977**, *45*, 1211–1219. [CrossRef]
226. Guzick, D.S.; Wing, R.; Smith, D.; Berga, S.L.; Winters, S.J. Endocrine consequences of weight loss in obese, hyperandrogenic, anovulatory women. *Fertil. Steril.* **1994**, *61*, 598–604. [CrossRef]
227. Hammoud, A.; Gibson, M.; Hunt, S.C.; Adams, T.D.; Carrell, D.T.; Kolotkin, R.L.; Meikle, A.W. Effect of Roux-en-Y Gastric Bypass Surgery on the Sex Steroids and Quality of Life in Obese Men. *J. Clin. Endocrinol. Metab.* **2009**, *94*, 1329–1332. [CrossRef]
228. Pitteloud, N.; Mootha, V.K.; Dwyer, A.A.; Hardin, M.; Lee, H.; Eriksson, K.-F.; Tripathy, D.; Yialamas, M.; Groop, L.; Elahi, D.; et al. Relationship between testosterone levels, insulin sensitivity, and mitochondrial function in men. *Diabetes Care* **2005**, *28*, 1636–1642. [CrossRef]
229. Kajaia, N.; Binder, H.; Dittrich, R.; Oppelt, P.G.; Flor, B.; Cupisti, S.; Beckmann, M.W.; Mueller, A. Low sex hormone-binding globulin as a predictive marker for insulin resistance in women with hyperandrogenic syndrome. *Eur. J. Endocrinol.* **2007**, *157*, 499–507. [CrossRef]
230. Laaksonen, D.E.; Niskanen, L.; Punnonen, K.; Nyyssönen, K.; Tuomainen, T.-P.; Salonen, R.; Rauramaa, R.; Salonen, J.T. Sex hormones, inflammation and the metabolic syndrome: A population-based study. *Eur. J. Endocrinol.* **2003**, *149*, 601–608. [CrossRef]
231. Brand, J.S.; Van Der Tweel, I.; Grobbee, D.E.; Emmelot-Vonk, M.H.; Van Der Schouw, Y.T. Testosterone, sex hormone-binding globulin and the metabolic syndrome: A systematic review and meta-analysis of observational studies. *Int. J. Epidemiol.* **2010**, *40*, 189–207. [CrossRef] [PubMed]
232. Jaruvongvanich, V.; Sanguankeo, A.; Riangwiwat, T.; Upala, S. Testosterone, Sex Hormone-Binding Globulin and Nonalcoholic Fatty Liver Disease: A Systematic Review and Meta-Analysis. *Ann. Hepatol.* **2017**, *16*, 382–394. [CrossRef] [PubMed]
233. Ding, E.L.; Song, Y.; Malik, V.S.; Liu, S. Sex differences of endogenous sex hormones and risk of type 2 diabetes: A systematic review and meta-analysis. *JAMA* **2006**, *295*, 1288–1299. [CrossRef] [PubMed]
234. Hu, J.; Zhang, A.; Yang, S.; Wang, Y.; Goswami, R.; Zhou, H.; Zhang, Y.; Wang, Z.; Li, R.; Cheng, Q.; et al. Combined effects of sex hormone-binding globulin and sex hormones on risk of incident type 2 diabetes. *J. Diabetes* **2015**, *8*, 508–515. [CrossRef]

235. Muka, T.; Nano, J.; Jaspers, L.; Meun, C.; Bramer, W.M.; Hofman, A.; Dehghan, A.; Kavousi, M.; Laven, J.S.; Franco, O.H. Associations of Steroid Sex Hormones and Sex Hormone–Binding Globulin With the Risk of Type 2 Diabetes in Women: A Population-Based Cohort Study and Meta-analysis. *Diabetes* **2016**, *66*, 577–586. [CrossRef]
236. Pugeat, M.; Crave, J.C.; Elmidani, M.; Nicolas, M.H.; Garoscio-Cholet, M.; Lejeune, H.; Déchaud, H.; Tourniaire, J. Pathophysiology of sex hormone binding globulin (SHBG): Relation to insulin. *J. Steroid Biochem. Mol. Biol.* **1991**, *40*, 841–849. [CrossRef]
237. Plymate, S.R.; Matej, L.A.; Jones, R.E.; Friedl, K.E. Inhibition of sex hormone-binding globulin production in the human hepatoma (Hep G2) cell line by insulin and prolactin. *J. Clin. Endocrinol. Metab.* **1988**, *67*, 460–464. [CrossRef]
238. Winters, S.J.; Gogineni, J.; Karegar, M.; Scoggins, C.; Wunderlich, C.A.; Baumgartner, R.; Ghooray, D.T. Sex Hormone-Binding Globulin Gene Expression and Insulin Resistance. *J. Clin. Endocrinol. Metab.* **2014**, *99*, E2780–E2788. [CrossRef] [PubMed]
239. Shin, J.Y.; Kim, S.-K.; Lee, M.Y.; Kim, H.S.; Ye, B.I.; Shin, Y.G.; Baik, S.K.; Chung, C.H. Serum sex hormone-binding globulin levels are independently associated with nonalcoholic fatty liver disease in people with type 2 diabetes. *Diabetes Res. Clin. Pr.* **2011**, *94*, 156–162. [CrossRef]
240. Flechtner-Mors, M.; Schick, A.; Oeztuerk, S.; Haenle, M.M.; Wilhelm, M.; Koenig, W.; Imhof, A.; Boehm, B.O.; Graeter, T.; Mason, R.A.; et al. Associations of Fatty Liver Disease and Other Factors Affecting Serum SHBG Concentrations: A Population Based Study on 1657 Subjects. *Horm. Metab. Res.* **2013**, *46*, 287–293. [CrossRef]
241. Hedderson, M.M.; Xu, F.; Darbinian, J.A.; Quesenberry, C.P.; Sridhar, S.; Kim, C.; Gunderson, E.P.; Ferrara, A. Prepregnancy SHBG Concentrations and Risk for Subsequently Developing Gestational Diabetes Mellitus. *Diabetes Care* **2014**, *37*, 1296–1303. [CrossRef] [PubMed]
242. Li, M.-Y.; Rawal, S.; Hinkle, S.N.; Zhu, Y.-Y.; Tekola-Ayele, F.; Tsai, M.Y.; Liu, S.-M.; Zhang, C.-L. Sex Hormone-binding Globulin, Cardiometabolic Biomarkers, and Gestational Diabetes: A Longitudinal Study and Meta-analysis. *Matern. Med.* **2020**, *2*, 2–9. [CrossRef]
243. Smirnakis, K.V.; Plati, A.; Wolf, M.; Thadhani, R.; Ecker, J.L. Predicting gestational diabetes: Choosing the optimal early serum marker. *Am. J. Obstet. Gynecol.* **2007**, *196*, 410.e1–410.e7. [CrossRef] [PubMed]
244. Bulletins–Obstetrics ACoOaGCoP. ACOG Practice Bulletin. Clinical management guidelines for obstetrician-gynecologists. Number 30, September 2001 (replaces Technical Bulletin Number 200, December 1994). Gestational diabetes. *Obstet. Gynecol.* **2001**, *98*, 525–538.
245. Siddiqui, K.; George, T.P.; Joy, S.S.; Nawaz, S.S. Association of sex hormone binding globulin with gestational age and parity in gestational diabetes mellitus. *J. Matern. Neonatal Med.* **2020**, *2020*, 1–6. [CrossRef]
246. Ajjan, R.; Carter, A.M.; Somani, R.; Kain, K.; Grant, P.J. Ethnic differences in cardiovascular risk factors in healthy Caucasian and South Asian individuals with the metabolic syndrome. *J. Thromb. Haemost.* **2007**, *5*, 754–760. [CrossRef]
247. McElduff, A.; Hitchman, R.; McElduff, P. Is sex hormone-binding globulin associated with glucose tolerance? *Diabet. Med.* **2006**, *23*, 306–312. [CrossRef]
248. Key, T.J.; Pike, M.C.; Moore, J.W.; Wang, D.Y.; Morgan, B. The relationship of free fatty acids with the binding of oestradiol to SHBG and to albumin in women. *J. Steroid Biochem.* **1990**, *35*, 35–38. [CrossRef]
249. Hamllton-Falrley, D.; White, D.; Griffiths, M.; Anyaoku, V.; Kolstlnen, R.; Seppälä, M.; Franks, S. Diurnal variation of sex hormone binding globulin and insulin-like growth factor binding protein-1 in women with polycystic ovary syndrome. *Clin. Endocrinol.* **1995**, *43*, 159–165. [CrossRef] [PubMed]
250. Catalano, P.M. Carbohydrate Metabolism and Gestational Diabetes. *Clin. Obstet. Gynecol.* **1994**, *37*, 25–38. [CrossRef]
251. Stefan, N.; Kantartzis, K.; Häring, H.-U. Causes and Metabolic Consequences of Fatty Liver. *Endocr. Rev.* **2008**, *29*, 939–960. [CrossRef]
252. Venugopal, S.K.; Devaraj, S.; Jialal, I. Macrophage conditioned medium induces the expression of C-reactive protein in human aortic endothelial cells: Potential for paracrine/autocrine effects. *Am. J. Pathol.* **2005**, *166*, 1265–1271. [CrossRef]
253. Ganter, U.; Arcone, R.; Toniatti, C.; Morrone, G.; Ciliberto, G. Dual control of C-reactive protein gene expression by interleukin-1 and interleukin-6. *EMBO J.* **1989**, *8*, 3773–3779. [CrossRef] [PubMed]
254. Sproston, N.R.; Ashworth, J.J. Role of C-Reactive Protein at Sites of Inflammation and Infection. *Front. Immunol.* **2018**, *9*, 754. [CrossRef] [PubMed]
255. Retnakaran, R.; Hanley, A.J.G.; Raif, N.; Connelly, P.W.; Sermer, M.; Zinman, B. C-Reactive Protein and Gestational Diabetes: The Central Role of Maternal Obesity. *J. Clin. Endocrinol. Metab.* **2003**, *88*, 3507–3512. [CrossRef]
256. Jabs, W.J.; Lögering, B.A.; Gerke, P.; Kreft, B.; Wolber, E.-M.; Klinger, M.H.F.; Fricke, L.; Steinhoff, J. The kidney as a second site of human C-reactive protein formation in vivo. *Eur. J. Immunol.* **2003**, *33*, 152–161. [CrossRef]
257. Kim, S.H.; Reaven, G.; Lindley, S. Relationship between insulin resistance and C-reactive protein in a patient population treated with second generation antipsychotic medications. *Int. Clin. Psychopharmacol.* **2011**, *26*, 43–47. [CrossRef]
258. Moran, A.; Steffen, L.M.; Jacobs, J.D.R.; Steinberger, J.; Pankow, J.S.; Hong, C.-P.; Tracy, R.P.; Sinaiko, A.R. Relation of C-Reactive Protein to Insulin Resistance and Cardiovascular Risk Factors in Youth. *Diabetes Care* **2005**, *28*, 1763–1768. [CrossRef]
259. Yan, Y.; Li, S.; Liu, Y.; Bazzano, L.; He, J.; Mi, J.; Chen, W. Temporal relationship between inflammation and insulin resistance and their joint effect on hyperglycemia: The Bogalusa Heart Study. *Cardiovasc. Diabetol.* **2019**, *18*, 1–10. [CrossRef] [PubMed]
260. Ridker, P.; Buring, J.; Cook, N.; Rifai, N. C-reactive protein, the metabolic syndrome, and risk of incident cardiovascular events. An 8-year follow-up of 14,719 initially healthy American women. *ACC Curr. J. Rev.* **2003**, *12*, 33–34. [CrossRef]

261. Aronson, D.; Bartha, P.; Zinder, O.; Kerner, A.; Markiewicz, W.; Avizohar, O.; Brook, G.J.; Levy, Y. Obesity is the major determinant of elevated C-reactive protein in subjects with the metabolic syndrome. *Int. J. Obes.* **2004**, *28*, 674–679. [CrossRef]
262. Visser, M.; Bouter, L.M.; McQuillan, G.M.; Wener, M.H.; Harris, T.B. Elevated C-Reactive Protein Levels in Overweight and Obese Adults. *JAMA* **1999**, *282*, 2131–2135. [CrossRef] [PubMed]
263. Kahn, S.E.; Zinman, B.; Haffner, S.M.; O'Neill, M.C.; Kravitz, B.G.; Yu, D.; Freed, M.I.; Herman, W.H.; Holman, R.R.; Jones, N.P.; et al. Obesity Is a Major Determinant of the Association of C-Reactive Protein Levels and the Metabolic Syndrome in Type 2 Diabetes. *Diabetes* **2006**, *55*, 2357–2364. [CrossRef] [PubMed]
264. Alamolhoda, S.H.; Yazdkhasti, M.; Namdari, M.; Zakariayi, S.J.; Mirabi, P. Association between C-reactive protein and gestational diabetes: A prospective study. *J. Obstet. Gynaecol.* **2019**, *40*, 349–353. [CrossRef]
265. Savvidou, M.; Nelson, S.M.; Makgoba, M.; Messow, C.-M.; Sattar, N.; Nicolaides, K. First-Trimester Prediction of Gestational Diabetes Mellitus: Examining the Potential of Combining Maternal Characteristics and Laboratory Measures. *Diabetes* **2010**, *59*, 3017–3022. [CrossRef] [PubMed]
266. Wolf, M.; Sandler, L.; Hsu, K.; Vossen-Smirnakis, K.; Ecker, J.L.; Thadhani, R. First-Trimester C-Reactive Protein and Subsequent Gestational Diabetes. *Diabetes Care* **2003**, *26*, 819–824. [CrossRef]
267. Alyas, S.; Roohi, N.; Ashraf, S.; Ilyas, S.; Ilyas, A. Early pregnancy biochemical markers of placentation for screening of gestational diabetes mellitus (GDM). *Diabetes Metab. Syndr. Clin. Res. Rev.* **2019**, *13*, 2353–2356. [CrossRef]
268. Korkmazer, E.; Solak, N. Correlation between inflammatory markers and insulin resistance in pregnancy. *J. Obstet. Gynaecol.* **2014**, *35*, 142–145. [CrossRef]
269. Corcoran, S.M.; Achamallah, N.; Loughlin, J.O.; Stafford, P.; Dicker, P.; Malone, F.D.; Breathnach, F. First trimester serum biomarkers to predict gestational diabetes in a high-risk cohort: Striving for clinically useful thresholds. *Eur. J. Obstet. Gynecol. Reprod. Biol.* **2018**, *222*, 7–12. [CrossRef]
270. Adam, S.; Pheiffer, C.; Dias, S.; Rheeder, P. Association between gestational diabetes and biomarkers: A role in diagnosis. *Biomarkers* **2018**, *23*, 386–391. [CrossRef]
271. Classification and diagnosis of diabetes mellitus and other categories of glucose intolerance. National Diabetes Data Group. *Diabetes* **1979**, *28*, 1039–1057. [CrossRef] [PubMed]
272. Amirian, A.; Rahnemaei, F.A.; Abdi, F. Role of C-reactive Protein(CRP) or high-sensitivity CRP in predicting gestational diabetes Mellitus:Systematic review. *Diabetes Metab. Syndr. Clin. Res. Rev.* **2020**, *14*, 229–236. [CrossRef]
273. Oh-I, S.; Shimizu, H.; Satoh, T.; Okada, S.; Adachi, S.; Inoue, K.; Eguchi, H.; Yamamoto, M.; Imaki, T.; Hashimoto, K.; et al. Identification of nesfatin-1 as a satiety molecule in the hypothalamus. *Nature* **2006**, *443*, 709–712. [CrossRef] [PubMed]
274. Su, Y.; Zhang, J.; Tang, Y.; Bi, F.; Liu, J.-N. The novel function of nesfatin-1: Anti-hyperglycemia. *Biochem. Biophys. Res. Commun.* **2010**, *391*, 1039–1042. [CrossRef]
275. Dong, J.; Xu, H.; Wang, P.-F.; Cai, G.-J.; Song, H.-F.; Wang, C.-C.; Dong, Z.-T.; Ju, Y.-J.; Jiang, Z.-Y. Nesfatin-1 Stimulates Fatty-Acid Oxidation by Activating AMP-Activated Protein Kinase in STZ-Induced Type 2 Diabetic Mice. *PLoS ONE* **2013**, *8*, e83397. [CrossRef] [PubMed]
276. Li, Q.-C.; Wang, H.-Y.; Chen, X.; Guan, H.-Z.; Jiang, Z.-Y. Fasting plasma levels of nesfatin-1 in patients with type 1 and type 2 diabetes mellitus and the nutrient-related fluctuation of nesfatin-1 level in normal humans. *Regul. Pept.* **2010**, *159*, 72–77. [CrossRef]
277. Zhai, T.; Li, S.-Z.; Fan, X.-T.; Tian, Z.; Lu, X.-Q.; Dong, J. Circulating Nesfatin-1 Levels and Type 2 Diabetes: A Systematic Review and Meta-Analysis. *J. Diabetes Res.* **2017**, *2017*, 1–8. [CrossRef]
278. Kucukler, F.K.; Gorkem, U.; Simsek, Y.; Kocabas, R.; Gulen, S.; Guler, S. Low level of Nesfatin-1 is associated with gestational diabetes mellitus. *Gynecol. Endocrinol.* **2016**, *32*, 759–761. [CrossRef]
279. Ademoglu, E.N.; Gorar, S.; Keskin, M.; Carlioglu, A.; Ucler, R.; Erdamar, H.; Culha, C.; Aral, Y. Serum nesfatin-1 levels are decreased in pregnant women newly diagnosed with gestational diabetes. *Arch. Endocrinol. Metab.* **2017**, *61*, 455–459. [CrossRef] [PubMed]
280. Mierzyński, R.; Poniedziałek-Czajkowska, E.; Dłuski, D.; Patro-Małysza, J.; Kimber-Trojnar, Ż.; Majsterek, M.; Leszczyńska-Gorzelak, B. Nesfatin-1 and Vaspin as Potential Novel Biomarkers for the Prediction and Early Diagnosis of Gestational Diabetes Mellitus. *Int. J. Mol. Sci.* **2019**, *20*, 159. [CrossRef]
281. Fialova, L.; Malbohan, I.M. Pregnancy-associated plasma protein A (PAPP-A): Theoretical and clinical aspects. *Bratisl Lek List.* **2002**, *103*, 194–205.
282. Dugoff, L.; Hobbins, J.C.; Malone, F.D.; Porter, T.F.; Luthy, D.; Comstock, C.H.; Hankins, G.; Berkowitz, R.L.; Merkatz, I.; Craigo, S.D.; et al. First-trimester maternal serum PAPP-A and free-beta subunit human chorionic gonadotropin concentrations and nuchal translucency are associated with obstetric complications: A population-based screening study (The FASTER Trial). *Am. J. Obstet. Gynecol.* **2004**, *191*, 1446–1451. [CrossRef] [PubMed]
283. Leguy, M.C.; Brun, S.; Pidoux, G.; Salhi, H.; Choiset, A.; Menet, M.C.; Gil, S.; Tsatsaris, V.; Guibourdenche, J. Pattern of secretion of pregnancy-associated plasma protein-A (PAPP-A) during pregnancies complicated by fetal aneuploidy, in vivo and in vitro. *Reprod. Biol. Endocrinol.* **2014**, *12*, 129. [CrossRef] [PubMed]
284. Pellitero, S.; Reverter, J.L.; Pizarro, E.; Pastor, M.C.; Granada, M.L.; Tàssies, D.; Reverter, J.-C.; Salinas, I.; Sanmartí, A. Pregnancy-associated plasma protein-a levels are related to glycemic control but not to lipid profile or hemostatic parameters in type 2 diabetes. *Diabetes Care* **2007**, *30*, 3083–3085. [CrossRef]

285. Resch, Z.T.; Chen, B.-K.; Bale, L.K.; Oxvig, C.; Overgaard, M.T.; Conover, C.A. Pregnancy-Associated Plasma Protein A Gene Expression as a Target of Inflammatory Cytokines. *Endocrinology* **2004**, *145*, 1124–1129. [CrossRef]
286. Donovan, B.M.; Nidey, N.L.; Jasper, E.A.; Robinson, J.G.; Bao, W.; Saftlas, A.F.; Ryckman, K.K. First trimester prenatal screening biomarkers and gestational diabetes mellitus: A systematic review and meta-analysis. *PLoS ONE* **2018**, *13*, e0201319. [CrossRef]
287. Wells, G.; Bleicher, K.; Han, X.; McShane, M.; Chan, Y.F.; Bartlett, A.; White, C.; Lau, S.M. Maternal Diabetes, Large for Gestational Age Births and First Trimester Pregnancy Associated Plasma Protein-A. *J. Clin. Endocrinol. Metab.* **2015**, *100*, 2372–2379. [CrossRef]
288. Jayabalan, N.; Lai, A.; Nair, S.; Guanzon, D.; Scholz-Romero, K.; Palma, C.; McIntyre, H.D.; Lappas, M.; Salomon, C. Quantitative Proteomics by SWATH-MS Suggest an Association Between Circulating Exosomes and Maternal Metabolic Changes in Gestational Diabetes Mellitus. *Proteomics* **2018**, *19*, e1800164. [CrossRef]
289. Alapatt, P.; Guo, F.; Komanetsky, S.M.; Wang, S.; Cai, J.; Sargsyan, A.; Díaz, E.R.; Bacon, B.T.; Aryal, P.; Graham, T.E. Liver Retinol Transporter and Receptor for Serum Retinol-binding Protein (RBP4). *J. Biol. Chem.* **2013**, *288*, 1250–1265. [CrossRef] [PubMed]
290. Majerczyk, M.; Olszanecka-Glinianowicz, M.; Puzianowska-Kuźnicka, M.; Chudek, J. Retinol-binding protein 4 (RBP4) as the causative factor and marker of vascular injury related to insulin resistance. *Postepy Hig. Med. Dosw.* **2016**, *70*, 1267–1275.
291. Yang, Q.; Graham, T.E.; Mody, N.; Preitner, F.; Peroni, O.D.; Zabolotny, J.M.; Kotani, K.; Quadro, L.; Kahn, B.B. Serum retinol binding protein 4 contributes to insulin resistance in obesity and type 2 diabetes. *Nature* **2005**, *436*, 356–362. [CrossRef]
292. Jin, C.; Lin, L.; Han, N.; Zhao, Z.; Liu, Z.; Luo, S.; Xu, X.; Liu, J.; Wang, H. Plasma retinol-binding protein 4 in the first and second trimester and risk of gestational diabetes mellitus in Chinese women: A nested case-control study. *Nutr. Metab.* **2020**, *17*, 1–7. [CrossRef]
293. Khovidhunkit, W.; Pruksakorn, P.; Plengpanich, W.; Tharavanij, T. Retinol-binding protein 4 is not associated with insulin resistance in pregnancy. *Metabolism* **2012**, *61*, 65–69. [CrossRef]
294. Huang, Q.-T.; Huang, Q.; Luo, W.; Li, F.; Hang, L.-L.; Yu, Y.-H.; Zhong, M. Circulating retinol-binding protein 4 levels in gestational diabetes mellitus: A meta-analysis of observational studies. *Gynecol. Endocrinol.* **2015**, *31*, 337–344. [CrossRef] [PubMed]
295. Hu, S.; Liu, Q.; Huang, X.; Tan, H. Serum level and polymorphisms of retinol-binding protein-4 and risk for gestational diabetes mellitus: A meta-analysis. *BMC Pregnancy Childbirth* **2016**, *16*, 52. [CrossRef] [PubMed]
296. Jia, J.; Bai, J.; Liu, Y.; Yin, J.; Yang, P.; Yu, S.; Ye, J.; Wang, N.; Yuan, G. Association between retinol-binding protein 4 and polycystic ovary syndrome: A meta-analysis. *Endocr. J.* **2014**, *61*, 995–1002. [CrossRef] [PubMed]
297. Kim, S.-H.; Im, J.-A.; Choi, H.-J. Retinol-binding protein 4 responses during an oral glucose tolerance testing in women with gestational diabetes mellitus. *Clin. Chim. Acta* **2008**, *391*, 123–125. [CrossRef]
298. Chan, T.-F.; Chen, H.-S.; Chen, Y.-C.; Lee, C.-H.; Chou, F.-H.; Chen, I.-J.; Chen, S.-Y.; Jong, S.-B.; Tsai, E.-M. Increased Serum Retinol-Binding Protein 4 Concentrations in Women With Gestational Diabetes Mellitus. *Reprod. Sci.* **2007**, *14*, 169–174. [CrossRef] [PubMed]
299. Zhaoxia, L.; Mengkai, D.; Qin, F.; Danqing, C. Significance of RBP4 in patients with gestational diabetes mellitus: A case-control study of Han Chinese women. *Gynecol. Endocrinol.* **2013**, *30*, 161–164. [CrossRef] [PubMed]
300. Su, Y.-X.; Hong, J.; Yan, Q.; Xu, C.; Gu, W.-Q.; Zhang, Y.-F.; Shen, C.-F.; Chi, Z.-N.; Dai, M.; Xu, M.; et al. Increased serum retinol-binding protein-4 levels in pregnant women with and without gestational diabetes mellitus. *Diabetes Metab.* **2010**, *36*, 470–475. [CrossRef]
301. Tepper, B.J.; Kim, Y.-K.; Shete, V.; Shabrova, E.; Quadro, L. Serum Retinol-Binding Protein 4 (RBP4) and retinol in a cohort of borderline obese women with and without gestational diabetes. *Clin. Biochem.* **2010**, *43*, 320–323. [CrossRef] [PubMed]
302. Krzyzanowska, K.; Zemany, L.; Krugluger, W.; Schernthaner, G.H.; Mittermayer, F.; Schnack, C.; Rahman, R.; Brix, J.; Kahn, B.B. Serum concentrations of retinol-binding protein 4 in women with and without gestational diabetes. *Diabetologia* **2008**, *51*, 1115–1122. [CrossRef]
303. Lewandowski, K.C.; Stojanovic, N.; Bienkiewicz, M.; Tan, B.K.; Prelevic, G.M.; Press, M.; Tuck, S.; O'Hare, P.J.; Randeva, H.S. Elevated concentrations of retinol-binding protein-4 (RBP-4) in gestational diabetes mellitus: Negative correlation with soluble vascular cell adhesion molecule-1 (sVCAM-1). *Gynecol. Endocrinol.* **2008**, *24*, 300–305. [CrossRef] [PubMed]
304. Abetew, D.F.; Qiu, C.; Fida, N.G.; Dishi, M.; Hevner, K.; Williams, M.A.; Enquobahrie, D.A. Association of retinol binding protein 4 with risk of gestational diabetes. *Diabetes Res. Clin. Pr.* **2013**, *99*, 48–53. [CrossRef]
305. Liu, M.; Chen, Y.; Chen, D. Association between transthyretin concentrations and gestational diabetes mellitus in Chinese women. *Arch. Gynecol. Obstet.* **2020**, *302*, 329–335. [CrossRef] [PubMed]
306. Graham, T.E.; Wason, C.J.; Blüher, M.; Kahn, B.B. Shortcomings in methodology complicate measurements of serum retinol binding protein (RBP4) in insulin-resistant human subjects. *Diabetologia* **2007**, *50*, 814–823. [CrossRef]
307. Idris, N.; Hatikah, C.C.; Murizah, M.; Rushdan, M. Universal Versus Selective Screening for Detection of Gestational Diabetes Mellitus in a Malaysian Population. *Malays Fam Physician* **2009**, *4*, 83–87. [PubMed]
308. Avalos, G.E.; Owens, L.A.; Dunne, F.; Collaborators, F.T.A.D. Applying Current Screening Tools for Gestational Diabetes Mellitus to a European Population: Is It Time for Change? *Diabetes Care* **2013**, *36*, 3040–3044. [CrossRef]
309. Alberico, S.; Strazzanti, C.; De Santo, D.; De Seta, F.; Lenardon, P.; Bernardon, M.; Zicari, S.; Guaschino, S. Gestational diabetes: Universal or selective screening? *J. Matern. Fetal. Neonatal. Med.* **2004**, *16*, 331–337. [CrossRef]
310. Kuo, C.-H.; Li, H.-Y. Diagnostic Strategies for Gestational Diabetes Mellitus: Review of Current Evidence. *Curr. Diabetes Rep.* **2019**, *19*, 155. [CrossRef]

311. Mo, X.; Tobe, R.G.; Takahashi, Y.; Arata, N.; Liabsuetrakul, T.; Nakayama, T.; Mori, R. Economic Evaluations of Gestational Diabetes Mellitus Screening: A Systematic Review. *J. Epidemiol.* **2021**, *31*, 220–230. [CrossRef]
312. Danyliv, A.; Gillespie, P.; O'Neill, C.; Tierney, M.; O'Dea, A.; McGuire, B.E.; Glynn, L.G.; Dunne, F.P. The cost-effectiveness of screening for gestational diabetes mellitus in primary and secondary care in the Republic of Ireland. *Diabetologia* **2015**, *59*, 436–444. [CrossRef] [PubMed]
313. Di Cianni, G.; Volpe, L.; Casadidio, I.; Bottone, P.; Marselli, L.; Lencioni, C.; Boldrini, A.; Teti, G.; Del Prato, S.; Benzi, L. Universal screening and intensive metabolic management of gestational diabetes: Cost-effectiveness in Italy. *Acta Diabetol.* **2002**, *39*, 69–73. [CrossRef]
314. Miailhe, G.; Kayem, G.; Girard, G.; Legardeur, H.; Mandelbrot, L. Selective rather than universal screening for gestational diabetes mellitus? *Eur. J. Obstet. Gynecol. Reprod. Biol.* **2015**, *191*, 95–100. [CrossRef]
315. Cosson, E.; Benbara, A.; Pharisien, I.; Nguyen, M.T.; Revaux, A.; Lormeau, B.; Sandre-Banon, D.; Assad, N.; Pillegand, C.; Valensi, P.; et al. Diagnostic and Prognostic Performances Over 9 Years of a Selective Screening Strategy for Gestational Diabetes Mellitus in a Cohort of 18,775 Subjects. *Diabetes Care* **2012**, *36*, 598–603. [CrossRef] [PubMed]
316. Wen, S.W.; Liu, S.; Kramer, M.S.; Joseph, K.S.; Levitt, C.; Marcoux, S.; Liston, R.M. Impact of Prenatal Glucose Screening on the Diagnosis of Gestational Diabetes and on Pregnancy Outcomes. *Am. J. Epidemiol.* **2000**, *152*, 1009–1014. [CrossRef] [PubMed]
317. Cosson, E.; Benchimol, M.; Carbillon, L.; Pharisien, I.; Pariès, J.; Valensi, P.; Lormeau, B.; Bolie, S.; Uzan, M.; Attali, J.R. Universal rather than selective screening for gestational diabetes mellitus may improve fetal outcomes. *Diabetes Metab.* **2006**, *32*, 140–146. [CrossRef]
318. Farrar, D.; Fairley, L.; Wright, J.; Tuffnell, D.; Whitelaw, D.; Lawlor, D.A. Evaluation of the impact of universal testing for gestational diabetes mellitus on maternal and neonatal health outcomes: A retrospective analysis. *BMC Pregnancy Childbirth* **2014**, *14*, 317. [CrossRef]
319. Griffin, M.E.; Coffey, M.; Johnson, H.; Scanlon, P.; Foley, M.; Stronge, J.; O'Meara, N.M.; Firth, R.G. Universal vs. risk factor-based screening for gestational diabetes mellitus: Detection rates, gestation at diagnosis and outcome. *Diabet. Med.* **2000**, *17*, 26–32. [CrossRef]
320. Sweeting, A.N.; Ross, G.P.; Hyett, J.; Molyneaux, L.; Constantino, M.; Harding, A.J.; Wong, J. Gestational Diabetes Mellitus in Early Pregnancy: Evidence for Poor Pregnancy Outcomes Despite Treatment. *Diabetes Care* **2015**, *39*, 75–81. [CrossRef] [PubMed]
321. Most, O.L.; Kim, J.H.; Arslan, A.A.; Klauser, C. Maternal and neonatal outcomes in early glucose tolerance testing in an obstetric population in New York city. *J. Périnat. Med.* **2009**, *37*, 114–117. [CrossRef] [PubMed]
322. Simmons, D.; Nema, J.; Parton, C.; Vizza, L.; Robertson, A.; Rajagopal, R.; Ussher, J.; Perz, J. The treatment of booking gestational diabetes mellitus (TOBOGM) pilot randomised controlled trial. *BMC Pregnancy Childbirth* **2018**, *18*, 1–8. [CrossRef] [PubMed]
323. Zhu, Z.; Cao, F.; Li, X. Epigenetic Programming and Fetal Metabolic Programming. *Front. Endocrinol.* **2019**, *10*, 764. [CrossRef]
324. Mayeux, R. Biomarkers: Potential uses and limitations. *NeuroRx* **2004**, *1*, 182–188. [CrossRef]
325. Mahdi, T.; Hänzelmann, S.; Salehi, A.; Muhammed, S.J.; Reinbothe, T.M.; Tang, Y.; Axelsson, A.S.; Zhou, Y.; Jing, X.; Almgren, P.; et al. Secreted Frizzled-Related Protein 4 Reduces Insulin Secretion and Is Overexpressed in Type 2 Diabetes. *Cell Metab.* **2012**, *16*, 625–633. [CrossRef]
326. Schuitemaker, J.H.N.; Beernink, R.H.J.; Franx, A.; Cremers, T.I.F.H.; Koster, M.P.H. First trimester secreted Frizzled-Related Protein 4 and other adipokine serum concentrations in women developing gestational diabetes mellitus. *PLoS ONE* **2020**, *15*, e0242423. [CrossRef] [PubMed]
327. Ipekci, S.; Baldane, S.; Kebapcilar, A.G.; Abuşoğlu, S.; Beyhekim, H.; Ilhan, T.T.; Unlu, A.; Kebapçılar, L. Prorenin and secreted frizzled-related protein-4 levels in women with gestational diabetes mellitus. *Endocr. Abstr.* **2018**, *119*, 450–453. [CrossRef]
328. Yuan, X.-S.; Zhang, M.; Wang, H.-Y.; Jiang, J.; Yu, B. Increased secreted frizzled-related protein 4 and ficolin-3 levels in gestational diabetes mellitus women. *Endocr. J.* **2018**, *65*, 499–508. [CrossRef] [PubMed]
329. Amini, M.; Kazemnejad, A.; Zayeri, F.; Montazeri, A.; Rasekhi, A.; Amirian, A.; Kariman, N. Diagnostic accuracy of maternal serum multiple marker screening for early detection of gestational diabetes mellitus in the absence of a gold standard test. *BMC Pregnancy Childbirth* **2020**, *20*, 1–9. [CrossRef]
330. Liu, L.; Hu, J.; Yang, L.; Wang, N.; Liu, Y.; Wei, X.; Gao, M.; Wang, Y.; Ma, Y.; Wen, D. Association of WISP1/CCN4 with Risk of Overweight and Gestational Diabetes Mellitus in Chinese Pregnant Women. *Dis. Markers* **2020**, *2020*, 1–10. [CrossRef]
331. Sahin Ersoy, G.; Altun Ensari, T.; Subas, S.; Giray, B.; Simsek, E.E.; Cevik, O. WISP1 is a novel adipokine linked to metabolic parameters in gestational diabetes mellitus. *J. Matern. Fetal. Neonatal. Med.* **2017**, *30*, 942–946. [CrossRef] [PubMed]
332. Al-Ghazali, M.J.; Ali, H.A.; Al-Rufaie, M.M. Serum irisin levels as a potential marker for diagnosis of gestational diabetes mellitus. *Acta Biomed.* **2020**, *91*, 56–63.
333. Onat, T.; Inandiklioglu, N. Circulating Myonectin and Irisin Levels in Gestational Diabetes Mellitus—A Case-control Study. *Z. Geburtshilfe Neonatol.* **2021**. [CrossRef]
334. Gutaj, P.; Sibiak, R.; Jankowski, M.; Awdi, K.; Bryl, R.; Mozdziak, P.; Kempisty, B.; Wender-Ozegowska, E. The Role of the Adipokines in the Most Common Gestational Complications. *Int. J. Mol. Sci.* **2020**, *21*, 9408. [CrossRef] [PubMed]
335. Zhong, L.; Long, Y.; Wang, S.; Lian, R.; Deng, L.; Ye, Z.; Wang, Z.; Liu, B. Continuous elevation of plasma asprosin in pregnant women complicated with gestational diabetes mellitus: A nested case-control study. *Placenta* **2020**, *93*, 17–22. [CrossRef]

336. Yavuzkir, S.; Ugur, K.; Deniz, R.; Ustebay, D.U.; Mirzaoglu, M.; Yardim, M.; Sahin, I.; Baykus, Y.; Karagoz, Z.K.; Aydin, S. Maternal and umbilical cord blood subfatin and spexin levels in patients with gestational diabetes mellitus. *Peptides* **2020**, *126*, 170277. [CrossRef]
337. Kang, L.; Li, H.-Y.; Ou, H.-Y.; Wu, P.; Wang, S.-H.; Chang, C.-J.; Lin, S.-Y.; Wu, C.-L.; Wu, H.-T. Role of placental fibrinogen-like protein 1 in gestational diabetes. *Transl. Res.* **2020**, *218*, 73–80. [CrossRef]
338. Liu, L.; Hu, J.; Wang, N.; Liu, Y.; Wei, X.; Gao, M.; Ma, Y.; Wen, D. A novel association of CCDC80 with gestational diabetes mellitus in pregnant women: A propensity score analysis from a case-control study. *BMC Pregnancy Childbirth* **2020**, *20*, 1–9. [CrossRef]
339. Deischinger, C.; Leitner, K.; Baumgartner-Parzer, S.; Bancher-Todesca, D.; Kautzky-Willer, A.; Harreiter, J. CTRP-1 levels are related to insulin resistance in pregnancy and gestational diabetes mellitus. *Sci. Rep.* **2020**, *10*, 1–9. [CrossRef]
340. The Top 10 Research Priorities for Diabetes in Pregnancy. Available online: https://www.jla.nihr.ac.uk/news/the-top-10-research-priorities-for-diabetes-in-pregnancy/26184 (accessed on 7 January 2021).

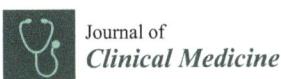

Journal of
Clinical Medicine

Review

Screening for Gestational Diabetes Mellitus in Early Pregnancy: What Is the Evidence?

Lore Raets [1], Kaat Beunen [1] and Katrien Benhalima [2,*]

1. Department of Clinical and Experimental Endocrinology, KU Leuven, Herestraat 49, 3000 Leuven, Belgium; lore.raets@kuleuven.be (L.R.); kaat.beunen@kuleuven.be (K.B.)
2. Department of Endocrinology, University Hospital Gasthuisberg, KU Leuven, Herestraat 49, 3000 Leuven, Belgium
* Correspondence: katrien.benhalima@uzleuven.be

Abstract: The incidence of gestational diabetes mellitus (GDM) is increasing worldwide. This has a significant effect on the health of the mother and offspring. There is no doubt that screening for GDM between 24 and 28 weeks is important to reduce the risk of adverse pregnancy outcomes. However, there is no consensus about diagnosis and treatment of GDM in early pregnancy. In this narrative review on the current evidence on screening for GDM in early pregnancy, we included 37 cohort studies and eight randomized controlled trials (RCTs). Observational studies have shown that a high proportion (15–70%) of women with GDM can be detected early in pregnancy depending on the setting, criteria used and screening strategy. Data from observational studies on the potential benefit of screening and treatment of GDM in early pregnancy show conflicting results. In addition, there is substantial heterogeneity in age and BMI across the different study populations. Smaller RCTs could not show benefit but several large RCTs are ongoing. RCTs are also necessary to determine the appropriate cut-off for HbA1c in pregnancy as there is limited evidence showing that an HbA1c $\geq 6.5\%$ has a low sensitivity to detect overt diabetes in early pregnancy.

Keywords: pregnancy; gestational diabetes mellitus; early screening; diabetes

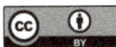

Citation: Raets, L.; Beunen, K.; Benhalima, K. Screening for Gestational Diabetes Mellitus in Early Pregnancy: What Is the Evidence?. *J. Clin. Med.* **2021**, *10*, 1257. https://doi.org/10.3390/jcm10061257

Academic Editor: Kei Nakajima

Received: 21 January 2021
Accepted: 16 March 2021
Published: 18 March 2021

Publisher's Note: MDPI stays neutral with regard to jurisdictional claims in published maps and institutional affiliations.

Copyright: © 2021 by the authors. Licensee MDPI, Basel, Switzerland. This article is an open access article distributed under the terms and conditions of the Creative Commons Attribution (CC BY) license (https://creativecommons.org/licenses/by/4.0/).

1. Introduction

Worldwide, the incidence of gestational diabetes mellitus (GDM) is increasing. This has a significant effect on the health of the mother and offspring. GDM is defined as diabetes diagnosed in the second or third trimester of pregnancy provided that overt diabetes early in pregnancy has been excluded [1]. There is no doubt that screening for GDM between 24 and 28 weeks is important to reduce the risk for adverse pregnancy outcomes such as large-for-gestational age infants (LGA) and preeclampsia [2,3]. There is a large variation in recommendations concerning screening for GDM in early pregnancy. The "American Diabetes Association" (ADA) recommends screening for overt diabetes at first prenatal visit, especially in women with risk factors. However, the ADA does not provide any specific recommendations concerning screening for GDM in early pregnancy [4]. "The International Association of the Diabetes and Pregnancy Study Groups" (IADPSG) initially recommended classification of GDM in early pregnancy when a fasting plasma glucose (FPG) ≥ 5.1 mmol/L occurs. However, the IADPSG criteria have not been validated for use in early pregnancy. Other associations such as the "International Federation of Gynecology and Obstetrics" (FIGO) recommend to screen universally in early pregnancy for diabetes and GDM [5]. In contrast, the "National Institute for Health and Care Excellence" recommends screening for early GDM if there are risk factors present, such as obesity, previous history of GDM, family history of diabetes (first-degree relative), previous macrocosmic baby or an ethnicity with a high prevalence of diabetes [6]. Early testing for overt diabetes will lead to the identification of hyperglycemia under the threshold of overt diabetes. These women could be labeled as early GDM based on IADPSG criteria, but there is a lack of evidence from randomized controlled trials (RCTs) on the potential benefits and harms of diagnosing and treating GDM in early pregnancy compared to treatment later in pregnancy. The ongoing controversy reflects in a lack of international consensus on screening for GDM in early pregnancy. The aim of this narrative review was therefore to evaluate the current evidence on screening and treatment for GDM in early pregnancy. In addition, we also reviewed pragmatic approaches to screening for glucose intolerance in pregnancy in a pandemic setting.

2. Materials and Methods

2.1. Data Sources and Search Strategies

Between November 2020 and December 2020, a literature search was conducted on PubMed. Cross-sectional studies, case–control studies, cohort studies, and RCTs were considered for this review. This is a narrative review. We did not perform a systematic review due to heterogeneity of studies and could therefore not perform a meta-analysis.

We used the following inclusion criteria:

1. The study population were pregnant women with early-onset GDM.
2. The control group could either be mothers with early GDM who were not treated or mothers with GDM diagnosed at 24–28 weeks of pregnancy (late-onset GDM).
3. The following comparisons were made: women with early GDM were compared to women with GDM diagnosed at 24–28 weeks or women with early GDM who received treatment before 24 weeks were compared to women with early GDM who did not receive treatment before 24 weeks.
4. The pregnancy outcomes studied were the development of GDM at 24–28 weeks, gestational weight gain, cesarean section, shoulder dystocia, preeclampsia, need for insulin treatment, LGA, neonatal intensive care unit (NICU) admission, neonatal hypoglycemia, preterm delivery and gestation age at delivery.

We excluded animal studies, descriptive designs (case series and case reports), studies with a low quality (no method section, no p-values mentioned), and articles written in a language other than English, French or Dutch. We did not limit our search to a specific population or ethnicity, or to a specific age category.

We used the following search strategies:

("diabetes, gestational"(MeSH Terms) OR "Gestational diabetes"(Title/Abstract) OR "diabetes mellitus"(MeSH Terms) OR "diabetes mellitus" (Title/Abstract)) AND ("Blood Glucose" (MeSH Terms) OR "Blood Glucose" (Title/Abstract) OR "Insulin Resistance" (MeSH Terms) OR "hyperglycemia/blood" (MeSH Terms) OR "hyperglycemia" (Title/Abstract) OR "Glucose Intolerance" (MeSH Terms) OR "Glucose Tolerance Test" (MeSH Terms) OR "Glucose Tolerance Test" (Title/Abstract) OR "early screening" (Title/Abstract)) AND ("pregnancy trimester, first" (MeSH Terms) OR "First trimester pregnancy"(Title/Abstract))

In addition, we searched the reference lists of the selected articles and relevant reviews by hand. We also did a manual search for articles on screening for GDM during the COVID-19 Pandemic. We focused on articles that proposed a pragmatic approach on screening for diabetes and GDM in early pregnancy during the COVID-19 pandemic and compared the rate of missed cases of GDM between different screening tests and strategies.

2.2. Data Synthesis and Analysis

The extracted data included the study design, country, number of study participants, the diagnostic criteria used for GDM, adjustments that were made and pregnancy outcomes. We reported our results in a descriptive manner. A p-value <0.05 was considered significant.

3. Results

3.1. Search Results

We identified 356 articles of which 137 articles were selected as possibly relevant. After examination of the full text, 46 studies were included in the current review (Figure 1).

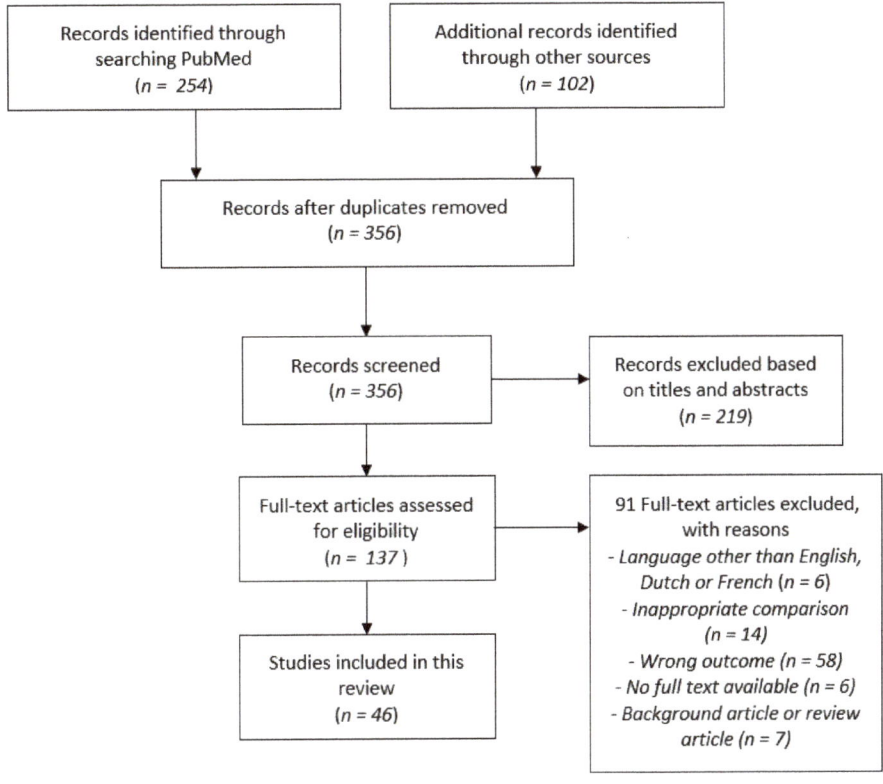

Figure 1. The literature search and selection process.

3.2. Study Characteristics

The study characteristics are shown in Tables 1–3. In total, there were seven prospective cohort studies (15.6%), 29 retrospective cohort studies (63.0%), eight RCTs (17.8%), one post-hoc analysis (2.2%) and one population-based cohort study (2.2%). Six studies were performed in Asia (13.3%), 18 in Europe (39.1%), seven in America (15.6%), three in the Middle East (6.7%), four in Australia (8.9%), two in New Zealand (4.5%) and six multi-national studies (13.3%). All but one study was performed from 2000 onwards. Forty-one studies (89.9%) were performed from 2010 onwards. Twelve studies used the IADPSG criteria (26.7%). In total, 16 studies (34.9%) performed selective screening based on risk factors, while 30 studies (77.7%) used universal screening. Appendix A gives an overview of the diagnostic criteria used in the different studies.

Table 1. Observational studies.

Author, Year/Country (Ref.)	Design	Subjects (N)	Study Population	Timeframe Testing (Weeks)	GDM Criteria	Comparison	Main Results
De Muylder, 1984/Belgium [7]	Prospective cohort study	139	Hi risk	<24 weeks	3 h OGTT/ O'Sullivan criteria	GDM diagnosis <24 weeks vs. GDM diagnosis 24–32 weeks vs. GDM diagnosis >32 weeks	Early GDM treated group had less complications such as preterm labor, preeclampsia and cesarean section
Bartha, 2000/Spain [8]	Prospective cohort study	3986	All pregnant women	First antenatal visit	50 g GCT and 3 h 100 g OGTT	Early-onset (most during 1st trimester) vs. late-onset GDM	Early GDM diagnosis represented a high-risk subgroup

Table 1. Cont.

Author, Year/Country (Ref.)	Design	Subjects (N)	Study Population	Timeframe Testing (Weeks)	GDM Criteria	Comparison	Main Results
Barahona, 2005/Spain [9]	Retrospective study	1708 offspring	Women with GDM	<24 weeks	50 g GCT and 3 h OGTT/2nd and 3rd Workshop Conference Criteria on GDM	GDM diagnosis <24 weeks vs. 24–30 weeks vs. >31 weeks	Early GDM diagnosis was a predictor of adverse maternal and neonatal outcome
Hawkins, 2008/US [10]	Retrospective cohort study	3334	All pregnant women	<24 weeks (Hi risk)	50 g GCT and 3 h 100 g OGTT/ NDDG criteria	Diet-treated GDM <24 weeks (early diagnosis in hi risk population) vs. ≥24 weeks (routine diagnosis)	Twofold increased risk of preeclampsia in women with early diagnosis of diet treated GDM
Riskin, 2009/Israel [11]	Retrospective study	6129	Singleton pregnancies >24 weeks in mothers without ODIP or 1st FTFPG ≥5.8 mmol/L	<13 weeks	FTFPG/C&C criteria	FPG categories (<4.2 mmol/L, 4.2–4.4 mmol/L, 4.5–4.7 mmol/L, 4.8–5.0 mmol/L, 5.1–5.2 mmol/L, 5.3–5.5 mmol/L and 5.6–5.8 mmol/L)	Higher FTFPG in early pregnancy increased the risk of adverse pregnancy outcomes
Plasencia, 2011/Spain [12]	Retrospective study	1716	Singleton pregnancies	6–14 weeks	50 g GCT and 3 h 100 g OGTT/ C&C criteria	GDM vs. non-GDM and GCT and OGTT results at 6–14 vs. 20–30 weeks	Effective diagnosis of GDM in the first trimester could be achieved by lowering the GCT and OGTT plasma glucose cut-offs
Corrado, 2012/Italy [13]	Retrospective study	738	Singleton pregnancies	<13 weeks	FTFPG/IADPSG criteria	FTFPG vs. 2 h 75 g OGTT early in the third trimester	FPG ≥5.1 mmol/L may be considered a highly predictive risk factor for GDM
Zhu W.W., 2013/China [14]	Retrospective cohort study	14,039	All pregnant women without ODIP	First antenatal visit (<24 weeks)	FPG/China GDM diagnosis criteria	6 FPG groups (<4.1, 4.1–4.59, 4.60–5.09, 5.10–5.59, 5.6–6.09, 6.10–6.99 mmol/L)	Only 30.3% of women who had an FPG of ≥5.1 mmol/L still had an FPG of ≥5.1 mmol/L at 24–28 weeks
Alunni, 2015/US [15]	Retrospective cohort study	2652	Singleton pregnancies in women without ODIP	≤24 weeks	HbA1c and FPG/HbA1c ≥5.7% or FPG ≥5.1 mmol/L at ≤24 weeks or C&C criteria	Early screening vs. standard two-step ACOG approach (1 h 50 g GCT followed by a 3 h 100 g OGTT/ C&C Criteria)	Implementing early screening for GDM gave no significant difference in neonatal outcomes
Amylidi, 2015/Switzerland [16]	Retrospective cohort study	208	Hi risk	<13 weeks	HbA1c/ADA and HAPO study guidelines	GDM vs. non-GDM (diagnosis based on one-step standardized 2 h 75 g OGTT between 24 and 28 weeks) and HbA1c ≥6% vs. <6%	Values HbA1c ≥6.0% in early pregnancy were predictive of GDM
Harreiter, 2016/International [17]	Retrospective study	1035	Pregnant women with BMI ≥ 29.0 kg/m²	Early pregnancy	2 h 75 g OGTT/ WHO 2013 criteria	NGT vs. early GDM vs. DIP	Pre-pregnancy BMI was a significant predictor of early GDM and the only predictor among nulliparous women
Mañé, 2016/Spain [18]	Prospective multi-ethnic cohort study	1228	Singleton pregnancies in women without ODIP	<13 weeks	HbA1c/≥5.9%	HbA1c ≥5.9% vs. HbA1c <5.9%	Early HbA1c ≥5.9% measurement identified women at high risk for poorer pregnancy outcomes
Osmundson, 2016/US [19]	Retrospective cohort study	2812	Singleton pregnancy >20 weeks	≤13^{6/7} weeks	HbA1c (prediabetes: 5.7–6.4%)	Prediabetic women (HbA1c of 5.7–6.4%) vs. women with a normal first trimester HbA1c (<5.7%)	HbA1c early in pregnancy was a poor test to identify women who will develop GDM

Table 1. Cont.

Author, Year/Country (Ref.)	Design	Subjects (N)	Study Population	Timeframe Testing (Weeks)	GDM Criteria	Comparison	Main Results
Sweeting, 2016/ Australia [20]	Retrospective cohort study	4873	Hi risk	<24 weeks	2 h 75 g OGTT/ADIPS diagnostic criteria	T2DM vs. GDM <12 weeks vs. GDM 12–23 weeks vs. GDM ≥24 weeks	Early GDM in high-risk women remains associated with poorer pregnancy outcomes
Sweeting, 2017/ Australia [21]	Retrospective cohort study	3098	Hi risk	<24 weeks	HbA1c measurement at time of GDM diagnosis	Early GDM (<24 weeks) vs. standard GDM (≥24 weeks)	HbA1c >5.9% early in pregnancy identified an increased risk of LGA, macrosomia, C-section, and hypertensive disorders in standard GDM
Hosseini, 2018/Iran [22]	Prospective population-based cohort study	929	Singleton pregnancies	6–14 weeks	FPG/IADPSG	Normal pregnancy vs. early-onset GDM (6–14 weeks) vs. late-onset GDM (24–28 weeks)	Early-onset GDM was associated with poorer pregnancy outcomes
Ryan, 2018/UK [23]	Retrospective clinical audit of prospectively maintained database	576	Hi risk singleton pregnancies	11–13 weeks	FPG/SIGN 2010 thresholds	Routine vs. early screening	Early screening improved the pregnancy outcomes, such as emergency cesarean section, neonatal hypoglycemia and macrosomia.
Salman, 2018/Israel [24]	Retrospective cohort study	5030	Singleton pregnancies of women without ODIP	<13 weeks	FTFPG cut-off 5.3 mmol/L	Women with FTFPG < 5.3 mmol/L and FTFPG ≥ 5.3 mmol/L	FTFPG ≥5.3 mmol/L was an independent risk factor for adverse perinatal outcome
Bianchi, 2019/Italy [25]	Retrospective study	290	Hi risk	16–18 weeks	2 h 75 g OGTT (and FPG)/ IADPSG criteria	Early (16–18 weeks) vs. standard (24–28 weeks) screening	Similar short-term maternal-fetal outcomes in both groups
Del Val López, 2019/ Spain [26]	Retrospective study	1425	All pregnant women without ODIP	<13 weeks	FTFPG/O'Sullivan criteria	FTFPG <5.1 and ≥5.1 mmol/L (FTFPG vs. classical 2-step OGTT)	FTFPG was not a good substitute for conventional diagnosis of GDM in the second trimester
Mañé, 2019/Spain [27]	Retrospective analysis of a prospective observational cohort study	1228	Women with singleton pregnancy without ODIP	<13 weeks	FPG and HbA1c/Criteria unknown	FPG vs. HbA1c cut-off values	FTFPG levels were not a better predictor of pregnancy complications than HbA1c
Benhalima, 2020/Belgium [28]	Multi-centric prospective cohort study	2006	All pregnant women	6–14 weeks	FPG/IADPSG criteria	FPG ≥5.1–5.5 mmol/L in early pregnancy vs. FPG <5.1 mmol/L in early pregnancy	Group with increased FPG in early pregnancy had significantly more NICU admissions
Boriboonhirunsarn/ Thailand, 2020 [29]	Retrospective cohort study	1200	All pregnant women	<24 weeks	50 g GCT and 100 g OGTT/ ADA and ACOG recommendation	No GDM vs. early-onset GDM vs. late-onset GDM	Significant lower gestational weight gain and higher rates of preeclampsia, LGA infants, and NICU admission despite treatment for early-onset GDM
Clarke, 2020/ Australia [30]	Retrospective cohort study	769	Hi risk with singleton pregnancy and without ODIP	<24 weeks	75 g 2 h OGTT/IADPSG criteria, as per the ADIPS guidelines	Early GDM (hi risk women diagnosed <24 weeks) vs. late GDM (women diagnosed ≥24 weeks)	Early pregnancy GDM was not associated with an adverse outcome
Cosson, 2020/France [31]	Retrospective study	523	Women with singleton pregnancy and without ODIP	<22 weeks	FPG/IADPSG criteria	Immediate care vs. no immediate care for early fasting hyperglycemia	Treating women with early fasting hyperglycemia, especially when FPG is ≥5.5 mmol/L, may improve pregnancy outcomes

Table 1. Cont.

Author, Year/Country (Ref.)	Design	Subjects (N)	Study Population	Timeframe Testing (Weeks)	GDM Criteria	Comparison	Main Results
Immanuel, 2020/ International [32]	Post-hoc analysis of DALI study	869	Women with BMI $\geq$29 kg/m^2 with singleton pregnancy and without ODIP	<20 weeks	HbA1c and 2 h 75 g OGTT/ IADPSG criteria	HbA1c $\geq$5.7% vs. <5.7% group (prediabetes threshold)	Limited use of early pregnancy HbA1c for predicting GDM or adverse outcomes in overweight/obese European women
Jokelainen, 2020/Finland [33]	Population-based cohort study	1401	All singleton pregnancies without ODIP	12–16 weeks	2 h 75 g OGTT/FCCG	Early- vs. late-GDM vs. no GDM	Of the women who had early GDM based on the IADPSG/ WHO criteria, 39.1% received the diagnosis of late GDM at the second OGTT
Liu, 2020/ China [34]	Prospective cohort study	522	Singleton pregnancies	18–20 weeks	2 h 75 g OGTT/ IADPSG-2015 guidelines	4 groups: NGT (no GDM diagnosis), EGDM (GDM diagnosis in only early OGTT), LGDM (GDM diagnosis in only standard OGTT) and GDM (GDM diagnosis in both OGTTs)	Early GDM diagnosis at 18–20 weeks is associated with adverse outcomes
Nakanishi, 2020/Japan [35]	Multicenter prospective cohort study	146	Hi risk without ODIP	<20 weeks	2 h 75 g OGTT/IADPSG criteria 2010	False-positive early GDM (early+/late-) vs. true GDM (early+/late+) (late = standard)	Of the 146 women diagnosed with early-onset GDM, 69 (47%) had normal 75 g OGTT values at 24–28 weeks of gestation.
Sesmilo, 2020/Spain [36]	Retrospective cohort study	6845	Singleton pregnancies in women without ODIP and available data	<13 weeks	FPG/NDDG criteria	FPG: $\leq$4.3, 4.4–4.6, 4.7–4.8 and $\geq$4.9 mmol/L	FTFPG is an early marker of GDM and LGA.

GDM: gestational diabetes mellitus; OGTT: oral glucose tolerance test; hi risk: high risk; GCT: glucose challenge test; NDDG: National Diabetes Data Group; ODIP: overt diabetes in pregnancy; FTFPG: first trimester fasting plasma glucose; HAPO: Hyperglycemia and Adverse Pregnancy Outcomes; C&C: Carpenter and Coustan; IADPSG: International Association of the Diabetes and Pregnancy Study Groups; FPG: fasting plasma glucose; HbA1c: hemoglobin A1C; ACOG: American Congress of Obstetricians and Gynecologists; ADA: American Diabetes Association; BMI: body mass index; WHO: World Health Organization; NGT: normal glucose tolerance; DIP: diabetes in pregnancy; ADIPS: Australian diabetes in pregnancy society; LGA: large-for-gestational age; C-section: cesarian section; SIGN: Scottish Intercollegiate Guidelines Network; NICU: neonatal intensive care unit; T2DM: type 2 diabetes mellitus; FCCG: Finnish Current Care Guideline; EGDM: early-onset gestational diabetes; LGDM: late-onset gestational diabetes; DALI: Diabetes and Pregnancy Vitamin D And Lifestyle Intervention for Gestational Diabetes Mellitus Prevention.

Table 2. Randomized controlled trials.

Author, Year/Country (Ref.)	Subjects (N)	Study Population	Timeframe Testing (Weeks)	GDM Criteria	Comparison	Main Results
Osmundson, 2016/US [37]	83	Women with singleton pregnancy and without ODIP	<14.0 weeks	HbA1c/between 5.7 and 6.4%	Usual care vs. early treatment for GDM with diet, BG monitoring, and insulin as needed	Early treatment did not significantly reduce the risk of GDM except in non-obese women
Hughes, 2018 (PINTO feasibility study)/New Zealand [38]	47	Women with singleton pregnancy and without ODIP	<14.0 weeks	HbA1c/between $\geq$5.9 and 6.4%/2 h 75 h OGTT New Zealand criteria	Standard care vs. early intervention in pregnancies complicated by prediabetes	First results expected in 2021
Simmons, 2018 (ToBOGM pilot study)/ Australia [39]	79	Hi risk women with singleton pregnancy	<20.0 weeks (4–19.6 weeks)	2 h 75 g OGTT/ IADPSG criteria	Women with booking GDM receiving immediate (clinical referral or ongoing treatment) vs. deferred (no) treatment vs. women without booking GDM ("decoys")	More NICU admission in the early GDM group with a tendency for more SGA but less LGA

Table 2. Cont.

Author, Year/Country (Ref.)	Subjects (N)	Study Population	Timeframe Testing (Weeks)	GDM Criteria	Comparison	Main Results
Simmons, 2018 (ToBOGM study protocol)/ International [40]	4000	Hi risk women with singleton pregnancy	<20.0 weeks (4–19.6 weeks)	2 h 75 g OGTT/2014 Australasian Diabetes-in-Pregnancy Society criteria for pregnant women with GA 24–28 weeks	Intervention (immediate treatment) vs. control (no treatment) vs. decoys (NGT but undergo all procedures) vs. non-active (NGT and records reviewed postnatally)	First results expected mid-2021
Vinter, 2018 (LiP study)/ Denmark [41]	90	Obese pregnant women (BMI 30–45 kg/m^2) with singleton pregnancy	12–15 weeks	2 h 75 g OGTT/ IADPSG Criteria	Lifestyle intervention vs. SoC	Lifestyle intervention was not effective in improving obstetric or metabolic outcomes
Roeder, 2019 (RCT)/ US [42]	157	Women with hyperglycemia and singleton pregnancy without ODIP	≤15.0 weeks	HbA1c and/or FPG, respectively, 5.7–6.4% and/or 5.1–6.9 mmol/L	Early pregnancy vs. 3rd trimester treatment of hyperglycemia	Treatment in early pregnancy did not improve maternal or neonatal outcomes significantly
Harper, 2020 (EGGO study)/ US [43]	922	Obese women (BMI ≥30 kg/m^2) without ODIP and history of bariatric surgery	14–20 weeks	2-step method: 1 h 50 g GCT followed by a 3 h 100 g OGTT/C&C criteria	Early GDM screening (14–20 weeks) vs. routine screening (24–28 weeks)	Early GDM screening in obese women did not reduce the composite perinatal outcomes, such as macrosomia, C-section and shoulder dystocia
Hung-Yuan Li (TESGO study)/ Taiwan (NCT03523143)	2068	Singleton pregnancy without ODIP	18–20 weeks	75 g 2 h OGTT/ IADPSG criteria	Early screening group (18–20 weeks) vs. standard screening group (24–28 weeks)	Results expected beginning of 2021

ODIP: overt diabetes in pregnancy; HbA1c: hemoglobin A1c; GDM: gestational diabetes mellitus; BG: blood glucose; PINTO: Pre diabetes in pregnancy, can early intervention improve outcomes; OGTT: oral glucose tolerance test; Hi risk: high risk; ToBOGM: Treatment of Booking Gestational diabetes Mellitus; IADPSG: International Association of the Diabetes and Pregnancy Study Groups; NICU: neonatal intensive care unit; SGA: small-for-gestational age; LGA: large-for-gestational age; GA: gestational age; NGT: normal glucose tolerance; LIP: Lifestyle in Pregnancy; BMI: body mass index; SoC: standard of care; FPG: fasting plasma glucose; GCT: glucose challenge test; C&C: Carpenter and Coustan; C-section: cesarean section; EGGO: Early Gestational Diabetes Screening in the Gravid Obese Woman; TESGO: The Effect of Early Screening and Intervention for Gestational Diabetes Mellitus on Pregnancy Outcomes.

3.3. Screening for Overt Diabetes in Early Pregnancy

The prevalence of type 2 diabetes (T2DM) in women of childbearing age is increasing. Since T2DM is often asymptomatic at the beginning and women with severe hyperglycemia early in pregnancy are at high risk for adverse pregnancy outcomes, timely detection and treatment of diabetes is needed. Most international associations such as the IADPSG, the ADA and the World Health Organization (WHO) recommend therefore to screen for overt diabetes at the first antenatal visit using an FPG, HbA1c or 75 g oral glucose tolerance test (OGTT) with the same cut-offs as for non-pregnant populations. The measurements of FPG and HbA1c should ideally be repeated twice to confirm the diagnosis of overt diabetes. HbA1c can be used to screen for diabetes but not to screen for GDM due to the very low sensitivity [44]. Measurement of fasting glycemia has a higher sensitivity than HbA1c to screen for diabetes. On the other hand, HbA1c has the advantage that it can be performed in the non-fasting state. An observational study from New Zealand [45] showed that an HbA1c ≥5.9% identified all women with diabetes who completed an OGTT before 20 weeks of pregnancy and this also identified a group at significantly increased risk for adverse pregnancy outcomes, such as preeclampsia and shoulder dystocia. In addition, the study demonstrated that an HbA1c ≥6.5% would have missed almost half of these women. These data suggest therefore that the currently recommended HbA1c is too high for screening purposes in pregnancy. However, large RCTs are required to confirm these results.

3.4. Screening for GDM in Early Pregnancy

As shown in Table 1, numerous observational studies were performed over the years. These studies show conflicting results. In general, most studies show that women with early GDM are at high risk for adverse pregnancy outcomes but treatment of GDM early in pregnancy compared to later in pregnancy does not always translate into improved outcomes. Seven studies reported an improved pregnancy outcome by treatment of early-onset GDM [7,9,10,29–31,34]. Barahona et al. [9] showed that diagnosing GDM early in pregnancy is a predictor of adverse maternal and neonatal outcomes, such as pregnancy-induced hypertension, insulin treatment during pregnancy, preterm birth, hyperbilirubinemia and perinatal mortality. More recently, Cosson et al. [31] reported that women who received initial care vs. those who did not, were more likely to be insulin-treated during pregnancy (58.0% vs. 20.9%, respectively; $p < 0.00001$), gained less gestational weight (8.6 ± 5.4 kg vs. 10.8 ± 6.1 kg, respectively; $p < 0.00001$), had a lower rate of preeclampsia (1.2% vs. 2.6%, respectively; adjusted odds ratio (aOR): 0.247 (0.082–0.759), $p = 0.01$), and similar rates of LGA infants and shoulder dystocia. A very recent study from Thailand showed that early GDM women had a high risk for adverse pregnancy outcomes with higher rates of preeclampsia, LGA infants, and NICU admission [29].

However, five studies described no beneficial effect of early diagnosing or treatment of GDM on maternal or neonatal outcomes [15,20,22,25,30]. Both Alluni et al. [15] and Bianchi et al. [25] showed that patients diagnosed and treated for early-onset GDM were more prone to be insulin-treated during pregnancy but showed no differences in neonatal outcomes such as small-for-gestational age (SGA) infants, cesarean sections, macrosomia, and LGA. An Australian study demonstrated also that early diagnosis and intervention had no effect on pregnancy outcomes [21]. This was confirmed by a recent Australian study showing no differences in pregnancy outcomes between early-onset GDM and late-onset GDM [30].

RCTs are needed to determine whether treating early-onset GDM improves pregnancy outcomes compared to standard treatment of GDM at 24–28 weeks of pregnancy. Table 2 gives an overview of the (ongoing) RCTs. The largest RCTs such as the "Prediabetes in pregnancy, can early intervention improve outcomes" PINTO study, the "Treatment of Booking Gestational diabetes Mellitus" (ToBOGM) study and the "Effect of Early Screening and Intervention for Gestational Diabetes Mellitus on Pregnancy Outcomes" (TESGO) study are still ongoing. Results are expected at the earliest in 2021. The ToBOGM study, the "Early Gestational Diabetes Screening in the Gravid Obese Woman" (EGGO) study and "Lifestyle in Pregnancy" (LiP) study focused on high-risk populations and obese women. In contrast, the TESGO and PINTO studies included also lower risk women.

A small RCT showed that early treatment of mild hyperglycemia (women with an HbA1c of 5.7–6.4%) did not reduce the risk of GDM, except for non-obese women [37]. The pilot study of ToBOGM [39] demonstrated that early treatment may have both benefits and harms for mother and offspring. NICU admission was highest in the treated early GDM group (36% vs. 0% $p = 0.043$), driven by a higher rate of SGA infants. Women who received no treatment for early-onset GDM had more LGA infants (0% vs. 33% $p = 0.030$). The LiP study [41] focused on the effect of lifestyle intervention vs. standard care for obese women with early GDM. They found that lifestyle intervention in early pregnancy did not improve obstetric or metabolic outcomes. In addition, the EGGO study [43] showed no effect on the composite perinatal outcomes in obese women who had early screening for GDM. Similarly, Roeder et al. [42] did not find any improvement in maternal and neonatal outcomes after treatment in early pregnancy.

3.5. Criteria to Define GDM in Early Pregnancy

Of all observational studies (Table 1), 15 studies discussed the diagnostic criteria for GDM early in pregnancy [11–14,16,18,21,24,26–28,31,32,35,36]. Riskin et al. showed that first trimester fasting glucose levels (FTFPG) in the non-diabetic range resulted in a higher risk for adverse pregnancy outcomes, such as more cesarian sections, LGA and macrosomia. These findings were confirmed by a recent Belgium study [28] demonstrating more NICU admissions in the high FTFPG group (FPG $\geq$ 5.1–5.5 mmol/L). A large Chinese study showed that an FTFPG of 6.1–7.0 mmol/L in early pregnancy is a strong predictor for GDM later in pregnancy [14]. In contrast, an FTFPG $\geq$ 5.1 mmol/L (GDM according to IADPSG criteria) was not a good predictor for GDM in their population. Several other studies (including studies in European populations) confirmed that ≥ 5.1 mmol/L is a poor predictor for GDM early in pregnancy [26,28]. A Belgium study [28] for instance demonstrated that only 37% of all women with an FTFPG ≥ 5.1–5.5 mmol/L, developed GDM based on the OGTT later in pregnancy. A French study proposed to use an FTFPG ≥ 5.5 mmol/L to start treatment for GDM in early pregnancy, as they demonstrated improved pregnancy outcomes in their population [31].

Few studies evaluated HbA1c in early pregnancy to diagnose GDM. These studies showed that an HbA1c ≥ 5.9% identifies women at high risk for adverse pregnancy outcomes independently of GDM diagnosis later in pregnancy [21,27].

A small RCT showed that early treatment of women with a first trimester HbA1c of 5.7–6.4% did not significantly reduce the risk of GDM, except in non-obese women [37]. Roeder et al. [42] used HbA1c ≥ 5.7% and/or an FTFPG ≥ 5.1 mmol/L to identify women with hyperglycemia early in pregnancy. Treatment in early pregnancy did not improve maternal or neonatal outcomes. Only 19% of this cohort developed GDM later in pregnancy [42]. In contrast, the ToBOGM pilot trial reported that 89% of untreated women (with an FPG ≥ 5.1 mmol/L early in pregnancy) had GDM at 24–28 weeks [39].

3.6. Screening for Diabetes and GDM in Early Pregnancy in COVID Times

Due to the COVID-19 pandemic, screening for GDM using OGTT's might lead to an increased risk for exposure to the virus. Six large observational studies describe how screening for GDM could be organized in a pragmatic way using blood tests, and risk calculators applied to underlying risk factors (Table 3).

Table 3. Screening for diabetes and GDM (early) in pregnancy in COVID times.

Article	Pragmatic Approach	Main Results
Thangaratinam, 2020 [49]	Test strategy: - Early GDM screening: additional tests at booking (HbA1c and RPG) to detect overt diabetes and identify those at highest risk for GDM Suggested thresholds and actions: - HbA1c ≥ 6.5% or RPG ≥ 11.1mmol/L: treat as preexisting diabetes. - HbA1c 5.9–6.5% or RPG 9–11 mmol/L: consider managing using the GDM pathway. - Avoid OGTT at 24–28 weeks and instead offer HbA1c along with FPG or RPG if fasting values are not availableSuggested thresholds and actions: Suggested thresholds and actions: HbA1c ≥ 5.7% or FPG ≥ 5.6 mmol/L or RPG ≥ 9 mmol/L: treat as GDM.	Using FPG alone will only pick up about half of all women with GDM, based on NICE or IADPSG criteria. Combining FPG with HbA1c may improve the detection rate. Maintaining existing FPG thresholds may be preferable, and services may consider lower thresholds consistent with the IADPSG diagnostic criteria (FPG ≥ 5.1), if resources allow.
Torlone, 2020 [50]	Screening for overt diabetes: - FPG ≥ 6.9 mmol/L - RPG ≥ 11.1 mmol/L - HbA1c ≥ 6.5% A single value can be considered valid during COVID-19 emergency Screening for GDM: risk factors assessment - Women at high risk for GDM: FPG ≥ 5.1 mmol/L at 16–18 weeks → GDM - Women at high risk for GDM: FPG ≤ 5.1 mmol/L at 16–18 weeks → FPG at 24–28 weeks ≥ 5.1 mmol/L → GDM - Women at medium risk for GDM: FPG ≥ 5.1 mmol/L at 24–28 weeks → GDM	A fasting glucose value can be considered diagnostic for GDM only when it is obtained at the gestational age when the OGTT should have been carried out, i.e., between 16 and 18 weeks in high-risk pregnant women or between 24 and 28 weeks in medium-risk women.

Table 3. *Cont.*

Article	Pragmatic Approach	Main Results
McIntyre, 2020 (Diagnosis and management GDM during COVID-19) [47]	Early in pregnancy: all guidelines: HbA1c $\geq$ 5.9% Standard screening (24–28 weeks): *UK:* at risk; GDM if HbA1c $\geq$ 5.7% and/or FVPG $\geq$ 5.6 mmol/L and/or Random VPG (not preferred) $\geq$ 9.0 mmol/L *CAN:* GDM if HbA1c $\geq$ 5.7% and/or Random VPG $\geq$ 11.1 mmol/L *AUS:* fasting VPG: Fasting VPG < 4.7 mmol/L = normal Fasting VPG 4.7–5.0 mmol/L = OGTT, WHO 2013 criteria Fasting VPG $\geq$ 5.1 mmol/L = GDM	Detecting only those with marked hyperglycemia
McIntyre, 2020 (Testing for GDM during COVID-19) [46]	*UK:* Risk factor based; no OGTT; GDM if HbA1c $\geq$ 5.7% and/or FVPG $\geq$ 5.6 mmol/L and/or Random VPG (not preferred) $\geq$ 9.0 mmol/L *CAN:* universal testing; no OGTT; GDM if HbA1c $\geq$ 5.7% and/or Random VPG $\geq$ 11.1 mmol/L *AUS:* fasting VPG: Fasting VPG < 4.7 mmol/L = normal Fasting VPG 4.7–5.0 mmol/L = OGTT, WHO 2013 criteria Fasting VPG $\geq$ 5.1 mmol/L = GDM	All post COVID-19 modified pathways reduced GDM frequency. Missed GDM's in Canadian women gave similar rates of pregnancy outcomes. Using UK modifications, missed GDM group was at slightly lower risk. Using the Australian modifications, missed GDM group was at substantially lower risk.
Meek, 2020 [48]	To evaluate the diagnostic and prognostic performance of alternative diagnostic strategies to 2 h 75 g OGTTs: HbA1c, RPG and FPG GDM diagnosis: criteria of the UK National Institute for Health and Care Excellence and IADPSG criteria	RPG at 12 weeks, and FPG or HbA1c at 28 weeks identify women with hyperglycemia at risk of suboptimal pregnancy outcomes.
Seshiah, 2020 [51]	The "single test procedure" for diagnosing GDM: 2 h PG $\geq$ 7.8 mmol/L with 75 g oral glucose administered to a pregnant woman in the fasting or non-fasting state, without regard to the time of the last meal (glucose load can also be taken at home and the pregnant woman can visit the hospital 2 h after the glucose ingestion to give a single sample for plasma glucose estimation)	The economical and evidence based "single test procedure" of DIPSI is most appropriate for screening during the COVID pandemic as performing OGTTs is resource intensive, the fasting state is impractical with very high dropout rate.

GDM: gestational diabetes mellitus; HbA1c: hemoglobin A1c; RPG: random plasma glucose; OGTT: oral glucose tolerance test; FPG: fasting plasma glucose; NICE: National Institute for Health and Care Excellence; IADPSG: International Association of the Diabetes and Pregnancy Study Groups; VPG: venous plasma glucose; UK: United Kingdom; CAN: Canada; AUS: Australia; WHO: World Health Organization; PG: plasma glucose; DIPSI: Diabetes in Pregnancy Study Group India.

McIntyre et al. [46,47] described the diagnosis and management of GDM during COVID-19 in Australia, Canada and the United Kingdom (UK). For early screening, the guidelines were similar in the different countries, with an HbA1c $\geq$ 5.9% considered as hyperglycemia. For diagnosing GDM at 24–28 weeks, each country had a slightly different approach. The UK invited only women at high risk. GDM was diagnosed if HbA1c $\geq$ 5.7% and/or fasting venous plasma glucose (FVPG) $\geq$ 5.6 mmol/L and/or random venous plasma glucose (VPG) (not preferred) $\geq$ 9.0 mmol/L. Canada recommended universal screening. GDM was diagnosed if HbA1c $\geq$ 5.7% and/or random VPG $\geq$ 11.1 mmol/L. Australia used universal testing with an initial FVPG. If FVPG was between 4.7 and 5.0 mmol/L, an OGTT was performed. If FVPG $\geq$ 5.1 mmol/L, then GDM was diagnosed immediately.

Meek et al. [48] reported that random plasma glucose (RPG) at 12 weeks, and FPG or HbA1c at 28 weeks identifies women with hyperglycemia at risk of suboptimal pregnancy outcomes. When an OGTT is not possible, as an alternative RPG, FPG and HbA1c are recommended. Thangaratinam et al. [49] suggested additional tests at booking to detect overt diabetes and identify those at highest risk for GDM. HbA1c $\geq$ 6.5% or RPG $\geq$ 11.1 mmol/L is considered as pre-existing diabetes. As the recommended antenatal routine booking blood tests are often not performed in the fasting state, a pragmatic approach was suggested with the use of RPG. GDM can be diagnosed by HbA1c 5.9–6.4% or RPG 9–11 mmol/L to diagnose diabetes. The following thresholds for diagnosing GDM were suggested: HbA1c $\geq$ 5.7%, FPG $\geq$ 5.6 mmol/L or RPG $\geq$ 9 mmol/L.

To conclude, Italian recommendations [50] propose that if an OGTT cannot be safely performed, screening for GDM should be based on risk factors and the FPG value. Women with high risk factors should be tested at 16–18 weeks and an FPG $\geq$5.1 mmol/L is diagnosed as GDM. Women with high risk factors and an FPG $\leq$5.1 mmol/L or women with medium risk factors should be tested at 24–28 weeks. If FPG $\geq$5.1 mmol/L at 24–28 weeks, the woman will be diagnosed with GDM.

4. Discussion

4.1. Summary of Findings

In this narrative review, we demonstrate that there is need for clear guidelines and criteria concerning overt diabetes and early screening for GDM. The HbA1c threshold of diabetes as currently recommended is probably too high to detect all women with overt diabetes in early pregnancy. Furthermore, observational studies show conflicting results on the effects of screening and treatment of GDM in early pregnancy. It is also not clear which diagnostic criteria should be used to define GDM in early pregnancy. Evidence from large RCTs is needed to evaluate whether treatment has a beneficial effect on maternal and neonatal outcomes, without increased risk for harm (such as increased risk for SGA infants). Large RCTs such as the TOBOGM study will also help to inform which diagnostic criteria are appropriate to use for GDM in early pregnancy.

The COVID-19 pandemic has brought us additional challenges. OGTT's could often not be performed as they involve high exposure risks and health service burden. Different guidelines have proposed pragmatic approached to screening with HbA1c, FPG or even RPG as an alternative during the pandemic.

4.2. Results in Relation to What We Already Know

Screening for overt diabetes in early pregnancy is necessary. At the moment, the threshold for diagnosing overt diabetes is an HbA1c $\geq$6.5%. However, there is limited data suggesting that in pregnancy the cut-off of HbA1c should be lowered to $\geq$5.9% to identify all women with diabetes as this identifies a population at high risk for adverse pregnancy outcomes. A threshold of $\geq$6.5% would have missed half of these women [45].

Screening and treatment of GDM between 24 and 28 weeks of pregnancy is widely accepted. This is beneficial to reduce adverse pregnancy outcomes. More women are identified with mild hyperglycemia in early pregnancy due to increased screening for overt diabetes. Observational studies show conflicting results as to whether screening and treatment of GDM in early pregnancy is beneficial compared to screening later in pregnancy. Some studies have shown that despite treatment, early-onset GDM women have more adverse pregnancy complications than late-onset GDM women, while other studies demonstrated similar short-term obstetrical outcomes in both groups and improved outcomes in the early screening group. At this moment, we can only speculate whether the fact that early treatment of GDM often only leads to similar pregnancy outcomes might represent success rather than failure. We cannot exclude that treatment of this group later in pregnancy might lead to more adverse pregnancy outcomes. In addition, studies had substantial heterogeneity in maternal age in pregnancy and BMI. In developed countries, increasing maternal age in pregnancy disposes to higher insulin resistance, whereas most pregnant women are younger in developing countries. Data are needed from well-designed RCTs. In the meantime, treatment of mild hyperglycemia in early pregnancy remains controversial due to lack of evidence from large RCTs supporting any benefit of treatment of GDM before 24 weeks of pregnancy. Moreover, a diagnosis of GDM could also be associated with increased medicalization of pregnancy (with more inductions and cesarean sections) and an increased risk for SGA infants due to overtreatment. Furthermore, it remains unclear which diagnostic criteria should be used to define GDM in early pregnancy, and whether universal or selective screening should be used to detect GDM before 24 weeks. Many studies evaluated high risk populations and there was also a high heterogeneity in the risk factors used across the different studies to screen for GDM in early pregnancy.

Several studies have shown that FPG in early pregnancy is a poor predictor for GDM later in pregnancy. The IADPSG criteria might therefore not be appropriate to use in early pregnancy.

4.3. Practical Implications

As for maternal and neonatal outcomes, smaller RCTs did not show benefits of early screening and treatment of GDM. The EGGO and LIP studies were performed in obese populations and showed no improvement in pregnancy outcomes in the group who received treatment early in pregnancy compared to treatment later in pregnancy. These data suggest that future studies should focus on interventions starting pre-pregnancy in obese women. The pilot study of the TOBOGM study showed both benefits and harms of early treatment of GDM in a high-risk population. The treated group had a lower LGA rate but more NICU admissions, mainly due to a higher SGA rate. SGA can be a consequence of overtreatment [52], or insufficient gestational weight gain [53]. This highlights the need for data from large RCTs. The results of several large ongoing RCTs are expected for mid-2021 at the earliest. Many studies were conducted in a high-risk population. It is therefore also important to have evidence on the potential benefit or harm of screening for early GDM in low-risk populations and when using a universal screening strategy.

As we are waiting for stronger evidence from RCT's, we do currently not recommend screening and treatment of GDM before 24–28 weeks of gestation in our center [54]. In line with the Flemish consensus of 2019 on screening for GDM [54], we recommend to universally screen for overt diabetes in early pregnancy. In addition, we propose a pragmatic approach for women who are diagnosed with mild hyperglycemia (FPG 5.5–6.9 mmol/L) in early pregnancy. We do not label these women as early GDM but advise follow-up with a dietician early in pregnancy (since these women are often overweight) and provide screening for GDM with an OGTT at 24 weeks of pregnancy [54].

The first results of the RCTs also show that treatment of women with HbA1c $\geq$ 5.7% and/or an FTFPG $\geq$ 5.1 mmol/L in early pregnancy, does not improve pregnancy outcomes [42]. HbA1c alone was not a good predictor for GDM early in pregnancy, because of the low sensitivity. It should always be used with other standard diagnostic tests for GDM, as was also demonstrated by the systematic review of Renz et al. [44]. FPG level generally further decreases by the end of the first trimester. Using FPG early in pregnancy, can lead to false positive results. Several studies have shown that an FPG level is a poor predictor for GDM with a sensitivity and specificity of 33–66% to predict GDM later in pregnancy. In contrast, the ToBOGM pilot study reported that 89% of the untreated women with early GDM in their study developed GDM at 24–28 weeks of gestation [39]. However, an OGTT was used in early pregnancy to screen for GDM (not only FTFPG) and this study evaluated a high-risk population.

Studies did not always report the pre-analytical method of collecting blood for FPG. Correct pre-analytic sampling of plasma glucose is important to prevent glycolysis and to prevent false negative results. A recent study of O'Malley showed that fluoride tubes must be stored on ice or must be centrifuged within 30 min to prevent glycolysis [55].

Since 2020, we have been faced with the impact of the COVID-19 pandemic on health care delivery. This might also impact screening for GDM and diabetes in pregnancy. There is a need to balance the sometimes-competing requirement of lowering the risk of direct viral transmission against the potential adverse impact of service changes. A pragmatic approach to screening for GDM is advised if an OGTT is not feasible. As an alternative, FPG, RPG and HbA1c, can be used. Women with a high-risk profile or with a history of GDM need to be closely monitored. It is important that usual guidelines and care will be re-evaluated as soon as possible [46–49,51].

4.4. Strengths and Limitations

A strength of this overview is that we performed an extensive narrative review including 45 studies evaluating the evidence on screening for GDM from both observational studies and RCTs. We provided an updated and detailed overview of the different observational and (ongoing) RCT's, including data on timing of screening, the diagnostic criteria used for GDM, the screening strategy and comparator used. In addition, we highlighted the heterogeneity in risk factors used for selective screening in early pregnancy. However, our review also has several limitations. We did not perform a systematic review and could therefore not perform a meta-analysis. We could therefore also not assess the risk of bias of individual studies and did not contact the authors for obtaining missing and unpublished data. In addition, we did not assess the pre-analytical method of collecting blood for FPG determination.

5. Conclusions

Observational studies show conflicting results as to whether screening and treatment of GDM in early pregnancy is beneficial. However, most studies show that women with early GDM are at high risk of adverse pregnancy outcomes. A slight majority of relevant observational studies report an improved pregnancy outcome by treatment of early-onset GDM. However, so far, RCTs have not provided conclusive evidence of the beneficial effects of early treatment. Evidence from large RCTs is urgently needed, also evaluating lower risk populations to determine appropriate early-pregnancy OGTT thresholds for the diagnosis of GDM, and to assess the impact of early treatment on obstetrical outcomes and long-term offspring health. RCTs are also necessary to determine the appropriate cut-off of HbA1c in early pregnancy to identify women at risk for adverse pregnancy outcomes. Therefore, we currently recommend a pragmatic approach for women diagnosed with mild hyperglycemia in early pregnancy. A pragmatic approach to screen for GDM can be implemented during the COVID-19 pandemic, using FPG, RPG or HbA1c. However, routine guidelines and care must be re-evaluated as soon as possible.

Author Contributions: L.R., K.B. (Kaat Beunen) and K.B. (Katrien Benhalima) wrote the manuscript. All authors have read and agreed to the published version of the manuscript.

Funding: Katrien Benhalima is the recipient of a "Fundamenteel Klinisch Navorserschap FWO Vlaanderen".

Data Availability Statement: No new data were created or analyzed in this study. Data sharing is not applicable to this article.

Conflicts of Interest: The authors declare no conflict of interest.

Appendix A

Table 1. This table gives an overview of the gestational diabetes mellitus diagnosis criteria used in this review.

Criteria	OGTT	FPG	1 h	2 h	3 h	Number of Abnormal Values
C&C	100 g	≥5.3 mmol/L	≥10 mmol/L	≥8.6 mmol/L	≥7.8 mmol/L	≥2
NDDG	100 g	≥5.8 mmol/L	≥10.5 mmol/L	≥9 mmol/L	≥8 mmol/L	≥2
IADPSG, WHO 2013	75 g	≥5.1 mmol/L	≥10 mmol/L	≥8.5 mmol/L		≥1
ADA	100 g	≥5.3 mmol/L	≥10 mmol/L	≥8.6 mmol/L	7.8 mmol/L	≥2
WHO 1999	75 g	≥6 mmol/L		≥7.8 mmol/L		≥1
Finnish Diabetes Association	75 g	>5.3 mmol/L	>10 mmol/L	>8.6 mmol/L		≥1
New-Zealand criteria	75 g	≥5.5 mmol/L		≥9 mmol/L		≥1
O'Sullivan criteria	100 g	≥5 mmol/L	≥9 mmol/L	≥7.8 mmol/L	≥6.9 mmol/L	≥2
Chinese GDM criteria	75 g	≥5.1 mmol/L	≥10 mmol/L	≥8.5 mmol/L		≥1
ADIPS	75 g	≥5.1 mmol/L	≥10 mmol/L	≥8.5 mmol/L		≥1

Table 1. Cont.

Criteria	OGTT	FPG	1 h	2 h	3 h	Number of Abnormal Values
Scottish Intercollegiate Guidelines Network	75 g	≥5.1 mmol/L	≥10 mmol/L	≥8.5 mmol/L		≥1
DIPSI	75 g			≥7.8 mmol/L		≥1

OGTT: oral glucose tolerance test; FPG: fasting plasma glucose; C&C: Carpenter and Coustan; NDDG: National Diabetes Data Group; IADPSG: International Association of the Diabetes and Pregnancy Study Groups; WHO: World Health Organization; ADA: American Diabetes Association; ADIPS: Australian Diabetes in Pregnancy society; DIPSI: Diabetes in Pregnancy Study Group India.

References

1. Standards of medical care in diabetes–2013. *Diabetes Care* **2013**, *36* (Suppl. 1), S11–S66. [CrossRef] [PubMed]
2. Crowther, C.A.; Hiller, J.E.; Moss, J.R.; McPhee, A.J.; Jeffries, W.S.; Robinson, J.S. Effect of treatment of gestational diabetes mellitus on pregnancy outcomes. *N. Engl. J. Med.* **2005**, *352*, 2477–2486. [CrossRef] [PubMed]
3. Landon, M.B.; Spong, C.Y.; Thom, E.; Carpenter, M.W.; Ramin, S.M.; Casey, B.; Wapner, R.J.; Varner, M.W.; Rouse, D.J.; Thorp, J.M., Jr.; et al. A multicenter, randomized trial of treatment for mild gestational diabetes. *N. Engl. J. Med.* **2009**, *361*, 1339–1348. [CrossRef] [PubMed]
4. American Diabetes Association. 14. Management of Diabetes in Pregnancy: Standards of Medical Care in Diabetes–2020. *Diabetes Care* **2020**, *43*, S183–S192. [CrossRef] [PubMed]
5. Hod, M.; Kapur, A.; Sacks, D.A.; Hadar, E.; Agarwal, M.; Di Renzo, G.C.; Roura, L.C.; McIntyre, H.D.; Morris, J.L.; Divakar, H. The International Federation of Gynecology and Obstetrics (FIGO) Initiative on gestational diabetes mellitus: A pragmatic guide for diagnosis, management, and care#. *Int. J. Gynecol. Obstet.* **2015**, *131*, S173–S211.
6. Webber, J.; Charlton, M.; Johns, N. Diabetes in pregnancy: Management of diabetes and its complications from preconception to the postnatal period (NG3). *Br. J. Diabetes* **2015**, *15*, 107–111. [CrossRef]
7. De Muylder, X. Perinatal complications of gestational diabetes: The influence of the timing of the diagnosis. *Eur. J. Obstet. Gynecol. Reprod. Biol.* **1984**, *18*, 35–42. [CrossRef]
8. Bartha, J.L.; Martinez-Del-Fresno, P.; Comino-Delgado, R. Gestational diabetes mellitus diagnosed during early pregnancy. *Am. J. Obstet. Gynecol.* **2000**, *182*, 346–350. [CrossRef]
9. Barahona, M.J.; Sucunza, N.; García-Patterson, A.; Hernández, M.; Adelantado, J.M.; Ginovart, G.; De Leiva, A.; Corcoy, R. Period of gestational diabetes mellitus diagnosis and maternal and fetal morbidity. *Acta Obstet. Gynecol. Scand.* **2005**, *84*, 622–627. [CrossRef]
10. Hawkins, J.S.; Lo, J.Y.; Casey, B.M.; McIntire, D.D.; Leveno, K.J. Diet-treated gestational diabetes mellitus: Comparison of early vs routine diagnosis. *Am. J. Obstet. Gynecol.* **2008**, *198*, 287.e1–287.e6. [CrossRef]
11. Riskin-Mashiah, S.; Younes, G.; Damti, A.; Auslender, R. First-trimester fasting hyperglycemia and adverse pregnancy outcomes. *Diabetes Care* **2009**, *32*, 1639–1643. [CrossRef] [PubMed]
12. Plasencia, W.; Garcia, R.; Pereira, S.; Akolekar, R.; Nicolaides, K.H. Criteria for screening and diagnosis of gestational diabetes mellitus in the first trimester of pregnancy. *Fetal Diagn. Ther.* **2011**, *30*, 108–115. [CrossRef] [PubMed]
13. Corrado, F.; D'Anna, R.; Cannata, M.L.; Interdonato, M.L.; Pintaudi, B.; Di Benedetto, A. Correspondence between first-trimester fasting glycaemia, and oral glucose tolerance test in gestational diabetes diagnosis. *Diabetes Metab.* **2012**, *38*, 458–461. [CrossRef] [PubMed]
14. Zhu, W.W.; Yang, H.X.; Wei, Y.M.; Yan, J.; Wang, Z.L.; Li, X.L.; Wu, H.R.; Li, N.; Zhang, M.H.; Liu, X.H.; et al. Evaluation of the value of fasting plasma glucose in the first prenatal visit to diagnose gestational diabetes mellitus in china. *Diabetes Care* **2013**, *36*, 586–590. [CrossRef] [PubMed]
15. Alunni, M.L.; Roeder, H.A.; Moore, T.R.; Ramos, G.A. First trimester gestational diabetes screening—Change in incidence and pharmacotherapy need. *Diabetes Res. Clin. Pract.* **2015**, *109*, 135–140. [CrossRef] [PubMed]
16. Amylidi, S.; Mosimann, B.; Stettler, C.; Fiedler, G.M.; Surbek, D.; Raio, L. First-trimester glycosylated hemoglobin in women at high risk for gestational diabetes. *Acta Obstet. Gynecol. Scand.* **2016**, *95*, 93–97. [CrossRef]
17. Harreiter, J.; Simmons, D.; Desoye, G.; Corcoy, R.; Adelantado, J.M.; Devlieger, R.; van Assche, A.; Galjaard, S.; Damm, P.; Mathiesen, E.R.; et al. IADPSG and WHO 2013 Gestational Diabetes Mellitus Criteria Identify Obese Women With Marked Insulin Resistance in Early Pregnancy: Table 1. *Diabetes Care* **2016**, *39*, e90–e92. [CrossRef]
18. Mañé, L.; Flores-Le Roux, J.A.; Benaiges, D.; Rodríguez, M.; Marcelo, I.; Chillarón, J.J.; Pedro-Botet, J.; Llauradó, G.; Gortazar, L.; Carreras, R.; et al. Role of first trimester HbA1c as a predictor of adverse obstetric outcomes in a multi-ethnic cohort. *J. Clin. Endocrinol. Metab.* **2016**. [CrossRef] [PubMed]
19. Osmundson, S.S.; Zhao, B.S.; Kunz, L.; Wang, E.; Popat, R.; Nimbal, V.C.; Palaniappan, L.P. First Trimester Hemoglobin A1c Prediction of Gestational Diabetes. *Amer. J. Perinatol.* **2016**, *33*, 977–982. [CrossRef]
20. Sweeting, A.N.; Ross, G.P.; Hyett, J.; Molyneaux, L.; Constantino, M.; Harding, A.J.; Wong, J. Gestational Diabetes Mellitus in Early Pregnancy: Evidence for Poor Pregnancy Outcomes Despite Treatment. *Diabetes Care* **2016**, *39*, 75–81. [CrossRef]

21. Sweeting, A.N.; Ross, G.P.; Hyett, J.; Molyneaux, L.; Tan, K.; Constantino, M.; Harding, A.J.; Wong, J. Baseline HbA1c to identify high-risk gestational diabetes: Utility in early vs standard gestational diabetes. *J. Clin. Endocrinol. Metab.* **2017**, *102*, 150–156. [CrossRef] [PubMed]
22. Hosseini, E.; Janghorbani, M.; Shahshahan, Z. Comparison of risk factors and pregnancy outcomes of gestational diabetes mellitus diagnosed during early and late pregnancy. *Midwifery* **2018**, *66*, 64–69. [CrossRef] [PubMed]
23. Ryan, D.K.; Haddow, L.; Ramaesh, A.; Kelly, R.; Johns, E.C.; Denison, F.C.; Dover, A.R.; Reynolds, R.M. Early screening and treatment of gestational diabetes in high-risk women improves maternal and neonatal outcomes: A retrospective clinical audit. *Diabetes Res. Clin. Pract.* **2018**, *144*, 294–301. [CrossRef]
24. Salman, L.; Arbib, N.; Borovich, A.; Shmueli, A.; Chen, R.; Wiznitzer, A.; Hadar, E. The impact of first trimester fasting glucose level on adverse perinatal outcome. *J. Perinatol.* **2018**, *38*, 451–455. [CrossRef]
25. Bianchi, C.; de Gennaro, G.; Romano, M.; Battini, L.; Aragona, M.; Corfini, M.; Del Prato, S.; Bertolotto, A. Early vs. standard screening and treatment of gestational diabetes in high-risk women—An attempt to determine relative advantages and disadvantages. *Nutr. Metab. Cardiovasc. Dis.* **2019**, *29*, 598–603. [CrossRef]
26. Del Val, T.L.; Lázaro, V.A.; Lacalle, C.G.; Moreno, B.T.; Carbajal, G.C.; Fernandez, B.A. Fasting glucose in the first trimester: An initial approach to diagnosis of gestational diabetes. *Endocrinol. Diabetes Nutr.* **2019**, *66*, 11–18.
27. Mañé, L.; Flores-Le Roux, J.A.; Pedro-Botet, J.; Gortazar, L.; Chillarón, J.J.; Llauradó, G.; Payà, A.; Benaiges, D. Is fasting plasma glucose in early pregnancy a better predictor of adverse obstetric outcomes than glycated haemoglobin? *Eur. J. Obstet. Gynecol. Reprod. Biol.* **2019**, *234*, 79–84. [CrossRef]
28. Benhalima, K.; Van Crombrugge, P.; Moyson, C.; Verhaeghe, J.; Vandeginste, S.; Verlaenen, H.; Vercammen, C.; Maes, T.; Dufraimont, E.; De Block, C.; et al. Women with mild fasting hyperglycemia in early pregnancy have more neonatal intensive care admissions. *J. Clin. Endocrinol. Metab.* **2020**. [CrossRef] [PubMed]
29. Boriboonhirunsarn, D.; Sunsaneevithayakul, P.; Pannin, C.; Wamuk, T. Prevalence of early-onset GDM and associated risk factors in a university hospital in Thailand. *J. Obstet. Gynaecol.* **2020**, 1–5. [CrossRef]
30. Clarke, E.; Cade, T.J.; Brennecke, S. Early Pregnancy Screening for Women at High-Risk of GDM Results in Reduced Neonatal Morbidity and Similar Maternal Outcomes to Routine Screening. *J. Pregnancy* **2020**, *2020*, 1–6. [CrossRef]
31. Cosson, E.; Vicaut, E.; Berkane, N.; Cianganu, T.L.; Baudry, C.; Portal, J.-J.; Boujenah, J.; Valensi, P.; Carbillon, L. Prognosis associated with initial care of increased fasting glucose in early pregnancy: A retrospective study. *Diabetes Metab.* **2020**. [CrossRef]
32. Immanuel, J.; Simmons, D.; Desoye, G.; Corcoy, R.; Adelantado, J.M.; Devlieger, R.; Lapolla, A.; Dalfra, M.G.; Bertolotto, A.; Harreiter, J.; et al. Performance of early pregnancy HbA1c for predicting gestational diabetes mellitus and adverse pregnancy outcomes in obese European women. *Diabetes Res. Clin. Pract.* **2020**, *168*, 108378. [CrossRef]
33. Jokelainen, M.; Stach-Lempinen, B.; Rönö, K.; Nenonen, A.; Kautiainen, H.; Teramo, K.; Klemetti, M.M. Oral glucose tolerance test results in early pregnancy: A Finnish population-based cohort study. *Diabetes Res. Clin. Pract.* **2020**, *162*, 108077. [CrossRef]
34. Liu, B.; Cai, J.; Xu, Y.; Long, Y.; Deng, L.; Lin, S.; Zhang, J.; Yang, J.; Zhong, L.; Luo, Y.; et al. Early Diagnosed Gestational Diabetes Mellitus Is Associated With Adverse Pregnancy Outcomes: A Prospective Cohort Study. *J. Clin. Endocrinol. Metab.* **2020**, *105*. [CrossRef] [PubMed]
35. Nakanishi, S.; Aoki, S.; Kasai, J.; Shindo, R.; Obata, S.; Hasegawa, Y.; Mochimaru, A.; Miyagi, E. High probability of false-positive gestational diabetes mellitus diagnosis during early pregnancy. *BMJ Open Diabetes Res. Care* **2020**, *8*, e001234. [CrossRef]
36. Sesmilo, G.; Prats, P.; Garcia, S.; Rodríguez, I.; Rodríguez-Melcón, A.; Berges, I.; Serra, B. First-trimester fasting glycemia as a predictor of gestational diabetes (GDM) and adverse pregnancy outcomes. *Acta Diabetol.* **2020**, *57*, 697–703. [CrossRef]
37. Osmundson, S.S.; Norton, M.E.; El-Sayed, Y.Y.; Carter, S.; Faig, J.C.; Kitzmiller, J.L. Early Screening and Treatment of Women with Prediabetes: A Randomized Controlled Trial. *Amer. J. Perinatol.* **2016**, *33*, 172–179. [CrossRef]
38. Hughes, R.C.E.; Rowan, J.; Williman, J. Prediabetes in pregnancy, can early intervention improve outcomes? A feasibility study for a parallel randomised clinical trial. *BMJ Open* **2018**, *8*, e018493. [CrossRef] [PubMed]
39. Simmons, D.; Nema, J.; Parton, C.; Vizza, L.; Robertson, A.; Rajagopal, R.; Ussher, J.; Perz, J. The treatment of booking gestational diabetes mellitus (TOBOGM) pilot randomised controlled trial. *BMC Pregnancy Childbirth* **2018**, *18*, 151. [CrossRef] [PubMed]
40. Simmons, D.; Hague, W.M.; Teede, H.J.; Cheung, N.W.; Hibbert, E.J.; Nolan, C.J.; Peek, M.J.; Girosi, F.; Cowell, C.T.; Wong, V.W.M.; et al. Hyperglycaemia in early pregnancy: The Treatment of Booking Gestational diabetes Mellitus (TOBOGM) study. A randomised controlled trial. *Med. J. Aust.* **2018**, *209*, 405–406. [CrossRef] [PubMed]
41. Vinter, C.A.; Tanvig, M.H.; Christensen, M.H.; Ovesen, P.G.; Jørgensen, J.S.; Andersen, M.S.; McIntyre, H.D.; Jensen, D.M. Lifestyle Intervention in Danish Obese Pregnant Women With Early Gestational Diabetes Mellitus According to WHO 2013 Criteria Does Not Change Pregnancy Outcomes: Results From the LiP (Lifestyle in Pregnancy) Study. *Diabetes Care* **2018**, *41*, 2079–2085. [CrossRef]
42. Roeder, H.A.; Moore, T.R.; Wolfson, M.T.; Gamst, A.C.; Ramos, G.A. Treating hyperglycemia in early pregnancy: A randomized controlled trial. *Am. J. Obstet. Gynecol. MFM* **2019**, *1*, 33–41. [CrossRef]
43. Harper, L.M.; Jauk, V.; Longo, S.; Biggio, J.R.; Szychowski, J.M.; Tita, A.T. Early gestational diabetes screening in obese women: A randomized controlled trial. *Am. J. Obstet. Gynecol.* **2020**, *222*, 495.e1–495.e8. [CrossRef]
44. Renz, P.B.; Chume, F.C.; Timm, J.R.T.; Pimentel, A.L.; Camargo, J.L. Diagnostic accuracy of glycated hemoglobin for gestational diabetes mellitus: A systematic review and meta-analysis. *Clin. Chem. Lab. Med.* **2019**, *57*, 1435–1449. [CrossRef] [PubMed]

45. Hughes, R.C.E.; Moore, M.P.; Gullam, J.E.; Mohamed, K.; Rowan, J. An early pregnancy HbA1c ≥5.9% (41 mmol/mol) is optimal for detecting diabetes and identifies women at increased risk of adverse pregnancy outcomes. *Diabetes Care* **2014**, *37*, 2953–2959. [CrossRef]
46. McIntyre, H.D.; Gibbons, K.S.; Ma, R.C.W.; Tam, W.H.; Sacks, D.A.; Lowe, J.; Madsen, L.R.; Catalano, P.M. Testing for gestational diabetes during the COVID-19 pandemic. An evaluation of proposed protocols for the United Kingdom, Canada and Australia. *Diabetes Res. Clin. Pract.* **2020**, *167*, 108353. [CrossRef] [PubMed]
47. McIntyre, H.D.; Moses, R.G. The Diagnosis and Management of Gestational Diabetes Mellitus in the Context of the COVID-19 Pandemic. *Diabetes Care* **2020**, *43*, 1433–1434. [CrossRef] [PubMed]
48. Meek, C.L.; Lindsay, R.S.; Scott, E.M.; Aiken, C.E.; Myers, J.; Reynolds, R.; Simmons, D.; Yamamoto, J.M.; McCance, D.R.; Murphy, H.R. Approaches to screening for hyperglycaemia in pregnant women during and after the COVID-19 pandemic. *Diabet. Med.* **2020**, e14380. [CrossRef]
49. Thangaratinam, S.; Cooray, S.D.; Sukumar, N.; Huda, M.S.B.; Devlieger, R.; Benhalima, K.; McAuliffe, F.; Saravanan, P.; Teede, H.J. ENDOCRINOLOGY IN THE TIME OF COVID-19: Diagnosis and management of gestational diabetes mellitus. *Eur. J. Endocrinol.* **2020**, *183*, G49–G56. [CrossRef]
50. Torlone, E.; Festa, C.; Formoso, G.; Scavini, M.; Sculli, M.A.; Succurro, E.; Sciacca, L.; Di Bartolo, P.; Purrello, F.; Lapolla, A. Italian recommendations for the diagnosis of gestational diabetes during COVID-19 pandemic: Position statement of the Italian Association of Clinical Diabetologists (AMD) and the Italian Diabetes Society (SID), diabetes, and pregnancy study group. *Nutr. Metab. Cardiovasc. Dis.* **2020**, *30*, 1418–1422. [CrossRef]
51. Seshiah, V.; Balaji, V.; Banerjee, S.; Sahay, R.; Divakar, H.; Jain, R.; Chawla, R.; Das, A.K.; Gupta, S.; Krishnan, D. Diagnosis and principles of management of gestational diabetes mellitus in the prevailing COVID-19 pandemic. *Int. J. Diabetes Dev. Ctries.* **2020**, *40*, 329–334. [CrossRef] [PubMed]
52. Langer, O.; Levy, J.; Brustman, L.; Anyaegbunam, A.; Merkatz, R.; Divon, M. Glycemic control in gestational diabetes mellitus—how tight is tight enough: Small for gestational age versus large for gestational age? *Am. J. Obstet. Gynecol.* **1989**, *161*, 646–653. [CrossRef]
53. Catalano, P.M.; Mele, L.; Landon, M.B.; Ramin, S.M.; Reddy, U.M.; Casey, B.; Wapner, R.J.; Varner, M.W.; Rouse, D.J.; Thorp, J.M., Jr.; et al. Inadequate weight gain in overweight and obese pregnant women: What is the effect on fetal growth? *Am. J. Obstet. Gynecol.* **2014**, *211*, 137.e1–137.e7. [CrossRef]
54. Benhalima, K.; Minschart, C.; Van Crombrugge, P.; Calewaert, P.; Verhaeghe, J.; Vandamme, S.; Theetaert, K.; Devlieger, R.; Pierssens, L.; Ryckeghem, H.; et al. The 2019 Flemish consensus on screening for overt diabetes in early pregnancy and screening for gestational diabetes mellitus. *Acta Clin. Belg.* **2020**, *75*, 340–347. [CrossRef] [PubMed]
55. O'Malley, E.G.; Reynolds, C.M.E.; O'Kelly, R.; Killalea, A.; Sheehan, S.R.; Turner, M.J. A Prospective Evaluation of Point-of-Care Measurements of Maternal Glucose for the Diagnosis of Gestational Diabetes Mellitus. *Clin. Chem.* **2020**, *66*, 316–323. [CrossRef] [PubMed]

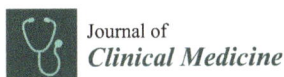

Review

Glucose Homeostasis, Fetal Growth and Gestational Diabetes Mellitus in Pregnancy after Bariatric Surgery: A Scoping Review

Ellen Deleus [1], Bart Van der Schueren [2,3], Roland Devlieger [4], Matthias Lannoo [1,3] and Katrien Benhalima [2,*]

1. Department of Abdominal Surgery, University Hospital Gasthuisberg, KU Leuven, Herestraat 49, 3000 Leuven, Belgium; ellen.deleus@uzleuven.be (E.D.); matthias.lannoo@uzleuven.be (M.L.)
2. Department of Endocrinology, University Hospital Gasthuisberg, KU Leuven, Herestraat 49, 3000 Leuven, Belgium; bart.vanderschueren@uzleuven.be
3. Department of Chronic Diseases, Metabolism and Ageing, KU Leuven, Herestraat, 49, 3000 Leuven, Belgium
4. Department of Obstetrics & Gynaecology, University hospital Gasthuisberg, KU Leuven, Herestraat 49, 3000 Leuven, Belgium; roland.devlieger@uzleuven.be
* Correspondence: katrien.benhalima@uzleuven.be

Received: 13 June 2020; Accepted: 19 August 2020; Published: 24 August 2020

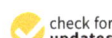

Abstract: Background: Pregnancies in women with a history of bariatric surgery are becoming increasingly prevalent. Surgically induced metabolic changes benefit mother and child, but can also lead to some adverse pregnancy outcomes. Knowledge about glucose homeostasis in these pregnancies could elucidate some of the mechanisms behind these outcomes. This review focusses on glucose homeostasis and birth weight. Methods: We considered papers dealing with glucose homeostasis, gestational diabetes mellitus (GDM) and/or small-for-gestational age infants (SGA) in pregnancies with a history of sleeve gastrectomy (SG) or Roux-en-y gastric bypass (RYGB). Results: Since an OGTT is unreliable to diagnose GDM in a pregnancy after bariatric surgery, the true incidence of GDM is unknown. Alternative screening strategies are needed. Furthermore, these pregnancies are marked by frequent hypoglycemic events as well as wide and rapid glycemic excursions, an issue that is very likely underreported. There is a lack of uniformity in reporting key outcomes and a large variation in study design and control population. Conclusion: Alteration of glucose homeostasis in a pregnancy after bariatric surgery should be further studied using unequivocal definition of key concepts. Glycemic control may prove to be a modifiable risk factor for adverse pregnancy outcomes such as the delivery of an SGA baby.

Keywords: bariatric surgery; pregnancy outcome; glucose homeostasis; gestational diabetes mellitus; gastric bypass; sleeve gastrectomy; small-for-gestational-age; self-monitoring of blood glucose; continuous glucose monitoring

1. Introduction

The prevalence of obesity continues to rise worldwide: in 2015 it was estimated to be 5% among children and 12% among adults. In every age group, women are more affected than men [1]. In a Belgian survey from 2018, 15.9% of the general population had obesity (body mass index (BMI) ≥30 kg/m^2), in comparison to 10.8% in 1997 [2]. Maternal obesity is also rising, with the Euro-Peristat (perinatal health information in Europe) survey indicating a median prevalence of maternal obesity of 13.2% [3]. Maternal obesity during pregnancy is associated with increased risk of miscarriage, congenital anomalies, gestational diabetes mellitus (GDM), macrosomia, caesarian section, hypertensive disorders and admission to neonatal intensive care unit (NICU) [4,5]. For women with a BMI of ≥40 kg/m^2 or a

BMI of ≥35 kg/m^2 with comorbidities, bariatric surgery is the most effective long-term treatment [6]. The International Federation for Surgery of Obesity and Metabolic Disorders (IFSO) global registry report showed that between the period 2014 and 2018, 73.7% of all patients undergoing bariatric surgery was female. Median age at the time of operation was 42 years [7]. This confirms other reports that show that more than 50% of bariatric surgeries are performed in women of childbearing age [8].

The most commonly performed bariatric surgeries are currently Roux-en-Y gastric bypass (RYGB) and sleeve gastrectomy (SG). Laparoscopic adjustable gastric banding (LAGB) has been largely abandoned because of high long-term failure and removal rate [9,10]. Bariatric surgery has historically been divided into malabsorptive and restrictive procedures. However, based on vast scientific evidence from both animal and human research, this labeling does not reflect the mechanisms of action [11]. Both RYGB and SG are associated with distinct glycemic patterns marked by postprandial hyperinsulinemic hypoglycemia, nightly hypoglycemia and wide glycemic variability [12,13]. Improvement in insulin sensitivity as marked by improvement in HOMA-IR index (homeostatic model assessment for insulin resistance index) contributes largely to an improved glucose homeostasis [14]. On the other hand, β-cell function does not seem to recover after RYGB [15]. The Swedish Obese Subjects (SOS) trial showed a 75% decrease in new onset type 2 diabetes mellitus 2 and 10 years after bariatric surgery [16]. Moreover, the improvement in glucose homeostasis occurs before significant weight loss. A prospective randomized trial from Switzerland in non-pregnant patients showed that HOMA-IR index was significantly reduced a week after surgery. The effect at one week postoperative was more pronounced after RYGB, however after three months most SG and RYGB subjects had similar insulin resistance to lean controls [17]. This improvement has been attributed to an improved glucose-mediated incretin release [18]. However, this comes with a price, since both RYGB and SG are marked by enhanced glycemic variability and frequent occurrence of hypoglycemia [13,19,20].

Pregnancy after maternal bariatric surgery is a specific entity; it holds benefits as well as possible harms for both mother and child. Four recent meta-analyses examined the specific risks and benefits of a pregnancy after bariatric surgery (Table 1). Pregnancies after bariatric surgery, as compared with non-surgical controls, were associated with lower risk of GDM (OR 0.20–0.47) [21–23]; lower risk of macrosomia/large-for-gestational age (LGA) infants (OR 0.31–0.46) [8,21–23] and lower risk of hypertensive disorders of pregnancy (HDP) (OR 0.38–0.45) [21–23]. However other outcomes were worse; all four meta-analyses reported a higher risk for small-for-gestational age (SGA) (OR 1.93–2.23) [8,21–23]. Three meta-analyses also reported a higher risk for preterm birth (PB) (OR 1,31–1,35) [8,21,22], and two reported a higher risk for perinatal death (PD) (OR 1.05–1.38) [8,21].

Table 1. Maternal and neonatal outcomes in a pregnancy after bariatric surgery.

Study Characteristics	Cases/Controls *	Control	Outcome •					
			LGA	GDM	HDP	SGA	PB	PD
Galazis et al., UK, 2014 [21]	5.361/160.773	obese ♀ or BMI matched	0.46 †	0.47 †	0.45 ‡	1.93 †	1.31 ‡	1.05~
Akhter et al., UK and Belgium, 2019 [8]	14.880/3.979.978	population	0.42 †	NR	NR	2.13 †	1.35 †	1.38 ‡
Kwong et al., Canada, 2018 [22]	8.364/2.780.717	population	0.31 °	0.21 °	0.38 °	2.18 °	1.33 °	ND
		pre-S		0.20 °		2.16 °		
		pre-P		1.04 °		2.23 °		
Yi et al., China, 2015 [23]	4.178/16.016	obese ♀	0.40 °	0.31 °	0.42 °	2.16 °	1.33 °	NR

BMI: body mass index, LGA: large for gestational age, GDM: gestational diabetes mellitus, HDP: hypertensive disorders of pregnancy, SGA: small for gestational age, PB: premature birth, PD: perinatal death, NR: not reported, ND: no difference * Cases represent number of pregnancies in women with a history of bariatric surgery/Controls are pregnancies in women without history of bariatric surgery, • odds ratios are reported for cases versus controls † p-value <0.001, ‡ p-value <0.05, ~no statistically significant difference, ° p-value not reported, ♀ BMI ≥ 30 kg/m^2, Pre-S: pre-surgery BMI matched, Pre-P: pre-pregnancy BMI matched.

In pregnancy, the effect of low glucose levels on unfavorable pregnancy outcomes are poorly studied. A different intrauterine environment may be responsible for an infant to be SGA [24,25]. In the 1970s and 1980s, several authors report on the association between maternal hypoglycemia during oral glucose tolerance test (OGTT) and intra uterine growth restriction [26–28]. A recent paper in a non-bariatric surgery population confirmed a significant association between low fasting plasma glucose and hypoglycemia during standard 2 h 75 gr OGTT and low birth weight [29].

Consequently, changes in glucose homeostasis after bariatric surgery may play an important role in observed outcomes. In a normal pregnancy, insulin sensitivity shifts during gestation. Early gestation is marked by an increased insulin sensitivity. When gestation progresses, a combination of maternal and placental hormones induce a state of insulin resistance [30]. As such, the fetus receives more glucose which, in turn, drives fetal production of insulin, an important growth factor in fetal live [31]. Since bariatric surgery improves insulin resistance, this may explain the improvement in GDM diagnosis. However, it could also be linked to the increased risk for SGA, since the level of insulin resistance in the later stages of gestation could be insufficient to provide enough glucose flux to the fetus.

About 80% of GDM cases in normal pregnancy are related to β-cell dysfunction on a background of chronic insulin resistance. The rate of GDM in the general population worldwide is about 16.5% [30]. However, there is a great variation in the diagnostic criteria for GDM worldwide [32,33]. In 2010, the 'International Association of Diabetes and Pregnancy Study Groups' (IADPSG) published recommendations for GDM screening during pregnancy. A 2 h 75 g OGTT between 24 and 28 weeks is recommended.

The purpose of this scoping review is to explore the existing evidence on the specific changes in glucose homeostasis as a result of the combined impact of pregnancy and altered gastro-intestinal physiology after RYGB and SG. In addition, data on the influence of altered glucose handling on fetal growth and diagnosis of GDM are analyzed.

2. Methods

2.1. Data Search

We applied the PRISMA guidelines for Scoping Reviews [34]. Between 15th January 2020 and 17th February 2020, a PubMed search was performed. The search was limited to research on humans, published after 2010. Studies on both singleton and multiple pregnancies were included. Since RYGB and SG are the most commonly performed bariatric surgery procedures, these search terms were used. However, data on other types of bariatric surgery were also included since it was often impossible to extract data specifically for SG and RYGB. The following search terms were used: ("Pregnancy"(Mesh) AND "Glucose"(Mesh) AND "Bariatric Surgery"(Mesh) OR "Gastric Bypass"(Mesh) OR "Gastrectomy"(Mesh) AND "Hypoglycemia"(Mesh) OR "Glucose"(Mesh)); ("Infant, Small for Gestational Age"(Mesh) AND "Bariatric Surgery (Mesh) OR "Gastric Bypass"(Mesh) OR "Gastrectomy"(Mesh) AND "Nutrient"(Mesh)); ("Bariatric Surgery"(Mesh) OR "Gastric Bypass"(Mesh) OR "Gastrectomy"(Mesh) AND "Diabetes, Gestational"(Mesh)). In addition, we hand-searched the reference lists of all selected articles and reviews. Exclusion criteria included no full text, full text not in English or Dutch, opinion, editorial, case report, not relevant or animal studies. Duplicates were removed. Certain clinical practice guidelines and narrative reviews were only used to underline arguments and were therefore not mentioned in the flow chart of included articles.

2.2. Data Analysis

We included original and review articles. Since this is not a systematic review, no quality analysis of the selected studies was done. We did not use a review protocol, data charting was done independently. We performed a descriptive analysis of all original articles using the following data: year, type of study, size of patient group, type of bariatric surgery performed, type of control group and outcome variables.

Numbers reported in tables represent total number of pregnancies after bariatric surgery. Glycemic values are reported in mg/dL.

All four systematic reviews with meta-analysis are summarized in Table 1 with odds ratios regarding: macrosomia/LGA, GDM, hypertensive disorders of pregnancy, SGA, preterm birth and perinatal death.

3. Literature Search and Overview of Selection

Initially, a total of 243 articles was found. After screening of titles and abstracts on relevance for the topic, we included 101 articles. We excluded 14 articles because of duplicate or publication before 2010. After applying exclusion criteria we retained 57 papers: 53 original articles and four meta-analyses (Figure 1).

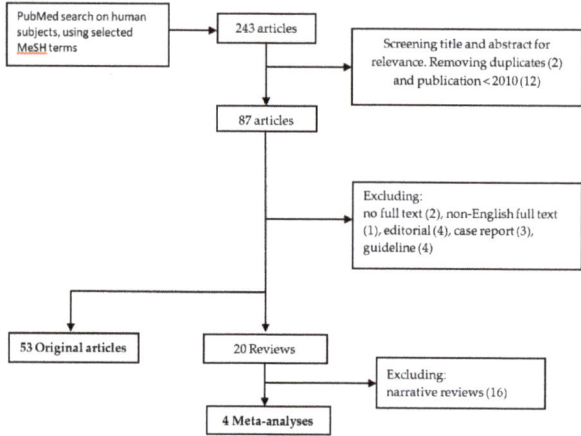

Figure 1. Literature search and selection process.

4. Results

4.1. Characteristics of Glucose Homeostasis in Pregnancy After Bariatric Surgery

We identified nine observational studies that report on glycemic levels during a pregnancy after bariatric surgery (Table 2). Seven studies had a study population of less than 50 participants.

The most common technique to evaluate maternal glucose homeostasis in a pregnancy after bariatric surgery was a 75 or 100 g OGTT [35,37–43]. Consistently, a high prevalence of hypoglycemic events during the OGTT was reported, ranging from 5.26% to 90% of all patients. A retrospective cohort study from 2016 described glucose levels during an OGTT in pregnant RYGB women and BMI-matched, lean and obese controls. Mean fasting glucose was significantly lower in pregnant women after RYGB (74.95 mg/dL). Pregnant women after RYGB had a glycemic rise at 60 min, followed by hypoglycemia (<60 mg/dL) at 120 min, occurring in 54.8% of cases. When considering glycemic levels at 120 min (and not at 60 min) only 1.6% met the IADPSG criteria for GDM. When considering glycemic levels at 60 min, 43.5% of the post-RYGB women met the IADPSG criteria for GDM, however 39.3% of these women developed hypoglycemia at 120 min. The control group of obese women had no hypoglycemic episodes [37]. The highest rates of hypoglycemic events were reported in a population of RYGB patients that underwent an extended and frequently sampled 3 h 75 g OGTT after at least 8 h of fasting. Ninety percent of these women developed hypoglycemia (<50 mg/dL). The mean plasma glucose nadir in the RYGB group was 42.5 mg/dL [39]. After a 3 h 100 g OGTT, another group confirmed that the nadir was reached in 2 h in 42.4% and only after 3 h in 57.6%. Hypoglycemia was most commonly seen after RYGB (83.3%) and SG (54.5%), and less after LAGB (11.8%) [43].

Table 2. Glucose profile in a pregnancy after bariatric surgery.

Author, Year	Design	Cases *	Type of BS	Control Group	Test †	Hypoglycemia	Symptoms	Conclusion ‡
Andrade, 2016 [35]	Case series	38	NR	Not-pregnant post-BS	OGTT	5.26% (≤ 50 mg/dL)	26.31%	Lower risk of hypoglycemia during pregnancy versus non-pregnant post BS control.
Bonis, 2016 [36]	Case series	35	RYGB	no	CGM	NR	NR	High mean maximum IG, low mean minimum IG.
Feichtinger, 2017 [37]	Retrospective cohort	76	RYGB	BMI matched ∞ / lean ∞ / obese ∞	OGTT	54.8% (≤ 60 mg/dL)	NR	Lower fasting glucose, glycemic rise at 60 min, followed by hypoglycemia. Trend to positive association between FG and BW.
Freitas, 2014 [38]	Case series	30	RYGB	no	OGTT	25% (≤ 50 mg/dL)	57.9%	New diagnostic criteria for GDM increase diagnosis of GDM after RYGB with 50%, but no change in pregnancy outcome.
Göbl, 2017 [39]	Retrospective cohort	25	RYGB	morbidly obese ∞ / lean ∞	OGTT (3 h) / IVGTT	90% (≤ 50 mg/dL)	NR	Positive association between FG and maternal glucose nadir level. IS during OGTT remained improved in RYGB versus BMI matched control.
Leutner, 2019 [40]	Prospective cohort	25	RYGB	obese ∞ / lean ∞	OGTT / IVGTT / CGM	76% (< 54 mg/dL, ADA guidelines)	NR	High risk of nightly hypoglycemia. Postprandial hypoglycemia is GLP-1 regulated.
Maric, 2019 [41]	Prospective cohort	41	LAGB, SG, RYGB	pre-P ∞	OGTT HOMA-IR	43.90% (< 60 mg/dL)	NR	Lower HOMA-IR, birthweight and body fat, same cord HOMA-IR. Positive association between postprandial glucose level and BW
Maric, 2020 [42]	Prospective cohort	47	20 SG and LAGB / 27 RYGB	pre-P ∞	OGTT	48.78% (< 60 mg/dL)	NR	Maternal glucose level at OGTT is positively associated with EFW and BW
Rottenstreich, 2018 [43]	Retrospective cohort	119	55 SG / 34 LAGB / 30 RYGB	no	OGTT (3 h, 100 gr)	49.6% (≤ 55 mg/dL)	NR	Hypoglycemia group: shorter surgery to conception interval, less GDM, more SGA. Hypoglycemia most prevalent after RYGB

BS: bariatric surgery, NR: not reported, OGTT: oral glucose tolerance test, RYGB: Roux-en-y gastric bypass, CGM: continuous glucose monitoring, IG: interstitial glucose, BMI: body mass index, FG: fetal growth, BW: birth weight, GDM: gestational diabetes mellitus, IVGTT: intravenous glucose tolerance test, IS: insulin sensitivity, ADA: American diabetes association, GLP-1: glucagon-like peptide 1, LAGB: laparoscopic adjustable gastric band, SG: sleeve gastrectomy, Pre-P: pre-pregnancy BMI matched, HOMA-IR: homeostasis model assessment of insulin resistance, EFW: estimated fetal weight, SGA: small for gestational age, * number of pregnant women with a history of bariatric surgery, ∞ control group without history of bariatric surgery, † standard OGTT is 2 h 75 gr, non-standard method is described between brackets, percentage of pregnant women with a history of bariatric surgery displaying hypoglycemia and/or symptoms. Cut-off values for hypoglycemia are mentioned between brackets, ‡ main conclusion regarding pregnancies with maternal history of bariatric surgery.

A prospective observational study from the UK compared maternal insulin resistance in pregnant women after bariatric surgery versus pregnant women with similar BMI. A reduced insulin resistance, as assessed by HOMA-IR index, was found in pregnancies after bariatric surgery. The authors conclude that the positive effect of bariatric surgery on insulin resistance cannot solely be explained by weight reduction [41].

Two studies performed an intravenous glucose tolerance test (IVGTT) [39,40]. In 2017, Göbl et al. showed that IVGTT-derived insulin response was comparable between post RYGB pregnant women and normal weight pregnant women. They concluded that reactive hypoglycemia noticed after OGTT must be attributed to the specific anatomical alterations after gastric bypass surgery. An IVGTT reflects only the effect of plasma glucose on insulin release by the β-cell, whereas an OGTT reflects the additional effect of the altered gastro-intestinal tract on insulin release [39]. Leutner et al. also described an exaggerated expression of GLP-1 just before the occurrence of a hypoglycemic event in pregnant women after RYGB. This suggests that GLP-1 might be the main driver of this postprandial hyperinsulinemic hypoglycemia [40].

There are only two observational studies available with data on continuous glucose monitoring (CGM) during pregnancy after bariatric surgery [36,40]. In addition, there is one case report on the subject [44]. All three studies reported on CGM during pregnancy after RYGB. Bonis et al. described CGM in 35 RYGB pregnant women at 26.2 ± 5 weeks and reported wide and rapid changes in postprandial interstitial glucose (IG), as well as frequent hypoglycemia. The authors compared there results with CGM data from other studies in non-operated pregnant women and found these profiles to be very different. They showed that pregnant women after bariatric surgery have a lower mean fasting IG, similar 1 h postprandial IG and significantly lower 2 h postprandial IG. The postprandial IG peak occurred earlier, and the value was higher compared to non-operated women. The authors suggest therefore that a 75 g OGTT is probably a poor diagnostic tool for GDM, since baseline and 2 h value will be lower, and 1 h value will not be representative of the highest value [36]. In a study by Leutner et al., it was shown that pregnant women with previous RYGB had both the highest and the lowest mean IG values when comparing with non-operated normal-weight and obese pregnant women on a week-long CGM. The CGM (iPro2, Medtronic MiniMed, Northridge, CA, USA) was blinded to the participants and only retrospectively analyzed by the investigators. Glucose profile in a pregnancy after RYGB was characterized by frequent hypoglycemic events overnight. Daytime was characterized by glycemic variations with large amplitude, postprandial hyperglycemic spikes and hypoglycemic events [40].

A 2019 prospective observational study investigated cord blood glucose and insulin levels in a pregnancy after bariatric surgery (41 women), compared to levels in a pregnancy without maternal bariatric surgery (82 women). The control group was matched according to early pregnancy BMI. Investigators found no difference in cord blood glucose or insulin levels between both groups. Moreover, no association between maternal and neonatal insulin resistance was found [41]. This is in contrast to a 2009 report from Cleveland, (Ohio, USA) demonstrating an association between maternal obesity and fetal insulin resistance in normal pregnancy [45].

There is no evidence that treatment of GDM diagnosed by an OGTT in this population leads to improved pregnancy outcomes. This is highlighted by the study of Freitas et al. When applying the IADPSG criteria instead of the Carpenter and Coustan criteria in 30 post-RYGB pregnant women they, found a 50% increase in diagnosis of GDM, however, there was no difference in outcomes [38].

4.2. Is Abnormal Glucose Homeostasis a Main Culprit for Fetal Growth Retardation in A Pregnancy After Bariatric Surgery?

We identified 28 studies on the prevalence of SGA in a pregnancy after bariatric surgery (Table 3). These studies included smaller cohorts or case series, and larger population-based cohort studies. There were three nationwide studies from Denmark [46–48], three from Sweden [49–51] and four from the USA [52–55].

Table 3. Prevalence of small-for-gestational-age infants (SGA) in a pregnancy after bariatric surgery.

Author, Year	Design	Cases *	Type of BS	Control Group ∞	SGA Definition •	SGA Prevalence
Adams, 2015 [52]	Cohort, population	764	RYGB	obese	≤ 10th percentile	OR: 2.16
Balestrin, 2019 [56]	Cohort, single center	93	Uncertain	obese	< 10th percentile	19.4% vs. 11.6%
Basbug, 2019 [57]	Case series, single center	23	SG	no	< 10th percentile	8.69%
Belogolovkin, 2012 [53]	Cohort, population	293	Uncertain	obese	< 10th percentile	2.69
Chevrot, 2016 [58]	Case control, single center	139	RYGB, SG, LAGB	pre-P	< 10th percentile	29% vs. 6% ~
				pre-S		17% vs. 9% ~
Costa, 2018 [59]	Case series, single center	39	RYGB, SG, LAGB	no	< 10th percentile	17.9%
Dolin, 2019 [60]	Cohort, single center	76	RYGB, SG, LAGB	no	< 10th percentile	0%
Ducarme, 2013 [61]	Cohort, multicenter	94	RYGB, LAGB	no	< 10th percentile	RYGB: 32.3%
						LAGB: 17.5%
Feichtinger, 2018 [62]	Case control, single center	43	RYGB	BMI matched	NR	26.2% vs. 4.7% ‡
Gascoin, 2017 [63]	Case control, single center	56	RYGB	lean	< 10th percentile	23% vs. 3.6%~
Gonzalez, 2015 [64]	Case series, multicenter	168	RYBG, SG, VBG, LAGB, BPD	no	< 3rd percentile	19.6%
Grandfils, 2019 [65]	Case series, multicenter	337	RYGB, SG, LAGB	no	< 10th percentile	25.81%
Hammeken, 2017 [66]	Cohort, single center	151	RYGB	pre-P	22% below average	2.67 OR
Hazart, 2017 [67]	Case series, single center	57	RYGB, LAGB, SG	no	< 10th percentile	36%
Johansson, 2015 [49]	Cohort, population	670	RYGB (98%), LAGB, other	pre-S	< 10th percentile	15.6% vs. 7.6% †, OR 2.20
Josefsson, 2011 [50]	Cohort, population	126	RYGB, VBG, LAGB	population	≥ 2 SD below mean	3.38% vs. 2.1% ~
Karadag, 2019 [68]	Cohort, single center	90	SG	obese	< 10th percentile	17.7% vs. 7.4%
Kjaer, feb 2013 [47]	Cohort, population	339	RYGB, LAGB	pre-P	≥ 2 SD below mean	OR: 2.29, RYGB: 2.78
Kjaer, mar 2013 [48]	Case series, population	286	RYGB	no	≥ 2 SD below mean	7.69%
Lesko, 2012 [69]	Cohort, single center	70	RYGB, LAGB	pre-P	NR	17.4% vs. 5.0% ~
				pre-S		(OR 3.94)
Norgaard, 2014 [46]	Cohort, population	387	RYGB	population	< 10th percentile	18.8%
Parent, 2017 [54]	Cohort, population	1859	RYGB, SG, LAGB, VBG	population	< 10th percentile	13.0% vs. 8.9% (RR 1.93 adjusted)
Parker, 2016 [55]	Cohort, population	1585	NR	obese population	< 10th percentile ••	5.7% vs. 2.2% †
Roos, 2013 [51]	Cohort, population	2562	RYGB, VBG, LAGB, other	BMI > 35	≥ 2SD below mean	5.2% vs. 3%†, OR 2
Rottenstreich, ma 2018 [70]	Case control, multicenter	119	SG	pre-S	< 10th percentile	14.3% vs. 4.2% ~
Rottenstreich, sep 2018 [71]	Case series, single center	154	SG	no	< 10th percentile	13.64%
Sancak, 2019 [72]	Case series, single center	44	SG	no	< 10th percentile	25%
Stentebjerg, 2017 [73]	Case series, single center	71	RYGB	no	≥ 2SD below mean	1.4%

BS: bariatric surgery, OR: odds ratio, RYGB: Roux-en-y gastric bypass, NR: not reported, LAGB: laparoscopic adjustable gastric band, VBG: vertical banded gastroplasty, SG: sleeve gastrectomy, Pre-P: pre-pregnancy BMI matched, Pre-S: pre-surgery BMI matched, BMI: body mass index, BPD: biliopancreatic diversion, SD: standard deviation, RR: relative risk, * number of pregnant women with a history of bariatric surgery, ∞ control group without history of bariatric surgery, † p-value < 0.001, ‡ p-value < 0.05, ~ no statistically significant difference, p-value not reported, • of mean birth weight, unless otherwise mentioned •• of mean weight during pregnancy.

There are several findings that point to an association between SGA and abnormal glycemic levels after bariatric surgery. An Austrian paper investigated differences in frequently sampled 3 h 75 g OGTT and IVGTT in RYGB patients compared to obese and normal-weight control pregnant women. The results were correlated with pregnancy outcomes. A positive association was found between fetal growth and maternal glucose nadir during the OGTT [39]. A 2019 observational study investigated glucose levels during 75 g OGTT, as well as cord blood analyses, neonatal weight and body composition. In this report, a positive correlation was found between birthweight and post OGTT glucose level [41]. In an Israeli study, evaluating pregnancy outcomes after bariatric surgery between a group with hypoglycemic events compared to a group without hypoglycemic events, the hypoglycemic group presented with less GDM, but more SGA [43].

The timing of growth retardation in these fetuses is a topic of debate. A 2017 Austrian study found more pronounced hypoglycemia during an OGTT to be associated with reduced fetal abdominal circumference during the second trimester of pregnancy [62]. A 2020 prospective longitudinal study from the UK showed reduced fetal growth velocity starting in the third trimester, when compared to non-operated women with similar pre-pregnancy BMI [42]. A Danish national cohort study investigating 387 women after RYGB found an overall SGA proportion of 18.8%. In contrast to other studies, they found that early fetal growth was significantly impaired when compared to a historical cohort of 9450 singleton pregnancies in Denmark [46].

A large cohort study from Sweden with 670 pregnancies after bariatric surgery of which 98% were RYGB, noted more SGA when there was a longer surgery to conception interval [49]. On the other hand, a Turkish retrospective study investigating outcome after SG, found more SGA with a shorter surgery to conception interval [68]. A Danish national cohort study found no significant difference in SGA depending on a short or long surgery to conception interval (before or after 18 months: 19.7% versus 18%), there was a trend to lower SGA rates with increasing maternal BMI [46].

4.3. Prevalence of GDM in a Pregnancy After Bariatric Surgery

We identified 35 studies on the prevalence of GDM in a pregnancy after bariatric surgery (Table 4). These studies include smaller cohorts or case series, and larger population-based cohort studies. There are three population studies from Denmark [47,48,74], three from the USA [52,53,55], two from Sweden [49,50] and one from Australia [75]. Only 15 studies reported on the method of diagnosis of GDM: oral glucose tolerance test (OGTT), capillary blood glucose monitoring (CBGM) or measurement of glycosylated hemoglobin (HbA1c) (Table 4).

Table 4. Prevalence of GDM in a pregnancy after bariatric surgery.

Author, Year	Design	Cases *	Type of BS	Control Group ∞	GDM Test •	GDM Prevalence
Adams, 2015 [52]	Cohort, population	764	RYGB	obese	NR	OR: 0.33 †
Amsalem, 2014 [76]	Retrospective cohort	109	LAGB, VBG	pregnancy before BS	NR	6.1% vs. 19% ~
Balestrin, 2019 [56]	Cohort, single center	93	Uncertain	obese	OGTT	12.9% vs. 26.5% ~
Basbug, 2019 [57]	Case series, single center	23	SG	no	OGTT	0%
Belogolovkin, 2012 [53]	Cohort, population	293	Uncertain	obese	NR	OR: 0.44
Berlac, 2014 [74]	Cohort, population	415	RYGB	pre-P	NR	9.2% vs. 8.1%
				lean		9.2% vs. 1.3% †
Burke, 2010 [77]	Retrospective cohort	354	87% RYGB	pregnancy before BS	NR	8% vs. 27%
						OR 0.23°
Chevrot, 2016 [58]	Case control, single center	139	RYGB, SG, LAGB	pre-P	NR	12 vs. 10% ~
				pre-S		12 vs. 23 % ~
Costa, 2018 [59]	Case series, single center	39	RYGB, SG, LAGB	no	NR	7.7%
De Alencar Costa, 2016 [78]	Retrospective case-control	63	RYGB	obese	NR	0% vs. 19.2% †
Dolin, 2019 [60]	Cohort, single center	76	RYGB, SG, LAGB	no	OGTT or CBGM	2.63%
Ducarme, 2013 [61]	Cohort, multicenter	94	RYGB, LAGB	no	OGTT (50 or 75 gr)	19.4%
Gascoin, 2017 [63]	Case control, single center	56	RYGB	lean	NR	1.78% vs. 0% ~
Gonzalez, 2015 [64]	Case series, multicenter	168	RYBG, SG, VBG, LAGB, BPD	no	OGTT (50 or 100 gr)	3%
Grandfils, 2019 [65]	Case series, multicenter	337	RYGB, SG, LAGB	no	NR	26.34%
Han, 2013 [79]	Case series	12	SG	no	NR	0%
Hazart, 2017 [67]	Case series, single center	57	RYGB, LAGB, SG	no	OGTT (50 gr)	18%
Ibiebele, 2019 [75]	Retrospective cross sectional	1484	RYGB, LAGB, SG	population	NR	10.8% vs. 8.3% †
Ibiebele, 2019 [75]	Retrospective cross sectional	1484	RYGB, LAGB, SG	population	NR	10.8% vs. 8.3% †
Johansson, 2015 [49]	Cohort, population	670	RYGB (98%), LAGB, other	pre-S	OGTT or CBGM	1.9% vs. 6.8% †
						OR 0.25
Josefsson, 2011 [50]	Cohort, population	126	RYGB, VBG, LAGB	population	NR	no difference
Karadag, 2019 [68]	Cohort, single center	90	SG	obese	OGTT	6.6% vs. 29.6%
Kjaer, feb 2013 [47]	Cohort, population	339	RYGB, LAGB	pre-P	NR	8.9% vs. 7.1% ~
Kjaer, mar 2013 [48]	Case series, population	286	RYGB	no	NR	9.44%
Lesko, 2012 [69]	Cohort, single center	70	RYGB, LAGB	pre-P	OGTT (3 h)	0% vs. 9.3%, OR 0.04 ~
				pre-S		0% vs. 16.4%, OR 0.07 ~
Malakauskiene, 2019 [80]	Retrospective cohort	130	RYGB, LAGB	no	OGTT	2.31%
Parker, 2016 [55]	Cohort, population	1585	NR	obese	NR	7.3% vs. 4.4% ~
Rasteiro, 2018 [81]	Case series	86	RYGB, LAGB	no	OGTT or CBGM	19.77%

Table 4. Cont.

Author, Year	Design	Cases *	Type of BS	Control Group ∞	GDM Test •	GDM Prevalence
Rottenstreich, ma 2018 [70]	Case control, multicenter	119	SG	pre-S	NR	3.4% vs. 17.6% †
Rottenstreich, sep 2018 [71]	Case series, single center	154	SG	no	OGTT (100 gr, 3 h) or CBGM	2.6%
Rottenstreich, 2019 [82]	Retrospective case control	22	RYGB, LAGB, SG	pre-S	OGTT (100 gr, 3 h) or CBGM	9.1% vs. 36.4% †
Shai, 2014 [83]	Retrospective cohort	326	NR	obese	NR	10.1% vs. 14.7% ‡
Sheiner, 2011 [84]	Case series	489	RYGB, LAGB, VBG	no	NR	7.98%
Stone, 2011 [85]	Case series	102	NR	no	NR	11.76%
Watanabe, 2019 [86]	Case series, single center	24	RYGB, SG, LAGB, BPD-DS	no	HbA1c ≥ 6.5%	8.33%
Yau, 2017 [87]	Case series	49	RYGB, LAGB, SG	no	OGTT	2.44%

BS: bariatric surgery, GDM: gestational diabetes mellitus, RYGB: Roux-en-y gastric bypass, NR: not reported, vs: versus, OR: odds ratio, LAGB: laparoscopic adjustable gastric band, VBG: vertical banded gastroplasty, OGTT: oral glucose tolerance test, SG: sleeve gastrectomy, Pre-P: pre-pregnancy BMI matched, Pre-S: pre-surgery BMI matched, BMI: body mass index, BPD: biliopancreatic diversion, CBGM: capillary blood glucose monitoring, BPD-DS: biliopancreatic diversion with duodenal switch, HbA1c: glycosylated hemoglobin, * number of pregnant women with a history of bariatric surgery, ∞ control group without history of bariatric surgery, • standard OGTT is 2 h 75 gr, non-standard method is described between brackets, † p-value < 0.001, ‡ p-value < 0.05, ~ no statistically significant difference, p-value not reported.

In most observational studies where a non-operated control group was used, bariatric surgery is associated with a lower prevalence of GDM (Table 4). Prevalence of GDM after bariatric surgery in these studies ranged from 0 to 12.9% [49,52,53,56,68–70,76–78,82,83]. Other studies comparing the GDM rate to a non-operated group showed a higher rate of GDM in women with a history of bariatric surgery [47,55,63,74,75]. There is significant heterogeneity in both case and control groups (Table 4).

The highest rate of GDM (26.34%) after bariatric surgery was found in a 2019 paper investigating the effect of gestational weight gain on pregnancy outcomes after bariatric surgery. A total of 337 pregnancies in women that underwent RYGB, SG and LAGB were studied. GDM diagnosis was based on patient charts, no information was available on the diagnostic method. Surprisingly, GDM was most prevalent in the group that had insufficient gestational weight gain (29.7%), whereas in the group of patients with excessive weight gain, a percentage of 22.1% was noted [65].

4.4. Impact of the Interval Between Bariatric Surgery And Pregnancy on the Prevalence of GDM

A recent Eurasian consensus paper recommends that pregnancy should be postponed until stable weight is achieved. In practice, this means 12 months after RYGB or SG [88]. The reason to delay a pregnancy is to prevent adverse outcome, mainly SGA. Several studies reported no difference in prevalence of GDM when comparing an interval shorter or longer than 1 year after bariatric surgery [48,60,68,80,84]. Other studies investigated longer intervals, of up to 2 years, and also showed no difference [49,57,71,81,87]. These effects were similar in different types of bariatric surgery including SG and RYGB.

There is however some evidence that a shorter interval between surgery and pregnancy is associated with a higher risk for hypoglycemia following a 100 g OGTT, as was shown by a study from Israel with patients after RYGB, SG and LAGB. In the hypoglycemia group, time from surgery to conception was significantly shorter (median 711 versus 1246 days, p = 0.002), risk of GDM tended to be lower (0% versus 10.9%, p-value: 0.3) and risk of SGA was higher (11.9% versus 1.7%, p-value: 0.3) [43]. A study investigating the effect of a 75 g OGTT in pregnant women with previous SG, compared women that became pregnant in the year after SG with women that conceived after twelve months. The early conception group reported more early (58%) and late (16%) dumping symptoms than the late conception group (14% and 9%, respectively) [68].

4.5. Impact of BMI After Bariatric Surgery on the Prevalence of GDM

In a case series of 102 post-bariatric-surgery pregnant women (type of surgery not reported), there was no difference in GDM prevalence between BMI ≥ 30 versus < 30 kg/m^2 [85]. A larger cohort study from Sweden confirmed this finding, showing that pre-pregnancy BMI and the amount of weight loss from bariatric surgery to early pregnancy does not modify the effect of bariatric surgery on the risk of developing GDM. In the bariatric surgery group with BMI < 42.1 versus ≥ 42.1 kg/m^2, GDM occurred in, respectively, 2.5% versus 1.5% of cases after bariatric surgery. In the bariatric surgery group with a decrease in BMI of ≥ 12.9 versus <12.9 kg/m^2, GDM occurred in 2.3% versus 1.6% of cases [49]. A French case series studied the effect of the amount of gestational weight gain in 337 pregnancies after bariatric surgery (RYGB, SG, LAGB), according to the 2009 Institute of Medicine (IOM) recommendations. Insufficient gestational weight gain (35%), as well as excessive gestational weight gain (38%) were frequent. The amount of gestational weight gain, however, had no statistically significant effect on the prevalence of GDM. GDM occurred in 29.7%, 28.1% and 22.1% of women with insufficient, adapted and excessive gestational weight gain, respectively (p-value: 0.36). There was no information on how GDM diagnosis was made. Insufficient gestational weight gain was positively correlated with low birth weight and SGA. Surgery to conception interval had no influence on the amount of gestational weight gain in this study [65].

4.6. Impact of Type of Bariatric Surgery on Prevalence of GDM

To our knowledge, there are no studies directly comparing the difference in GDM prevalence between SG and RYGB. Few studies have looked specifically at the prevalence of GDM after SG and report a percentage of 0–6.6% [57,68,71]. These studies used OGTT or CBGM. GDM prevalence in these studies was low when compared to studies in RYGB patients. A prospective observational study from the UK investigated pregnancy outcomes after restrictive versus malabsorptive bariatric surgery. The malabsorptive group consisted solely of women with RYGB; the restrictive group consisted of patients after SG or LAGB. GDM diagnosis was made with a 75 g OGTT. In the RYGB group, 0% of GDM was recorded in the SG-LAGB group, 21.1%. However, maternal post-prandial hypoglycemia was significantly more prevalent in the RYGB group (70%) compared with the SG-LAGB group (22%) [41]. The effect of SG on the development of postprandial hypoglycemia may be blunted by mixing LAGB with SG in one combined group, as a cohort study with 30 RYGB, 55 SG and 34 LAGB pregnant women showed postprandial hypoglycemia percentages of 83.3%, 54.5% and 11.8%, respectively [43].

5. Discussion

5.1. Summary of Findings

In this scoping review, we show that hypoglycemia as well as large and rapid glycemic excursions are underreported in pregnancies after bariatric surgery. These changes in glucose homeostasis may be responsible for adverse pregnancy outcomes such as SGA. The diagnosis of GDM in a pregnancy after bariatric surgery is challenging. Most studies reporting on GDM prevalence are based on an OGTT, although this test is considered unreliable.

5.2. Results in Relation to What We Already Know

Clinical practice recommendations on the diagnosis of GDM were published by the American Diabetes Association (ADA) in 2020 [89]. Screening for overt diabetes should be done at first prenatal contact using standard diagnostic criteria. In women without pre-existing diabetes mellitus, a test for GDM is advised at 24–28 weeks of gestation. GDM diagnosis can be made with one of two methods: a one-step 75 g OGTT (IADPSG criteria), or a two-step approach with a 50 glucose challenge test (GCT) followed by a 100 g OGTT in case of positive screening (Carpenter-Coustan criteria) [89]. A one-step 2 h 75 g OGTT is the gold standard test [90]. There is no evidence that treatment of GDM diagnosed by an OGTT in a population after bariatric surgery, leads to improved pregnancy outcomes. Since an OGTT is an unreliable and poorly tolerated test in women with a history of bariatric surgery, an alternative screening strategy for GDM is needed. Our research group recommended using CBGM daily before and after meals during 3–7 days at 24–28 weeks of pregnancy. Glycemic targets were based on American Diabetes Association (ADA) recommendations [91]. More research is needed to define optimal glycemic targets in this population. Each type of bariatric surgery has a specific glycemic footprint [17,20]. Both RYGB and SG are marked by postprandial hyperinsulinemic hypoglycemia, nightly hypoglycemia and wide glycemic variability [12,13]. This is influenced by specific anatomical alterations to the gastro-intestinal tract that alter glucose handling [19].

When examining SGA in a pregnancy after bariatric surgery, confounders such as smoking, lower socio-economic status and paternal BMI must be taken into account. Several studies note that patients after bariatric surgery are more likely to be smokers and have a lower socio-economic status [46,50]. A recent systematic review and meta-analysis showed that high paternal BMI can lead to distortion of fetal growth, leading to both SGA and LGA in normal pregnancies [92]. Levels of micronutrients, lipids, amino-acids and leptin have been shown to influence fetal growth. Micronutrient deficiencies are found to be more frequent after bariatric surgery, however, evidence linking these deficiencies to adverse pregnancy outcomes is weak [93]. The most common deficiencies after bariatric surgery are vitamin B12, vitamin D and other fat-soluble vitamins, folate, calcium, iron, proteins and fat [94]. Cord blood micronutrient levels in infants after RYGB showed deficiencies in calcium, zinc, iron and vitamin A when compared with neonates from lean, healthy mothers [63]. Maternal lipids and amino-acid levels have been linked to disturbed fetal growth [95]. Metabolomic and lipidomic research has shown a disturbed lipid profile in mothers and fetuses with intra-uterine growth restriction [96]. Low maternal leptin levels in mid pregnancy have been linked to SGA, a finding that persisted when adjusting for pre-pregnancy BMI [97].

In pregnancies after bariatric surgery, the impact of pre-pregnancy BMI on pregnancy outcomes is unclear. All three systematic reviews with meta-analysis report significant decrease in GDM prevalence after bariatric surgery. Subgroup analysis with matching for pre-pregnancy BMI no longer showed a significant improvement in GDM prevalence after bariatric surgery, concluding that the improvement in GDM is mainly weight-loss-driven [21,22]. On the other hand, other studies reported that pre-pregnancy BMI and the amount of weight loss from bariatric surgery to early pregnancy does not modify the effect of bariatric surgery on GDM improvement [49,85]. A recent prospective observational study from the UK compared maternal insulin resistance in pregnant women after RYGB versus pregnant women with similar BMI. A reduced insulin resistance, as assessed by HOMA-IR, was found in pregnancies after bariatric surgery [41]. In addition, a recent Austrian study found a significant reduction in HOMA-IR and liver fat in post-pregnancy NMR-spectroscopy in a RYGB group in comparison to an obese control group [40]. These results suggest that the positive effect of bariatric surgery on glucose homeostasis cannot solely be explained by weight reduction, but also by weight-independent improvement in insulin sensitivity [41]. Improved insulin sensitivity after SG and RYGB is present well before significant weight loss occurs [17,98]. Bariatric surgery has been proven to resolve or improve pre-existing type 2 diabetes mellitus during 3- to 5-year follow-up periods [99] and preoperative fasting insulin levels are shown to drop by 45% and 50% in the first 3 months after SG and RYGB, respectively [17]. These insights into the mechanisms of substantial insulin sensitivity improvement after bariatric surgery question the high rate of GDM in a pregnancy after bariatric surgery. On the other hand, we would expect insulin resistance during pregnancy to attenuate the severity of reactive hypoglycemia.

The reported dramatic changes in glucose homeostasis after bariatric surgery are variable depending on the timing after surgery [17]. In a pregnancy after bariatric surgery, the length of the interval does not seem to have an effect on the incidence of GDM. However, a shorter interval is related to more frequent occurrence of hypoglycemic events and symptoms consistent with dumping syndrome [43].

5.3. Novelty and Practical Implications

Most research groups divide bariatric surgery in malabsorptive versus restrictive types. SG and LAGB are therefore often considered as a similar operation. This is an archaic differentiation that does not take into account the current insights in the working mechanism of these complex metabolic surgeries [11]. For most bariatric surgery experts, LAGB is no longer considered as one of the gold standard bariatric interventions, since one out of three patients develops band erosions, and almost 50% of patients require band removal [10,100]. On the other hand, SG has proven to have metabolic effects that go well beyond the effect of restriction [101,102]. Since the efficacy of procedures improves, decision making on type of surgery is complex and is often still based on surgeons' preference and experience. An ongoing prospective cohort study comparing the two major types of bariatric surgery will provide more accurate data [103].

Recent data suggest a correlation between hypoglycemia and reduced birthweight in a pregnancy after bariatric surgery [39,41,43]. Wide glycemic excursions and repeated periods of hypoglycemia could lead to the birth of an SGA baby. CGM could provide more detailed insight in glucose homeostasis during a pregnancy after bariatric surgery [36,40]. CGM should be blinded when used as a diagnostic tool, since misinterpretation can lead to aggravation of symptoms and glycemic excursions due to intake of foods with a high glycemic index [44]. Poor glycemic control is a known modifiable risk factor for GDM. In a pregnancy after bariatric surgery, optimizing glycemic time in range through targeted diet recommendations could further prevent adverse outcomes such as fetal growth impairment. Guidelines for adequate weight gain in a pregnancy after bariatric surgery should be reviewed [65].

5.4. Strengths and Limitations

We performed an extensive scoping review on the current knowledge of glucose homeostasis in a pregnancy after bariatric surgery. We specifically addressed the possible association with the development of SGA, as well as the positive impact on GDM prevalence. Because of the heterogeneity and scarcity of existing data, we did not perform a systematic review.

Research on glucose homeostasis after bariatric surgery consists of case-control and cohort studies. Larger, population-based studies have the disadvantage of using hospital or national register data, which makes accurate reporting of key concepts difficult. Most reports use a historical database, where often only ICD9 or ICD10 coding is available. Information on the type of bariatric surgery is not always available. SG and LAGB are often merged into one group of restrictive procedures. This is contrary to progresses made in the understanding of the working mechanism of these two very different operations [11]. In addition, different definitions of SGA were used across different studies. SGA is most commonly defined as a birthweight beneath the 10th percentile, however, some authors define SGA as below the 3rd percentile or less than two standard deviations below mean. The most commonly used diagnostic tool for GDM is a standard 2 h 75 g OGTT, however some studies used different amounts of glucose load. Different hypoglycemic cut-off values are used (50–60 mg/dL) as well as different timings of the glucose measurements. Furthermore, it is well established that an OGTT is unreliable to make a GDM diagnosis in this patient population [91].

5.5. Future Research

In the last 10 years, research has focused on the prevalence of improved and adverse pregnancy outcomes after bariatric surgery. There is now a growing interest and need to investigate the pathophysiology behind these outcomes. There is strong evidence that bariatric surgery induces a substantial shift in the intestinal microbiome [104]. In addition, these alterations have been linked to improved glucose homeostasis in both animal and human research [104]. Indeed, the intestinal microbiome has an important role in the pathophysiology of type 2 diabetes mellitus [105]. Evidence from metabolomics research and intestinal bacterial profiling in a pregnant population that underwent bariatric surgery is currently very limited. Very recently, a small study in pregnant women after bariatric surgery (25 with RYBG and eight with SG), showed that the subgroup with RYBG had significantly lower serum concentrations of branched-chain amino acids (leucine and isoleucine) and branched-chain fatty acids (isobutyrate) in the third trimester of pregnancy [106]. Furthermore, these changes were associated with a shift in the intestinal microbiome. Data from this research also suggest an association with reduced maternal insulin resistance, as well as the risk of delivery of an SGA infant [106]

Another mechanism might be through epigenetic changes. In 2013, a group from Canada and the US reported on differences in DNA methylation profile in offspring of women before versus after biliopancreatic diversion. Improved insulin sensitivity in offspring after biliopancreatic diversion was maintained through childhood [107].

6. Conclusions

Since an OGTT is unreliable to diagnose GDM in a pregnancy after bariatric surgery, the true incidence of GDM is unknown and future research is needed. Data from CBGM and CGM can give more accurate insights in glucose homeostasis in a pregnancy after bariatric surgery. More research is needed to develop accurate guidelines on gestational weight gain, ideal pre-pregnancy BMI, screening strategy and treatment of GDM in this specific population.

Author Contributions: Conceptualization, K.B. and E.D.; methodology, E.D.; resources, E.D.; M.L. and K.B.; writing—original draft preparation, E.D.; writing—review and editing, E.D.; K.B.; M.L.; R.D.; B.V.d.S. All authors have read and agreed to the published version of the manuscript.

Funding: This research received no external funding.

Acknowledgments: K.B., B.v.D. and R.D. are the recipient of a 'Fundamenteel Klinisch Navorserschap FWO Vlaanderen'.

Conflicts of Interest: The authors declare no conflict of interest.

References

1. Afshin, A.; Forouzanfar, M.H.; Reitsma, M.B.; Sur, P.; Estep, K.; Lee, A.; Marczak, L.; Mokdad, A.H.; Moradi-Lakeh, M.; Naghavi, M.; et al. Health effects of overweight and obesity in 195 countries over 25 years. *N. Engl. J. Med.* **2017**, *377*, 13–27. [CrossRef]
2. Drieskens, R.C.S.; Gisle, L. Gezondheidsenquête 2018: Voedingsstatus. Brussel, België: Sciensano; Rapportnummer: D/2019/14.440/53. Available online: https://his.wiv-isp.be/nl/SitePages/Introductiepagina.aspx (accessed on 18 May 2020).
3. Euro-Peristat. Euro-Peristat Project. European Perinatal Health Report. Core Indicators of the Health and Care of Pregnant Women and Babies in Europe in 2015. Available online: www.europeristat.com (accessed on 18 May 2020).
4. Devlieger, R.; Benhalima, K.; Damm, P.; Van Assche, A.; Mathieu, C.; Mahmood, T.; Dunne, F.; Bogaerts, A. Maternal obesity in Europe: Where do we stand and how to move forward? A scientific paper commissioned by the European Board and College of Obstetrics and Gynaecology (EBCOG). *Eur. J. Obstet. Gyn. Reprod. B* **2016**, *201*, 203–208. [CrossRef]
5. Catalano, P.M.; Shankar, K. Obesity and pregnancy: Mechanisms of short term and long term adverse consequences for mother and child. *BMJ* **2017**, *356*, j1. [CrossRef]
6. Adams, T.D.; Davidson, L.E.; Hunt, S.C. Weight and metabolic outcomes 12 years after gastric bypass. *N. Engl. J. Med.* **2018**, *378*, 93–96. [CrossRef] [PubMed]
7. Welbourn, R.; Hollyman, M.; Kinsman, R.; Dixon, J.; Liem, R.; Ottosson, J.; Ramos, A.; Vage, V.; Al-Sabah, S.; Brown, W.; et al. Bariatric surgery worldwide: Baseline demographic description and one-year outcomes from the fourth IFSO global registry report 2018. *Obes. Surg.* **2019**, *29*, 782–795. [CrossRef] [PubMed]
8. Akhter, Z.; Rankin, J.; Ceulemans, D.; Ngongalah, L.; Ackroyd, R.; Devlieger, R.; Vieira, R.; Heslehurst, N. Pregnancy after bariatric surgery and adverse perinatal outcomes: A systematic review and meta-analysis. *PLoS Med.* **2019**, *16*, e1002866. [CrossRef] [PubMed]
9. Angrisani, L.; Lorenzo, M.; Borrelli, V. Laparoscopic adjustable gastric banding versus Roux-en-Y gastric bypass: 5-Year results of a prospective randomized trial. *Surg. Obes. Relat. Dis.* **2007**, *3*, 127–132. [CrossRef] [PubMed]
10. Himpens, J.; Cadiere, G.B.; Bazi, M.; Vouche, M.; Cadiere, B.; Dapri, G. Long-term outcomes of laparoscopic adjustable gastric banding. *Arch. Surg.* **2011**, *146*, 802–807. [CrossRef]

11. Batterham, R.L.; Cummings, D.E. Mechanisms of diabetes improvement following bariatric/metabolic surgery. *Diabetes Care* **2016**, *39*, 893–901. [CrossRef]
12. Cavin, J.B.; Bado, A.; Le Gall, M. Intestinal adaptations after bariatric surgery: Consequences on glucose homeostasis. *Trends Endocrinol. Metab.* **2017**, *28*, 354–364. [CrossRef]
13. Kefurt, R.; Langer, F.B.; Schindler, K.; Shakeri-Leidenmuhler, S.; Ludvik, B.; Prager, G. Hypoglycemia after Roux-En-Y gastric bypass: Detection rates of continuous glucose monitoring (CGM) versus mixed meal test. *Surg. Obes. Relat. Dis.* **2015**, *11*, 564–569. [CrossRef] [PubMed]
14. Schauer, P.R.; Kashyap, S.R.; Wolski, K.; Brethauer, S.A.; Kirwan, J.P.; Pothier, C.E.; Thomas, S.; Abood, B.; Nissen, S.E.; Bhatt, D.L. Bariatric surgery versus intensive medical therapy in obese patients with diabetes. *N. Engl. J. Med.* **2012**, *366*, 1567–1576. [CrossRef] [PubMed]
15. Dutia, R.; Brakoniecki, K.; Bunker, P.; Paultre, F.; Homel, P.; Carpentier, A.C.; Mcginty, J.; Laferrère, B. Limited recovery of b-cell function after gastric bypass despite clinical diabetes remission. *Diabetes* **2014**, *63*, 1214–1223. [CrossRef] [PubMed]
16. Sjostrom, L. Review of the key results from the Swedish Obese Subjects (SOS) trial—A prospective controlled intervention study of bariatric surgery. *J. Intern. Med.* **2013**, *273*, 219–234. [CrossRef]
17. Peterli, R.; Wolnerhanssen, B.; Peters, T.; Devaux, N.; Kern, B.; Christoffel-Courtin, C.; Drewe, J.; von Flue, M.; Beglinger, C. Improvement in glucose metabolism after bariatric surgery: Comparison of laparoscopic Roux-en-Y gastric bypass and laparoscopic sleeve gastrectomy: A prospective randomized trial. *Ann. Surg.* **2009**, *250*, 234–241. [CrossRef]
18. Mingrone, G.; Panunzi, S.; De Gaetano, A.; Ahlin, S.; Spuntarelli, V.; Bondia-Pons, I.; Barbieri, C.; Capristo, E.; Gastaldelli, A.; Nolan, J.J. Insulin sensitivity depends on the route of glucose administration. *Diabetologia* **2020**, *63*, 1382–1395. [CrossRef]
19. Tharakan, G.; Behary, P.; Wewer Albrechtsen, N.J.; Chahal, H.; Kenkre, J.; Miras, A.D.; Ahmed, A.R.; Holst, J.J.; Bloom, S.R.; Tan, T. Roles of increased glycaemic variability, GLP-1 and glucagon in hypoglycaemia after Roux-en-Y gastric bypass. *Eur. J. Endocrinol.* **2017**, *177*, 455–464. [CrossRef]
20. Capristo, E.; Panunzi, S.; De Gaetano, A.; Spuntarelli, V.; Bellantone, R.; Giustacchini, P.; Birkenfeld, A.L.; Amiel, S.; Bornstein, S.R.; Raffaelli, M.; et al. Incidence of Hypoglycemia After Gastric Bypass vs. Sleeve Gastrectomy: A Randomized Trial. *J. Clin. Endocrinol. Metab.* **2018**, *103*, 2136–2146. [CrossRef]
21. Galazis, N.; Docheva, N.; Simillis, C.; Nicolaides, K.H. Maternal and neonatal outcomes in women undergoing bariatric surgery: A systematic review and meta-analysis. *Eur. J. Obstet. Gynecol. Reprod. Biol.* **2014**, *181*, 45–53. [CrossRef]
22. Kwong, W.; Tomlinson, G.; Feig, D.S. Maternal and neonatal outcomes after bariatric surgery; a systematic review and meta-analysis: Do the benefits outweigh the risks? *Am. J. Obstet. Gynecol.* **2018**, *218*, 573–580. [CrossRef]
23. Yi, X.Y.; Li, Q.F.; Zhang, J.; Wang, Z.H. A meta-analysis of maternal and fetal outcomes of pregnancy after bariatric surgery. *Int. J. Gynaecol. Obstet.* **2015**, *130*, 3–9. [CrossRef]
24. Wang, J.; Shen, S.; Price, M.J.; Lu, J.; Sumilo, D.; Kuang, Y.; Manolopoulos, K.; Xia, H.; Qiu, X.; Cheng, K.K.; et al. Glucose, insulin, and lipids in cord blood of neonates and their association with birthweight: Differential metabolic risk of large for gestational age and small for gestational age babies. *J. Pediatr.* **2020**, *220*, 64–72.e2. [CrossRef] [PubMed]
25. Scholl, T.O.; Sowers, M.; Chen, X.; Lenders, C. Maternal glucose concentration influences fetal growth, gestation, and pregnancy complications. *Am. J. Epidemiol.* **2001**, *154*, 514–520. [CrossRef] [PubMed]
26. Abell, D.A.; Beischer, N.A. Relationship between maternal glucose-tolerance and fetal size at birth. *Aust. Nz. J. Obstet. Gyn.* **1976**, *16*, 1–4. [CrossRef]
27. Khouzami, V.A.; Ginsburg, D.S.; Daikoku, N.H.; Johnson, J.W. The glucose tolerance test as a means of identifying intrauterine growth retardation. *Am. J. Obstet. Gynecol.* **1981**, *139*, 423–426. [CrossRef]
28. Langer, O.; Damus, K.; Maiman, M.; Divon, M.; Levy, J.; Bauman, W. A link between relative hypoglycemia-hypoinsulinemia during oral glucose tolerance tests and intrauterine growth retardation. *Am. J. Obstet. Gynecol.* **1986**, *155*, 711–716. [CrossRef]
29. Nayak, A.U.; Vijay, A.M.A.; Indusekhar, R.; Kalidindi, S.; Katreddy, V.M.; Varadhan, L. Association of hypoglycaemia in screening oral glucose tolerance test in pregnancy with low birth weight fetus. *World J. Diabetes* **2019**, *10*, 304–310. [CrossRef]

30. Plows, J.F.; Stanley, J.L.; Baker, P.N.; Reynolds, C.M.; Vickers, M.H. The pathophysiology of gestational diabetes mellitus. *Int. J. Mol. Sci.* **2018**, *19*, 3342. [CrossRef]
31. Rogne, T.; Jacobsen, G.W. Association between low blood glucose increase during glucose tolerance tests in pregnancy and impaired fetal growth. *Acta Obstet. Gyn. Scan.* **2014**, *93*, 1160–1169. [CrossRef]
32. Capula, C.; Chiefari, E.; Vero, A.; Arcidiacono, B.; Iiritano, S.; Puccio, L.; Pullano, V.; Foti, D.P.; Brunetti, A.; Vero, R. Gestational diabetes mellitus: Screening and outcomes in southern Italian pregnant women. *ISRN Endocrinol.* **2013**, *2013*, 387495. [CrossRef]
33. Gopalakrishnan, V.; Singh, R.; Pradeep, Y.; Kapoor, D.; Rani, A.K.; Pradhan, S.; Bhatia, E.; Yadav, S.B. Evaluation of the prevalence of gestational diabetes mellitus in North Indians using the International Association of Diabetes and Pregnancy Study groups (IADPSG) criteria. *J. Postgrad. Med.* **2015**, *61*, 155–158. [CrossRef] [PubMed]
34. Tricco, A.C.; Lillie, E.; Zarin, W.; O'Brien, K.K.; Colquhoun, H.; Levac, D.; Moher, D.; Peters, M.D.J.; Horsley, T.; Weeks, L.; et al. PRISMA Extension for Scoping Reviews (PRISMA-ScR): Checklist and Explanation. *Ann. Intern. Med.* **2018**, *169*, 467–473. [CrossRef] [PubMed]
35. Andrade, H.F.; Pedrosa, W.; Diniz Mde, F.; Passos, V.M. Adverse effects during the oral glucose tolerance test in post-bariatric surgery patients. *Arch. Endocrinol. Metab.* **2016**, *60*, 307–313. [CrossRef] [PubMed]
36. Bonis, C.; Lorenzini, F.; Bertrand, M.; Parant, O.; Gourdy, P.; Vaurs, C.; Cazals, L.; Ritz, P.; Hanaire, H. Glucose Profiles in Pregnant Women After a Gastric Bypass: Findings from Continuous Glucose Monitoring. *Obes. Surg.* **2016**, *26*, 2150–2155. [CrossRef]
37. Feichtinger, M.; Stopp, T.; Hofmann, S.; Springer, S.; Pils, S.; Kautzky-Willer, A.; Kiss, H.; Eppel, W.; Tura, A.; Bozkurt, L.; et al. Altered glucose profiles and risk for hypoglycaemia during oral glucose tolerance testing in pregnancies after gastric bypass surgery. *Diabetologia* **2017**, *60*, 153–157. [CrossRef] [PubMed]
38. Freitas, C.; Araujo, C.; Caldas, R.; Lopes, D.S.; Nora, M.; Monteiro, M.P. Effect of new criteria on the diagnosis of gestational diabetes in women submitted to gastric bypass. *Surg. Obes. Relat. Dis.* **2014**, *10*, 1041–1046. [CrossRef]
39. Gobl, C.S.; Bozkurt, L.; Tura, A.; Leutner, M.; Andrei, L.; Fahr, L.; Husslein, P.; Eppel, W.; Kautzky-Willer, A. Assessment of glucose regulation in pregnancy after gastric bypass surgery. *Diabetologia* **2017**, *60*, 2504–2513. [CrossRef]
40. Leutner, M.; Klimek, P.; Gobl, C.; Bozkurt, L.; Harreiter, J.; Husslein, P.; Eppel, W.; Baumgartner-Parzer, S.; Pacini, G.; Thurner, S.; et al. Glucagon-like peptide 1 (GLP-1) drives postprandial hyperinsulinemic hypoglycemia in pregnant women with a history of Roux-en-Y gastric bypass operation. *Metabolism* **2019**, *91*, 10–17. [CrossRef]
41. Maric, T.; Kanu, C.; Johnson, M.R.; Savvidou, M.D. Maternal, neonatal insulin resistance and neonatal anthropometrics in pregnancies following bariatric surgery. *Metabolism* **2019**, *97*, 25–31. [CrossRef]
42. Maric, T.; Kanu, C.; Muller, D.C.; Tzoulaki, I.; Johnson, M.R.; Savvidou, M.D. Fetal growth and feto-placental circulation in pregnancies following bariatric surgery: A prospective study. *BJOG* **2020**, *127*, 847. [CrossRef]
43. Rottenstreich, A.; Elazary, R.; Ezra, Y.; Kleinstern, G.; Beglaibter, N.; Elchalal, U. Hypoglycemia during oral glucose tolerance test among post–bariatric surgery pregnant patients: Incidence and perinatal significance. *Surg. Obes. Relat. Dis.* **2018**, *14*, 347–353. [CrossRef] [PubMed]
44. Novodvorsky, P.; Walkinshaw, E.; Rahman, W.; Gordon, V.; Towse, K.; Mitchell, S.; Selvarajah, D.; Madhuvrata, P.; Munir, A. Experience with Freestyle libre flash glucose monitoring system in management of refractory dumping syndrome in pregnancy shortly after bariatric surgery. *Endocrinol. Diabetes. Metab. Case Rep.* **2017**, *2017*. [CrossRef] [PubMed]
45. Catalano, P.M.; Presley, L.; Minium, J.; Hauguel-de Mouzon, S. Fetuses of obese mothers develop insulin resistance in utero. *Diabetes Care* **2009**, *32*, 1076–1080. [CrossRef] [PubMed]
46. Norgaard, L.N.; Gjerris, A.C.; Kirkegaard, I.; Berlac, J.F.; Tabor, A. Fetal growth in pregnancies conceived after gastric bypass surgery in relation to surgery-to-conception interval: A Danish national cohort study. *PLoS ONE* **2014**, *9*, e90317. [CrossRef] [PubMed]
47. Kjaer, M.M.; Lauenborg, J.; Breum, B.M.; Nilas, L. The risk of adverse pregnancy outcome after bariatric surgery: A nationwide register-based matched cohort study. *Am. J. Obstet. Gynecol.* **2013**, *208*, 464.e1–464.e4645. [CrossRef] [PubMed]
48. Kjaer, M.M.; Nilas, L. Timing of pregnancy after gastric bypass-a national register-based cohort study. *Obes. Surg.* **2013**, *23*, 1281–1285. [CrossRef]

49. Johansson, K.; Cnattingius, S.; Näslund, I.; Roos, N.; Lagerros, Y.T.; Granath, F.; Stephansson, O.; Neovius, M. Outcomes of pregnancy after bariatric surgery. *N. Engl. J. Med.* **2015**, *372*, 814–824. [CrossRef]
50. Josefsson, A.; Blomberg, M.; Bladh, M.; Frederiksen, S.G.; Sydsjo, G. Bariatric surgery in a national cohort of women: Sociodemographics and obstetric outcomes. *Am. J. Obstet. Gynecol.* **2011**, *205*, 206.e201–208. [CrossRef]
51. Roos, N.; Neovius, M.; Cnattingius, S.; Trolle Lagerros, Y.; Saaf, M.; Granath, F.; Stephansson, O. Perinatal outcomes after bariatric surgery: Nationwide population based matched cohort study. *BMJ* **2013**, *347*, f6460. [CrossRef]
52. Adams, T.D.; Hammoud, A.O.; Davidson, L.E.; Laferrere, B.; Fraser, A.; Stanford, J.B.; Hashibe, M.; Greenwood, J.L.; Kim, J.; Taylor, D.; et al. Maternal and neonatal outcomes for pregnancies before and after gastric bypass surgery. *Int. J. Obes.* **2015**, *39*, 686–694. [CrossRef]
53. Belogolovkin, V.; Salihu, H.M.; Weldeselasse, H.; Biroscak, B.J.; August, E.M.; Mbah, A.K.; Alio, A.P. Impact of prior bariatric surgery on maternal and fetal outcomes among obese and non-obese mothers. *Arch. Gynecol. Obstet.* **2012**, *285*, 1211–1218. [CrossRef] [PubMed]
54. Parent, B.; Martopullo, I.; Weiss, N.S.; Khandelwal, S.; Fay, E.E.; Rowhani-Rahbar, A. Bariatric surgery in women of childbearing age, timing between an operation and birth, and associated perinatal complications. *JAMA Surg.* **2017**, *152*, 128–135. [CrossRef] [PubMed]
55. Parker, M.H.; Berghella, V.; Nijjar, J.B. Bariatric surgery and associated adverse pregnancy outcomes among obese women. *J. Matern. Fetal Neonatal Med.* **2016**, *29*, 1747–1750. [CrossRef] [PubMed]
56. Balestrin, B.; Urbanetz, A.A.; Barbieri, M.M.; Paes, A.; Fujie, J. Pregnancy After Bariatric Surgery: A comparative study of post-bariatric pregnant women versus non-bariatric obese pregnant women. *Obes. Surg.* **2019**, *29*, 3142–3148. [CrossRef] [PubMed]
57. Basbug, A.; Ellibes Kaya, A.; Dogan, S.; Pehlivan, M.; Goynumer, G. Does pregnancy interval after laparoscopic sleeve gastrectomy affect maternal and perinatal outcomes? *J. Matern. Fetal Neonatal Med.* **2019**, *32*, 3764–3770. [CrossRef]
58. Chevrot, A.; Kayem, G.; Coupaye, M.; Lesage, N.; Msika, S.; Mandelbrot, L. Impact of bariatric surgery on fetal growth restriction: Experience of a perinatal and bariatric surgery center. *Am. J. Obstet. Gynecol.* **2016**, *214*, 655.e1–655.e6557. [CrossRef]
59. Costa, M.M.; Belo, S.; Souteiro, P.; Neves, J.S.; Magalhaes, D.; Silva, R.B.; Oliveira, S.C.; Freitas, P.; Varela, A.; Queiros, J.; et al. Pregnancy after bariatric surgery: Maternal and fetal outcomes of 39 pregnancies and a literature review. *J. Obstet. Gynaecol. Res.* **2018**, *44*, 681–690. [CrossRef]
60. Dolin, C.D.; Chervenak, J.; Pivo, S.; Ude Welcome, A.; Kominiarek, M.A. Association between time interval from bariatric surgery to pregnancy and maternal weight outcomes. *J. Matern. Fetal Neonatal Med.* **2019**, *13*, 1–7. [CrossRef]
61. Ducarme, G.; Parisio, L.; Santulli, P.; Carbillon, L.; Mandelbrot, L.; Luton, D. Neonatal outcomes in pregnancies after bariatric surgery: A retrospective multi-centric cohort study in three French referral centers. *J. Matern. Fetal Neonatal Med.* **2013**, *26*, 275–278. [CrossRef]
62. Feichtinger, M.; Falcone, V.; Schoenleitner, T.; Stopp, T.; Husslein, P.W.; Eppel, W.; Chalubinski, K.M.; Gobl, C.S. Intrauterine fetal growth delay during late pregnancy after maternal gastric bypass surgery. *Ultraschall Med.* **2018**, *41*, 52–59. [CrossRef]
63. Gascoin, G.; Gerard, M.; Salle, A.; Becouarn, G.; Rouleau, S.; Sentilhes, L.; Coutant, R. Risk of low birth weight and micronutrient deficiencies in neonates from mothers after gastric bypass: A case control study. *Surg. Obes. Relat. Dis.* **2017**, *13*, 1384–1391. [CrossRef] [PubMed]
64. Gonzalez, I.; Rubio, M.A.; Cordido, F.; Breton, I.; Morales, M.J.; Vilarrasa, N.; Monereo, S.; Lecube, A.; Caixas, A.; Vinagre, I.; et al. Maternal and perinatal outcomes after bariatric surgery: A Spanish multicenter study. *Obes. Surg.* **2015**, *25*, 436–442. [CrossRef] [PubMed]
65. Grandfils, S.; Demondion, D.; Kyheng, M.; Duhamel, A.; Lorio, E.; Pattou, F.; Deruelle, P. Impact of gestational weight gain on perinatal outcomes after a bariatric surgery. *J. Gynecol. Obstet. Hum. Reprod.* **2019**, *48*, 401–405. [CrossRef] [PubMed]
66. Hammeken, L.H.; Betsagoo, R.; Jensen, A.N.; Sorensen, A.N.; Overgaard, C. Nutrient deficiency and obstetrical outcomes in pregnant women following Roux-en-Y gastric bypass: A retrospective Danish cohort study with a matched comparison group. *Eur. J. Obstet. Gynecol. Reprod. Biol.* **2017**, *216*, 56–60. [CrossRef]

67. Hazart, J.; Le Guennec, D.; Accoceberry, M.; Lemery, D.; Mulliez, A.; Farigon, N.; Lahaye, C.; Miolanne-Debouit, M.; Boirie, Y. Maternal Nutritional Deficiencies and Small-for-Gestational-Age Neonates at Birth of Women Who Have Undergone Bariatric Surgery. *J. Pregnancy* **2017**, *2017*, 4168541. [CrossRef]
68. Karadag, C.; Demircan, S.; Caliskan, E. Effects of laparoscopic sleeve gastrectomy on obstetric outcomes within 12 months after surgery. *J. Obstet. Gynaecol. Res.* **2019**, *46*, 266–271. [CrossRef]
69. Lesko, J.; Peaceman, A. Pregnancy outcomes in women after bariatric surgery compared with obese and morbidly obese controls. *Obstet. Gynecol.* **2012**, *119*, 547–554. [CrossRef]
70. Rottenstreich, A.; Elchalal, U.; Kleinstern, G.; Beglaibter, N.; Khalaileh, A.; Elazary, R. Maternal and Perinatal outcomes after laparoscopic sleeve gastrectomy. *Obstet. Gynecol.* **2018**, *131*, 451–456. [CrossRef]
71. Rottenstreich, A.; Levin, G.; Kleinstern, G.; Rottenstreich, M.; Elchalal, U.; Elazary, R. The effect of surgery-to-conception interval on pregnancy outcomes after sleeve gastrectomy. *Surg. Obes. Relat. Dis.* **2018**, *14*, 1795–1803. [CrossRef]
72. Sancak, S.; Celer, O.; Cirak, E.; Karip, A.B.; Tumicin Aydin, M.; Esen Bulut, N.; Mahir Fersahoglu, M.; Altun, H.; Memisoglu, K. Timing of gestation After Laparoscopic Sleeve Gastrectomy (LSG): Does it influence obstetrical and neonatal outcomes of pregnancies? *Obes. Surg.* **2019**, *29*, 1498–1505. [CrossRef]
73. Stentebjerg, L.L.; Andersen, L.L.T.; Renault, K.; Stoving, R.K.; Jensen, D.M. Pregnancy and perinatal outcomes according to surgery to conception interval and gestational weight gain in women with previous gastric bypass. *J. Matern. Fetal Neonatal Med.* **2017**, *30*, 1182–1188. [CrossRef] [PubMed]
74. Berlac, J.F.; Skovlund, C.W.; Lidegaard, O. Obstetrical and neonatal outcomes in women following gastric bypass: A Danish national cohort study. *Acta Obstet. Gynecol. Scand.* **2014**, *93*, 447–453. [CrossRef] [PubMed]
75. Ibiebele, I.; Gallimore, F.; Schnitzler, M.; Torvaldsen, S.; Ford, J.B. Perinatal outcomes following bariatric surgery between a first and second pregnancy: A population data linkage study. *BJOG* **2020**, *127*, 345–354. [CrossRef] [PubMed]
76. Amsalem, D.; Aricha-Tamir, B.; Levi, I.; Shai, D.; Sheiner, E. Obstetric outcomes after restrictive bariatric surgery: What happens after 2 consecutive pregnancies? *Surg. Obes. Relat. Dis.* **2014**, *10*, 445–449. [CrossRef] [PubMed]
77. Burke, A.E.; Bennett, W.L.; Jamshidi, R.M.; Gilson, M.M.; Clark, J.M.; Segal, J.B.; Shore, A.D.; Magnuson, T.H.; Dominici, F.; Wu, A.W.; et al. Reduced incidence of gestational diabetes with bariatric surgery. *J. Am. Coll. Surg.* **2010**, *211*, 169–175. [CrossRef]
78. de Alencar Costa, L.A.; Araujo Junior, E.; de Lucena Feitosa, F.E.; Dos Santos, A.C.; Moura Junior, L.G.; Costa Carvalho, F.H. Maternal and perinatal outcomes after bariatric surgery: A case control study. *J. Perinat. Med.* **2016**, *44*, 383–388. [CrossRef]
79. Han, S.M.; Kim, W.W.; Moon, R.; Rosenthal, R.J. Pregnancy outcomes after laparoscopic sleeve gastrectomy in morbidly obese Korean patients. *Obes. Surg.* **2013**, *23*, 756–759. [CrossRef]
80. Malakauskiene, L.; Nadisauskiene, R.J.; Ramasauskaite, D.; Bartuseviciene, E.; Ramoniene, G.; Maleckiene, L. Is it necessary to postpone pregnancy after bariatric surgery: A national cohort study. *J. Obstet. Gynaecol.* **2020**, *40*, 614–618. [CrossRef]
81. Rasteiro, C.; Araujo, C.; Cunha, S.; Caldas, R.; Mesquita, J.; Seixas, A.; Augusto, N.; Ramalho, C. Influence of time interval from bariatric surgery to conception on pregnancy and perinatal outcomes. *Obes. Surg.* **2018**, *28*, 3559–3566. [CrossRef]
82. Rottenstreich, A.; Levin, G.; Rottenstreich, M.; Ezra, Y.; Elazary, R.; Elchalal, U. Twin pregnancy outcomes after metabolic and bariatric surgery. *Surg. Obes. Relat. Dis.* **2019**, *15*, 759–765. [CrossRef]
83. Shai, D.; Shoham-Vardi, I.; Amsalem, D.; Silverberg, D.; Levi, I.; Sheiner, E. Pregnancy outcome of patients following bariatric surgery as compared with obese women: A population-based study. *J. Matern. Fetal Neonatal Med.* **2014**, *27*, 275–278. [CrossRef] [PubMed]
84. Sheiner, E.; Edri, A.; Balaban, E.; Levi, I.; Aricha-Tamir, B. Pregnancy outcome of patients who conceive during or after the first year following bariatric surgery. *Am. J. Obstet. Gynecol.* **2011**, *204*, 50.e1–50.e6. [CrossRef] [PubMed]
85. Stone, R.A.; Huffman, J.; Istwan, N.; Desch, C.; Rhea, D.; Stanziano, G.; Joy, S. Pregnancy outcomes following bariatric surgery. *J. Womens Health* **2011**, *20*, 1363–1366. [CrossRef] [PubMed]
86. Watanabe, A.; Seki, Y.; Haruta, H.; Kikkawa, E.; Kasama, K. Maternal impacts and perinatal outcomes after three types of bariatric surgery at a single institution. *Arch. Gynecol. Obstet.* **2019**, *300*, 145–152. [CrossRef] [PubMed]

87. Yau, P.O.; Parikh, M.; Saunders, J.K.; Chui, P.; Zablocki, T.; Welcome, A.U. Pregnancy after bariatric surgery: The effect of time-to-conception on pregnancy outcomes. *Surg. Obes. Relat. Dis.* **2017**, *13*, 1899–1905. [CrossRef] [PubMed]
88. Shawe, J.; Ceulemans, D.; Akhter, Z.; Neff, K.; Hart, K.; Heslehurst, N.; Stotl, I.; Agrawal, S.; Steegers-Theunissen, R.; Taheri, S.; et al. Pregnancy after bariatric surgery: Consensus recommendations for periconception, antenatal and postnatal care. *Obes. Rev.* **2019**, *20*, 1507–1522. [CrossRef]
89. American Diabetes, A. 2. Classification and diagnosis of diabetes: Standards of medical care in diabetes-2020. *Diabetes Care* **2020**, *43*, S14–S31. [CrossRef]
90. Benhalima, K.; Minschart, C.; Van Crombrugge, P.; Calewaert, P.; Verhaeghe, J.; Vandamme, S.; Theetaert, K.; Devlieger, R.; Pierssens, L.; Ryckeghem, H.; et al. The 2019 Flemish consensus on screening for overt diabetes in early pregnancy and screening for gestational diabetes mellitus. *Acta Clin. Belg.* **2019**, *1*, 1–8. [CrossRef]
91. Benhalima, K.; Minschart, C.; Ceulemans, D.; Bogaerts, A.; Van Der Schueren, B.; Mathieu, C.; Devlieger, R. Screening and management of gestational diabetes mellitus after bariatric surgery. *Nutrients* **2018**, *10*, 1479. [CrossRef]
92. Campbell, J.M.; McPherson, N.O. Influence of increased paternal BMI on pregnancy and child health outcomes independent of maternal effects: A systematic review and meta-analysis. *Obes. Res. Clin. Pract.* **2019**, *13*, 511–521. [CrossRef]
93. Jans, G.; Matthys, C.; Bogaerts, A.; Lannoo, M.; Verhaeghe, J.; Van der Schueren, B.; Devlieger, R. Maternal micronutrient deficiencies and related adverse neonatal outcomes after bariatric surgery: A systematic review. *Adv. Nutr.* **2015**, *6*, 420–429. [CrossRef] [PubMed]
94. Mechanick, J.I.; Youdim, A.; Jones, D.B.; Garvey, W.T.; Hurley, D.L.; McMahon, M.M.; Heinberg, L.J.; Kushner, R.; Adams, T.D.; Shikora, S.; et al. Clinical practice guidelines for the perioperative nutritional, metabolic, and nonsurgical support of the bariatric surgery patient—2013 update: Cosponsored by American Association of Clinical Endocrinologists, The Obesity Society, and American Society for Metabolic & Bariatric Surgery. *Obesity* **2013**, *21* (Suppl. 1), S1–S27. [CrossRef] [PubMed]
95. Barbour, L.A.; Hernandez, T.L. Maternal non-glycemic contributors to fetal growth in obesity and gestational diabetes: Spotlight on lipids. *Curr. Diab. Rep.* **2018**, *18*, 37. [CrossRef] [PubMed]
96. Miranda, J.; Simoes, R.V.; Paules, C.; Canueto, D.; Pardo-Cea, M.A.; Garcia-Martin, M.L.; Crovetto, F.; Fuertes-Martin, R.; Domenech, M.; Gomez-Roig, M.D.; et al. Metabolic profiling and targeted lipidomics reveals a disturbed lipid profile in mothers and fetuses with intrauterine growth restriction. *Sci. Rep.* **2018**, *8*, 13614. [CrossRef]
97. Shroff, M.R.; Holzman, C.; Tian, Y.; Evans, R.W.; Sikorskii, A. Mid-pregnancy maternal leptin levels, birthweight for gestational age and preterm delivery. *Clin. Endocrinol.* **2013**, *78*, 607–613. [CrossRef]
98. Pories, W.J.; Swanson, M.S.; MacDonald, K.G.; Long, S.B.; Morris, P.G.; Brown, B.M.; Barakat, H.A.; deRamon, R.A.; Israel, G.; Dolezal, J.M.; et al. Who would have thought it? An operation proves to be the most effective therapy for adult-onset diabetes mellitus. *Ann. Surg.* **1995**, *222*, 339–350. [CrossRef]
99. Osland, E.; Yunus, R.M.; Khan, S.; Memon, B.; Memon, M.A. Diabetes improvement and resolution following laparoscopic vertical sleeve gastrectomy (LVSG) versus laparoscopic Roux-en-Y gastric bypass (LRYGB) procedures: A systematic review of randomized controlled trials. *Surg. Endosc.* **2017**, *31*, 1952–1963. [CrossRef]
100. Magouliotis, D.E.; Tasiopoulou, V.S.; Svokos, A.A.; Svokos, K.A.; Sioka, E.; Zacharoulis, D. Roux-En-Y gastric bypass versus sleeve gastrectomy as revisional procedure after adjustable gastric band: A systematic review and meta-analysis. *Obes. Surg.* **2017**, *27*, 1365–1373. [CrossRef]
101. Peterli, R.; Wolnerhanssen, B.K.; Peters, T.; Vetter, D.; Kroll, D.; Borbely, Y.; Schultes, B.; Beglinger, C.; Drewe, J.; Schiesser, M.; et al. Effect of laparoscopic sleeve gastrectomy vs laparoscopic Roux-en-Y Gastric bypass on weight loss in patients with morbid obesity: The SM-BOSS randomized clinical trial. *JAMA* **2018**, *319*, 255–265. [CrossRef]
102. Salminen, P.; Helmio, M.; Ovaska, J.; Juuti, A.; Leivonen, M.; Peromaa-Haavisto, P.; Hurme, S.; Soinio, M.; Nuutila, P.; Victorzon, M. Effect of laparoscopic sleeve gastrectomy vs laparoscopic Roux-en-Y gastric bypass on weight loss at 5 years among patients with morbid obesity: The sleevepass randomized clinical trial. *JAMA* **2018**, *319*, 241–254. [CrossRef]

103. Jans, G.; Matthys, C.; Bel, S.; Ameye, L.; Lannoo, M.; Van der Schueren, B.; Dillemans, B.; Lemmens, L.; Saey, J.P.; van Nieuwenhove, Y.; et al. Aurora: Bariatric surgery registration in women of reproductive age—A multicenter prospective cohort study. *BMC Pregnancy Childbirth* **2016**, *16*, 195. [CrossRef] [PubMed]
104. Guo, Y.; Huang, Z.P.; Liu, C.Q.; Qi, L.; Sheng, Y.; Zou, D.J. Modulation of the gut microbiome: A systematic review of the effect of bariatric surgery. *Eur. J. Endocrinol.* **2018**, *178*, 43–56. [CrossRef] [PubMed]
105. Kahn, S.E.; Cooper, M.E.; Del Prato, S. Pathophysiology and treatment of type 2 diabetes: Perspectives on the past, present, and future. *Lancet* **2014**, *383*, 1068–1083. [CrossRef]
106. West, K.A.; Kanu, C.; Maric, T.; McDonald, J.A.K.; Nicholson, J.K.; Li, J.V.; Johnson, M.R.; Holmes, E.; Savvidou, M.D. Longitudinal metabolic and gut bacterial profiling of pregnant women with previous bariatric surgery. *Gut* **2020**, *69*, 1452–1459. [CrossRef] [PubMed]
107. Guenard, F.; Deshaies, Y.; Cianflone, K.; Kral, J.G.; Marceau, P.; Vohl, M.C. Differential methylation in glucoregulatory genes of offspring born before vs. after maternal gastrointestinal bypass surgery. *Proc. Natl. Acad. Sci. USA* **2013**, *110*, 11439–11444. [CrossRef] [PubMed]

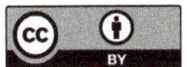

© 2020 by the authors. Licensee MDPI, Basel, Switzerland. This article is an open access article distributed under the terms and conditions of the Creative Commons Attribution (CC BY) license (http://creativecommons.org/licenses/by/4.0/).

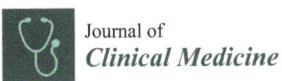

Article

Limiting the Use of Oral Glucose Tolerance Tests to Screen for Hyperglycemia in Pregnancy during Pandemics

Charlotte Nachtergaele [1], Eric Vicaut [1], Sopio Tatulashvili [2], Sara Pinto [3], Hélène Bihan [2], Meriem Sal [2], Narimane Berkane [2], Lucie Allard [2], Camille Baudry [2], Jean-Jacques Portal [1], Lionel Carbillon [4] and Emmanuel Cosson [2,5,*]

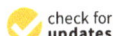

Citation: Nachtergaele, C.; Vicaut, E.; Tatulashvili, S.; Pinto, S.; Bihan, H.; Sal, M.; Berkane, N.; Allard, L.; Baudry, C.; Portal, J.-J.; et al. Limiting the Use of Oral Glucose Tolerance Tests to Screen for Hyperglycemia in Pregnancy during Pandemics. *J. Clin. Med.* **2021**, *10*, 397. https://doi.org/10.3390/jcm10030397

Received: 18 December 2020
Accepted: 17 January 2021
Published: 21 January 2021

Publisher's Note: MDPI stays neutral with regard to jurisdictional claims in published maps and institutional affiliations.

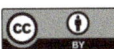

Copyright: © 2021 by the authors. Licensee MDPI, Basel, Switzerland. This article is an open access article distributed under the terms and conditions of the Creative Commons Attribution (CC BY) license (https://creativecommons.org/licenses/by/4.0/).

[1] AP-HP, Unité de Recherche Clinique St-Louis-Lariboisière, Université Denis Diderot, 75009 Paris, France; nachtergaele.charlotte@yahoo.fr (C.N.); eric.vicaut@aphp.fr (E.V.); jean-jacques.portal@aphp.fr (J.-J.P.)
[2] AP-HP, Department of Endocrinology-Diabetology-Nutrition, Avicenne Hospital, Paris 13 University, Sorbonne Paris Cité, CRNH-IdF, CINFO, 93 000 Bobigny, France; sopio.tatulashvili@aphp.fr (S.T.); helene.bihan@aphp.fr (H.B.); meriem.sal@aphp.fr (M.S.); narimane.berkane@aphp.fr (N.B.); lucie.allard@aphp.fr (L.A.); camille.baudry@aphp.fr (C.B.)
[3] AP-HP, Department of Endocrinology-Diabetology-Nutrition, Jean Verdier Hospital, Paris 13 University, Sorbonne Paris Cité, CRNH-IdF, CINFO, 93 143 Bondy, France; sara.pinto@aphp.fr
[4] AP-HP, Department of Obstetrics and Gynecology, Jean Verdier Hospital, Paris 13 University, Sorbonne Paris Cité, 93 000 Bondy, France; lionel.carbillon@aphp.fr
[5] Paris 13 University, Sorbonne Paris Cité, UMR U557 INSERM/U11125 INRAE/CNAM/Université Paris13, Unité de Recherche Epidémiologique Nutritionnelle, 93 000 Bobigny, France
* Correspondence: emmanuel.cosson@aphp.fr; Tel.: +33-1-48-95-59-47; Fax: +33-1-48-95-55-60

Abstract: We aimed to evaluate each proposal of Australian–New Zealand Societies to limit the number of oral glucose tolerance tests (OGTTs) to diagnose hyperglycemia in pregnancy (HIP) during the coronavirus disease 2019 (COVID-19) pandemic. At our university hospital (2012–2016), we retrospectively applied in 4245 women who had OGTT between 22 and 30 weeks of gestation (reference standard: WHO criteria) the proposals in which OGTT is performed only in high-risk women; in all (Option 1) or high-risk (Option 1-Sel) women with fasting plasma glucose (FPG) 4.7–5.0 mmol/L; in all (Option 2) or high-risk (Option 2-Sel) women without history of HIP and with FPG 4.7–5.0 mmol/L. We also tested FPG measurement alone in all high-risk women. Measuring FPG alone had a sensitivity of 49% (95% confidence interval 45–54) applying universal screening. Option 2 appeared to have the best balance considering the needed OGTT (17.3%), sensitivity (72% (67–76)) and rates of a composite outcome (true negative cases: 10.6%, false positive cases: 24.4%; true positive cases: 19.5%; false negative cases: 10.2%). Consideration of a history of HIP and measuring first FPG can avoid more than 80% of OGTTs and identify women with the highest risk of adverse HIP-related events.

Keywords: Australian Diabetes in Pregnancy Society (ADIPS); Australian Diabetes Society (ADS); COVID-19; gestational diabetes mellitus; oral glucose tolerance test; pandemic; hyperglycemia in pregnancy; pregnancy outcomes; Royal Australian and New Zealand College of Obstetricians and Gynaecologists (RANZOG)

1. Introduction

Hyperglycemia in pregnancy (HIP) refers to gestational diabetes mellitus (GDM) and diabetes in pregnancy (DIP) [1–6]. DIP is considered as unknown pregravid diabetes and is usually screened using fasting plasma glucose (FPG) or HbA1c measurement in early pregnancy. DIP is associated with increased risk of stillbirth rate [7]. Early-diagnosed HIP is usually immediately treated. If early screening is normal, a new screening is performed in the late second trimester or early third trimester. Diagnosis is based on the oral glucose tolerance test (OGTT, the reference standard), with measurements of FPG, and one-hour

(1h-PG), two-hour (2h-PG) and sometimes three-hour plasma glucose [1–6]. Identifying and treating HIP diagnosed at that time reduces maternal and neonatal events [8,9].

Considering the current coronavirus disease 2019 (COVID-19) pandemic, pregnant women are advised to be stringent with public health measures such as social distancing and self-isolation to lower their risk of exposure. However, OGTT measurements require long times spent at OGTT testing centers. Therefore, temporary changes to the process of diagnostic testing for HIP need to be considered [10]. As proposed in Australia and New Zealand [11–13], such a perspective is to reduce the percentage of women who need to undergo an OGTT, whereby OGTTs may be indicated only in women with intermediate FPG values [11]. OGTTs may also be avoided in women with history of HIP who would be considered to have current HIP [11]. HIP might also be based on FPG measurement alone [12]. Finally, selective rather than universal screening could be applied. However, a poor sensitivity of such strategies could be deleterious, because unidentified women with HIP would not be managed. On the contrary, a poor specificity could lead to care for women without HIP.

We had the opportunity in our large retrospective cohort of women [14,15] to evaluate for seven options: (i) the percentage of women who would be selected to undergo OGTTs if these proposals would have been applied; (ii) the percentage of HIP who would have been diagnosed or not; and (iii) the occurrence of adverse outcomes if the women would have been correctly diagnosed or not, with a special interest for false negative and false positive cases of HIP.

2. Materials and Methods

2.1. Data Collection

This observational study was conducted in our university hospital in a suburban area of Paris, France, and was based on routine electronic medical records of maternal and neonatal events at birth between January 2012 and October 2016 [14,15]. In addition, we have collected data on HIP screening in all women. Women were informed that their medical records could be used for research, unless they opposed [14,15]. The data were analyzed anonymously. Our database was declared to the French Committee for computerized data (CNIL: Commission Nationale de l'Informatique et des Libertés, number 1704392v0).

2.2. Screening for Hyperglycemia in Pregnancy

We follow the French recommendations in our center [3], except that our policy is to universally screen women, both at the beginning of pregnancy and after 24 weeks of gestation (WG) if prior screening was normal or not done. Early screening during pregnancy is based on FPG measurement. Women with FPG levels $\geq$5.1 mmol/L are diagnosed with HIP. Those without early-diagnosed HIP undergo a 75 g OGTT between 24 and 28 WG, with measurements of FPG, 1h-PG and 2h-PG [3]. The International Association of Diabetes Pregnancy Study Group (IADPSG) [1] and World Health Organization (WHO) recommendations [2] are considered for HIP diagnosis, because these guidelines have been endorsed in France [3]. Accordingly, GDM was defined as FPG 5.1–6.9 mmol/L and/or 1h-PG $\geq$ 10.0 mmol/L and/or 2h-PG 8.5–11.0 mmol/L in the OGTT, whereas DIP was defined as FPG $\geq$ 7.0 and/or 2h-PG $\geq$ 11.1 mmol/L.

2.3. Selection Criteria for Our Study

Inclusion criteria were woman who had an OGTT between 22 and 30 WG, were 18 to 50 years old, single fetus pregnancies, and had no personal history of either diabetes or bariatric surgery. We considered OGTT results between 22 and 30 WG rather than between 24 and 28 WG because OGTTs were often used during this period of time [14]. We then selected the women whose risk factor for HIP status was known, and applied Australian–New Zealand risk factors [11]. They include any of the following factors: previous history of HIP or neonatal death; previously elevated blood glucose level (not available in our data set (NA)); maternal age $\geq$40 years; family history of diabetes; pre-pregnancy obesity (body mass index > 30 kg/m^2); previous baby with macrosomia; polycystic ovarian syndrome (NA); corticosteroids and antipsychotics medication (NA) and finally ethnicity. We have previously shown that North African, Indian, Pakistani, Sri Lankan, and Asian ethnicities were at high risk in our cohort [16]. We finally selected women who had no HIP in early pregnancy, defined as FPG levels <5.1 mmol/L (Flow chart in Figure S1).

2.4. Description of Tested Algorithms

The reference standard testing was the results of OGTTs between 22 and 30 WG according to IADPSG/WHO criteria applying universal screening. Figure 1 shows the seven tested algorithms (termed as "Options") in which:

- OGTTs would be performed only in women with risk factor for HIP, i.e., applying selective screening (Option Sel);
- OGTTs would be performed in women with FPG 4.7–5.0 mmol/L between 22 and 30 WG, applying universal (Option 1) or selective screening (Option 1-Sel) [11];
- OGTTs would be performed in women without history of HIP (those with previous HIP are considered to have GDM) and with FPG 4.7–5.0 mmol/L between 22 and 30 WG, applying universal (Option 2) or selective screening (Option 2-Sel) [11];
- FPG alone would be measured, applying universal (Option 3) or selective screening (Option 3-Sel) [12].

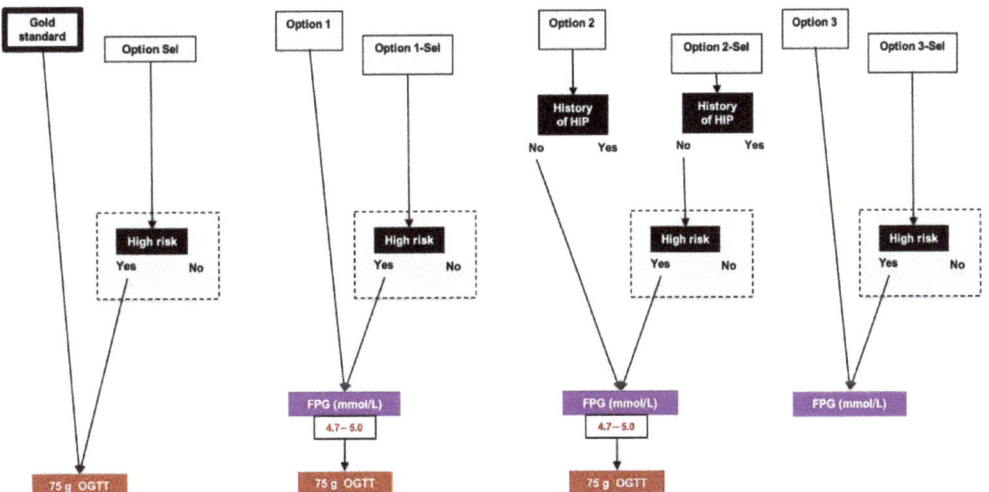

Figure 1. Reference standard and options that were evaluated after 22 weeks of gestation. Reference standard refers to universal screening with oral glucose tolerance test between 22 and 30 weeks of gestation (75 g oral glucose tolerance test, IADPSG/WHO criteria). We evaluated seven options, applying universal (Options 1, 2 and 3) or selective screening (Options Sel, 1-Sel, 2-Sel and 3-Sel). Women were considered at high risk according to Australian–New Zealand risk factors (please see text). OGTT: oral glucose tolerance test; 1h-PG and 2h-PG: plasma glucose value 1 and 2 h after 75 g oral glucose tolerance test, respectively; DIP: diabetes in pregnancy; FPG: fasting plasma glucose; GDM: gestational diabetes mellitus; HIP: hyperglycemia in pregnancy.

If the new proposals were applied, the women would be classified as:

- True negative: women who have no HIP (IADPSG/WHO criteria, universal screening) and would be correctly diagnosed as having no HIP with the tested proposal;
- False positive: women who have no HIP (IADPSG/WHO criteria, universal screening) but would be diagnosed as having HIP with the tested proposal;
- True positive: women who have HIP (IADPSG/WHO criteria, universal screening) and would be correctly diagnosed as having HIP with the tested proposal;

- False negative: women who have HIP (IADPSG/WHO criteria, universal screening) but would be misdiagnosed with the tested proposal.

2.5. Adverse Outcomes

The main predefined endpoint was the occurrence of a composite adverse outcome, which included at least one of the following events: (i) preeclampsia (blood pressure $\geq$ 140/90 mmHg on two recordings four hours apart and proteinuria of at least 300 mg/24 h or 3+ on dipstick testing in a random urine sample); (ii) an infant large for the gestational age (LGA: birth weight greater than the 90th percentile for a standard French population [14,15]); (iii) shoulder dystocia, defined as the use of obstetrical maneuvers (McRoberts maneuver, episiotomy after delivery of the fetal head, suprapubic pressure, posterior arm rotation to an oblique angle, rotation of the infant by 180 degrees, or delivery of the posterior arm); and (iv) neonatal hypoglycemia, defined as at least one blood glucose value less than 36 mg/dL during the first two days of life [14,15].

We also considered each of the previous events separately, and additionally infants small for the gestational age (birth weight lower than the 10th percentile for a standard French population [14,15]; selective and emergency (before or during delivery) caesarean sections; preterm delivery (delivery before 37 completed weeks); admission to a neonatal intensive care unit; respiratory distress syndrome (based on the clinical course, chest X-ray findings, blood gas and acid–base values); and finally intrauterine fetal or neonatal death (in the first 24 h of life). We also considered the need for insulin at the time of delivery [17].

To note, all women with HIP were referred to our multidisciplinary team including a diabetologist, an obstetrician, a midwife, a dietician, and a nurse educator, and managed according to French recommendations. They received individualized dietary advice, instructions on how to perform self-monitoring of blood glucose levels six times a day, and were seen by the diabetologist every 2–4 weeks. They received insulin therapy when pre-prandial and 2 h post-prandial glucose levels were greater than 5.0 and 6.7 mmol/L respectively, according to the French guidelines [3]. Obstetrical care also followed the French recommendations [3]. Timing and mode of delivery was discussed with the patient and obstetrical staff according to fetal weight estimation during ultrasound scans at 37 WG and considering glucose control. At 39 WG, labor induction (using prostaglandin E2 or oxytocin infusion) or even caesarean section was possibly decided according to obstetric history, maternal condition, and estimated fetal weight. Continuous fetal cardiotocography was routinely used during labor. Overall, it must be considered that, in our cohort, false negative cases of HIP were cared for, whereas false positive cases were not.

2.6. Statistics

Baseline continuous variables were expressed as the mean ± standard deviation (SD). Categorical variables were expressed as frequencies (percentages). First, we evaluated the proportions of women selected to undergo OGTTs according to each screening option. We then evaluated the performance of each option for screening for HIP after 22 WG. The reference standard was the results of the OGTT between 22 and 30 WG, applying universal screening. We considered sensitivity, specificity, positive (PPV), and negative predictive value (NPV) of each option.

We therefore compared characteristics and adverse outcome rates of true negative, false positive, true positive and false negative cases of HIP according to each option. To compare continuous variables by the different groups of patients (True negative, False positive, True positive and False negative), we used ANOVA. To compare categorical variables, we used the Chi-squared (χ^2) test or Fisher's exact test. Values were considered significant at a probability level of 0.05. For the difference between each group of patients by each other, we performed a post-hoc analysis for multiplicity by Bonferroni method and adjusted the *p*-value depending on the number of tests made in each option evaluated. All tests were two-sided. Analyses were conducted using R 3.6.3 software (R Foundation, Vienna, Austria, https://cran.r-project.org).

3. Results

3.1. Population Characteristics

We included 4245 women (Flow chart in Figure S1). Their baseline characteristics are shown in Table 1.

Table 1. Characteristics of the women by true/false positive/negative cases considering Option 2.

	Total	True Negative Cases	False Positive Cases	True Positive Cases	False Negative Cases	p
	$n = 4245$	$n = 3678$	$n = 86$	$n = 344$	$n = 137$	
OGTT between 22 and 30 WG						
Fasting plasma glucose (mmol/L)	4.38 (0.45)	4.30 (0.36) [a,b]	4.46 (0.37) [d,e]	5.23 (0.47) [f]	4.29 (0.26)	<0.001
1-h plasma glucose (mmol/L)	6.76 (1.76)	6.42 (1.46) [a,b,c]	7.48 (1.42) [d,e]	9.17 (2.02) [f]	9.61 (1.24)	<0.001
2-h plasma glucose (mmol/L)	5.96 (1.43)	5.67 (1.10) [a,b,c]	6.34 (1.20) [d,e]	7.93 (1.93) [f]	8.58 (1.34)	<0.001
Gestational age at time of OGTT (WG)	26.22 (1.89)	26.21 (1.88)	26.19 (2.03)	26.29 (1.91)	26.40 (1.85)	NS
Characteristics						
Age (years)	30.25 (5.32)	29.93 (5.25) [a,b,c]	32.38 (4.74)	32.42 (5.28)	32.01 (5.60)	<0.001
Preconception body mass index (kg/m^2)	24.36 (4.48)	24.15 (4.36) [b]	25.31 (4.55)	26.30 (5.14) [f]	24.57 (4.46)	<0.001
Obesity	493 (11.7)	388 (10.6) [b]	14 (16.7)	76 (22.2) [f]	15 (10.9)	<0.001
Preconception hypertension	28 (0.7)	19 (0.5) [b]	1 (1.2)	7 (2.0)	1 (0.7)	0.01
Family history of diabetes	824 (19.4)	671 (18.2) [a,b]	28 (32.6)	94 (27.3)	31 (22.6)	<0.001
Employment	1883 (44.4)	1649 (44.9)	28 (32.6)	148 (43.1)	58 (42.3)	NS
Smoking before pregnancy	493 (11.6)	447 (12.2)	3 (3.5)	34 (9.9)	9 (6.6)	0.012
Parity	2.03 (1.18)	2.00 (1.17)	2.90 (1.05)	2.28 (1.23)	1.83 (1.12)	
Previous pregnancy(ies)						
History of hyperglycemia in pregnancy						<0.001 *
First child	1769 (41.7)	1589 (43.2)	0 (0.0)	108 (31.4)	72 (52.6)	
No	2324 (54.7)	2089 (56.8)	0 (0.0)	170 (49.4)	65 (47.4)	
Yes	152 (3.6)	0 (0.0) [a,b]	86 (100.0) [d,e]	66 (19.2) [f]	0 (0.0)	
History of macrosomia						<0.001 *
First child	1769 (41.7)	1589 (43.2)	0 (0.0)	108 (31.4)	72 (52.6)	
No	2378 (56.0)	2022 (55.0)	77 (89.5)	218 (63.4)	61 (44.5)	
Yes	98 (2.3)	67 (1.8) [a,b]	9 (10.5)	18 (5.2)	4 (2.9)	

Table 1. Cont.

	Total	True Negative Cases	False Positive Cases	True Positive Cases	False Negative Cases	p
History of hypertensive disorders						NS *
First pregnancy	1226 (28.9)	1108 (30.1)	0 (0.0)	68 (19.8)	50 (36.5)	
No	2941 (69.3)	2504 (68.1)	84 (97.7)	268 (77.9)	85 (62.0)	
Yes	78 (1.8)	66 (1.8)	2 (2.3)	8 (2.3)	2 (1.5)	
History of fetal death						0.04 *
First pregnancy	1226 (28.9)	1108 (30.1)	0 (0.0)	68 (19.8)	50 (36.5)	
No	2964 (69.8)	2528 (68.7)	84 (97.7)	266 (77.3)	86 (62.8)	
Yes	55 (1.3)	42 (1.1) [b]	2 (2.3)	10 (2.9)	1 (0.7)	
Ethnicity						<0.01
North African	866 (20.4)	694 (18.9)	29 (33.7)	108 (31.5)	35 (25.5)	
European	1509 (35.6)	1353 (36.8)	16 (18.6)	93 (27.1)	47 (34.3)	
Sub-Saharan African	888 (20.9)	793 (21.6)	15 (17.4)	69 (20.1)	11 (8.0)	
Indian-Pakistan-Sri Lankan	342 (8.1)	267 (7.3)	15 (17.4)	44 (12.8)	16 (11.7)	
Caribbean	281 (6.6)	260 (7.1)	3 (3.5)	13 (3.8)	5 (3.6)	
Asian	72 (1.7)	59 (1.6)	2 (2.3)	3 (0.9)	8 (5.8)	
Other	285 (6.7)	251 (6.8)	6 (7.0)	13 (3.8)	15 (10.9)	
High-risk women	2050 (48.3)	1649 (44.8)	86 (100.0)	229 (66.6)	86 (62.8)	
Glycemic status (reference standard: IADPSG/WHO criteria)						<0.001
Normal	3764 (88.7)	3678 (100.0)	86 (100.0)	0 (0.0)	0 (0.0)	
Gestational diabetes mellitus	459 (10.8)	0 (0.0)	0 (0.0)	326 (94.8)	133 (97.1)	
Diabetes in pregnancy	22 (0.5)	0 (0.0)	0 (0.0)	18 (5.2)	4 (2.9)	
Events during pregnancy						
Composite adverse outcome	492 (11.6)	390 (10.6) [a,b]	21 (24.4) [e]	67 (19.5)	14 (10.2)	<0.001
Preeclampsia	71 (1.7)	59 (1.6)	1 (1.2)	6 (1.7)	5 (3.6)	0.29
LGA age infant	400 (9.4)	318 (8.6) [a,b]	20 (23.3) [e]	54 (15.7) [f]	8 (5.8)	<0.001
Shoulder dystocia	6 (0.1)	4 (0.1)	1 (1.2)	0 (0.0)	1 (0.7)	0.06
Neonatal hypoglycemia	27 (0.6)	15 (0.4) [b]	0 (0.0)	11 (3.2)	1 (0.7)	<0.001
Ceasarean section	862 (20.3)	721 (19.6) [b]	23 (26.7)	90 (26.2)	28 (20.4)	0.014
Preterm delivery (<37 weeks)	229 (5.4)	193 (5.2)	3 (3.5)	24 (7.0)	9 (6.6)	0.42
Offspring hospitalization	812 (19.1)	677 (18.4)	21 (24.4)	81 (23.5)	33 (24.1)	0.026
Respiratory distress syndrome	202 (4.8)	166 (4.5)	7 (8.1)	18 (5.2)	11 (8.0)	0.11

Table 1. *Cont.*

	Total	True Negative Cases	False Positive Cases	True Positive Cases	False Negative Cases	p
Intrauterine fetal or neonatal death	13 (0.3)	11 (0.3)	1 (1.2)	1 (0.3)	0 (0.0)	0.39
SGA infant	417 (9.8)	366 (10.0)	2 (2.3) [e]	30 (8.7)	19 (13.9)	0.04
Insulin therapy during	172 (4.1)	0 (0.0) [b,c]	0 (0.0) [d,e]	140 (40.7) [f]	32 (23.4)	<0.001

Date are n (%) or mean (standard deviation). HIP: hyperglycemia in pregnancy; IADPSG: International Association of Diabetes Pregnancy Study Group; LGA: large for gestational age; OGTT: oral glucose tolerance test; SGA: small for gestational age; WG: weeks of gestation; WHO: World Health Organization. Composite adverse outcome: preeclampsia or LGA infant or shoulder dystocia or neonatal hypoglycemia. Symbols indicate whether values are significant ($p < 0.05$) after Bonferroni adjustment for multiplicity: [a] True negative versus False positive, [b] True negative versus True positive, [c] True negative versus False negative, [d] False positive versus True positive, [e] False positive versus False negative, [f] True positive versus False negative; * yes versus no comparison; NS: non-significant.

3.2. Limiting the Percentage of Women Who Undergo OGTTs

The percentage of women who would have had OGTTs in our series was the highest for Option Sel (48.3%), then progressively decreased from Option 1 (18.5%), to Option 2 (17.3%), Option 1-Sel (9.7%) then Option 2-Sel (8.5%). There were no OGTTs performed for Options 3 and 3-Sel (Table 2).

Table 2. Percentage of women who underwent oral glucose tolerance test and performance of to diagnose hyperglycemia in pregnancy, by each option.

	Number of OGTTs	Sensitivity	Specificity	PPV	NPV
Option Sel	2050 (48.3)	0.65 (0.61–0.70)	1.00 (1.00–1.00)	1.00 (0.99–1.00)	0.96 (0.95–0.96)
Option 1	786 (18.5)	0.69 (0.65–0.73)	1.00 (1.00–1.00)	1.00 (0.99–1.00)	0.96 (0.96–0.97)
Option 1-Sel	413 (9.7)	0.45 (0.41–0.50)	1.00 (1.00–1.00)	1.00 (0.98–1.00)	0.93 (0.93–0.94)
Option 2	735 (17.3)	0.72 (0.67–0.76)	0.98 (0.97–0.98)	0.80 (0.76–0.97)	0.96 (0.96–0.97)
Option 2-Sel	362 (8.5)	0.48 (0.43–0.52)	0.98 (0.97–0.98)	0.73 (0.67–0.78)	0.94 (0.93–0.97)
Option 3	0	0.49 (0.45–0.54)	1.00 (1.00–1.00)	1.00 (0.98–1.00)	0.94 (50.93–0.95)
Option 3-Sel	0	0.33 (0.28–0.37)	1.00 (1.00–1.00)	1.00 (0.98–1.00)	0.92 (0.91–0.93)

Data are n (%) or unit (95% confidence interval). NPV: negative predictive value; OGTT: oral glucose tolerance test; PPV: positive predictive value.

3.3. Performance of Each Option to Diagnose HIP Cases

Table 2 shows the sensitivity, specificity, PPV and NPV of each option. Globally, sensitivities were around 70% for Option Sel, Options 1 and 2; around 50% for Options 1-Sel, 2-Sel and 3; and 33% for Option 3-Sel. Specificities were 98–100% for all options. PPV was 100% for all options (meaning there were no false positive cases), except for Option 2 and 2-Sel. In Option 2, the PPV was 80% (76–97%) and in Option 2-Sel, it was 73% (67–78%). Finally, NPV was higher than 90% for all options.

3.4. Characteristics of True Negative, False Positive, True Positive of False Negative Cases of HIP, and Their Prognosis

True/false negative/positive cases of HIP defined by each option are compared in a specific table by option: Option Sel (Supplementary Table S1), Option 1 (Supplementary Table S2), Option 1-Sel (Supplementary Table S3), Option 2 (Table 1), Option 2-Sel (Supplementary Table S4), Option 3 (Supplementary Table S5), Option 3-Sel (Supplementary Table S6). We chose to especially show results for Option 2, because this option appeared to have the best balance between the reduction in the percentage of OGTTs (by 82.7%) and identification of the women with the highest risk of adverse outcomes.

Globally, false negative cases as compared to true positive cases of HIP had a significantly lower preconception body mass index, with statistically different glucose values during the OGTTs. Additionally, in the options where selective screening was applied, false negative cases had fewer risk factors than true positive cases.

For Option 2 and 2-Sel, false positive cases had a personal history of HIP. As compared to true negative cases, they had higher FPG, 1h-PG, and 2h-PG values during OGTTs, were older, and were more prone to have, in addition to personal history of HIP, personal history of macrosomic infants or a family history of diabetes.

3.5. Prognosis Associated with True Negative, False Positive, True Positive and False Negative Cases of HIP

The same tables and Figure 2 show the rate of the composite adverse outcome in each group. Especially, the false negative cases, as compared to the true positive cases of HIP, had fewer adverse events during pregnancy—especially HIP-related events, LGA infants, and neonatal hypoglycemia.

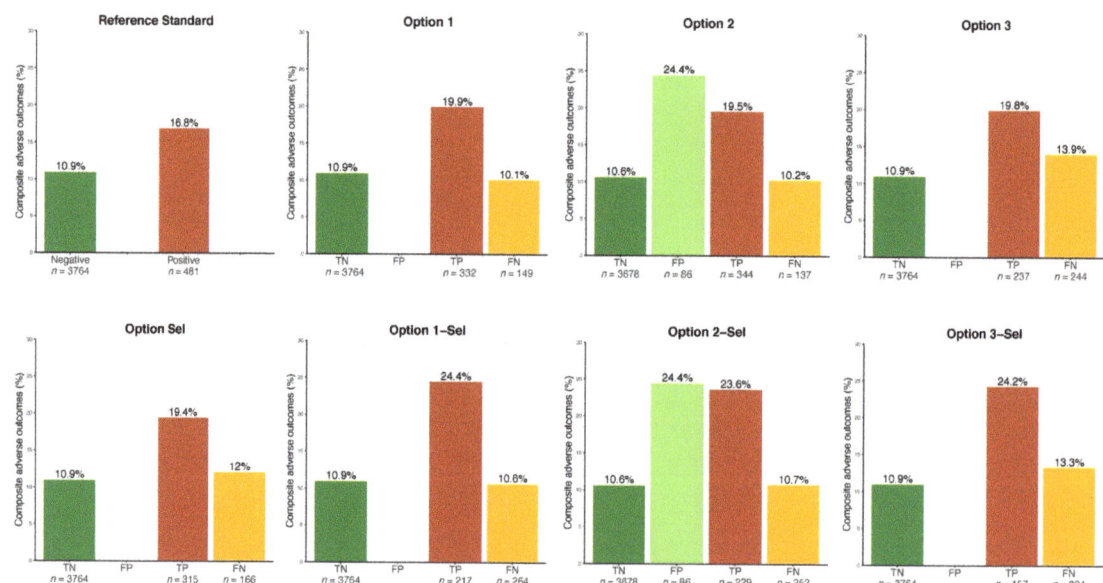

Figure 2. Rate of hyperglycemia in pregnancy-related events by true/false positive/negative cases by each option. Please see description of each option in Figure 1. TN, FP, TP, FN: true negative, false positive, true positive, false negative of hyperglycemia in pregnancy, respectively. HIP-related events: hyperglycemia in pregnancy-related events (composite: preeclampsia or large for gestational age infant or shoulder dystocia or neonatal hypoglycemia). Note that TP and FN cases had been treated for HIP in this observational cohort, whereas TN and FP cases had not.

Finally, the false positive cases as compared to the true negative cases (Option 2 and Option 2-Sel only) had significantly more composite adverse outcomes. This was driven by a higher rate of LGA infants.

4. Discussion

In the current study, we compared the diagnostic performance of various screening strategies for HIP diagnosis and to identify the women more prone to experience HIP-related events, with the aim to prevent a large proportion of pregnant women from undergoing an OGTT. This is particularly crucial during the COVID-19 pandemic. One option (Option 2) appears to offer a good compromise because it reduces the rate of women undergoing OGTTs by more than 80%, while it identifies around 70% of the women with HIP, especially those (both false positive and true positive cases) with the highest risk of adverse outcomes.

The sensitivity of selective rather than universal screening to identify women with HIP defined according to the IADPSG/WHO criteria has been shown to be between 60% and 95% [15,18–21]. We show here that performing OGTTs only in high-risk women had a sensitivity of 65%. In our series, 48.3% of women would have had an OGTT if selective screening had been applied. This rate would depend on locally considered risk factors and their prevalence. Whatever the options, a selective policy led to reduction by around one-half of the rate of screening. Using alternative options would lead to preventing more women from performing OGTTs.

In this perspective, several strategies have been suggested. Some include HbA1c measurement [11,22]. However, the use of HbA1c for diagnosing HIP has been disappointing because there is substantial overlap between women with normoglycemia and women with HIP. This has particularly been shown for HIP defined according to IADPSG/WHO criteria [23–29]. Some other strategies include a single random glucose measurement [30,31]. However this was considered to be inadequate to screen for HIP in a systematic review [32], due to its low sensitivity [33].

As shown in our study, FPG measurement alone is also not highly sensitive [34–36]. For example, in the Hyperglycemia Adverse Outcomes in Pregnancy (HAPO) study, one-half of GDM cases were detected through elevated 1h- and/or 2h-PG, whereas FPG levels were normal [34]. However, studies using IADPSG/WHO criteria showed FPG to be useful for simplifying the screening process and reducing the number of OGTTs [34–36]. Indeed, FPG thresholds of ≤4.4 mmol/L have been reported to rule out HIP in 50–65% of women with a sensitivity of 80–95% [34–37]. As proposed by one guidance [11], we used a FPG level <4.7 mmol/L to rule out women with HIP in this series. Sensitivities of such options were around 70% applying universal screening and 45% applying selective screening, which appears imperfect.

According to Australian–New Zealand guidance [11], women with a history of HIP might be considered as presenting current GDM (Options 2 and 2-Sel). In fact, as previously reviewed [38], the HIP recurrence rate is around 50%, and therefore leads to false positive cases of HIP. Over-management of these women might induce infants small for the gestational age, and will result in more testing, monitoring and contact with hospital services throughout their pregnancy. Similarly, not caring for women with HIP because they are not diagnosed might also be associated with adverse outcomes [8,9]. We therefore compared prognoses associated with false positive vs true negative cases of HIP and with false negative vs true positive cases.

We report for the first time that false positive cases of HIP, i.e., women with a history of HIP but a normal OGTT (Options 2 and 2-Sel), had a worse prognosis than true negative cases. One explanation is that: (i) they had higher glucose levels during OGTTs which correlates with more adverse outcomes [34]; and (ii) they had more risk factors for HIP, including history of personal HIP, also associated with a poor prognosis [15]. On the one hand, this suggests that management of these women with diet, exercise and possibly insulin treatment might be useful to reduce the number of HIP-related events. On the other hand, this implies more contact with hospital services throughout pregnancy.

Additionally, we have shown that the prognosis of false negative cases was better than that for true positive cases, but this is only partly reassuring. Indeed, these cases were actually managed for HIP, as observed in this study. Moreover, around one-quarter of false negative cases of HIP were insulin-treated in our series. One retrospective study based on the HAPO data suggested that missed diagnosed GDM with the COVID-19 proposal could present fewer events than those who are not missed, even when they are not treated [39]. This especially completes our data because the women included in the HAPO study were not treated. Overall, we do not know what the loss of treatment benefit would be if these women had not been managed, and randomized studies would be necessary to draw definitive conclusions. Indeed, not caring for HIP in low-risk women might lead to a doubling of the rate of adverse events during pregnancy [8,9].

The strengths of our study include the large numbers of subjects and a multiethnic cohort likely to be translatable to different populations, and a pragmatic guidance-based approach. The prospectively collected standardized data provide for a robust investigational data set and we could investigate several options in the same series of women. We excluded women who had no FPG measurements or had FPG levels ≥ 5.1 mmol/L in early pregnancy, whereas some guidance proposes to screen for HIP in early pregnancy with random plasma glucose and/or HbA1c measurement [11]. We limited our evaluation for women who underwent OGTTs in the late second and early third trimesters (22–30 WG). We could not consider preanalytical issues for FPG measurement: the time interval between sampling and spinning fasting glucose measurements can double or half the diagnoses of GDM [40]. Finally, an additional strength was the evaluation of the prognosis of true/false negative/positive cases, although while interpreting the results, we had to consider that false negative cases were managed for HIP in our series.

5. Conclusions

To conclude, during current and future pandemics, consideration that every pregnant woman should undergo an OGTT at the end of the second trimester is an important issue. We show here that FPG measurement first can avoid 80–90% of OGTTs. The sensitivity of such an option is around 70% and 50% applying universal and selective screening, respectively. In both cases, however, the women at the highest risk of adverse HIP-related events during pregnancy are identified and therefore would be managed during pregnancy. Any changes to international guidelines before the pandemic could be replaced by some options tested in this study only temporarily, pending resolution of the COVID-19 pandemic, and in any case with the awareness of exposing some women with HIP to the risk of not being identified and therefore not being treated. However, such a screening regimen may be applicable in countries where OGTTs are difficult to perform.

Supplementary Materials: The following are available online at https://www.mdpi.com/2077-0383/10/3/397/s1. Table S1: Characteristics of the women by true/false positive/negative cases considering Option Sel; Table S2: Characteristics of the women by true/false positive/negative cases considering Option 1; Table S3: Characteristics of the women by true/false positive/negative cases considering Option 1-Sel; Table S4: Characteristics of the women by true/false positive/negative cases considering Option 2-Sel; Table S5: Characteristics of the women by true/false positive/negative cases considering Option 3; Table S6: Characteristics of the women by true/false positive/negative cases considering Option 3-Sel; Figure S1: Flow chart of the study.

Author Contributions: C.N. prepared and analyzed the statistics and wrote the manuscript; E.V. co-directed research and reviewed/edited the manuscript; S.T. prepared the statistics and wrote the manuscript; S.P., H.B., M.S., N.B., L.A., C.B., and L.C. contributed to discussions and reviewed/edited the manuscript; J.-J.P. validated the statistical analyses; E.C. directed the research and wrote the manuscript. All authors have read and agreed to the published version of the manuscript.

Funding: The authors do not report any disclosure. Lilly France part-funded this study. Apart from funding, Lilly France did not participate in any part of this study (collection, analysis, and interpretation of data; writing of the report; the decision to submit the report for publication).

Institutional Review Board Statement: Not applicable.

Informed Consent Statement: Patient consent was not waived due to observational study. In Jean Verdier hospital and in general in the various Public Assistance Hospitals in Paris, all patients are informed at admission that their medical records may be used for research, unless they indicate their opposition. For the present study, no patient indicated opposition. Data were analyzed anonymously.

Data Availability Statement: The datasets generated during and/or analyzed during the current study are not publicly available but are available from the corresponding author on reasonable request.

Acknowledgments: Emmanuel Cosson and Lionel Carbillon are the guarantors of this work. We thank Didier André, AP-HP, Unité de Recherche Clinique GHU-SSPD, for data management.

Conflicts of Interest: The authors declare no conflict of interest.

Abbreviations

OGTT: 75 g oral glucose tolerance test; 1h-PG: plasma glucose value 1 h after 75 g oral glucose tolerance test; 2h-PG: plasma glucose value 1 h after 75 g oral glucose tolerance test; BMI: body mass index; DIP: diabetes in pregnancy; FPG: fasting plasma glucose; GDM: gestational diabetes mellitus; HIP: hyperglycemia in pregnancy; IADPSG: International Association of Diabetes Pregnancy Study Group; NA: not available in our dataset; NPP: negative predictive value; PPV: positive predictive value; WG: weeks of gestation; WHO: World Health Organization.

References

1. International Association of Diabetes and Pregnancy Study Groups Consensus Panel; Metzger, B.E.; Gabbe, S.G.; Persson, B.; Buchanan, T.A.; Catalano, P.A.; Damm, P.; Dyer, A.R.; de Leiva, A.; Hod, M.; et al. International Association of Diabetes and Pregnancy Study Groups Recommendations on the Diagnosis and Classification of Hyperglycemia in Pregnancy. *Diabetes Care* **2010**, *33*, 676–682. [CrossRef] [PubMed]
2. World Health Organization. Diagnostic Criteria and Classification of Hyperglycaemia First Detected in Pregnancy: A World Health Organization Guideline. *Diabetes Res. Clin. Pract.* **2014**, *103*, 341–363. [CrossRef] [PubMed]
3. Vambergue, A. Expert Consensus on Gestational Diabetes Mellitus. Summary of Expert Consensus. *Diabetes Metab.* **2010**, *36*, 695–699. [CrossRef] [PubMed]
4. Benhalima, K.; Mathieu, C.; Van Assche, A.; Damm, P.; Devlieger, R.; Mahmood, T.; Dunne, F. Survey by the European Board and College of Obstetrics and Gynaecology on Screening for Gestational Diabetes in Europe. *Eur. J. Obstet. Gynecol. Reprod. Biol.* **2016**, *201*, 197–202. [CrossRef]
5. Hod, M.; Kapur, A.; Sacks, D.A.; Hadar, E.; Agarwal, M.; Di Renzo, G.C.; Cabero Roura, L.; McIntyre, H.D.; Morris, J.L.; Divakar, H. The International Federation of Gynecology and Obstetrics (FIGO) Initiative on Gestational Diabetes Mellitus: A Pragmatic Guide for Diagnosis, Management, and Care. *Int. J. Gynaecol. Obstet. Off. Organ Int. Fed. Gynaecol. Obstet.* **2015**, *131* (Suppl. 3), S173–S211. [CrossRef]
6. American Diabetes Association. 2. Classification and Diagnosis of Diabetes: Standards of Medical Care in Diabetes—2020. *Diabetes Care* **2020**, *43*, S14–S31. [CrossRef]
7. Stacey, T.; Tennant, P.; McCowan, L.; Mitchell, E.A.; Budd, J.; Li, M.; Thompson, J.; Martin, B.; Roberts, D.; Heazell, A. Gestational Diabetes and the Risk of Late Stillbirth: A Case-Control Study from England, UK. *BJOG Int. J. Obstet. Gynaecol.* **2019**, *126*, 973–982. [CrossRef]
8. Landon, M.B.; Spong, C.Y.; Thom, E.; Carpenter, M.W.; Ramin, S.M.; Casey, B.; Wapner, R.J.; Varner, M.W.; Rouse, D.J.; Thorp, J.M.; et al. A Multicenter, Randomized Trial of Treatment for Mild Gestational Diabetes. *N. Engl. J. Med.* **2009**, *361*, 1339–1348. [CrossRef]
9. Crowther, C.A.; Hiller, J.E.; Moss, J.R.; McPhee, A.J.; Jeffries, W.S.; Robinson, J.S.; Australian Carbohydrate Intolerance Study in Pregnant Women (ACHOIS) Trial Group. Effect of Treatment of Gestational Diabetes Mellitus on Pregnancy Outcomes. *N. Engl. J. Med.* **2005**, *352*, 2477–2486. [CrossRef]
10. McIntyre, H.D.; Moses, R.G. The Diagnosis and Management of Gestational Diabetes Mellitus in the Context of the COVID-19 Pandemic. *Diabetes Care* **2020**, dci200026. [CrossRef]
11. Available online: https://www.Adips.org/Documents/ADIPSADSCOVID-19GDMDiagnosisUpdated250420Website.Pdf (accessed on 26 April 2020).
12. RANZCOG—COVID-19 and Gestational Diabetes Screening, Diagnosis and Management. Available online: https://ranzcog.edu.au/news/covid-19-and-gestational-diabetes-screening,-diagn (accessed on 1 May 2020).
13. Simmons, D.; Rudland, V.L.; Wong, V.; Flack, J.; Mackie, A.; Ross, G.P.; Coat, S.; Dalal, R.; Hague, B.M.; Cheung, N.W. Options for Screening for Gestational Diabetes Mellitus during the SARS-CoV-2 Pandemic. *Aust. N. Z. J. Obstet. Gynaecol.* **2020**. [CrossRef] [PubMed]
14. Cosson, E.; Vicaut, E.; Sandre-Banon, D.; Gary, F.; Pharisien, I.; Portal, J.-J.; Banu, I.; Bianchi, L.; Cussac-Pillegand, C.; Dina, R.; et al. Early Screening for Gestational Diabetes Mellitus Is Not Associated with Improved Pregnancy Outcomes: An Observational Study Including 9795 Women. *Diabetes Metab.* **2019**, *45*, 465–472. [CrossRef] [PubMed]

15. Cosson, E.; Vicaut, E.; Sandre-Banon, D.; Gary, F.; Pharisien, I.; Portal, J.-J.; Baudry, C.; Cussac-Pillegand, C.; Costeniuc, D.; Valensi, P.; et al. Performance of a Selective Screening Strategy for Diagnosis of Hyperglycaemia in Pregnancy as Defined by IADPSG/WHO Criteria. *Diabetes Metab.* **2019**. [CrossRef] [PubMed]
16. Cosson, E.; Cussac-Pillegand, C.; Benbara, A.; Pharisien, I.; Jaber, Y.; Banu, I.; Nguyen, M.T.; Valensi, P.; Carbillon, L. The Diagnostic and Prognostic Performance of a Selective Screening Strategy for Gestational Diabetes Mellitus According to Ethnicity in Europe. *J. Clin. Endocrinol. Metab.* **2014**, *99*, 996–1005. [CrossRef] [PubMed]
17. The INSPIRED Research Group; Egan, A.M.; Bogdanet, D.; Griffin, T.P.; Kgosidialwa, O.; Cervar-Zivkovic, M.; Dempsey, E.; Allotey, J.; Alvarado, F.; Clarson, C.; et al. A Core Outcome Set for Studies of Gestational Diabetes Mellitus Prevention and Treatment. *Diabetologia* **2020**, *63*, 1120–1127. [CrossRef]
18. Miailhe, G.; Kayem, G.; Girard, G.; Legardeur, H.; Mandelbrot, L. Selective Rather than Universal Screening for Gestational Diabetes Mellitus? *Eur. J. Obstet. Gynecol. Reprod. Biol.* **2015**, *191*, 95–100. [CrossRef]
19. Avalos, G.E.; Owens, L.A.; Dunne, F.; ATLANTIC DIP Collaborators. Applying Current Screening Tools for Gestational Diabetes Mellitus to a European Population: Is It Time for Change? *Diabetes Care* **2013**, *36*, 3040–3044. [CrossRef]
20. Corrado, F.; Pintaudi, B.; Di Vieste, G.; Interdonato, M.L.; Magliarditi, M.; Santamaria, A.; D'Anna, R.; Di Benedetto, A. Italian Risk Factor-Based Screening for Gestational Diabetes. *J. Matern.-Fetal Neonatal Med.* **2014**, *27*, 1445–1448. [CrossRef]
21. Pintaudi, B.; Di Vieste, G.; Corrado, F.; Lucisano, G.; Pellegrini, F.; Giunta, L.; Nicolucci, A.; D'Anna, R.; Di Benedetto, A. Improvement of Selective Screening Strategy for Gestational Diabetes through a More Accurate Definition of High-Risk Groups. *Eur. J. Endocrinol.* **2014**, *170*, 87–93. [CrossRef]
22. Vambergue, A.; Jacqueminet, S.; Lamotte, M.-F.; Lamiche-Lorenzini, F.; Brunet, C.; Deruelle, P.; Vayssière, C.; Cosson, E. Three Alternative Ways to Screen for Hyperglycaemia in Pregnancy during the COVID-19 Pandemic. *Diabetes Metab.* **2020**. [CrossRef]
23. Ye, M.; Liu, Y.; Cao, X.; Yao, F.; Liu, B.; Li, Y.; Wang, Z.; Xiao, H. The Utility of HbA1c for Screening Gestational Diabetes Mellitus and Its Relationship with Adverse Pregnancy Outcomes. *Diabetes Res. Clin. Pract.* **2016**, *114*, 43–49. [CrossRef] [PubMed]
24. Pastakia, S.D.; Njuguna, B.; Onyango, B.A.; Washington, S.; Christoffersen-Deb, A.; Kosgei, W.K.; Saravanan, P. Prevalence of Gestational Diabetes Mellitus Based on Various Screening Strategies in Western Kenya: A Prospective Comparison of Point of Care Diagnostic Methods. *BMC Pregnancy Childbirth* **2017**, *17*, 226. [CrossRef] [PubMed]
25. Renz, P.B.; Cavagnolli, G.; Weinert, L.S.; Silveiro, S.P.; Camargo, J.L. HbA1c Test as a Tool in the Diagnosis of Gestational Diabetes Mellitus. *PLoS ONE* **2015**, *10*, e0135989. [CrossRef] [PubMed]
26. Rajput, R.; Rajput, M.; Nanda, S. Utility of HbA1c for Diagnosis of Gestational Diabetes Mellitus. *Diabetes Res. Clin. Pract.* **2012**, *98*, 104–107. [CrossRef] [PubMed]
27. Soumya, S.; Rohilla, M.; Chopra, S.; Dutta, S.; Bhansali, A.; Parthan, G.; Dutta, P. HbA1c: A Useful Screening Test for Gestational Diabetes Mellitus. *Diabetes Technol. Ther.* **2015**, *17*, 899–904. [CrossRef]
28. Odsæter, I.H.; Åsberg, A.; Vanky, E.; Mørkved, S.; Stafne, S.N.; Salvesen, K.Å.; Carlsen, S.M. Hemoglobin A1c as Screening for Gestational Diabetes Mellitus in Nordic Caucasian Women. *Diabetol. Metab. Syndr.* **2016**, *8*. [CrossRef]
29. Nachtergaele, C.; Vicaut, E.; Pinto, S.; Tatulashvili, S.; Bihan, H.; Sal, M.; Berkane, N.; Allard, L.; Baudry, C.; Carbillon, L.; et al. COVID-19 Pandemic: Can Fasting Plasma Glucose and HbA1c Replace the Oral Glucose Tolerance Test to Screen for Hyperglycaemia in Pregnancy? *Diabetes Res. Clin. Pract.* **2020**, 108640. [CrossRef]
30. Gestational Diabetes Screening During COVID-19 Pandemic. Available online: https://www.sogc.org/en/content/featured-news/Gestational-Diabetes-Screening-During-COVID-19-Pandemic.aspx (accessed on 1 May 2020).
31. *Gestational Diabetes and COVID-19 • Gestational Diabetes UK*; Gestational Diabetes UK: London, UK, 2020.
32. van Leeuwen, M.; Opmeer, B.C.; Yilmaz, Y.; Limpens, J.; Serlie, M.J.; Mol, B.W.J. Accuracy of the Random Glucose Test as Screening Test for Gestational Diabetes Mellitus: A Systematic Review. *Eur. J. Obstet. Gynecol. Reprod. Biol.* **2011**, *154*, 130–135. [CrossRef]
33. Agbozo, F.; Abubakari, A.; Narh, C.; Jahn, A. Accuracy of Glycosuria, Random Blood Glucose and Risk Factors as Selective Screening Tools for Gestational Diabetes Mellitus in Comparison with Universal Diagnosing. *BMJ Open Diabetes Res. Care* **2018**, *6*, e000493. [CrossRef]
34. Agarwal, M.M.; Weigl, B.; Hod, M. Gestational Diabetes Screening: The Low-Cost Algorithm. *Int. J. Gynaecol. Obstet.* **2011**, *115* (Suppl. 1), S30–S33. [CrossRef]
35. Agarwal, M.M.; Dhatt, G.S.; Shah, S.M. Gestational Diabetes Mellitus: Simplifying the International Association of Diabetes and Pregnancy Diagnostic Algorithm Using Fasting Plasma Glucose. *Diabetes Care* **2010**, *33*, 2018–2020. [CrossRef] [PubMed]
36. Rüetschi, J.R.; Jornayvaz, F.R.; Rivest, R.; Huhn, E.A.; Irion, O.; Boulvain, M. Fasting Glycaemia to Simplify Screening for Gestational Diabetes. *BJOG Int. J. Obstet. Gynaecol.* **2016**, *123*, 2219–2222. [CrossRef] [PubMed]
37. van Gemert, T.E.; Moses, R.G.; Pape, A.V.; Morris, G.J. Gestational Diabetes Mellitus Testing in the COVID-19 Pandemic: The Problems with Simplifying the Diagnostic Process. *Aust. N. Z. J. Obstet. Gynaecol.* **2020**. [CrossRef] [PubMed]
38. Schwartz, N.; Nachum, Z.; Green, M.S. The Prevalence of Gestational Diabetes Mellitus Recurrence–Effect of Ethnicity and Parity: A Metaanalysis. *Am. J. Obstet. Gynecol.* **2015**, *213*, 310–317. [CrossRef]

39. McIntyre, H.D.; Gibbons, K.S.; Ma, R.C.W.; Tam, W.H.; Sacks, D.A.; Lowe, J.; Madsen, L.R.; Catalano, P.M. Testing for Gestational Diabetes during the COVID-19 Pandemic. An Evaluation of Proposed Protocols for the United Kingdom, Canada and Australia. *Diabetes Res. Clin. Pract.* **2020**, *167*, 108353. [CrossRef]
40. Potter, J.M.; Hickman, P.E.; Oakman, C.; Woods, C.; Nolan, C.J. Strict Preanalytical Oral Glucose Tolerance Test Blood Sample Handling Is Essential for Diagnosing Gestational Diabetes Mellitus. *Diabetes Care* **2020**, *43*, 1438–1441. [CrossRef]

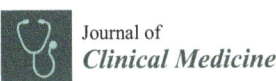

Review

Recurrent Gestational Diabetes Mellitus: A Narrative Review and Single-Center Experience

Aoife M. Egan [1,*], Elizabeth Ann L. Enninga [2], Layan Alrahmani [2,3], Amy L. Weaver [4], Michael P. Sarras [5] and Rodrigo Ruano [2]

1. Department of Endocrinology, Mayo Clinic, Rochester, MN 55905, USA
2. Department of Obstetrics and Gynecology, Mayo Clinic, Rochester, MN 55905, USA; Enninga.ElizabethAnn@mayo.edu (E.A.L.E.); layan.md@gmail.com (L.A.); ruano.rodrigo@mayo.edu (R.R.)
3. Department of Obstetrics and Gynecology, Loyola University Medical Center, Maywood, IL 60153, USA
4. Department of Health Sciences Research, Mayo Clinic, Rochester, MN 55905, USA; weaver@mayo.edu
5. Department of Cell Biology and Anatomy, Rosalind Franklin University of Medicine and Science, Chicago, IL 60064, USA; michael.sarras@rosalindfranklin.edu
* Correspondence: egan.aoife@mayo.edu; Tel.: +1-507-284-5211

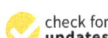

Citation: Egan, A.M.; Enninga, E.A.L.; Alrahmani, L.; Weaver, A.L.; Sarras, M.P.; Ruano, R. Recurrent Gestational Diabetes Mellitus: A Narrative Review and Single-Center Experience. *J. Clin. Med.* **2021**, *10*, 569. https://doi.org/10.3390/jcm10040569

Academic Editor: Katrien Benhalima
Received: 18 December 2020
Accepted: 29 January 2021
Published: 3 February 2021

Publisher's Note: MDPI stays neutral with regard to jurisdictional claims in published maps and institutional affiliations.

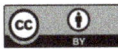

Copyright: © 2021 by the authors. Licensee MDPI, Basel, Switzerland. This article is an open access article distributed under the terms and conditions of the Creative Commons Attribution (CC BY) license (https://creativecommons.org/licenses/by/4.0/).

Abstract: Gestational diabetes mellitus (GDM) is a frequently observed complication of pregnancy and is associated with an elevated risk of adverse maternal and neonatal outcomes. Many women with GDM will go on to have future pregnancies, and these pregnancies may or may not be affected by GDM. We conducted a literature search, and based on data from key studies retrieved during the search, we describe the epidemiology of GDM recurrence. This includes a summary of the observed clinical risk factors of increasing maternal age, weight, ethnicity, and requirement for insulin in the index pregnancy. We then present our data from Mayo Clinic (January 2013–December 2017) which identifies a GDM recurrence rate of 47.6%, and illustrates the relevance of population-based studies to clinical practice. Lastly, we examine the available evidence on strategies to prevent GDM recurrence, and note that more research is needed to evaluate the effect of interventions before, during and after pregnancy.

Keywords: gestational diabetes; GDM; recurrence; pregnancy; glucose intolerance

1. Introduction

Gestational diabetes mellitus (GDM) is defined as carbohydrate intolerance resulting in hyperglycemia of variable severity with onset or first recognition during pregnancy [1]. It excludes those who likely had overt diabetes prior to gestation, and it is one of the most common medical complications of pregnancy, with a prevalence of up to 30% depending on the population studied [2,3]. GDM develops when insulin synthesis and secretion are insufficient to overcome the physiologic insulin resistance that increases during all pregnancies. It is associated with an increased risk of adverse maternal outcomes such as pre-eclampsia [4] and cesarean delivery [5], and undesirable infant outcomes including macrosomia and neonatal hypoglycemia [6]. Although GDM tends to resolve after the pregnancy, up to 60% of affected women develop type 2 diabetes in the subsequent 10–20 years [7,8]. While causality has not been fully established, children born to women with GDM are more likely to have disorders of glucose metabolism and adiposity in later life [9,10].

Established risk factors for GDM include increasing body mass index (BMI), advanced maternal age, non-white ethnicity, and family history of diabetes mellitus [11,12]. Having GDM in a prior pregnancy is also accepted as a strong risk factor for GDM in a subsequent pregnancy [13]. Reports on GDM recurrence rates are highly variable and influenced by the GDM diagnostic criteria used as well as baseline population characteristics. For example, one meta-analysis of 18 cross-sectional studies revealed recurrence rates ranging from 29% to 80% [14]. In addition to clarifying the prevalence of GDM recurrence, an understanding of which women are at highest risk of GDM recurrence is of significant clinical importance. It will potentially allow targeted interventions to address modifiable risk factors and decrease the chance of recurrence, along with facilitating earlier assessment and intervention in a subsequent pregnancy.

The aim of this review is to outline the epidemiology of GDM recurrence, drawing on data from large population-based studies. We will then present single-center data from a tertiary hospital to illustrate how information from these larger studies can relate to individual clinical practice. Finally, we will discuss strategies that may reduce the risk of GDM recurrence.

2. Materials and Methods

2.1. Comprehensive Literature Review

Between May 2020 and September 2020, a literature search was conducted on PubMed and Embase. The following search terms were used alone and in combination: "gestational diabetes", "GDM", "recurrence", "pregnancy", and "glucose intolerance". All studies published in the English language were considered, and a date restriction was not applied. Results were reviewed by the authors and selected for inclusion based on relevance to the topic. This was based on the judgment and agreement of the contributing authors. Additional articles were identified by manually searching reference lists of included articles.

2.2. Retrospective Study at Mayo Clinic

The retrospective cohort study included pregnant women who had their first pregnancy and were diagnosed with GDM between 1 January 2013 and 31 December 2017 at Mayo Clinic Rochester, Minnesota, U.S.A. It forms part of a series of studies aiming to better understand the molecular mechanisms underlying GDM and its relationship to future vascular complications [15]. The Mayo Clinic Investigational Review Board approved this retrospective study (Protocol: 17-009957). Searching the electronic medical records by the following ICD-9 and ICD-10 codes identified the cohort: 648.8, O24.410, O24.414, O24.419, O24.420, O24.424 and O24.343. Included women were between 18–45 years of age at the index pregnancy. Women with higher order pregnancies were excluded, as were women with established diabetes or a first trimester HbA1c >6.4%. This cohort was then followed until the end of 2018 to record whether or not they had a second pregnancy diagnosed with GDM.

The American College of Obstetricians and Gynecologists (ACOG) Clinical Management Practice Guidelines were used to diagnose GDM [16]. All women underwent a 50 g glucose challenge at 24–28 weeks gestation at Mayo Clinic (non-fasting). Following an overnight fast, women with a 1 h glucose of $\geq$140 mg/dL proceeded to a 3 h, 100 g oral glucose tolerance test. GDM was diagnosed if 2 or more of the following glucose thresholds were breached: fasting 95 mg/dL, 1 h 180 mg/dL, 2 h 155 mg/dL and 3 h 140 mg/dL.

A broad spectrum of clinical variables was collected for each pregnancy, including age, body mass index (BMI) at initial obstetric visit (<20 weeks in all cases), race, smoking history, family history, and GDM management. Abstracted data were collected in a secure online database. Comparisons between the two groups who did versus did not have GDM in their 2nd pregnancy were evaluated using the chi-squared test or Fisher's exact test, as appropriate, for categorical variables and the two-sample t-test for continuous variables. All calculated p-values were two-sided.

3. Epidemiology of GDM Recurrence

The majority of GDM risk factors will persist or become worse in subsequent pregnancies; therefore, it is reasonable to anticipate a relatively high GDM recurrence rate. Table 1 summarizes key studies in the area of GDM recurrence. In 2007, Kim et al. published a systematic literature review including 13 studies—11 retrospective cohorts and two case-control studies [17]. The number of participants in the included studies ranged from 19 to 1322. In the retrospective studies, the rate of GDM recurrence ranged from 30% to 84%. In the case-control studies, the risk of recurrent GDM was calculated using an odds ratio (OR), comparing the odds of a previous GDM pregnancy in women with a current GDM pregnancy versus women with a normal current pregnancy. This OR was calculated at 15.0 and 23.0 for the two included studies [18,19]. One of the included studies ($n = 651$) noted a 2.4% risk of pre-gestational diabetes in the subsequent pregnancy [20]. One of the major difficulties in comparing these studies is the differing criteria used to diagnose GDM. However, despite these differences, those with predominantly non-Hispanic white populations had a recurrence rate of <40%. On the other hand, studies containing predominantly minority populations including African Americans, Latinas and Asians had recurrence rates of >50%. No other risk factors were consistently identified across the studies.

Table 1. Key cited papers: epidemiology of gestational diabetes mellitus recurrence with identified clinical risk factors (in index pregnancy unless otherwise specified).

Meta-Analyses	N (with GDM in Index Pregnancy)	GDM Recurrence	Clinical Risk Factors for Recurrence
Kim et al., 2007 [17]	13 studies—11 retrospective cohorts, 2 case-control studies; 3790 women	30–84% in retrospective cohorts; OR 15–23 for case control studies	Minority populations: African American, Latina, Asian
Schwartz et al., 2016 [14]	14 cross-sectional cohort studies; 9211 women	30–80%	Maternal age Maternal BMI Inter-pregnancy weight gain OGTT glucose concentrations Use of insulin Multiparity Fetal macrosomia
Individual Studies	N (with GDM in Index Pregnancy), Location of Study	GDM Recurrence	Clinical Risk Factors for Recurrence
Getahun et al., 2010 [21]	2351, USA	52%	Ethnicity: Hispanic & Asian/Pacific Islanders
Ehrlich et al., 2011 [22]	1028, USA	38%	Inter-pregnancy weight gain
England et al., 2015 [23]	4102, USA	34–48%	Maternal age Born outside of United States
Wong et al., 2019 [24]	3587, Australia	73%	Maternal BMI OGTT glucose concentrations Inter-pregnancy weight gain
Wang et al., 2019 [25]	143, China	55%	OGTT glucose concentrations First trimester triglycerides

BMI: body mass index; GDM: gestational diabetes mellitus; OGTT: oral glucose tolerance testing; OR: odds ratio; USA: United States of America.

In 2016, Schwartz et al. conducted a further systematic review and found recurrence rates ranging from 30–80% [14]. They included 14 studies that examined risk factors for GDM recurrence, including two studies containing >1000 participants that were published subsequent to the aforementioned review by Kim et al. [17]. A meta-analysis was conducted in order to estimate the variability of risk factors for GDM recurrence and pooled effects. They found that increasing maternal age was a risk factor for GDM recurrence; however, the estimated difference in age between those with and without GDM recurrence was minimal at 1.32 years (95% confidence interval (CI) 0.89–1.76, $p < 0.0001$). Increasing maternal body mass index (BMI) was also identified as a risk factor with a weighted mean difference of 1.82 kg/m^2 (0.39–3.26, $p = 0.013$). The authors examined the oral glucose tolerance test (OGTT) glucose concentrations in six studies that presented the mean and standard deviation of the fasting measurement for each group [14]. For post-glucose load measurements, they included four studies that used a 100 g, three-hour OGTT for diagnosis. Although the effect side was not large, there was an increased risk of GDM recurrence with increasing OGTT values, and the first three measurements had the largest impact (fasting glucose standardized mean difference (SMD) = 0.41, glucose one-hour post-load SMD = 0.32 and glucose two-hour post-load SMD = 0.41). Although the inter-pregnancy interval was not found to effect GDM recurrence, inter-pregnancy weight gain had a large effect (SMD = 0.78; $p = 0.015$). Use of insulin therapy (pooled OR 6.3 (95% CI 3.9–10.2), $p < 0.001$), multiparity (pooled OR 1.88 (95% CI 1.09–3.24), $p < 0.02$) and fetal macrosomia (pooled OR 1.63 (95% CI 1.25–2.13), $p < 0.001$) were also noted to increase the risk of GDM recurrence in a subsequent pregnancy [14].

A number of additional important publications were not included in these systematic reviews. Population-based data from Kaiser Permanente Southern California, USA. found that, compared to women without GDM in their first pregnancies ($n = 65{,}132$), women with a first pregnancy complicated by GDM ($n = 2351$) were at a significantly increased risk of GDM in their second pregnancy (OR 13.2, 95% CI 12.0–14.6) [21]. Overall, they reported a 52% recurrence rate of GDM. Compared to non-Hispanic white women, Hispanic women (OR 1.6, 95% CI 1.4–1.7) and Asian/Pacific Islanders (OR 2.1, 95% CI 1.8–2.3) had a higher GDM recurrence risk. This disparity was not explained when women were stratified according to inter-pregnancy interval.

A study from Kaiser Permanente, Northern California, including a total cohort of 22,351 women, of which 4.6% had GDM in the first pregnancy, noted that the age-adjusted risk of recurrent GDM in a second pregnancy was 38.19% (95% CI 34.9–41.42) [22]. This compared to a 3.52% (95% CI 3.27–3.76) risk in those whose first pregnancy was not complicated by GDM. In an analysis adjusted for multiple baseline variables, women with GDM in the first pregnancy had a 17-fold higher risk of developing GDM again in the second pregnancy (OR = 16.55 (95% CI 14.08–19.45)) as compared to those without GDM in their first pregnancy [22]. The risk of GDM recurrence did not differ between women with a BMI <25.0 kg/m^2 and those with BMI ≥ 25.0 kg/m^2. Pregnancy BMI was calculated in each pregnancy at the mean gestational age of 16.9 weeks. It was noted that women who had GDM in the first pregnancy, but not the second pregnancy, gained fewer BMI units between pregnancies than those who had GDM in both pregnancies, particularly those women with a BMI of ≥ 25.0 kg/m^2 in the first pregnancy.

Another population-based study in the United States. included 4102 women with two sequential deliveries between 1998 and 2007, and GDM in the first pregnancy [23]. Depending on the method used to categorize maternal glucose status (birth certificate data versus hospital discharge records), the authors found a GDM recurrence rate of 34–48%. The authors also noted that estimates of progression from GDM in the first pregnancy to pregestational diabetes in the second pregnancy were 2.4–5.1%. Women with recurrent GDM were slightly older at the time of the first pregnancy than those who did not have GDM in the second pregnancy (29.7 versus 28.7 years, $p < 0.001$), and were more likely to have been born outside of the United States. (28.2 versus 25.3%, $p < 0.05$). BMI or weight gain data were not available for this study.

Outside of the United States, a retrospective review of women with GDM based in Australia noted a high rate of GDM recurrence (73.1%) [24]. Logistic regression analysis revealed pre-pregnancy BMI (aOR for BMI >30.0 kg/m^2: 3.8 (95% CI 1.7–8.6) compared to BMI 18.5–25.0 kg/m^2), fasting glucose concentration on OGTT (aOR for fasting glucose >5.2 mmol/L: 1.9 (95% CI 1.1–3.4) compared to ≤ 5.2 mmol/L), 2 h glucose concentration on OGTT (aOR for 2 h glucose >8.4 mmol/L: 2.7 (95% CI 1.6–4.7) compared to ≤ 8.4), and increasing categories of inter-pregnancy weight gain to be associated with recurrent GDM [24]. In fact, the OR for recurrent GDM among those who gained more than 8 kg was 20.5 (95% CI 5.0–84.5), compared with those who lost over 5 kg between the two pregnancies. In this cohort, recurrence of GDM was independent of ethnic backgrounds. Finally, a case control study based in China included 143 primiparous women who experienced GDM in their first pregnancy and went on to have a second pregnancy [25]. The authors observed a frequency of recurrent GDM of 55% and following adjustment for a number of factors, they identified the following risk factors for GDM recurrence: lower first trimester fasting plasma glucose (aOR 0.24 (95% CI 0.10–0.63)) and higher 1 h glucose (75 g OCTT) in the first pregnancy (aOR 1.43 (95% CI 1.09–1.87)) and higher first trimester triglyceride in the subsequent pregnancy (aOR 1.89 (95% CI 1.13–3.16)) [25].

4. Single-Center Experience of GDM Recurrence

4.1. Results

We identified 150 women who had their first delivery (live or still birth) between January 1, 2013, and December 31, 2017, and were diagnosed with GDM at Mayo Clinic. The majority of women were White (113/150, 75%), consistent with the background population in Rochester, Minnesota. Of these, 42 women had a subsequent delivery by the time of data collection, of which 20 (47.6%) were also diagnosed with GDM. The time between the two deliveries ranged from 0.8 to 3.6 years, with a mean of 1.9 (standard deviation 0.6) years.

Women with recurrent GDM were older at the time of the first pregnancy (mean age, 30.0 vs. 27.3 years; $p = 0.03$) (Table 2). A higher proportion of women with recurrent GDM required pharmacological therapy for GDM during the first pregnancy (45.0% (9/20) vs. 31.8% (7/22); $p = 0.38$) and a greater percentage of their first offspring had neonatal hypoglycemia (62.5% (10/16) vs. 36.8% (7/19); $p = 0.13$). However, these differences were not statistically significant. In addition, there was a tendency towards higher rates of pre-existing infertility in women who developed recurrent GDM (13.6% (3/22) vs. (35% (7/20); $p = 0.15$) (Table 3). Other variables including maternal weight, medical complications and mode of delivery were not associated with recurrent GDM (Tables 2 and 3).

Table 2. Maternal Characteristics.

Characteristic at Time of 1st Pregnancy	GDM in 2nd Pregnancy	
	No (n = 22)	Yes (n = 20)
Maternal race		
Asian	0 (0.0%)	1 (5.0%)
Black or African American	2 (9.1%)	0 (0.0%)
White	20 (90.9%)	18 (90.0%)
Unknown/Not Reported	0 (0.0%)	1 (5.0%)
Maternal Age (years), Mean (SD)	27.3 (3.8) *	30.0 (4.0) *
BMI (kg/m^2) (<20/40 gestation), Mean (SD)	30.0 (8.8)	30.3 (5.9)
Current smoking	2 (9.1%)	1 (5.0%)
History of Infertility	3 (13.6%)	7 (35.0%)
First degree relatives with diabetes		
No	13 (59.1%)	19 (95.0%)
Yes	6 (27.3%)	0 (0.0%)
Unknown	3 (13.6%)	1 (5.0%)
Characteristic at Time of 2nd Pregnancy		
Maternal Age (years), Mean (SD)	29.1 (3.9)	32.1 (4.1)
BMI (kg/m^2) (<20/40 gestation), Mean (SD)	29.8 (8.3)	30.2 (5.6)
Months between deliveries, Mean (SD)	20.9 (6.1)	24.2 (8.4)

Significant differences between groups are marked with * indicating $p < 0.05$.

Figure 1 outlines the difference in maternal weight between the start of the first pregnancy and the start of the secondary pregnancy (inter-pregnancy weight gain). There was no difference between women with and without recurrent GDM.

Table 3. Pregnancy outcomes (first pregnancy).

Maternal Outcomes	GDM in 2nd Pregnancy	
	No (n = 22)	Yes (n = 20)
Gestational age at GDM diagnosis, Mean (SD)	28.4 (1.6)	27.0 (1.9)
Diabetes Management		
Diet and lifestyle modifications	15 (68.2%)	11 (55.0%)
Glyburide	7 (31.8%)	9 (45.0%)
Insulin	0	0
Pregnancy-induced hypertension	3 (13.6%)	4 (20.0%)
Pre-eclampsia	3 (13.6%)	2 (10.0%)
Type of Labor		
Spontaneous onset of labor at term	6 (27.3%)	11 (55.0%)
Induction	14 (63.6%)	8 (40.0%)
Preterm onset of labor (PTL)	2 (9.1%)	1 (5.0%)
Method of Delivery		
Vaginal Delivery	12 (54.5%)	14 (70.0%)
Cesarean	10 (45.5%)	6 (30.0%)
Infant Outcomes		
Birth Outcome		
Live Birth—Term (greater than 37 weeks gest.)	16 (72.7%)	15 (75.0%)
Live Birth—Preterm (less than 37 weeks gest.)	6 (27.3%)	4 (20.0%)
Stillbirth	0 (0.0%)	1 (5.0%)
Gestational age at delivery (weeks)		
Mean (SD)	38.5 (2.4)	38.8 (1.9)
Infants with research authorization	(N = 19)	(N = 16)
Admission to neonatal intensive care unit	0	1 (6.3%)
Admission to high dependency unit	9 (47.4%)	7 (43.8%)
Shoulder dystocia	1 (5.3%)	0
Neonatal hypoglycemia	7 (36.8%)	10 (62.5%)
Neonatal death	0	1 (6.3%)

There were no significant between group differences.

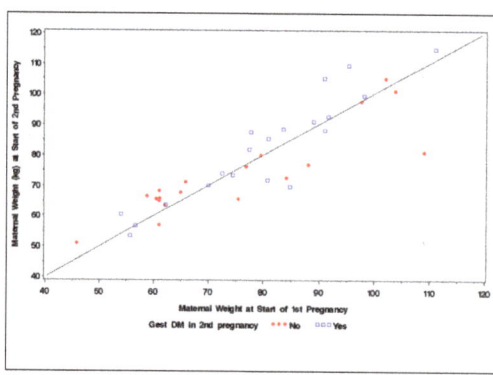

Figure 1. Scatter plot demonstrating interpregnancy weight change in women with and without recurrent gestational diabetes mellitus.

4.2. Discussion

At Mayo Clinic, the GDM recurrence rate of 47.6% was in-keeping with the pooled recurrence reported in a previous meta-analysis [14]. Our cohort contained detailed individual patient data, and women with pre-existing diabetes were excluded. Within this cohort, older maternal age was a significant risk factor for GDM recurrence. In addition, a higher proportion of women with GDM recurrence required pharmacological therapy during their index pregnancy, and their infants were more likely to have had neonatal hypoglycemia. This suggests that women with more severe GDM may be at higher risk of recurrence in a subsequent pregnancy. It is interesting that a history of infertility is associated with GDM recurrence. This may relate to the fact that fertility challenges are more common in older women [26] and hormone therapies used during fertility treatments are associated with increases in insulin resistance [27]. In addition, the underlying cause of the infertility may be associated with GDM—for example, polycystic ovarian syndrome [28]. Additional predictors noted in prior studies were not observed in our cohort. This may be related to our relatively small sample size or differences in baseline population characteristics.

Large, population-based studies identify clinical characteristics associated with GDM recurrence; however, our data highlights the difficulty in applying this information to a clinical practice serving populations with different demographics, and women with several combinations of risk factors. Despite this, it would seem that GDM is more likely to occur if it was more severe in the index pregnancy, and in the setting of higher maternal age. While this information will help inform patient counselling, we recommend that all women with GDM are advised on their relatively high risk of recurrence in a subsequent pregnancy.

5. Prevention of Recurrent GDM

Many trials have examined the effect of various lifestyle interventions in the prenatal setting to prevent GDM. While they have typically included women with risk factors for GDM, they have not specifically targeted those with previous GDM. Some of these studies demonstrated modest effects on GDM prevention [29,30], but many more have shown no effect [31–34]. One exception in terms of target population was a 2016 randomized controlled trial by Guelfi et al. [35]. This trial involved a 14-week supervised, home-based, exercise program starting at 14 weeks of gestation. Unfortunately, while it was associated with important benefits for maternal fitness and psychological well-being, it did not prevent the recurrence of GDM [35]. The failure of this intervention, and indeed many of the GDM lifestyle prevention trials, is possibly due to their initiation at a relatively late stage in the pregnancy (typically the second trimester) and not taking into account patient heterogeneity including variations in BMI and insulin resistance [31]. The RADIEL study (Gestational Diabetes Mellitus Can Be Prevented by Lifestyle Intervention: The Finnish Gestational Diabetes Prevention Study), enriched by women with previous GDM, is another important study in this area [29]. This trial was based in Finland and recruited women <20 weeks gestation with a history of GDM and/or a pre-pregnancy BMI ≥ 25 kg/m^2. Women were randomized to either a complex intervention (individual counseling on diet and physical activity), or standard antenatal care that included written information on diet and physical activity. The incidence of GDM was 13.9% in the intervention group versus 21.6% in the control group. The unadjusted analysis revealed this difference to be non-significant ($p = 0.097$), but it became significant following adjustment for a number of variables including age, pre-pregnancy BMI, previous GDM status, and number of weeks of gestation at time of oral glucose tolerance testing ($p = 0.044$). This study indicated that some women with previous GDM do respond favorably to a lifestyle intervention to reduce their risk of recurrence. We therefore await with interest the results of an ongoing randomized controlled trial in China, evaluating the efficacy of a dietary intervention in preventing the recurrence of GDM, with an estimated completion date of December 2021 [36]. In this study, women are enrolled in the first trimester of pregnancy. This approach is supported by a meta-analysis of 29 antenatal randomized controlled lifestyle trials by Song et al., involving 11,487 women [37]. The overall relative risk of GDM was 0.82 (95% CI 0.70–0.95), but this was due to a significant reduction in GDM among women where the intervention commenced at less than 15 weeks gestation (relative risk 0.78; 95% CI 0.64–0.96), with no significant reduction if the intervention commenced after this point (relative risk 0.97; 95% CI 0.82–1.13) [37].

There are no published trials that have evaluated pharmacological interventions to prevent recurrent GDM. The effect of metformin (initiated during pregnancy) on GDM prevention has been evaluated in two major trials, the 2015 EMPOWaR (effect of metformin on maternal and fetal outcomes in obese pregnant women) study [38] and the 2016 MOP (metformin versus placebo in obese pregnant women without diabetes mellitus) study [39]. Use of metformin for GDM prevention seems logical due to its positive effects on insulin sensitivity, lack of associated weight gain or hypoglycemia, and apparent safety in pregnancy. However, neither of these studies showed a reduction in the incidence of GDM. Data from the Diabetes Prevention Program Outcomes Study suggest that metformin can reduce progression to type 2 diabetes in women with a history of GDM and prediabetes [40]. However, in this study, there was an average interval of 12 years between the GDM pregnancy and initiation of metformin, and it remains unclear if metformin initiated postnatally in women with a history of GDM might lead to reduced risk of recurrent GDM. The TRIPOD (troglitazone in prevention of diabetes) [41] and the PIPOD (pioglitazone in prevention of diabetes) [42] studies demonstrated that thiazolidinediones may preserve β-cell function among women with a recent history of GDM. Although theoretically this may reduce the risk of recurrent GDM, this class of medications are not deemed safe in pregnancy and cannot be used in those who are actively planning to become pregnant. A double-blind, randomized controlled trial examining probiotics for the prevention of GDM in overweight and obese women found that this intervention was not effective, with similar rates of GDM in both arms of the trial (placebo 12.3% (25 of 204) versus 18.4% (38 of 207), $p = 0.10$) [43].

In those women who meet criteria based on BMI with/without medical comorbidities, the significant weight loss associated with bariatric surgery has been clearly linked with a reduction in risk of GDM [44,45]. As an illustrative example, Burke et al. examined 346 obese women who had a delivery before bariatric surgery (predominantly bypass procedures), and 354 who had a delivery after bariatric surgery. Women with a delivery after bariatric surgery had lower incidences of GDM (8% vs. 27%, OR 0.23, (95% CI 0.15–0.36)) [45]. While these studies tend not to focus on women with prior GDM specifically, one can assume that, in the appropriate clinical context, bariatric surgery will be associated with a reduction in risk of recurrent GDM.

Overall, there is a dearth of high-quality clinical evidence on how to reduce the risk of recurrent GDM. Until further information becomes available, it is reasonable to draw on the evidence from the broader GDM prevention studies, which suggest that intensive lifestyle interventions and significant inter-pregnancy weight loss may be effective in reducing risk. Indeed, women with a recent history of GDM may derive extra motivation from the potential of avoiding another high-risk pregnancy.

6. Conclusions

The GDM recurrence rate is high, with approximately 50% of women experiencing this same diagnosis in their subsequent pregnancy. Examination of large datasets suggests that the risk factors for GDM recurrence are similar to those for GDM itself, and include increasing maternal age, weight and certain ethnicities. In addition, women who require insulin to treat GDM in the index pregnancy seem more likely to experience recurrence. In practice, it is difficult to precisely determine an individual's risk based on their clinical characteristics, and it is therefore reasonable to consider all women with previous GDM as being at high risk of recurrence. These women should receive appropriate counselling; weight loss is the intervention most likely to reduce recurrence risk; therefore, it should be supported when clinically indicated. Although not without challenges, future studies should seek to implement interventions before conception and extend through pregnancy and delivery to assess the maximum effect on GDM recurrence risk and pregnancy outcomes.

Author Contributions: A.M.E. contributed to data analysis and manuscript writing and editing; E.A.L.E. contributed to data analysis and manuscript editing; L.A. contributed to data analysis and manuscript editing; A.L.W. contributed to statistical analysis; R.R. contributed to study design and manuscript editing; and M.P.S. contributed to data analysis and manuscript writing and editing. All authors have read and agreed to the published version of the manuscript.

Funding: This research was funded by the National Institutes of Health (NIH), grant numbers DK092721 and HD065987.

Institutional Review Board Statement: The study was conducted according to the guidelines of the Declaration of Helsinki, and approved by the Mayo Clinic Investigational Review Board on 17 November 2017 (Protocol: 17-009957).

Informed Consent Statement: Patient consent was waived because this was a chart review study.

Data Availability Statement: All data for this study are available via Mayo's RedCap system which can be accessed via email communication with the first author for an Excel Spreadsheet.

Acknowledgments: The authors wish to thank Maureen Lemens and Heather LaBrec for their help in study coordination and database design.

Conflicts of Interest: The authors declare no conflict of interest.

References

1. Diagnostic criteria and classification of hyperglycaemia first detected in pregnancy: A World Health Organization Guideline. *Diabetes Res. Clin. Pract.* **2014**, *103*, 341–363. [CrossRef] [PubMed]
2. American Diabetes Association. 2. Classification and Diagnosis of Diabetes. *Diabetes Care* **2019**, *42* (Suppl. 1), S13–S28. [CrossRef] [PubMed]
3. Zhu, Y.; Zhang, C. Prevalence of Gestational Diabetes and Risk of Progression to Type 2 Diabetes: A Global Perspective. *Curr. Diabetes Rep.* **2016**, *16*, 7. [CrossRef] [PubMed]
4. Yogev, C.; Hod, C.; Oats, M.; Metzger, L.; Dyer, D.; Trimble, M.; Rogers, H.P.; McIntyre, H.D.; Hyperglycemia and Adverse Pregnancy Outcome (HAPO) Study Cooperative Research Group. Hyperglycemia and Adverse Pregnancy Outcome (HAPO) study: Preeclampsia. *Am. J. Obstet. Gynecol.* **2010**, *202*, 255.e1–255.e7. [CrossRef] [PubMed]
5. O'Sullivan, E.P.; Avalos, G.; O'reilly, M.; Dennedy, M.C.; Gaffney, G.; Dunne, F. Atlantic Diabetes in Pregnancy (DIP): The prevalence and outcomes of gestational diabetes mellitus using new diagnostic criteria. *Diabetologia* **2011**, *54*, 1670–1675. [CrossRef]
6. Metzger, B.E.; Contreras, M.; Sacks, D.A.; Watson, W.; Dooley, S.L.; Foderaro, M.; Niznik, C.; Bjaloncik, J.; Catalano, P.M.; Dierker, L.; et al. Hyperglycemia and adverse pregnancy outcomes. *N. Engl. J. Med.* **2008**, *358*, 1991–2002. [PubMed]
7. Metzger, B.E.; Bybee, D.E.; Freinkel, N.; Phelps, R.L.; Radvany, R.M.; Vaisrub, N. Gestational diabetes mellitus. Correlations between the phenotypic and genotypic characteristics of the mother and abnormal glucose tolerance during the first year postpartum. *Diabetes* **1985**, *34* (Suppl. 2), 111–115. [CrossRef]
8. O'Sullivan, J. Long term follow up of gestational diabetics. In *Early Diabetes*; Academic Press: Cambridge, MA, USA, 1975.
9. Guerrero-Romero, F.; Aradillas-García, C.; Simental-Mendia, L.E.; Monreal-Escalante, E.; De la Cruz Mendoza, E.; Rodríguez-Moran, M. Birth weight, family history of diabetes, and metabolic syndrome in children and adolescents. *J. Pediatr.* **2010**, *156*, 719–723. [CrossRef]
10. Lowe, W.L.; Scholtens, D.M.; Lowe, L.P.; Kuang, A.; Nodzenski, M.; Talbot, O.; Catalano, P.M.; Linder, B.; Brickman, W.J.; Clayton, P.; et al. Association of Gestational Diabetes with Maternal Disorders of Glucose Metabolism and Childhood Adiposity. *JAMA* **2018**, *320*, 1005–1016. [CrossRef]
11. Avalos, G.E.; Owens, L.A.; Dunne, F.; Collaborators, A.D. Applying current screening tools for gestational diabetes mellitus to a European population: Is it time for change? *Diabetes Care* **2013**, *36*, 3040–3044. [CrossRef]
12. Farrar, D.; Simmonds, M.; Bryant, M.; Lawlor, D.A.; Dunne, F.; Tuffnell, D.; Sheldon, T.A. Risk factor screening to identify women requiring oral glucose tolerance testing to diagnose gestational diabetes: A systematic review and meta-analysis and analysis of two pregnancy cohorts. *PLoS ONE* **2017**, *12*, e0175288. [CrossRef] [PubMed]
13. National Institute for Health and Care Excellence. Diabetes in Pregnancy: Management from Preconception to the Postnatal Period. 2015. Available online: https://www.nice.org.uk/guidance/ng3 (accessed on 12 January 2021).
14. Schwartz, N.; Nachum, Z.; Green, M.S. Risk factors of gestational diabetes mellitus recurrence: A meta-analysis. *Endocrine* **2016**, *53*, 662–671. [CrossRef]
15. Enninga, E.A.L.; Egan, A.M.; Alrahmani, L.; Leontovich, A.A.; Ruano, R.; Sarras, M.P. Frequency of Gestational Diabetes Mellitus Reappearance or Absence during the Second Pregnancy of Women Treated at Mayo Clinic between 2013 and 2018. *J Diabetes Res.* **2019**, *2019*, 9583927. [CrossRef] [PubMed]
16. ACOG Practice Bulletin No. 190 Summary: Gestational Diabetes Mellitus. *Obstet. Gynecol.* **2018**, *131*, 406–408.
17. Kim, C.; Berger, D.K.; Chamany, S. Recurrence of gestational diabetes mellitus: A systematic review. *Diabetes Care* **2007**, *30*, 1314–1319. [CrossRef] [PubMed]

18. McGuire, V.; Rauh, M.J.; Mueller, B.A.; Hickock, D. The risk of diabetes in a subsequent pregnancy associated with prior history of gestational diabetes or macrosomic infant. *Paediatr. Perinat. Epidemiol.* **1996**, *10*, 64–72. [CrossRef] [PubMed]
19. Cheung, N.W.; Wasmer, G.; Al-Ali, J. Risk factors for gestational diabetes among Asian women. *Diabetes Care* **2001**, *24*, 955–956. [CrossRef]
20. MacNeill, S.; Dodds, L.; Hamilton, D.C.; Armson, B.A.; VandenHof, M. Rates and risk factors for recurrence of gestational diabetes. *Diabetes Care* **2001**, *24*, 659–662. [CrossRef] [PubMed]
21. Getahun, D.; Fassett, M.J.; Jacobsen, S.J. Gestational diabetes: Risk of recurrence in subsequent pregnancies. *Am. J. Obstet. Gynecol.* **2010**, *203*, 467.e1–467.e6. [CrossRef] [PubMed]
22. Ehrlich, S.F.; Hedderson, M.M.; Feng, J.; Davenport, E.R.; Gunderson, E.P.; Ferrara, A. Change in body mass index between pregnancies and the risk of gestational diabetes in a second pregnancy. *Obstet. Gynecol.* **2011**, *117*, 1323–1330. [CrossRef]
23. England, L.; Kotelchuck, M.; Wilson, H.G.; Diop, H.; Oppedisano, P.; Kim, S.Y.; Cui, X.; Shapiro-Mendoza, C.K. Estimating the Recurrence Rate of Gestational Diabetes Mellitus (GDM) in Massachusetts 1998–2007: Methods and Findings. *Matern. Child Health J.* **2015**, *19*, 2303–2313. [CrossRef] [PubMed]
24. Wong, V.W.; Chong, S.; Chenn, R.; Jalaludin, B. Factors predicting recurrence of gestational diabetes in a high-risk multi-ethnic population. *Aust. N. Z. J. Obstet. Gynaecol.* **2019**. [CrossRef] [PubMed]
25. Wang, Y.Y.; Liu, Y.; Li, C.; Lin, J.; Liu, X.M.; Sheng, J.Z.; Huang, H.F. Frequency and risk factors for recurrent gestational diabetes mellitus in primiparous women: A case control study. *BMC Endocr. Disord.* **2019**, *19*, 22. [CrossRef] [PubMed]
26. American College of Obstetricians and Gynecologists Committee on Gynecologic Practice and Practice Committee. Female age-related fertility decline. Committee Opinion No. 589. *Fertil. Steril.* **2014**, *101*, 633–634. [CrossRef] [PubMed]
27. Coussa, A.; Hasan, H.A.; Barber, T.M. Impact of contraception and IVF hormones on metabolic, endocrine, and inflammatory status. *J. Assist. Reprod Genet.* **2020**, *37*, 1267–1272. [CrossRef] [PubMed]
28. Teede, H.J.; Misso, M.L.; Costello, M.F.; Dokras, A.; Laven, J.; Moran, L.; Piltonen, T.; Norman, R.J. Recommendations from the international evidence-based guideline for the assessment and management of polycystic ovary syndrome. *Fertil. Steril.* **2018**, *110*, 364–379. [CrossRef]
29. Koivusalo, S.B.; Rönö, K.; Klemetti, M.M.; Roine, R.P.; Lindström, J.; Erkkola, M.; Kaaja, R.J.; Pöyhönen-Alho, M.; Tiitinen, A.; Huvinen, E.; et al. Gestational Diabetes Mellitus Can Be Prevented by Lifestyle Intervention: The Finnish Gestational Diabetes Prevention Study (RADIEL): A Randomized Controlled Trial. *Diabetes Care* **2016**, *39*, 24–30. [CrossRef]
30. Wang, C.; Wei, Y.; Zhang, X.; Zhang, Y.; Xu, Q.; Su, S.; Zhang, L.; Liu, C.; Feng, Y.; Shou, C.; et al. Effect of Regular Exercise Commenced in Early Pregnancy on the Incidence of Gestational Diabetes Mellitus in Overweight and Obese Pregnant Women: A Randomized Controlled Trial. *Diabetes Care* **2016**, *39*, e163–e164. [CrossRef]
31. Egan, A.M.; Simmons, D. Lessons learned from lifestyle prevention trials in gestational diabetes mellitus. *Diabetes Med.* **2019**, *36*, 142–150. [CrossRef]
32. Stafne, S.N.; Salvesen, K.; Romundstad, P.R.; Eggebø, T.M.; Carlsen, S.M.; Mørkved, S. Regular exercise during pregnancy to prevent gestational diabetes: A randomized controlled trial. *Obstet. Gynecol.* **2012**, *119*, 29–36. [CrossRef]
33. Poston, L.; Bell, R.; Croker, H.; Flynn, A.C.; Godfrey, K.M.; Goff, L.; Hayes, L.; Khazaezadeh, N.; Nelson, S.M.; Oteng-Ntim, E.; et al. Effect of a behavioural intervention in obese pregnant women (the UPBEAT study): A multicentre, randomised controlled trial. *Lancet Diabetes Endocrinol.* **2015**, *3*, 767–777. [CrossRef]
34. Simmons, D.; Devlieger, R.; Van Assche, A.; Jans, G.; Galjaard, S.; Corcoy, R.; Adelantado, J.M.; Dunne, F.; Desoye, G.; Harreiter, J.; et al. Effect of Physical Activity and/or Healthy Eating on GDM Risk: The DALI Lifestyle Study. *J. Clin. Endocrinol. Metab.* **2017**, *102*, 903–913. [CrossRef] [PubMed]
35. Guelfi, K.J.; Ong, M.J.; Crisp, N.A.; Fournier, P.A.; Wallman, K.E.; Grove, J.R.; Doherty, D.A.; Newnham, J.P. Regular Exercise to Prevent the Recurrence of Gestational Diabetes Mellitus: A Randomized Controlled Trial. *Obstet. Gynecol.* **2016**, *128*, 819–827. [CrossRef] [PubMed]
36. ClinicalTrials.gov. Lifestyle Intervention to Prevent the Recurrence of Gestational Diabetes Mellitus. Available online: https://clinicaltrials.gov/ct2/show/NCT03062475 (accessed on 17 November 2020).
37. Song, C.; Li, J.; Leng, J.; Ma, R.C.; Yang, X. Lifestyle intervention can reduce the risk of gestational diabetes: A meta-analysis of randomized controlled trials. *Obes. Rev.* **2016**, *17*, 960–969. [CrossRef] [PubMed]
38. Chiswick, C.; Reynolds, R.M.; Denison, F.; Drake, A.J.; Forbes, S.; Newby, D.E.; Walker, B.R.; Quenby, S.; Wray, S.; Weeks, A.; et al. Effect of metformin on maternal and fetal outcomes in obese pregnant women (EMPOWaR): A randomised, double-blind, placebo-controlled trial. *Lancet Diabetes Endocrinol.* **2015**, *3*, 778–786. [CrossRef]
39. Syngelaki, A.; Nicolaides, K.H.; Balani, J.; Hyer, S.; Akolekar, R.; Kotecha, R.; Pastides, A.; Shehata, H. Metformin versus Placebo in Obese Pregnant Women without Diabetes Mellitus. *N. Engl. J. Med.* **2016**, *374*, 434–443. [CrossRef]
40. Aroda, V.R.; Christophi, C.A.; Edelstein, S.L.; Zhang, P.; Herman, W.H.; Barrett-Connor, E.; Delahanty, L.M.; Montez, M.G.; Ackermann, R.T.; Zhuo, X.; et al. The effect of lifestyle intervention and metformin on preventing or delaying diabetes among women with and without gestational diabetes: The Diabetes Prevention Program outcomes study 10-year follow-up. *J. Clin. Endocrinol. Metab.* **2015**, *100*, 1646–1653. [CrossRef]
41. Buchanan, T.A.; Xiang, A.H.; Peters, R.K.; Kjos, S.L.; Marroquin, A.; Goico, J.; Ochoa, C.; Tan, S.; Berkowitz, K.; Hodis, H.N.; et al. Preservation of pancreatic beta-cell function and prevention of type 2 diabetes by pharmacological treatment of insulin resistance in high-risk hispanic women. *Diabetes* **2002**, *51*, 2796–2803. [CrossRef]

42. Xiang, A.H.; Peters, R.K.; Kjos, S.L.; Marroquin, A.; Goico, J.; Ochoa, C.; Kawakubo, M.; Buchanan, T.A. Effect of pioglitazone on pancreatic beta-cell function and diabetes risk in Hispanic women with prior gestational diabetes. *Diabetes* **2006**, *55*, 517–522. [CrossRef]
43. Callaway, L.K.; McIntyre, H.D.; Barrett, H.L.; Foxcroft, K.; Tremellen, A.; Lingwood, B.E.; Tobin, J.M.; Wilkinson, S.; Kothari, A.; Morrison, M.; et al. Probiotics for the Prevention of Gestational Diabetes Mellitus in Overweight and Obese Women: Findings from the SPRING Double-Blind Randomized Controlled trial. *Diabetes Care* **2019**, *42*, 364–371. [CrossRef]
44. Johansson, K.; Cnattingius, S.; Näslund, I.; Roos, N.; Trolle Lagerros, Y.; Granath, F.; Stephansson, O.; Neovius, M. Outcomes of pregnancy after bariatric surgery. *N. Engl. J. Med.* **2015**, *372*, 814–824. [CrossRef] [PubMed]
45. Burke, A.E.; Bennett, W.L.; Jamshidi, R.M.; Gilson, M.M.; Clark, J.M.; Segal, J.B.; Shore, A.D.; Magnuson, T.H.; Dominici, F.; Wu, A.W.; et al. Reduced incidence of gestational diabetes with bariatric surgery. *J. Am. Coll. Surg.* **2010**, *211*, 169–175. [CrossRef] [PubMed]

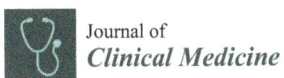

Article

Secretagogin is Related to Insulin Secretion but Unrelated to Gestational Diabetes Mellitus Status in Pregnancy

Carola Deischinger [1,†], Jürgen Harreiter [1,†,*], Karoline Leitner [1], Dagmar Bancher-Todesca [2], Sabina Baumgartner-Parzer [1] and Alexandra Kautzky-Willer [1]

1 Clinical Division of Endocrinology and Metabolism, Department of Internal Medicine III, Gender Medicine Unit, Medical University of Vienna, Waehringer Guertel 18–20, 1090 Vienna, Austria; carola.deischinger@meduniwien.ac.at (C.D.); karoline.leitner@meduniwien.ac.at (K.L.); sabina.baumgartner-parzer@meduniwien.ac.at (S.B.-P.); alexandra.kautzky-willer@meduniwien.ac.at (A.K.-W.)
2 Department of Obstetrics and Gynecology, Medical University of Vienna, Waehringer Guertel 18–20, 1090 Vienna, Austria; dagmar.bancher-todesca@meduniwien.ac.at
* Correspondence: juergen.harreiter@meduniwien.ac.at; Tel.: +43-(0)1-40400-22290
† These authors contributed equally to this work.

Received: 15 June 2020; Accepted: 15 July 2020; Published: 17 July 2020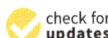

Abstract: Secretagogin (SCGN) is a calcium binding protein related to insulin release in the pancreas. Although SCGN is not co-released with insulin, plasma concentrations have been found to be increased in type 2 diabetes mellitus patients. Until now, no study on SCGN levels in pregnancy or patients with gestational diabetes mellitus (GDM) has been published. In 93 women of a high-risk population for GDM at the Medical University of Vienna, secretagogin levels of 45 GDM patients were compared to 48 women with a normal glucose tolerance (NGT). Glucose tolerance, insulin resistance and secretion were assessed with oral glucose tolerance tests (OGTT) between the 10th and 28th week of gestation (GW) and postpartum. In all women, however, predominantly in women with NGT, there was a significant positive correlation between SCGN levels and Stumvoll first ($r_p = 0.220$, $p = 0.032$) and second phase index ($r_p = 0.224$, $p = 0.028$). SCGN levels were not significantly different in women with NGT and GDM. However, SCGN was higher postpartum than during pregnancy (postpartum: 88.07 ± 35.63 pg/mL; pregnancy: 75.24 ± 37.90 pg/mL, $p = 0.004$). SCGN was directly correlated with week of gestation ($r_p = 0.308$; $p = 0.021$) and triglycerides ($r_p = 0.276$; $p = 0.038$) in women with GDM. Therefore, SCGN is related to insulin secretion and hyperinsulinemia during pregnancy; however, it does not display differences between women with NGT and GDM.

Keywords: biomarker; gestational diabetes mellitus; insulin secretion; pregnancy; secretagogin

1. Introduction

Secretagogin (SCGN) is a calcium-binding protein, which was discovered in the pancreas in 1998 [1]. Many interactions of SCGN have not yet been fully understood; however, they are assumed to be of importance to the function of secretory cells [2–7]. Besides neuroendocrine cells such as the islets of Langerhans and developing or adult neurons, SCGN can be found in the thyroid, gastrointestinal tract, adrenal medulla, adrenal gland and brain [1]. Its involvement with vesicle trafficking and exocytosis has already been proven for insulin release in pancreatic islet cells and corticotropin-releasing hormone (CRH) mediated stress responses [8–10]. The exact mechanism of secretagogin's influence on insulin release has only been understood rather recently and involves SCGN-interacting proteins which are either actin-binding proteins, involved in insulin granule trafficking and exocytosis [11] or have a regulatory function towards the actin cytoskeleton by facilitating vesicle transport to the periphery during insulin release [12]. SCGN further binds insulin and improves insulin signaling when compared to insulin action alone by increasing insulin-induced phosphorylation of Akt [13]. Accordingly, SCGN was recently found to be elevated in patients with type 2 diabetes [14] and has been related to beta-cell proliferation and insulin secretion [9]. In pregnancy, insulin resistance increases to ensure the glucose supply of the fetus, which is countered by a higher level of insulin production and secretion [15,16]. The pancreatic islets adapt to cope with the increased insulin production and secretion. Islet cell mass increases 1.4–2-fold during gestation [17,18], whereas adult islet cell mass remains steady and proliferates slowly outside of pregnancy [19]. If these adaptions are insufficient and the insulin supply fail to match tissue demand, pregnant women develop gestational diabetes mellitus (GDM) [20]. GDM is a form of hyperglycemia with its onset or first detection during pregnancy and has a prevalence of 2 to 6% in Europe [21]. Not only is GDM associated with an increased risk for complications for both mother and child during pregnancy and childbirth [22] but also have women who suffer from gestational diabetes a 3.44 elevated risk for developing type 2 diabetes mellitus postpartum [23]. Up to this day, no studies on SCGN and its possible roles during pregnancy have been published. Previously, SCGN was associated with beta-cell proliferation, insulin secretion and was increased in patients with diabetes mellitus. Therefore, we hypothesized SCGN might be similarly involved in GDM and aimed at investigating SCGN as a marker of insulin secretion in the context of pregnancy, postpartum and the development of GDM.

2. Materials and Methods

2.1. Study Participants and Design

The study population included 93 pregnant women (48 women with normal glucose tolerance (NGT), 45 with GDM) of all body mass index (BMI) categories recruited for two prospective longitudinal studies conducted at the Medical University of Vienna between 2010 and 2014. Both studies were approved by the local ethics committee (Ethics Committee of the Medical University of Vienna, EK Nr. 2022/2012 & 771/2008) and was performed in accordance with the Declaration of Helsinki. All subjects gave written informed consent for participation in the study [24]. Inclusion criteria were a singleton pregnancy and age ≥ 18 years. Exclusion criteria were pre-existing diabetes, chronic and/or infectious diseases, significant psychiatric disorders or inability to follow instructions related to the studies due to language difficulties. All study subjects were monitored and treated during their pregnancy following the national guidelines [25,26]. As a tertiary health care center taking care of higher risk pregnancies, a high number of cases with GDM is represented in our cohort. GDM was assessed according to IADPSG WHO guidelines [27]. Oral glucose tolerance tests and further clinical evaluations were performed at week of gestation (GW) 10–28 and postpartum (mean = 8 ± 6 months after delivery), respectively, with blood samples taken at baseline, 30, 60, 90 and 120 min for the measurement of glucose, insulin and c-peptide. Hemoglobin A1c according to the International Federation of Clinical Chemistry working group (HbA1c-IFCC) and levels of triglycerides, cholesterol, creatine and bioavailable estradiol were analyzed in our ISO 9001 certified central laboratory at the General Hospital in Vienna (AKH Wien, Austria, www.kimcl.at). Weight was measured on calibrated electronic scales (SECA 877/888, SECA, Hamburg, Germany) wearing no shoes and light clothes. Waist circumference was measured twice at the midpoint between the lower border of the rib cage and the iliac crest and hip circumference at the widest portion of the buttocks. Systolic and diastolic blood pressure and heart rate were measured on the left arm with an appropriate-sized cuff with an BOSO medicus device (Bosch + Sohn, Jungingen, Germany).

2.2. Calculation of Insulin Secretion and Sensitivity Indices

Approximations of insulin sensitivity and insulin secretion were calculated (Matsuda Index, Stumvoll first and second phase index, insulin secretion sensitivity index (ISSI-2), disposition index, area under the curve (AUC) insulin and glucose) for each oral glucose tolerance tests (OGTT). The Matsuda Index is an estimate of peripheral and hepatic insulin sensitivity (liver, muscle and adipose tissue). Due to the complexity of the formula, an online calculator was used [28]. Stumvoll first phase index for insulin secretion was calculated as $1.283 + 1.829 \times$ Insulin 30min $- 138.7 \times$ Glucose 30min $+ 3.772 \times$ Insulin 0 min for estimated first phase beta cell function. Stumvoll second phase index was calculated with the formula $287 + 0.4164 \times$ Insulin 30 min $- 26.07 \times$ Glucose 30min $+ 0.9226 \times$ Insulin 0 min [29]. Oral disposition index is the product of the Matsuda Index and Δ Insulin $0 - 30/\Delta$ Glucose $0 - 30$ [30,31]. To improve the assessment of beta-cell reserve, ISSI-2, the product of the Matsuda Index and the ratio of the area-under-the-insulin curve to the area-under-the-glucose curve, was used [32]. AUC insulin and AUC glucose were calculated using the trapezoidal method.

2.3. SCGN Assay

For the serum SCGN analysis, a human ELISA kit (BioVendor, Brno, Czech Republic) was used (https://www.biovendor.com/secretagogin-human-elisa?d=114). The detection range of this kit is 62.5–2000 pg/mL with an inter-assay coefficient of variability (CV) of 6.5% and an intra-assay CV of 6%. Samples were diluted 1 + 1 with dilution buffer (provided in the assay kit), internal control samples were analyzed in each assay and the measured concentrations were in the expected range. As internal controls gave almost identical results in three different assays adjustment for inter-assay bias was not done.

2.4. Statistical Analysis

Descriptive data analysis was performed for all parameters. Continuous variables were summarized by mean ± SD and categorical variables by counts and percentages. Assumption of Gaussian distribution of parameters was decided by visual assessment of histograms and calculation of skewness using Kolmogorov–Smirnov test. Consequently, the non-parametrically distributed parameter SCGN was log transformed. All women with SCGN values outside the reference range of the SCGN kit (62.5–2000 pg/mL) and outliers with $2 \times 1,5$ IQR were excluded from the analysis. An independent samples T-Test was used to investigate differences in SCGN levels between NGT and GDM in pregnancy. Due to missing values, postpartum SCGN values were not available for all women. In a subgroup of women with both pregnancy and postpartum SCGN values ($n = 34$), a paired T-test was performed. To assess SCGN levels over the course of an OGTT, a repeated measure ANOVA (with Greenhouse–Geisser correction due to rejected sphericity assumption) was calculated. Pearson's correlation was used for a correlation analysis. As this is a post hoc analysis, a power analysis was omitted. For the statistical analysis, SPSS 25.0 (SPSS Inc, Chicago, USA) was used. A two-sided p-value ≤ 0.05 was considered statistically significant.

3. Results

3.1. Baseline Characteristics

Characteristics of the study population are presented in Table 1 and show significant differences between the groups in anthropometric, glycemic and metabolic parameters. The AUC insulin ($p = 0.024$) and AUC glucose ($p < 0.001$) were elevated in women with GDM compared to NGT. Matsuda index ($p = 0.013$), ISSI-2 ($p < 0.001$), disposition index ($p < 0.001$), Stumvoll first phase ($p = 0.003$) and second phase index ($p = 0.020$) were lower; HbA1c ($p = 0.002$) and triglycerides ($p = 0.014$) higher in GDM than in NGT. Postpartum, none of the glycemic and metabolic parameters differed between NGT and those who had had GDM during pregnancy. Fetal parameters such as fetal weight, length, abdominal and head circumference did not differ between the groups either.

Table 1. Baseline characteristics and glycemic and metabolic parameters of oral glucose tolerance tests (OGTT) at GW 10–28 and postpartum for NGT and GDM.

	All	NGT	GDM	
	Mean (± SD)	Mean (± SD)	Mean (± SD)	*p*-Values
Maternal Indices at GW 10–28				
Number	93	48	45	
GDM in previous pregnancy	48.8%	40.9%	57.9%	0.094
Birth weight > 4000 g in previous pregnancy	23.5%	20.5%	27.0%	0.486
BMI before pregnancy (in kg/m^2)	28.59 (± 7.06)	27.88 (± 6.69)	29.34 (± 7.44)	0.243
Waist (in cm)	114.8 (± 10.8)	114.7 (± 9.1)	115.0 (± 12.4)	0.795
Hip (in cm)	123.6 (± 11.5)	124.1 (± 8.7)	123.0 (± 14.0)	0.833
Age (in years)	33 (± 5)	32 (± 5)	33 (± 5)	0.632
Blood pressure systolic (in mmHg)	114 (± 11)	114 (± 10)	114 (± 12)	0.809
Blood pressure diastolic (in mmHg)	69 (± 8)	68 (± 8)	70 (± 9)	0.177
Pregnancy (GW 10–28)				
SCGN (in pg/mL)	75.24 (± 37.90)	71.57 (± 34.47)	79.15 (± 41.28)	0.514
AUC insulin	70.36 (± 45.96)	59.77 (± 33.87)	85.06 (± 56.12)	0.024
AUC glucose	131.43 (± 29.26)	110.60 (± 12.85)	160.32 (± 19.18)	<0.001
Matsuda Index	5.77 (± 4.13)	6.68 (± 4.20)	4.49 (± 3.73)	0.013
Stumvoll first phase index (in pmol/L)	1171.65 (± 605.86)	1307.64 (± 626.24)	974.24 (± 523.90)	0.003
Stumvoll second phase index (in pmol/L)	343.24 (± 159.76)	371.18 (± 168.12)	302.68 (± 139.57)	0.020
Disposition Index	5.79 (± 5.30)	7.88 (± 5.75)	2.57 (± 1.89)	<0.001
ISSI-2	292.85 (± 127.09)	354.40 (± 111.32)	207.47 (± 94.81)	<0.001
HbA1c (in mmol/mol Hb)	32.22 (± 2.6)	30.03 (± 1.9)	33.32 (± 3.24)	0.002
Triglycerides (in mg/dL)	170 (± 58)	153 (± 55)	188 (± 56)	0.014
Cholesterol (in mg/dL)	224 (± 45)	221 (± 43)	228 (± 47)	0.667
Bioavailable estradiol (pg/mL)	1231 (± 685)	1117 (± 659)	1350 (± 698)	0.100
Postpartum				
Number	34	19	15	
SCGN (in pg/mL)	88.07 (± 35.63)	83.88 (± 24.65)	93.37 (± 46.45)	0.683
AUC insulin	39.98 (± 27.15)	29.09 (± 11.76)	44.34 (± 30.73)	0.363
AUC glucose	118.04 (± 18.01)	111.13 (± 19.46)	120.81 (± 17.67)	0.384
Matsuda Index	8.92 (± 5.89)	10.33 (± 5.65)	8.35 (± 6.18)	0.591
Stumvoll first phase index (in pmol/L)	862.12 (± 488.50)	883.31 (± 615.93)	853.65 (± 466.86)	0.923
Stumvoll second phase index (in pmol/L)	259.71 (± 129.43)	260.98 (± 154.27)	259.20 (± 127.52)	0.983
Disposition Index	4.70 (± 2.36)	6.41 (± 3.06)	3.94 (± 1.66)	0.080
ISSI-2	273.65 (± 99.19)	304.15 (± 135.65)	261.46 (± 86.60)	0.489

Table 1. *Cont.*

	All	NGT	GDM	
	Mean (± SD)	Mean (± SD)	Mean (± SD)	*p*-Values
HbA1c (in mmol/mol Hb)	32.24 (± 1.9)	34.41 (± 1.9)	32.24 (± 1.9)	0.157
Triglycerides (in mg/dL)	90 (± 45)	84 (± 44)	97 (± 47)	0.389
Cholesterol (in mg/dL)	193 (± 34)	189 (± 38)	197 (± 29)	0.466
Bioavailable estradiol (in pg/mL)	39 (± 55)	49 (± 69)	26 (± 22)	0.228

Continuous variables were summarized by mean ± standard deviation (SD) and categorical variables by counts and percentages. To assess differences between NGT and GDM and GDM subgroups, a T-Test was performed. NGT: normal glucose tolerance; GDM: gestational diabetes mellitus; GW: week of gestation; AUC: area under the curve; BMI: body mass index; SCGN: secretagogin; HbA1c: hemoglobin A1c; ISSI-2: insulin secretion sensitivity index.

3.2. SCGN Levels in NGT and GDM During Pregnancy and Postpartum

In the whole cohort, SCGN levels were significantly lower during pregnancy (mean = 75.24 pg/mL, SD = 37.90 pg/mL) compared to postpartum (mean = 88.07 pg/mL, SD = 35.63 pg/mL, *p* = 0.004). As illustrated in Figure 1, SCGN levels were higher postpartum in NGT (*p* = 0.034). SCGN levels displayed the same trend in women who had had GDM during gestation, albeit not significant (*p* = 0.067).

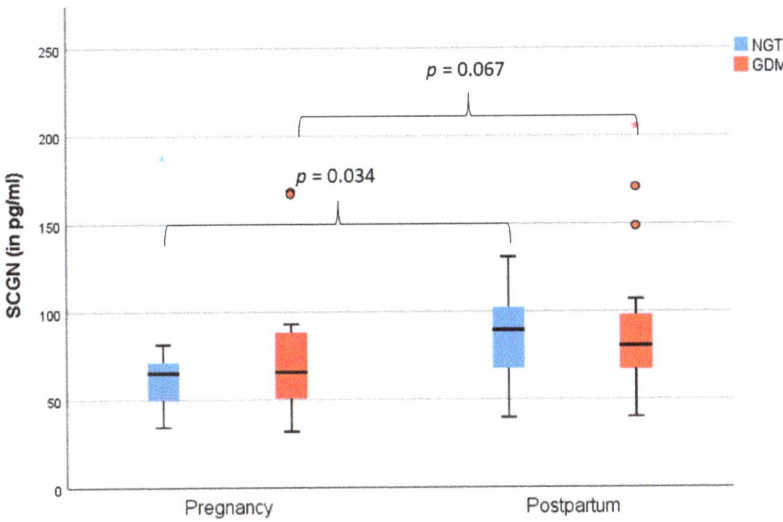

Figure 1. Clustered boxplot of secretagogin (SCGN) levels in normal glucose tolerance (NGT) (*n* = 19) and gestational diabetes mellitus (GDM) (*n* = 15) during pregnancy and postpartum.

Unlike in type 2 diabetes mellitus patients, there was no difference in SCGN levels between NGT and GDM (pregnancy: *p* = 0.514; postpartum: *p* = 0.683). When investigating SCGN over the course of an OGTT in a small subgroup of 9 women (5 NGT, 4 GDM), SCGN did not change significantly (*p* = 0.100) from 77.9 pg/mL (± 55.0 pg/mL) at baseline, 74.83 pg/mL (± 52.0 pg/mL) after 60 min to 80.1 pg/mL (± 52.5 pg/mL) at 120 min.

3.3. Correlation of SCGN with Covariates in Pregnancy and Postpartum

As demonstrated in Figure 2 and Table 2, there was a direct correlation between SCGN levels and Stumvoll first (r_p = 0.220, *p* = 0.032) and second phase index (r_p = 0.224, *p* = 0.028), parameters of insulin secretion, in all women during pregnancy, however, predominantly in women with NGT. In women with NGT, SCGN correlated positively with Stumvoll first (r_p = 0.390, *p* = 0.004) and second phase index ($r_p = 0.395$, $p = 0.003$), AUC insulin ($r_p = 0.380$, $p = 0.005$) and HbA1c ($r_p = -0.391$, $p = 0.002$) and negatively with the Matsuda index ($r_p = -0.273$, $p = 0.050$). Postpartum, these glycemic indices ceased to correlate with SCGN. Furthermore, SCGN was directly correlated with creatine ($r_p = 0.194$, $p = 0.012$) in the whole cohort and with triglycerides ($r_p = 0.276$, $p = 0.038$) in women with GDM during pregnancy (see Figure 3 and Table 2).

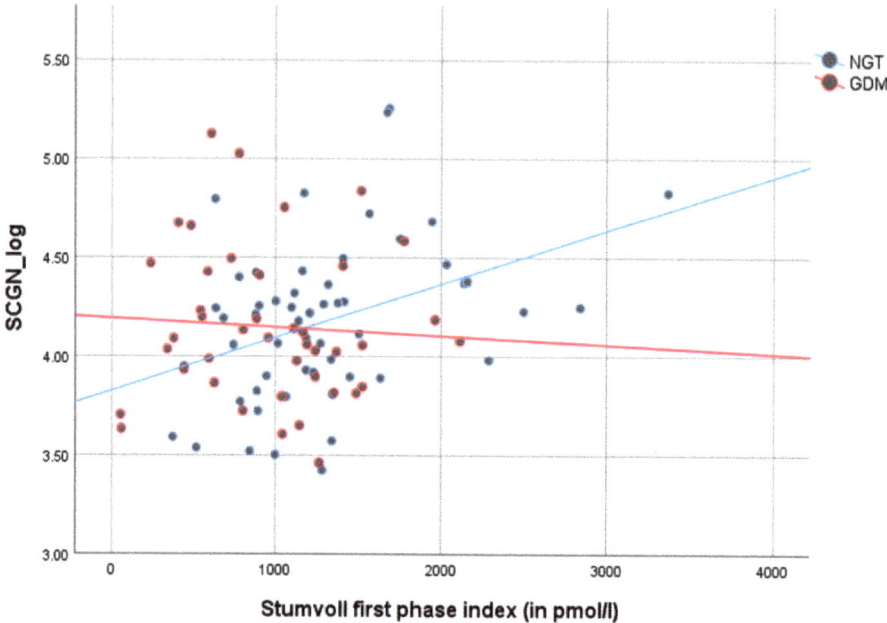

Figure 2. Grouped scatter dot plot according to glucose tolerance (blue = NGT, red = GDM) of the correlation between secretagogin (SCGN) (log-transformed) and Stumvoll first phase index during pregnancy. SCGN correlated directly with Stumvoll first phase index in women with NGT ($r_p = 0.390$, $p = 0.004$), an effect which was not present in GDM ($r_p = -0.056$, $p = 0.724$). NGT: normal glucose tolerance; GDM: gestational diabetes mellitus.

Table 2. Pearson's correlation analysis SCGN during pregnancy in all women, women with NGT and GDM. The significance level is $p \leq 0.05$.

Pearson' Correlation	All (in Pregnancy)		NGT (in Pregnancy)		GDM (in Pregnancy)	
	r_p	p	r_p	p	r_p	p
Week of gestation	0.172	0.068	0.035	0.791	0.308	0.021
BMI of visit	−0.069	0.470	0.055	0.686	−0.174	0.203
Blood pressure systolic	0.193	0.043	0.221	0.105	0.172	0.210
Blood pressure diastolic	0.121	0.209	0.219	0.108	0.030	0.829
Matsuda Index	−0.104	0.320	−0.273	0.050	0.093	0.563
Stumvoll first phase index	0.220	0.032	0.390	0.004	−0.056	0.724
Stumvoll second phase index	0.224	0.028	0.395	0.003	−0.058	0.714
Disposition index	0.107	0.316	0.002	0.987	0.316	0.057
ISSI-2	0.082	0.436	−0.026	0.856	0.163	0.310

Table 2. Cont.

Pearson' Correlation	All (in Pregnancy)		NGT (in Pregnancy)		GDM (in Pregnancy)	
	r_p	p	r_p	p	r_p	p
AUC insulin	0.132	0.206	0.380	0.005	−0.028	0.861
AUC glucose	−0.029	0.782	0.019	0.893	0.035	0.827
HbA1c	−0.158	0.092	−0.391	0.002	−0.028	0.836
Triglycerides	0.171	0.067	0.041	0.761	0.276	0.038
Cholesterol	0.169	0.072	0.078	0.560	0.246	0.065
Creatine	0.194	0.012	0.191	0.068	0.223	0.057
Bioavailable estradiol	0.139	0.139	0.151	0.263	0.113	0.402

SGGN: secretagogin; NGT: normal glucose tolerance; GDM: gestational diabetes mellitus; AUC: area under the curve; BMI: body mass index; ISSI-2: insulin secretion sensitivity index; HbA1c: hemoglobin A1c.

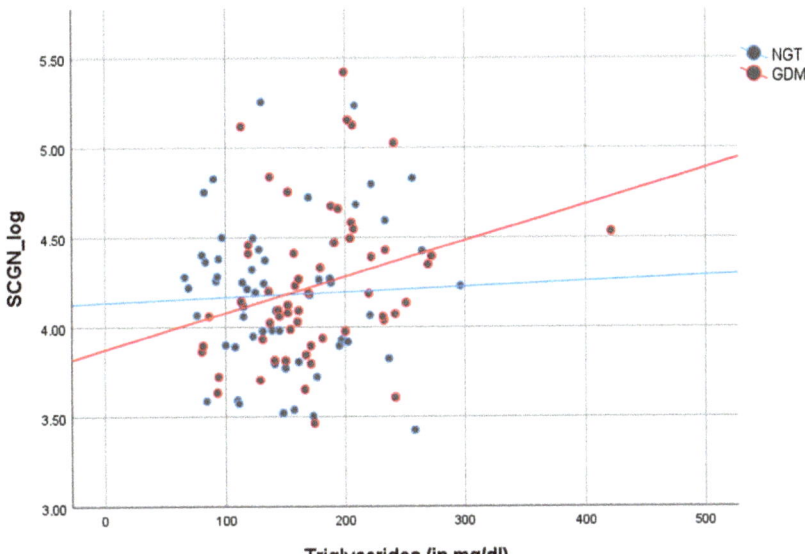

Figure 3. Grouped scatter dot plot according to glucose tolerance (blue = NGT, red = GDM) of the correlation between secretagogin (SCGN) (log-transformed) triglycerides during pregnancy. SCGN correlated positively with triglycerides (TG) in women with GDM (r_p = 0.276, p = 0.038). In NGT, a similar trend, albeit not significant, is visible (r_p = 0.041, p = 0.761). NGT: normal glucose tolerance; GDM: gestational diabetes mellitus; TG: triglycerides.

SCGN levels increased marginally during pregnancy; SCGN levels correlated positively with GW in women with GDM (r_p = 0.308, p = 0.021); in NGT, the correlation was not significant (see Figure 4 and Table 2).

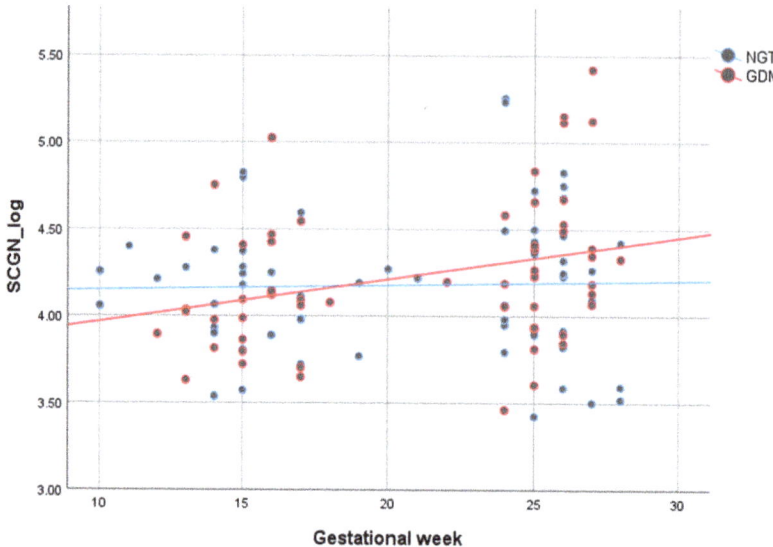

Figure 4. Grouped scatter dot plot according to glucose tolerance (blue = NGT, red = GDM) depicting the correlation of secretagogin (SCGN) (log-transformed) with week of gestation during pregnancy between week of gestation (GW) 10 and 28. In women with GDM, SCGN correlated positively with week of gestation ($r_p = 0.308$, $p = 0.021$). NGT displays the same trend, albeit not statistically significant ($r_p = 0.035$, $p = 0.791$). NGT: normal glucose tolerance; GDM: gestational diabetes mellitus.

4. Discussion

In the present study, SCGN was related to insulin secretion in all pregnant women, predominantly in women with NGT. SCGN correlated positively with the Stumvoll first and second phase index, which corresponds to previous studies supporting a connection between SCGN and insulin secretion. Furthermore, SCGN increased significantly postpartum compared to pregnancy. SCGN levels did not show a difference between NGT and GDM in our cohort of high-risk pregnant women in any of the visits during pregnancy and postpartum, although SCGN was elevated in type 2 diabetes mellitus patients in a previous study [14]. However, the cohort (NGT and GDM) is homogeneous in respect to GDM risk factors such as age and BMI. Furthermore, pregnancy is per se associated with increasing insulin resistance and insulin secretion [15,16]. The status of GDM, in contrast to type 2 diabetes mellitus, might, thus, not be the determining factor for differences in SCGN levels. To our best knowledge, no evaluation in pregnancy or of women with gestational diabetes mellitus has been done until now.

With regard to pancreatic islet cells, secretagogin has so far been related to insulin release in loss-of-function studies and the regulation of beta-cell proliferation [2,9,12,33]. SCGN binds insulin and improves insulin signaling when compared to insulin action alone and, accordingly, dropped over the course of an OGTT in one study [13]. We were not able to replicate these results in our OGTTs, most probably due to the low number of patients for whom these values were available. SCGN's involvement in insulin metabolism was further supported by research on SCGN knock-out mice, which demonstrated progressing glucose intolerance most likely due to loss of beta-cell mass [2] and in vivo studies showing differences in SCGN levels between type 2 diabetes mellitus patients and controls [14]. Recent studies came to the conclusion that type 2 diabetes mellitus could be a state of SCGN deficiency [2,34,35]. Exact mechanisms remain hypothetical at this point, especially considering the heterogeneity in insulin secretion of pre-diabetes and type 2 diabetes mellitus, ranging from hyperinsulinemia to varying degrees of beta-cell dysfunction [36].

SCGN might play a different role in insulin secretion in patients with type 2 diabetes than in pregnancy and women with gestational diabetes. SCGN levels did not differ between women with GDM and NGT in the present cohort. However, SCGN is intrinsically linked to insulin secretion and involved in weight control [1,13]. The pregnant women in both groups displayed similar characteristics in terms of BMI and age. Moreover, pregnancy is a state of hyperinsulinemia and insulin resistance [15,16]. Due to these similarities between NGT and GDM, the diagnosis GDM might not be reflected in SCGN levels.

SCGN levels were significantly higher postpartum than during pregnancy. This trend was visible in both women with NGT and GDM, albeit only significant in NGT. SCGN's ability to bind insulin [13] might offer an explanation for the lower values in pregnancy compared to postpartum due to the pregnancy-related hyperinsulinemia. Pregnancy is a state of progressing insulin resistance and hyperinsulinemia to supply the fetus with glucose [15,16]. Accordingly, SCGN correlated negatively with the Matsuda Index in women with NGT, and SCGN levels increased marginally during pregnancy in all pregnant women in this cohort. Furthermore, as SCGN is critical in neuronal growth and brain development [37], it might be involved in fetal neural development. Hypothetically, if SCGN was transferred via the maternal placenta to the fetus, it could explain the lower levels in mothers during pregnancy. However, the possibility of placental transfer is speculative at this point as SCGN has, to the best of our knowledge, not been investigated in the context of pregnancy before. Another potential explanation for the discrepancy between pregnancy and postpartum is changes in maternal kidney clearance during pregnancy [38]. These physiological adaptions might impact and heighten the renal clearance of SCGN. In support of this theory, SCGN correlated positively with creatine during pregnancy in our cohort. A noteworthy observation is the positive correlation of triglyceride levels with SCGN in women with GDM, which might indicate a compensatory mechanism to reduce triglyceride content. Accordingly, SCGN treatment reduced triglycerides and cholesterol in high-fat diet fed mice [13].

A limitation of this study is that postpartum SCGN values were not available for all women due to a high postpartum drop-out rate. Therefore, the assessment of changes from pregnancy to postpartum was limited to a restricted number of patients. Moreover, the conclusions on the relationship between insulin secretion and SCGN is based on correlations rather than causation.

Being the first study on SCGN in pregnancy and GDM, we were able to demonstrate a potential connection of SCGN to insulin secretion in pregnancy. SCGN was predominantly associated with insulin secretion in women with NGT, which suggests an involvement in the physiological increase in insulin secretion during gestation. It remains unclear whether the lower SCGN levels in pregnancy compared to postpartum are the actuator or the result of pregnancy-related changes in insulin metabolism. A larger cohort, non-pregnant controls and the addition of pre-pregnancy SCGN levels in future studies would allow for a better judgement on changes during gestation and postpartum. The discrepancy between studies in patients with type 2 diabetes mellitus compared to GDM indicate the necessity for further research. To ameliorate the understanding of the functions of this biomarker, studies in other models of insulin resistance and changing insulin secretion are imperative, for instance, in patients with impaired glucose tolerance or normal lean pregnancies.

Author Contributions: Data curation, K.L., J.H. and S.B.-P.; formal analysis, A.K.-W.; investigation, K.L., J.H. and S.B.-P.; methodology, C.D.; resources, K.L. and S.B.-P.; supervision, J.H. and A.K.-W.; visualization, C.D.; writing—original draft, C.D. and J.H.; writing—review and editing, J.H., K.L., D.B.-T., S.B.-P. and A.K.-W. All authors have read and agreed to the published version of the manuscript.

Funding: This research was funded by the Medical Scientific Fund of the Mayor of Vienna, project 09063 and project 15205.

Conflicts of Interest: The authors declare no conflicts of interest. The funding source had no role in conception of the study, study conduct or analysis and interpretation of data.

References

1. Maj, M.; Wagner, L.; Tretter, V. 20 Years of Secretagogin: Exocytosis and Beyond. *Front. Mol. Neurosci.* **2019**, *12*, 1–10. [CrossRef]
2. Malenczyk, K.; Girach, F.; Szodorai, E.; Storm, P.; Segerstolpe, Å.; Tortoriello, G.; Schnell, R.; Mulder, J.; Romanov, R.A.; Borók, E.; et al. A TRPV1-to-secretagogin Regulatory Axis Controls Pancreatic B-cell Survival by Modulating Protein Turnover. *EMBO J.* **2017**, *36*, 2107–2125. [CrossRef]
3. Malenczyk, K.; Szodorai, E.; Schnell, R.; Lubec, G.; Szabó, G.; Hökfelt, T.; Harkany, T. Secretagogin Protects Pdx1 from Proteasomal Degradation to Control a Transcriptional Program Required for β Cell Specification. *Mol. Metab.* **2018**, *14*, 108–120. [CrossRef]
4. Huttlin, E.L.; Ting, L.; Bruckner, R.J.; Gebreab, F.; Gygi, M.P.; Szpyt, J.; Tam, S.; Zarraga, G.; Colby, G.; Baltier, K.; et al. The BioPlex Network: A Systematic Exploration of the Human Interactome. *Cell* **2015**, *162*, 425–440. [CrossRef]
5. Huttlin, E.L.; Bruckner, R.J.; Paulo, J.A.; Cannon, J.R.; Ting, L.; Baltier, K.; Colby, G.; Gebreab, F.; Gygi, M.P.; Parzen, H.; et al. Architecture of the Human Interactome Defines Protein Communities and Disease Networks. *Nature* **2017**, *545*, 505–509. [CrossRef]
6. Romanov, R.A.; Alpár, A.; Zhang, M.-D.; Zeisel, A.; Calas, A.; Landry, M.; Fuszard, M.; Shirran, S.L.; Schnell, R.; Dobolyi, Á.; et al. A Secretagogin Locus of the Mammalian Hypothalamus Controls Stress Hormone Release. *EMBO J.* **2015**, *34*, 36–54. [CrossRef]
7. Hanics, J.; Szodorai, E.; Tortoriello, G.; Malenczyk, K.; Keimpema, E.; Lubec, G.; Hevesi, Z.; Lutz, M.I.; Kozsurek, M.; Puskár, Z.; et al. Secretagogin-Dependent Matrix Metalloprotease-2 Release from Neurons Regulates Neuroblast Migration. *Proc. Natl. Acad. Sci. USA* **2017**, *114*, E2006–E2015. [CrossRef]
8. Mulder, J.; Spence, L.; Tortoriello, G.; Dinieri, J.A.; Uhlén, M.; Shui, B.; Kotlikoff, M.I.; Yanagawa, Y.; Aujard, F.; Hökfelt, T.; et al. Secretagogin Is a Ca2+-Binding Protein Identifying Prospective Extended Amygdala Neurons in the Developing Mammalian Telencephalon. *Eur. J. Neurosci.* **2010**, *31*, 2166–2177. [CrossRef] [PubMed]
9. Wagner, L.; Oliyarnyk, O.; Gartner, W.; Nowotny, P.; Groeger, M.; Kaserer, K. Cloning and Expression of Secretagogin, a Novel Neuroendocrine and Pancreatic Islet of Langerhans-Specific Ca2+-Binding Protein. *J. Biol. Chem.* **2000**, *275*, 24740–24751. [CrossRef] [PubMed]
10. Gartner, W.; Lang, W.; Leutmetzer, F.; Domanovits, H.; Waldhäusl, W.; Wagner, L. Cerebral Expression and Serum Detectability of Secretagogin, a Recently Cloned EF-Hand Ca2+-Binding Protein. *Cereb. Cortex* **2001**, *11*, 1161–1169. [CrossRef] [PubMed]
11. Ferdaoussi, M.; Fu, J.; Dai, X.; Manning Fox, J.E.; Suzuki, K.; Smith, N.; Plummer, G.; MacDonald, P.E. SUMOylation and Calcium Control Syntaxin-1A and Secretagogin Sequestration by Tomosyn to Regulate Insulin Exocytosis in Human β Cells. *Sci. Rep.* **2017**, *7*, 248. [CrossRef] [PubMed]
12. Yang, S.-Y.; Lee, J.-J.; Lee, J.-H.; Lee, K.; Oh, S.H.; Lim, Y.-M.; Lee, M.-S.; Lee, K.-J. Secretagogin Affects Insulin Secretion in Pancreatic β-Cells by Regulating Actin Dynamics and Focal Adhesion. *Biochem. J.* **2016**, *473*, 1791–1803. [CrossRef] [PubMed]
13. Sharma, A.K.; Khandelwal, R.; Kumar, M.J.M.; Ram, N.S.; Chidananda, A.H.; Raj, T.A.; Sharma, Y. Secretagogin Regulates Insulin Signaling by Direct Insulin Binding. *iScience* **2019**, *21*, 736–753. [CrossRef]
14. Hansson, S.F.; Zhou, A.-X.; Vachet, P.; Eriksson, J.W.; Pereira, M.J.; Skrtic, S.; Jongsma Wallin, H.; Ericsson-Dahlstrand, A.; Karlsson, D.; Ahnmark, A.; et al. Secretagogin Is Increased in Plasma from Type 2 Diabetes Patients and Potentially Reflects Stress and Islet Dysfunction. *PLoS ONE* **2018**, *13*, e0196601. [CrossRef]
15. Banerjee, R.R. Piecing Together the Puzzle of Pancreatic Islet Adaptation in Pregnancy. *Ann. N. Y. Acad. Sci.* **2018**, *1411*, 120–139. [CrossRef] [PubMed]
16. Butte, N.F. Carbohydrate and Lipid Metabolism in Pregnancy: Normal Compared with Gestational Diabetes Mellitus. *Am. J. Clin. Nutr.* **2000**, *71*, 1256S–1261S. [CrossRef] [PubMed]
17. Butler, A.E.; Cao-Minh, L.; Galasso, R.; Rizza, R.A.; Corradin, A.; Cobelli, C.; Butler, P.C. Adaptive Changes in Pancreatic Beta Cell Fractional Area and Beta Cell Turnover in Human Pregnancy. *Diabetologia* **2010**, *53*, 2167–2176. [CrossRef]
18. Van Assche, F.A.; Aerts, L.; De Prins, F. A Morphological Study of the Endocrine Pancreas. *Br. J. Obs. Gynecol.* **1978**, *85*, 818–820. [CrossRef]

19. Kushner, J.A. The Role of Aging upon β Cell Turnover. *J. Clin. Invest.* **2013**, *123*, 990–995. [CrossRef]
20. Buchanan, T.A.; Xiang, A.; Kjos, S.L.; Watanabe, R. What Is Gestational Diabetes? *Diabetes Care* **2007**, *30* Suppl. 2. [CrossRef]
21. Buckley, B.S.; Harreiter, J.; Damm, P.; Corcoy, R.; Chico, A.; Simmons, D.; Vellinga, A.; Dunne, F. Gestational Diabetes Mellitus in Europe: Prevalence, Current Screening Practice and Barriers to Screening. A Review. *Diabetes Med.* **2012**, *29*, 844–854. [CrossRef] [PubMed]
22. The HAPO Study Cooperative Research Group. Hyperglycemia and Adverse Pregnancy Outcomes. *N. Engl. J. Med.* **2008**, *358*, 1991–2002. [CrossRef]
23. Lowe, W.L. Jr.; Scholtens, D.M.; Lowe, L.P.; Kuang, A.; Nodzenski, M.; Talbot, O.; Catalano, P.M.; Linder, B.; Brickman, W.J.; Clayton, P.; et al. Association of Gestational Diabetes With Maternal Disorders of Glucose Metabolism and Childhood Adiposity. *JAMA* **2018**, *320*, 1005–1016. [CrossRef]
24. Jelsma, J.; van Poppel, M.; Galjaard, S.; Desoye, G.; Corcoy, R.; Devlieger, R.; van Assche, A.; Timmerman, D.; Jans, G.; Harreiter, J.; et al. Dali: Vitamin D and Lifestyle Intervention for Gestational Diabetes Mellitus (GDM) Prevention: An European Multicentre, Randomised Trial—Study Protocol. *BMC Pregnancy Childbirth* **2013**, 13. [CrossRef] [PubMed]
25. Österreichische Diabetes Gesellschaft. Diabetes Mellitus—Anleitungen Für Die Praxis. *Wien. Klin. Wochenschr.* **2019**, *131*, 1–246.
26. Kautzky-Willer, A.; Harreiter, J.; Bancher-Todesca, D.; Berger, A.; Repa, A.; Lechleitner, M.; Weitgasser, R. Gestationsdiabetes (GDM). *Wien. Klin. Wochenschr.* **2016**, *128*, 103–112. [CrossRef]
27. Egan, A.M.; Vellinga, A.; Harreiter, J.; Simmons, D.; Desoye, G.; Corcoy, R.; Adelantado, J.M.; Devlieger, R.; Van Assche, A.; Galjaard, S.; et al. Epidemiology of Gestational Diabetes Mellitus According to IADPSG/WHO 2013 Criteria among Obese Pregnant Women in Europe. *Diabetologia* **2017**, *60*, 1913–1921. [CrossRef]
28. Matsuda, M.; DeFronzo, R. Insulin Sensitivity Indices Obtained from Oral Glucose Tolerance Testing: Comparison with the Euglycemic Insulin Clamp. *Diabetes Care* **1999**, *22*, 1462–1470. [CrossRef]
29. Stumvoll, M.; Van Haeften, T.; Fritsch, A.; Gerich, J. Oral Glucose Tolerance Test Indexes for Insulin Sensitivity and Secretion Based on Various Availabilities of Sampling Times. *Diabetes Care* **2001**, *24*, 794–797. [CrossRef] [PubMed]
30. Utzschneider, K.M.; Prigeon, R.L.; Faulenbach, M.V.; Tong, J.; Carr, D.B.; Boyko, E.J.; Leonetti, D.L.; McNeely, M.J.; Fujimoto, W.Y.; Kahn, S.E. Oral Disposition Index Predicts the Development of Future Diabetes above and beyond Fasting and 2-h Glucose Levels. *Diabetes Care* **2009**, *32*, 335–341. [CrossRef]
31. Kim, D.L.; Kim, S.D.; Kim, S.K.; Park, S.; Song, K.H. Is an Oral Glucose Tolerance Test Still Valid for Diagnosing Diabetes Mellitus? *Diabetes Metab. J.* **2016**, *40*, 118–128. [CrossRef] [PubMed]
32. Saisho, Y.; Miyakoshi, K.; Tanaka, M.; Shimada, A.; Ikenoue, S.; Kadohira, I.; Yoshimura, Y.; Itoh, H. Beta Cell Dysfunction and Its Clinical Significance in Gestational Diabetes. *Endocr. J.* **2010**, *57*, 973–980. [CrossRef] [PubMed]
33. Maj, M.; Milenkovic, I.; Bauer, J.; Berggård, T.; Veit, M.; Ilhan-Mutlu, A. Novel Insights into the Distribution and Functional Aspects of the Calcium Binding Protein Secretagogin from Studies on Rat Brain and Primary Neuronal Cell Culture. *Front. Mol. Neurosci.* **2012**, 5. [CrossRef] [PubMed]
34. Hasegawa, K.; Wakino, S.; Kimoto, M.; Minakuchi, H.; Fujimura, K.; Hosoya, K.; Komatsu, M.; Kaneko, Y.; Kanda, T.; Tokuyama, H.; et al. The Hydrolase DDAH2 Enhances Pancreatic Insulin Secretion by Transcriptional Regulation of Secretagogin through a Sirt1-Dependent Mechanism in Mice. *FASEB J.* **2013**, 2301–2315. [CrossRef]
35. Westwood, S.; Liu, B.; Baird, A.L.; Anand, S.; Nevado-holgado, A.J.; Newby, D.; Pikkarainen, M.; Hallikainen, M.; Kuusisto, J.; Streffer, J.R.; et al. The Influence of Insulin Resistance on Cerebrospinal Fluid and Plasma Biomarkers of Alzheimer's Pathology. *Alzheimer's Res. Ther.* **2017**, 1–11. [CrossRef]
36. Ferrannini, E.; Gastaldelli, A.; Miyazaki, Y.; Matsuda, M.; Mari, A.; Defronzo, R.A. β-Cell Function in Subjects Spanning the Range from Normal Glucose Tolerance to Overt Diabetes: A New Analysis. *JCEM* **2005**, *90*, 493–500. [CrossRef]

37. Qin, J.; Liu, Q.; Liu, Z.; Pan, Y.Z.; Sifuentes-Dominguez, L.; Stepien, K.P.; Wang, Y.; Tu, Y.; Tan, S.; Wang, Y.; et al. Structural and Mechanistic Insights into Secretagogin-Mediated Exocytosis. *Proc. Natl. Acad. Sci. USA* **2020**, *117*, 6559–6570. [CrossRef]
38. Lopes van Balen, V.A.; van Gansewinkel, T.A.G.; de Haas, S.; Spaan, J.J.; Ghossein-Doha, C.; van Kuijk, S.M.J.; van Drongelen, J.; Cornelis, T.; Spaanderman, M.E.A. Maternal Kidney Function during Pregnancy: Systematic Review and Meta-Analysis. *Ultrasound Obs. Gynecol.* **2019**, *54*, 297–307. [CrossRef]

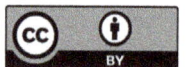

© 2020 by the authors. Licensee MDPI, Basel, Switzerland. This article is an open access article distributed under the terms and conditions of the Creative Commons Attribution (CC BY) license (http://creativecommons.org/licenses/by/4.0/).

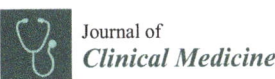

Article

Pregnancy Outcomes and Maternal Insulin Sensitivity: Design and Rationale of a Multi-Center Longitudinal Study in Mother and Offspring (PROMIS)

Anoush Kdekian [1], Maaike Sietzema [2], Sicco A. Scherjon [3], Helen Lutgers [2] and Eline M. van der Beek [1,*]

[1] Laboratory of Pediatrics, University Medical Centre Groningen, University of Groningen, Hanzeplein 1, 9713 GZ Groningen, The Netherlands; A.Kdekian@umcg.nl
[2] Clinical Endocrinology, Medical Centre Leeuwarden, Henri Dunantweg 2, 8934 AD Leeuwarden, The Netherlands; m.sietzema@umcg.nl (M.S.); Helen.lutgers@mcl.nl (H.L.)
[3] Department of Gynaecology and Obstetrics, University Medical Centre Groningen, Hanzeplein 1, 9713 GZ Groningen, The Netherlands; s.a.scherjon@umcg.nl
* Correspondence: e.m.van.der.beek@umcg.nl

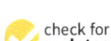

Citation: Kdekian, A.; Sietzema, M.; Scherjon, S.A.; Lutgers, H.; van der Beek, E.M. Pregnancy Outcomes and Maternal Insulin Sensitivity: Design and Rationale of a Multi-Center Longitudinal Study in Mother and Offspring (PROMIS). *J. Clin. Med.* 2021, 10, 976. https://doi.org/10.3390/jcm10050976

Academic Editor: Katrien Benhalima

Received: 30 January 2021
Accepted: 19 February 2021
Published: 2 March 2021

Publisher's Note: MDPI stays neutral with regard to jurisdictional claims in published maps and institutional affiliations.

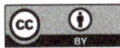

Copyright: © 2021 by the authors. Licensee MDPI, Basel, Switzerland. This article is an open access article distributed under the terms and conditions of the Creative Commons Attribution (CC BY) license (https://creativecommons.org/licenses/by/4.0/).

Abstract: The worldwide prevalence of overweight and obesity in women of reproductive age is rapidly increasing and a risk factor for the development of gestational diabetes (GDM). Excess adipose tissue reduces insulin sensitivity and may underlie adverse outcomes in both mother and child. The present paper describes the rationale and design of the PRegnancy Outcomes and Maternal Insulin Sensitivity (PROMIS) study, an exploratory cohort study to obtain detailed insights in insulin sensitivity and glucose metabolism during pregnancy and its relation to pregnancy outcomes including early infancy growth. We aim to recruit healthy pregnant women with a body mass index (BMI) ≥ 25 kg/m^2 before 12 weeks of gestation in Northern Netherlands. A total of 130 woman will be checked on fasted (≤ 7.0 mmol/L) or random (≤ 11.0 mmol/L) blood glucose to exclude pregestational diabetes at inclusion. Subjects will be followed up to six months after giving birth, with a total of nine contact moments for data collection. Maternal data include postprandial measures following an oral meal tolerance test (MTT), conducted before 16 weeks and repeated around 24 weeks of gestation, followed by a standard oral glucose tolerance test before 28 weeks of gestation. The MTT is again performed around three months postpartum. Blood analysis is done for baseline and postprandial glucose and insulin, baseline lipid profile and several biomarkers of placental function. In addition, specific body circumferences, skinfold measures, and questionnaires about food intake, eating behavior, physical activity, meal test preference, mental health, and pregnancy complications will be obtained. Fetal data include assessment of growth, examined by sonography at week 28 and 32 of gestation. Neonatal and infant data consist of specific body circumferences, skinfolds, and body composition measurements, as well as questionnaires about eating behavior and complications up to 6 months after birth. The design of the PROMIS study will allow for detailed insights in the metabolic changes in the mother and their possible association with fetal and postnatal infant growth and body composition. We anticipate that the data from this cohort women with an elevated risk for the development of GDM may provide new insights to detect metabolic deviations already in early pregnancy. These data could inspire the development of new interventions that may improve the management of maternal, as well as offsrping complications from already early on in pregnancy with the aim to prevent adverse outcomes for mother and child.

Keywords: pregnancy; insulin sensitivity; (early) pregnancy; pregnancy outcomes; growth; glucose; overweight; obesity; LGA; maternal health; child health; gestational diabetes mellitus; OGTT; meal tolerance test; postprandial

1. Introduction

Insulin sensitivity normally decreases by the end of the second trimester due to the effect of placental hormones, such as human placental lactogen (HPL), progesterone, and human placental growth hormone, to ensure a continuous supply of nutrients to the growing fetus [1,2]. Decreased insulin sensitivity leads to beta-cell proliferation and a larger volume of individual beta-cells, returning to non-pregnant levels after parturition. Hyperglycemia may develop due to insufficient beta-cell proliferation [3–6]. However, the mechanism behind insulin resistance is multifactorial. Women with a body mass index (BMI) $\geq$ 25 kg/m^2 have excess adipose tissue which is known to reduce insulin sensitivity and may explain the correlation with adverse outcomes of pregnancy for both mother and child [7]. The worldwide prevalence of overweight and obesity during pregnancy is rapidly increasing, with a prevalence of nearly 54 million worldwide [8]. In the Netherlands, the prevalence of overweight women age 30–40 years was 39% in 2017 and around 44% in 2019 [9], suggesting that many women are already overweight when becoming pregnant. The physiological insulin resistance during pregnancy in combination with overweight or obesity could increase the risk for hyperglycemia. The hyperglycemia and pregnancy outcomes (HAPO) study has shown that already small increases in maternal glucose levels show a linear relationship with adverse outcomes [10].

Insulin resistance during pregnancy increases the risk of pregnancy complications such as pregnancy induced hypertension, pre-eclampsia, caesarian section and gestational diabetes mellitus (GDM), and excessive pregnancy weight gain during pregnancy and weight retention postpartum, while longer term it also increases the risk of cardiovascular diseases and diabetes mellitus (DM) type 2 and other non-communicable diseases. Adverse outcomes of pregnancy hyperglycemia in infants could be macrosomia and large for gestational age (LGA), as well as neonatal complications on the short term and a higher risk on childhood obesity and non-communicable diseases longer term [7].

Maintaining euglycemia despite the developing insulin resistance over the course of pregnancy is critical. Deviations in maternal glucose metabolism could potentially already be detected early in pregnancy [7,10,11]. Yet, potential hyperglycemia is currently standardly examined at the end of the second trimester by an oral glucose tolerance test (OGTT), and in the Netherlands only in an at-risk population defined as BMI $\geq$ 30 kg/m^2 [12]. This test, taking baseline and 2-h blood glucose levels as a result, is not suitable to detect mild hyperglycemia in early pregnancy and shows considerable within subject variability [13]. Markers of insulin sensitivity and related metabolic adaptations, for instance in lipid metabolism, may be a more straightforward measure in which deviations could potentially be detected earlier [14]. An integration of postprandial responses of glucose and insulin combined with lipid markers following a challenge test would provide clearer insights in maternal metabolic function. To this end, a meal tolerance test (MTT), which contains a well-defined balanced macro- and micronutrient composition may be much more sensitive than the standard OGTT. Assessing glucose homeostasis based on glucose concentrations only is not reliable as there are numerous perturbations where glucose production and its utilization increases or decreases to the same extent without any changes in blood concentrations [15]. For the understanding of the physiology and pathophysiology of glucose uptake and metabolism during pregnancy, glucose tracers could be used [16].

The design of the Pregnancy Outcomes and Maternal Insulin Sensitivity (PROMIS) study will allow collection of detailed insights in insulin sensitivity and glucose metabolism during (early) pregnancy in women with overweight and obesity and assess its possible relation to growth and body composition during of the offspring during the fetal and early infancy period. We hypothesize that using an MTT, disturbed insulin sensitivity in overweight pregnant women could be identified much earlier in pregnancy. Early detection could help to better predict the risk of possible adverse outcomes short term and reduce the risk of non-communicable diseases on the longer term.

2. Materials and Methods

2.1. Overall Study Design

The PROMIS study is a multi-center exploratory prospective cohort-based study in the two Northern provinces of the Netherlands (Groningen and Friesland). The study has been approved by the medical ethical committee University Medical Centre Groningen prior to the start of the study (NL68845.042.19) and is registered at ClinicalTrials.gov (NCT04315545). Healthy pregnant women with a BMI ≥ 25 kg/m^2 are eligible for participation. Weight and height of women as well as fasting glucose levels will be confirmed via measurements by study staff at inclusion. Study duration will be from 12 weeks of gestation up to 6 months after giving birth with a total of nine contact moments when data will be collected. The MTT will be performed between weeks 12 and 16 and repeated between weeks 24 and 28 of gestation and three months postpartum. A standard OGTT will be performed after the second MTT, also between weeks 24 and 28 of gestation. In addition, maternal anthropometrics will be assessed at the time of the MTT challenges. Additional sonographies will be made during gestation at week 28 and 32 to assess fetal growth. Neonatal and infant anthropometrics will be obtained after birth and at 1, 2, 3, 4, and 6 months of age from the records of the baby clinic visits. Body composition measurements using an air displacement plethysmography (Pea Pod, COSMED, Rome, Italy) [17] will be performed at 1, 3, and 6 months of age. Questionnaires about nutrition and lifestyle will also be collected at several time points throughout the study. A study overview is depicted in Figure 1.

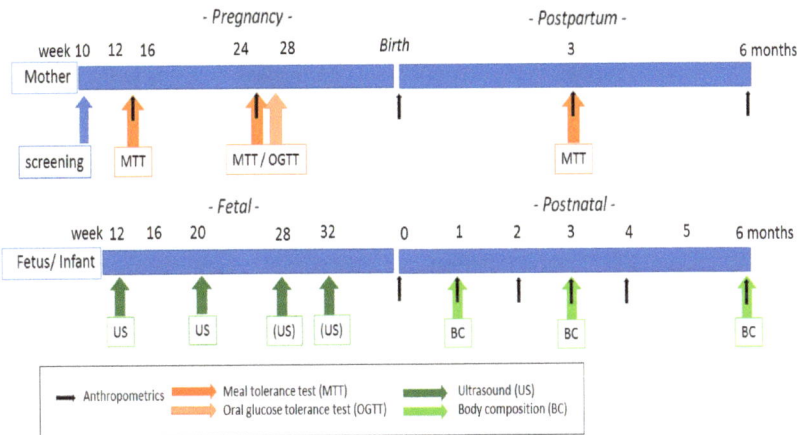

Figure 1. Schematic representation of the prospective cohort indicating readouts and proposed timing of measurement between early pregnancy up to 6 months postpartum in both mother (upper panel) and offspring (lower panel).

2.2. In-and Exclusion Criteria

Inclusion criteria are singleton pregnancy, BMI ≥ 25 kg/m^2, fasted (≤ 7.0 mmol/L) or random (≤ 11.0 mmol/L) blood glucose level, aged ≥ 18 years, and written informed consent. Women will be excluded from the study if they have pre-existing DM type 1 or 2, serious health complications (hypertension, hyperlipidemia, asthma, haemochromatosis) or medication use that influences the glucose metabolism or fetal growth (e.g., chronic use of corticosteroids). In addition, women who are participating in any other studies involving investigation of medication or nutritional products, have a severe illness, psychological dysfunctions, used antibiotics two weeks prior to participation, have HIV or hepatitis, expected to not comply to the study protocol (e.g., fear of needles), known allergies or intolerances for one or more nutritional ingredient used in the MTT will also be excluded.

2.3. Recruitment

Women will be recruited in the provinces of Groningen and Friesland from a diverse range of socio-economic and ethnic backgrounds. Hospitals, midwife practices, ultrasound practices, and family doctor's practices are involved in recruitment. To optimize recruitment, flyers were made, and social media accounts set up. Information sheets explaining aspects of the study, as well as a short video explaining the study set up will be provided to eligible participants. Women will have the opportunity to consider participation and to ask questions to the researchers and can terminate participation at any time within the study without affecting their usual care. The privacy of the participant will be ensured via protected data collection and processing by the researchers and will be saved anonymously. Written informed consent will be obtained prior to the first baseline measurement. Women are requested to give consent for (1) participation in the study, including taking of blood samples, collecting associated measurements, and extraction of relevant data from medical records; (2) storage of blood in a bio bank and (3) participation of their child in this study including gathering protocol specified measurements.

2.4. Meal Tolerance and Oral Glucose Tolerance Testing

To conduct the MTT, a non-investigational product, Nutridrink Compact, will be used. Nutridrink Compact is a liquid product for medical use to treat malnutrition. It provides energy and nutrients in a relatively compact volume and contains a suitable combination and levels of macro- and micronutrients, largely comparable to the energy and nutrient composition of a standard breakfast. The product volume will be standardized to 50 gr carbohydrates and contains 24 g of protein and 9 g of fat, equivalent to 404 kcal in a total volume of 169 mL. The study participants are asked not to eat or drink (except for water) anything from 11 pm before the test day to arrive in the fasted state. For regular OGTT testing, a standard 75 gr glucose solution of 200 mL will be used. Participants will be diagnosed with GDM when plasma blood glucose is ≥ 7.0 mmol/L in fasted state or ≥ 7.8 mmol/L 2 h after the OGTT. These guidelines are according to the Dutch Association of Obstetrics and Gynecology (NVOG) [18]. In a subgroup of participants (estimate $n = 20$) we will add 2% of the total amount of carbohydrates in the MTT as glucose tracers. In total, 1.25 g of D-(6,6-D2, 99%)-glucose, used as the tracer, will be added to the MTT, as well as to the OGTT, selected to ensure participant and experimental safety [19]. The solution will be prepared by the research pharmacy in special units that require only the addition of the required MTT or OGTT volume. In both the MTT and the OGTT, the participant should ingest the drink within 5 min.

2.5. Sample Size Calculation

The primary outcome of the PROMIS study is to detect changes in blood glucose- and insulin levels following an MTT, containing 50 g of carbohydrates next to other nutrients. The null hypothesis is that early pregnancy assessment of maternal glucose-insulin metabolism with an MTT will identify more mothers at risk for pregnancy complications compared to a standard OGTT conducted at the end of the second trimester. The current prevalence of GDM, a state of reduced insulin sensitivity leading to hyperglycemia based on standard OGTT testing, is estimated to be 3–5% in the Netherlands, as diagnosed between 24–28 weeks of gestation. Given the reported linear relationship between blood glucose and adverse outcomes [10] and higher rates of insulin resistance with increased BMI [20], more heterogeneity, disturbances in blood glucose, and insulin values are expected in our study population than the indicated 3–5% [21] for the total population of pregnant women in the Netherlands. In addition, we anticipate that the first abnormal blood values, in particular signs of insulin resistance might already be detected in early gestation using this more physiological testing paradigm. To be able to reject the null hypothesis, we estimate that a total of 130 pregnant women are needed to participate in the PROMIS study, allowing for a dropout rate of 20%. This is based on an expected sensitivity of 74% and a minimal lower confidence limit of 0.62 in OGTT's containing 50 g of carbohydrates, given before

32 weeks of gestation for observational studies [22,23]. Given the exploratory nature of the study, the sample size will be re-estimated after the first OGTT has been completed in 25 subjects based on available sensitivity and specificity data.

2.6. Interim Analysis

After including a total of 5 participants that completed the first MTT, a first interim analysis will be performed to see if the added amount of glucose tracer is indeed sufficient to trace glucose fate following the MTT. If the amount of glucose tracer is insufficient for analysis, the size of the subgroup and the percentage of added glucose tracer can be adjusted. The first interim will also be used to assess possible unexpected adverse events. A second interim analysis will be done after the completion of the OGTT in the first 25 subjects to recalculate the sample size by sensitivity and specificity after confirmation of GDM incidence based on blood glucose levels. It is expected that the final number for inclusion will be lower than the calculated 130 participants given the detailed data collection to assess glucose-insulin metabolism.

2.7. Data Collection

An overview of all the parameters measured during pregnancy in the mother and fetus (Table 1) and postpartum in mother and child (Table 2) is provided below.

Table 1. Timing of data collection during pregnancy up to 2 weeks postpartum in mother and fetus-infant.

	Screening	Week 12–16	Week 20	Week 24–26	Week 28	Week 32	Week 36	Birth
Visit number	Visit 1	Visit 2	Routine [1]	Visits 3 and 4	Visit 5	Visit 6	Phone call	Routine [2]
Visit window	≤12 weeks	±1 week	±2 weeks	±1 week	±1 week	±1 week	±1 week	+2 weeks
Informed consent	X							
Inclusion/exclusion criteria	X							
Baseline and demographics		X						
Maternal anthropometrics	X	X		X			X	
Fasting or random blood glucose	X							
Blood parameters (for MTT)		X		X				
Blood parameters (for OGTT)				X				
Maternal skinfolds and fundal height		X		X				
Fetal sonography			X		X	X		
FFQ		X		X				
PPAQ		X		X		X		
Sensory questionnaire				X				
EQ-5D		X		X		X		
AEBQ		X		X				
Birth outcomes								X
Neonatal adiposity and anthropometrics								X
Intake drugs, alcohol, smoking	X			X				
Maternal complications	X	X		X			X	X
Neonatal complications								X

[1] Routine care includes standard sonography measure, [2] Routine postpartum care is performed at home or at the neonatal clinic, OGTT: oral glucose tolerance test, MTT: mixed meal tolerance test, PPAQ: pregnancy physical activity questionnaire, EQ-5D: euroQol-5D, AEBQ: adult eating behavior questionnaire, FFQ: food frequency questionnaire, method to assess dietary intake in mothers, IPAQ: international physical activity questionnaire.

Table 2. Timing of data collection up to 6 months postpartum.

	1 Month Postpartum	2 Months Postpartum	3 Months Postpartum	4 Months Postpartum	6 Months Postpartum
Visit number	Visit 7	Routine [1]	Visit 8	Routine [1]	Visit 9
Visit window (days)	±1 week	±3 days	±1 week	±3 days	±1 week
Maternal anthropometrics			X		X
Blood parameters MTT			X		
Skinfolds			X		X
Food Frequency Questionnaire	X		X		X
IPAQ			X		X
EQ-D5	X		X		X
AEBQ	X		X		X
BEBQ	X		X		X
Infant adiposity and anthropometrics	X	X	X	X	X
Peapod/skinfolds	X		X		X
Maternal complications	X	X	X	X	X

[1] Routine care postpartum is performed at home or the neonatal clinic, MTT: mixed meal tolerance test, PPAQ: pregnancy physical activity questionnaire, EQ-5D: euroQol-5D, AEBQ: adult eating behavior questionnaire, 24-h recall: method to assess dietary intake in mothers, IPAQ: international physical activity questionnaire, BEBQ: baby eating behavior questionnaire.

2.7.1. Maternal Measurements

Basal ($t = 0$), as well as postprandial blood samples, will be collected at the following time points; 10, 20, 30, 45, 60, 90, and 120 min after consumption of the test meal. In fasted state, the following blood parameters will be measured; glucose, labeled glucose, insulin, hbA1c, triglycerides, free fatty acids, total cholesterol, HDL-cholesterol, HPL, c-peptide, and cortisol. Postprandial blood measures include glucose, glucose tracers, and insulin. Several blood parameters will be directly analyzed by the routine laboratory available in the hospitals, while other blood collection tubes will be directly centrifuged for 10 min at $1300\times g$, divided into aliquots varying from 500 uL to 2 mL and stored in a $-80\ °C$ freezer for later analysis. Glucose, total cholesterol, and HDL-cholesterol will be analyzed by photometrics, insulin, and cortisol will be analyzed by luminescent-immuno-assay, HbA1c will be analyzed by liquid chromatography, leptin, free fatty acids, and HPL will be analyzed by the ELISA method and C-peptide will be analyzed by Immuno-assay. To measure the labeled glucose, blood spots of 75–80 uL will be taken to onto 903 protein saver cards (Whatman [24]). Fractional contributions of glucose tracer in blood will be measured by gas chromatography mass spectrometry (GCMS) according to van Dijk et al. (2003) [16]. The collected data will be used in the minimal model adapted from Cobelli et al. (2009) [15]. This mathematical model allows estimation of endogenous glucose production and clearance rates at fasting as well as postprandial states. The fractional absorption rate, delay time, and apparent volumes of distribution of the administered bolus can be estimated. For the utilization parameters, peripheral insulin sensitivity, and glucose effectiveness will be estimated, as well as hepatic insulin sensitivities.

From the postprandial time points, the area under the curve (AUC), peak, insulin sensitivity index and deltas can be calculated. The calculation of the homeostatic model assessment for insulin resistance (HOMA-IR) will be made based on the fasting plasma glucose (FPG) and insulin (FPI) values (FPG × FPI/22.5). The quantitative insulin sensitivity check index (QUICKI) is based on fasting blood samples and is calculated using the following formula QUICKI = $1/(\log(I0) + \log(G0))$, in which I0 is the fasting insulin, where G0 is the fasting glucose value.

Maternal anthropometric measures that will be collected include height, weight, pre-pregnancy weight, (self-reported) pre-pregnancy weight, gestational weight gain, circumferences, and maternal fat mass. BMI is calculated as weight divided by square heights. Measured circumferences include neck, waist, thigh, hip, wrist, and upper arm. The hip–waist ratio will also be calculated. Maternal fat mass will be estimated using skinfold thickness measurements by Harpenden Skinfold Caliper (Baty international [25]. Skinfold thickness measurements will be done at one side of the body for three times. The average of those three skinfolds will be used. The skinfolds will be obtained twice during pregnancy at the time of the challenge tests, between 12–16 weeks and between 24–28 weeks, and postpartum after 3 and 6 months. Skinfolds to assess adiposity have been validated in pregnant women and will be measured at 4 locations; (1) triceps, (2) biceps, (3) subscapular skinfold, and (4) suprailiac skinfold [26]. Skinfolds will be calculated by the equations of Durnin and Womersley [27].

2.7.2. Fetal Measurements

Fetal growth characteristics including crown and rump length, biparietal diameter (BPD), head circumference (HC), abdominal circumference (AC), Femur Length (FL), and occipito-frontal diameter (OFD) will be obtained through sonography by trained professionals in weeks 28 and 32 of gestation. The INTERGROWTH-21 [28] provides additional data to the standard growth standards of the world health organization (WHO) [29] and will be used for the estimation fetal growth by filling in the calculator of gestational age and estimated weight of fetus. The ultrasounds will be performed in certified ultrasound (midwifery) centers by their own certified staff.

2.7.3. Neonatal and Infant Measurements

Neonatal and infant data collection consists out of birth weight taken from antenatal records, anthropometrics (height, weight), circumferences (head, upper arm, wrist, thigh, neck, waste), and skinfolds (biceps, triceps, supra-illiac, thigh) at 1, 2, 3, 4, and 6 months of age. Body composition measurements will be performed using air displacement plethysmography at 1, 3, and 6 months of age. Data output will include calculated estimates of fat mass and fat free mass, as well as body volume and body density.

2.7.4. Diet and Behavioral Data

Specific validated questionnaires will be given to the participants to gain insight in different diet and behavioral data at different times throughout the pregnancy and postpartum period. A food frequency questionnaire (FFQ) which consist out of items related to different food groups, will be used to measure food intake, and calculate energy and macronutrient intake in the mother over the last month [30]. The adult eating behavior questionnaire (AEBQ) will be given to study eating habits, it consists out of 34 items with five answer options ranging from strongly disagree to strongly agree [31]. The EuroQol-5D (EQ-5D) which consist of five dimensions regarding mobility, self-care, daily activities, pain, and mood to measure quality of life will be measured [32]. The pregnancy physical activity questionnaire (PPAQ) will be used to measure overall activity duration and intensity during pregnancy. It consists out of 34 items with six answering options [33]. After pregnancy, the international physical activity questionnaire (IPAQ) will be used, which consists out of 7 items where participants can fill in a certain number of hours and minutes [34]. In addition, we will use a short questionnaire to collect data on the consumption of the MTT and OGTT. This 'sensory questionnaire' is used to determine which challenge test is preferred. It consists out of 34 items ranging in different variables. For the infant we use a questionnaire about the type of feeding the baby is receiving (e.g., breastfed vs. formula fed), as well as the baby eating behavior questionnaire (BEBQ). This questionnaire consists out of 18 items with five answer options ranging from never to always [35].

2.7.5. Other Outcomes

Social demographics recorded include marital status, household composition, occupation, ethnicity, financial household income, level of education, and paternal information.

The questionnaire used includes family history of DM, previous GDM diagnosis, birth weight of previous pregnancy (if any), more detailed questions about previous child or children born, polycystic ovary syndrome (PCOS), medication use, pregnancy eclampsia, and pre-pregnancy hypertension. In addition, obstetrical and perinatal complications during and after pregnancy will be registered, such as spontaneous or induced abortion, intrauterine death, preeclampsia, pre-term delivery (<37 weeks), need for labor induction, assisted vaginal delivery, shoulder dystocia, caesarian section. Finally, adverse events related to the neonate/infant such as macrosomia, large for gestational age, small for gestational age, hypoglycemia, respiratory distress, neonatal hospitalization, and other complications (if any) will be recorded.

2.8. Statistical Analysis

Data will be expressed as mean ± Standard Deviation (SD) or ranges for continuous variables. Categorical variables will be presented as percentages. All statistical comparisons are considered significant at $p \leq 0.05$ (two-sided). Descriptive statistics will present averages and differences at baseline between medium (BMI ≥ 25 kg/m^2), and high risk (BMI ≥ 30 kg/m^2) groups in our study population. The significance of the mean differences will be tested using analysis of variance (ANOVA). Differences between categorical variables will be tested using the k^2 test when appropriate. Associations will be tested and corrected for selected confounders and multiple testing where appropriate. Mixed models will be used to measure postprandial responses. A statistical analysis plan will be made for each interim analysis as well as for more detailed analysis of all collected parameters before data base closure.

2.9. Database

All participant data will be entered into Research electronic data capture (REDCap, Vanderbilt University) [24]. Operatory entry is password protected. Pages are in English and consist of drop-down menu's, pick lists, and text boxes. No personal study subject identifiers can be found in the database, data will be entered under study ID number, wherein the first number identifies the study location.

3. Discussion

The PROMIS study is an exploratory cohort study wherein the primary outcome is the association between fasting and postprandial glucose and insulin, using the AUC in relation to fetal growth and birth weight. Secondary parameters including plasma lipids and (placental) hormones, growth and adiposity will be analyzed in relation to glucose-insulin outcomes in different stages during and after pregnancy. Exploratory study parameters to assess glucose- and insulin metabolism include analysis of glucose tracers and modeling glucose disappearance rates, as well as lifestyle parameters and the food-and behavior questionnaires.

The PROMIS study investigates early insulin resistance during pregnancy focusing on healthy women with an increased risk of adverse outcomes. The WHO guidelines already consider women with a BMI ≥ 25 kg/m^2 to have an increased risk of developing GDM [36]. In the Netherlands, however, only overweight defined as BMI equal or above 30 is considered as a risk factor for GDM [18], excluding specifically women with a BMI between 25 and 30 from screening for GDM during the second trimester of pregnancy. This is one of the first studies to focus on assessment of metabolic parameters in early pregnancy as possible predictors for adverse outcomes in both mother and child.

Current guidelines for the diagnosis of GDM focus on the inability of the maternal metabolism to cope with changes in insulin sensitivity and insulin demand. From the HAPO study results it is clear that the linear relationship between blood glucose levels in the second trimester of pregnancy and different short term (birth weight, C-section), as well as long term (child growth, insulin sensitivity) outcomes may advocate a different approach if we aim to prevent some of these pregnancy complications in a following study [10]. The focus on glucose rather than on the underlying adaptations in insulin production that are needed to compensate for the changes in insulin sensitivity, make it impossible to diagnose those at risk for adverse outcomes earlier in pregnancy, unless the metabolic deviations are severe. As insulin sensitivity also strongly influences the nutrient flow of the placenta to the fetus, diagnosis around the second trimester may simply be too late to prevent adverse consequences for the growing fetus. In most countries, GDM is diagnosed between week 24–28 of gestation only in women with agreed risk factors, such as obesity (BMI $\geq$ 30 kg/m^2), previous GDM, LGA, small for gestational age (SGA), first family relative with diabetes, ethnic background, or PCOS [18]. The standardly used OGTT containing 75 gr of glucose dissolved in water has been subject of much debate [37,38]. By using an MTT in the present study, which contains a balanced macronutrient composition of proteins and fats besides carbohydrates, we will challenge the glucose metabolism, as well as the insulin production and the response of the lipid metabolism. In this way, we hope to collect more accurate and reliable insights in metabolic function already much earlier in pregnancy and generate more reliable data using a much lower and physiological metabolic load challenge test.

The design of the PROMIS study has some potential weaknesses. First, we intend to recruit women with a risk factor for metabolic deviations in a cohort like approach rather than using a randomized trial design directly comparing groups from different BMI classes. Although the latter may use accepted standard definitions, BMI may not adequately represent body adiposity, the major driver of insulin sensitivity. The choice for focus on more detailed assessment in women with a clear risk for increased adiposity may reduce the total number of women we need to include for adequate analysis of the results. The current power estimate, however, which is based on glucose data only, may not allow for powered analysis for many of the secondary outcomes. Secondly, the detailed and repeated measurements may form a burden for participants increasing the risk of drop out. We hope to overcome this hurdle by offering specific assessments with attention for health of mother and her infant next to the routine care these women receive during and after pregnancy. The detailed assessment of glucose, as well as insulin values using multiple time points during the postprandial phase, as well as the addition of stable labelled glucose to assess other glucose parameters, i.e., glucose production and disappearance rates, is a clear strength of this study. The repeated assessment will allow for longitudinal assessment of pregnancy related changes in glucose-insulin metabolism, as well as within subject comparison of results between MTT and OGTT, where the MTT provides a more physiological challenge compared to the standard OGTT. Finally, the detailed measurements of fetal as well as early postnatal growth and body composition in the infants may generate insights in early growth trajectories in relation to maternal glycemia and other metabolic markers. These data may help to develop markers for early detection of metabolic deviations and improve the diagnostic toolbox, as well as inform the development of new interventions, although these would require in depth validation in new clinical studies.

4. Conclusions

The design of the PROMIS study will generate insight in early pregnancy metabolic changes in overweight and obese women that may predict later pregnancy and postpartum maternal outcomes and possible associations with offspring growth and body composition outcomes. These data may provide a starting point for future design of focused intervention studies to prevent and manage maternal as well as fetal and infant complications.

Author Contributions: Conceptualization and methodology A.K., M.S., S.A.S., H.L., and E.M.v.d.B., writing—original draft preparation, A.K., E.M.v.d.B., and M.S.; writing—review and editing, A.K., M.S., H.L., S.A.S., and E.M.v.d.B., funding acquisition, E.M.v.d.B. and A.K. All authors have read and agreed to the published version of the manuscript.

Funding: This investigator-initiated study received financial support from Danone Nutricia Research, Utrecht, the Netherlands and the Top Sector Agri and Food (www.tki-agrifood.nl, (assessed on 23

February 2021), ref nr AF17068), as well as a small contribution from a hospital-based research fund, e.g., "kleine vis—grote vis'. These sponsors have no role in the design of the study nor in execution, interpretation, and in writing.

Institutional Review Board Statement: The study has been approved by the medical ethical committee of the UMC Groningen prior to the start of the study (NL68845.042.19) and is registered at ClinicalTrials.gov (NCT04315545).

Informed Consent Statement: Informed consent will be obtained from all subjects involved in the study.

Data Availability Statement: No new data were created or analyzed in this study. Data sharing is not applicable to this article.

Conflicts of Interest: The authors declare no conflicts of interest. E.M.v.d.B. was a part-time employee of Danone Nutricia Research at the time of study protocol development.

References

1. Sonagra, A.D.; Biradar, S.M.; Dattatreya, K.; Murthy, D.S.J. Normal pregnancy—A state of insulin resistance. *J. Clin. Diagn. Res.* **2014**, *8*, CC01–CC03. [CrossRef]
2. Marcinkevage, J.A.; Narayan, K.V. Gestational diabetes mellitus: Taking it to heart. *Prim. Care Diabetes* **2011**, *5*, 81–88. [CrossRef] [PubMed]
3. Devlieger, R.; Casteels, K.; Van Assche, F.A. Reduced adaptation of the pancreatic B cells during pregnancy is the major causal factor for gestational diabetes: Current knowledge and metabolic effects on the offspring. *Acta Obstet. Gynecol. Scand.* **2008**, *87*, 1266–1270. [CrossRef] [PubMed]
4. Bellmann, O.; Hartmann, E. Influence of pregnancy on the kinetics of insulin. *Am. J. Obstet. Gynecol.* **1975**, *122*, 829–833. [CrossRef]
5. Baeyens, L.; Hindi, S.; Sorenson, R.L.; German, M.S. β-Cell adaptation in pregnancy. *Diabetes Obes. Metab.* **2016**, *18*, 63–70. [CrossRef] [PubMed]
6. Rieck, S.; Kaestner, K.H. Expansion of β-cell mass in response to pregnancy. *Trends Endocrinol. Metab.* **2010**, *21*, 151–158. [CrossRef] [PubMed]
7. Catalano, P.A.; Ehrenberg, H. The short-and long-term implications of maternal obesity on the mother and her offspring. *BJOG Int. J. Obstet. Gynaecol.* **2006**, *113*, 1126–1133. [CrossRef] [PubMed]
8. Chen, C.; Xu, X.; Yan, Y. Estimated global overweight and obesity burden in pregnant women based on panel data model. *PLoS ONE* **2018**, *13*, e0202183. [CrossRef]
9. Lengte en gewicht van personen, ondergewicht en overgewicht; vanaf 1981. Available online: https://www.cbs.nl/nl-nl/cijfers/detail/81565NED?dl=35805 (assessed on 23 February 2021).
10. HAPO Study Cooperative Research Group. Hyperglycemia and adverse pregnancy outcomes. *N. Engl. J. Med.* **2008**, *358*, 1991–2002. [CrossRef]
11. Seshiah, V.; Cynthia, A.; Balaji, V.; Balaji, M.S.; Ashalata, S.; Sheela, R.; Thamizharasia, M.; Arthia, T. Detection and care of women with gestational diabetes mellitus from early weeks of pregnancy results in birth weight of newborn babies appropriate for gestational age. *Diabetes Res. Clin. Pract.* **2008**, *80*, 199–202. [CrossRef]
12. Phillips, P.J. Oral glucose tolerance testing. *Aust. Fam. Physician* **2012**, *41*, 391. [PubMed]
13. Ko, G.T.; Chan, J.C.; Woo, J.; Lau, E.; Yeung, V.T.; Chow, C.; Cockram, C.S. The reproducibility and usefulness of the oral glucose tolerance test in screening for diabetes and other cardiovascular risk factors. *Ann. Clin. Biochem.* **1998**, *35*, 62–67. [CrossRef] [PubMed]
14. Benhalima, K.; Van Crombrugge, P.; Moyson, C.; Verhaeghe, J.; Vandeginste, S.; Verlaenen, H.; Vercammen, C.; Maes, T.; Dufraimont, E.; De Block, C.; et al. Characteristics and pregnancy outcomes across gestational diabetes mellitus subtypes based on insulin resistance. *Diabetologia* **2019**, *62*, 2118–2128. [CrossRef] [PubMed]
15. Cobelli, C.; Dalla Man, C.; Sparacino, G.; Magni, L.; De Nicolao, G.; Kovatchev, B.P. Diabetes: Models, signals, and control. *IEEE Rev. Biomed. Eng.* **2009**, *2*, 54–96. [CrossRef]
16. Van Dijk, T.H.; Boer, T.S.; Havinga, R.; Stellaard, F.; Kuipers, F.; Reijngoud, D. Quantification of hepatic carbohydrate metabolism in conscious mice using serial blood and urine spots. *Anal. Biochem.* **2003**, *322*, 1–13. [CrossRef] [PubMed]
17. Cosmed the metabolic company. PEAPOD, the world's gold standard for non-invasive Infant body composition assessment. Available online: https://www.cosmed.com/en/products/body-composition/pea-pod (assessed on 23 February 2021).
18. DIABETES MELLITUS EN ZWANGERSCHAP versie 3.0. de Otterlo werkgroep en Cie Kwaliteitsdocumenten NVOG. 2018. Available online: https://www.nvog.nl (assessed on 23 February 2021).
19. Muscogiuri, G.; Sarno, G.; Gastaldelli, A.; Savastano, S.; Ascione, A.; Colao, A.; Orio, F. The good and bad effects of statins on insulin sensitivity and secretion. *Endocr. Res.* **2014**, *39*, 137–143. [CrossRef] [PubMed]
20. Catalano, P.M. Obesity, insulin resistance, and pregnancy outcome. *Reproduction* **2010**, *140*, 365–371. [CrossRef] [PubMed]
21. van Leeuwen, M.; Prins, S.M.; de Valk, H.W.; Evers, I.M.; Visser, G.H.A.; Mol, B.J.M. Stand van zaken Diabetes gravidarum. Behandeling vermindert kans op complicaties. *Ned. Tijdschr. Geneeskd.* **2011**, *155*, A2291.

22. Van Leeuwen, M.; Louwerse, M.; Opmeer, B.; Limpens, J.; Serlie, M.; Reitsma, J.; Mol, B.W.J. Glucose challenge test for detecting gestational diabetes mellitus: A systematic review. *BJOG Int. J. Obstet. Gynaecol.* **2012**, *119*, 393–401. [CrossRef]
23. Flahault, A.; Cadilhac, M.; Thomas, G. Sample size calculation should be performed for design accuracy in diagnostic test studies. *J. Clin. Epidemiol.* **2005**, *58*, 859–862. [CrossRef]
24. Research Electronic Data Capture (REDCap). Available online: https://redcap.vanderbilt.edu (accessed on 23 February 2021).
25. Harpenden Skinfold Caliper. Available online: http://www.harpenden-skinfold.com/measurements.html (accessed on 23 February 2021).
26. Marshall, N.E.; Murphy, E.J.; King, J.C.; Haas, E.K.; Lim, J.Y.; Wiedrick, J.; Thornburg, K.L.; Purnell, J.Q. Comparison of multiple methods to measure maternal fat mass in late gestation, 2. *Am. J. Clin. Nutr.* **2016**, *103*, 1055–1063. [CrossRef]
27. Durnin, J.; Rahaman, M.M. The assessment of the amount of fat in the human body from measurements of skinfold thickness. *Br. J. Nutr.* **1967**, *21*, 681–689. [CrossRef]
28. Villar, J.; Ismail, L.C.; Victora, C.G.; O Ohuma, E.; Bertino, E.; Altman, D.G.; Lambert, A.; Papageorghiou, A.T.; Carvalho, M.; A Jaffer, Y.; et al. International standards for newborn weight, length, and head circumference by gestational age and sex: The Newborn Cross-Sectional Study of the INTERGROWTH-21st Project. *Lancet* **2014**, *384*, 857–868. [CrossRef]
29. World Health Organization. *WHO Child Growth Standards: Methods and Development: Head Circumference-for-Age, Arm Circumference-for-Age, Triceps Skinfold-for-Age and Subscapular Skinfold-for-Age*; World Health Organization: Geneva, Switzerland, 2007.
30. Molag, M. Towards Transparent Development of Food Frequency Questionnaires: Scientific Basis of the Dutch FFQ-TOOL tm: A Computer System to Generate, Apply and Process FFQs. Ph.D. Thesis, Wageningen University, Wageningen, The Netherland, 2010.
31. Hunot, C.; Fildes, A.; Croker, H.; Llewellyn, C.H.; Wardle, J.; Beeken, R.J. Appetitive traits and relationships with BMI in adults: Development of the Adult Eating Behaviour Questionnaire. *Appetite* **2016**, *105*, 356–363. [CrossRef] [PubMed]
32. Rabin, R.; Charro, F.D. EQ-SD: A measure of health status from the EuroQol Group. *Ann. Med.* **2001**, *33*, 337–343. [CrossRef] [PubMed]
33. Chasan-taber, L.; Schmidt, M.D.; Roberts, D.E.; Hosmer, D.; Markenson, G.; Freedson, P.S. Development and validation of a pregnancy physical activity questionnaire. *Med. Sci. Sports Exerc.* **2004**, *36*, 1750–1760. [CrossRef]
34. Hagströmer, M.; Oja, P.; Sjöström, M. The International Physical Activity Questionnaire (IPAQ): A study of concurrent and construct validity. *Public Health Nutr.* **2006**, *9*, 755–762. [CrossRef]
35. Llewellyn, C.H.; van Jaarsveld, C.H.; Johnson, L.; Carnell, S.; Wardle, J. Development and factor structure of the Baby Eating Behaviour Questionnaire in the Gemini birth cohort. *Appetite* **2011**, *57*, 388–396. [CrossRef]
36. World Health Organization. *Global Report on Diabetes.* 2016; WHO: Geneva, Switzerland, 2017.
37. Maegawa, Y.; Sugiyama, T.; Kusaka, H.; Mitao, M.; Toyoda, N. Screening tests for gestational diabetes in Japan in the 1st and 2nd trimester of pregnancy. *Diabetes Res. Clin. Pract.* **2003**, *62*, 47–53. [CrossRef]
38. Rijkelijkhuizen, J.M.; Girman, C.J.; Mari, A.; Alssema, M.; Rhodes, T.; Nijpels, G.; Kostense, P.J.; Stein, P.P.; Eekhoff, E.M.; Heine, R.J.; et al. Classical and model-based estimates of beta-cell function during a mixed meal vs. an OGTT in a population-based cohort. *Diabetes Res. Clin. Pract.* **2009**, *83*, 280–288. [CrossRef]

Article

Trends in Prevalence of Diabetes among Twin Pregnancies and Perinatal Outcomes in Catalonia between 2006 and 2015: The DIAGESTCAT Study

Lucia Gortazar [1,2], Juana Antonia Flores-Le Roux [1,2,3], David Benaiges [1,2,3,4,*], Eugènia Sarsanedas [5], Humberto Navarro [1,2], Antonio Payà [6], Laura Mañé [1,2], Juan Pedro-Botet [1,2,3] and Albert Goday [1,2,3]

1. Department of Endocrinology and Nutrition, Hospital del Mar, Passeig Marítim, 25-29, E-08003 Barcelona, Spain; lucia.gortazar@gmail.com (L.G.); 94066@parcdesalutmar.cat (J.A.F.-L.R.); humberto20192@gmail.com (H.N.); laurams47112@gmail.com (L.M.); 86620@parcdesalutmar.cat (J.P.-B.); Agoday@parcdesalutmar.cat (A.G.)
2. Department of Medicine, Universitat Autònoma de Barcelona, 08139 Barcelona, Spain
3. Institut Hospital del Mar d'Investigacions Mèdiques, 08003 Barcelona, Spain
4. Consorci Sanitari de l'Alt Penedès Garraf, 08720 Vilafranca del Penedès, Spain
5. Health Information Management Department, Hospital del Mar, 08003 Barcelona, Spain; esarsanedas@parcdesalutmar.cat
6. Department of Gynecology and Obstetrics, Hospital del Mar, 08003 Barcelona, Spain; apaya@parcdesalutmar.cat
* Correspondence: DBenaiges@parcdesalutmar.cat or 96002@parcdesalutmar.cat; Tel.: +34-932483902; Fax: +34-932483254

Abstract: The aims of our study were to evaluate the trends in the prevalence of diabetes among twin pregnancies in Catalonia, Spain between 2006 and 2015, to assess the influence of diabetes on perinatal outcomes of twin gestations and to ascertain the interaction between twin pregnancies and glycaemic status. A population-based study was conducted using the Spanish Minimum Basic Data Set. Cases of gestational diabetes mellitus (GDM) and pre-existing diabetes were identified using ICD-9-CM codes. Data from 743,762 singleton and 15,956 twin deliveries between 2006 and 2015 in Catalonia was analysed. Among twin pregnancies, 1088 (6.82%) were diagnosed with GDM and 83 (0.52%) had pre-existing diabetes. The prevalence of GDM among twin pregnancies increased from 6.01% in 2006 to 8.48% in 2015 ($p < 0.001$) and the prevalence of pre-existing diabetes remained stable (from 0.46% to 0.27%, $p = 0.416$). The risk of pre-eclampsia was higher in pre-existing diabetes (15.66%, $p = 0.015$) and GDM (11.39%, $p < 0.001$) than in normoglycaemic twin pregnancies (7.55%). Pre-existing diabetes increased the risk of prematurity (69.62% vs. 51.84%, $p = 0.002$) and large-for-gestational-age (LGA) infants (20.9% vs. 11.6%, $p = 0.001$) in twin gestations. An attenuating effect on several adverse perinatal outcomes was found between twin pregnancies and the presence of GDM and pre-existing diabetes. As a result, unlike in singleton pregnancies, diabetes did not increase the risk of all perinatal outcomes in twins and the effect of pre-existing diabetes on pre-eclampsia and LGA appeared to be attenuated. In conclusion, prevalence of GDM among twin pregnancies increased over the study period. Diabetes was associated with a higher risk of pre-eclampsia, prematurity and LGA in twin gestations. However, the impact of both, pre-existing diabetes and GDM, on twin pregnancy outcomes was attenuated when compared with its impact on singleton gestations.

Keywords: epidemiology; twins; gestational diabetes; pre-existing diabetes; prevalence; trends; perinatal outcomes

1. Introduction

Diabetes mellitus (DM) is the most frequent metabolic complication of pregnancy. Pre-existing diabetes and gestational diabetes mellitus (GDM) affect around 0.3–0.6% and 2–10% of pregnancies, respectively, in Europe [1–5], and there is evidence that the prevalence of diabetes in pregnancy is rising worldwide [6–8]. Women with GDM and pre-existing diabetes are at increased risk of adverse maternal and neonatal outcomes including congenital malformations, caesarean section, pre-eclampsia, macrosomia and neonatal hypoglycaemia [9,10]. The risk of perinatal complications appears to be greater in pre-existing diabetes than in GDM [11].

Twin pregnancies are also at high risk of maternal and neonatal morbidity and their incidence has increased worldwide in recent decades in association with increasing maternal age and the use of assisted reproductive technology (ART) [12].

It is therefore not surprising that both conditions are more likely to coincide and diabetes might add additional risk to twin gestations. However, evidence of the effect of diabetes on maternal and perinatal outcomes in twin pregnancies is conflicting. In this respect, population-based studies evaluating epidemiological data in twin pregnancies complicated by diabetes in Southern Europe are scant and few have focused on pre-existing diabetes.

Moreover, it has suggested that an interaction between twin pregnancies and glycaemic status might be present. Hiersch et al. reported that unlike in singleton pregnancies, GDM was not associated with hypertensive complications, neonatal intensive care unit admission and neonatal hypoglycaemia in twins [13]. Diabetes might differently influence outcomes in twin and singleton pregnancy, therefore affecting clinical care in women with diabetes and twin gestations.

Thus, our study was aimed to assess trends in prevalence of GDM and pre-existing diabetes among twin pregnancies between 2006 and 2015 in Catalonia, Spain; to evaluate the influence of both diabetic conditions on adverse gestational and perinatal outcomes in twin gestations and to ascertain the interaction between twin pregnancies and glycaemic status.

2. Materials and Methods

A retrospective cohort study was conducted using the Minimum Basic Data Set for Hospital Discharge (CMBD-AH). All maternal hospital discharge records of singleton and multiple deliveries in Catalonia from January 2006 to December 2015 were collected. The CMBD-AH database covers more than 95% of private and public hospital deliveries in Spain and is managed by the Spanish Ministry of Health which conducts periodic audits to ensure coding reliability.

Catalonia is an autonomous community in the northeast of Spain. It is the second largest in terms of population (7.7 million inhabitants) and Barcelona, its capital, is the second most populated city in Spain (1.6 million inhabitants) [14].

Women between 15 and 45 years of age with Diagnostic Related Groups codes 370–375 (caesarean and vaginal deliveries) were included. Deliveries occurring before 22 week's gestation were excluded. Among all discharge reports, women with multiple pregnancies were identified using International Classification of Diseases, Ninth Revision, Clinical Modification (ICD-9-CM) codes (651.0x, 651.1x, 651.2x, 651.3x, 651.4x, 651.5x, 651.6x, 651.7x, 651.8x, 651.9x, V27.2, V27.3, V27.4, V27.5, V27.6 and V27.7). In particular, twin pregnancies were identified using 651.0x, 651.3x and V27.2, V27.3 and V27.4 ICD-9-CM codes.

Cases of GDM were established using ICD-9-CM code 648.8x. Throughout the study period, universal screening for GDM in Spain was based on a two-step strategy (O'Sullivan test and 100 g OGTT) following the recommendations of the Spanish College of Obstetricians and Gynecologists, Spanish Diabetes Society and Spanish Paediatrics Association [15]. The pre-existing diabetes group included women with type 1 diabetes mellitus (ICD-9-CM codes 250.x1 or 250.x3) and those with "type 2 diabetes mellitus and other pre-existing diabetes" (counting women with type 2 diabetes ICD-9-CM codes 250.x0 or 250.x2 and women with "diabetes mellitus, pre-pregnancy" codes 648.0x).

Maternal characteristics included age, chronic hypertension (ICD-9-CM codes 642.0–642.2 or 401–405), dyslipidaemia (ICD-9-CM code 272) and smoking status (ICD-9-CM code 649.0 or 305.1). In relation to obstetric complications, pre-eclampsia was defined by ICD-9 codes 642.4–642.6 and caesarean section by ICD-9-CM codes 74.0, 74.4, 74.9, 74.91, 74.99, 669.7 and 669.71 listed anywhere on the discharge report.

Perinatal outcomes analysed included stillbirth, preterm birth, mean birth weight, macrosomia, large-for-gestational-age (LGA) and small-for-gestational-age (SGA). Stillbirth or foetal mortality was considered if one or both twins (>22 week's gestation) died in utero and was defined by ICD-9-CM codes V27.3 and V27.4 in twins and by V27.1 code in singleton pregnancies. Preterm delivery was defined as birth before 37 weeks' gestation according to the World Health Organization (WHO) and the American College of Obstetricians and Gynecologists (ACOG). Macrosomia was defined according to the American College of Obstetricians and Gynecologists as newborns with a birthweight ≥4000 g. LGA and SGA were defined as neonatal birth weight >90th and <10th centiles for gestational age, respectively, based on singleton or twin birth weights standardised for foetal sex and gestational age using Catalonian population standards [16]. The prevalence of outcomes that included birth weight was calculated from the total of newborns.

Data from all delivery reports remained anonymous and therefore informed consent was not recorded. The study was conducted according to the principles of the Declaration of Helsinki and approved by the Clinical Research Ethics Committee of our institution (CEIC-Parc de Salut MAR, number 2017/7209/I).

Statistical Analysis

Maternal and perinatal characteristics were reported using descriptive analysis. Chi-square test was used to compare prevalences of GDM and pre-existing diabetes among singleton and twin pregnancies. ANOVA was used to compare continuous variables among the three different glycaemic status groups. Maternal characteristics and perinatal outcomes of different study groups were compared using multivariate logistic regression models. Perinatal outcomes were adjusted for maternal age, hypertension, dyslipidaemia, year of delivery and smoking status. To study the interaction between singleton/twin pregnancies and glycaemic status on adverse outcomes the following analysis was undertaken. Firstly, adjusted Odds Ratio (OR) for each outcome in singleton vs. twin pregnancies regardless of glycaemic status, adjusted OR for GDM vs. non-DM and adjusted OR for pre-existing DM vs. non-DM in twin and singleton pregnancies were calculated. Secondly, a cross-product term between twin pregnancies and glycaemic status was included in multivariate models to assess the interaction effect of both factors and the risk of perinatal outcomes. In order to analyse the effect of each factor and its interaction on a specific adverse outcome, a B coefficient (and his statistical significance) was reported. Crude and age-adjusted annual GDM and pre-existing diabetes prevalences among twin pregnancies were calculated using direct standardisation to the maternal age structure of the whole study population. Time trends in twin pregnancies and the prevalence of GDM and pre-existing diabetes were assessed using a Poisson regression model. All p-values were two-tailed and statistical significance was accepted at 5% level. Data were analysed with the statistical software package IBM SPSS Statistics V.25.0.

3. Results

A total of 760,209 women gave birth in Catalonia between January 2006 and December 2015. Of these, 743,762 (97.8%) had singleton pregnancies. Data on singleton pregnancies, regarding prevalence and trends in perinatal outcomes of women with GDM, pre-existing diabetes and without diabetes, have been published elsewhere [3,4].

The vast majority of multiple deliveries (16,447 (2.16%)) corresponded to twin pregnancies (15,956 (2.10%)). We therefore analysed data on twin pregnancies, excluding other multiple deliveries. The rate of twin deliveries rose from 1.75% in 2006 to 2.22% in 2015 ($p < 0.001$).

Women with twin pregnancies were older than women with singleton gestations (33.7 ± 5.1 years vs. 31.4 ± 5.4 years, $p < 0.001$). Mothers of twins showed higher rates of chronic hypertension (0.9% vs. 0.6%, $p < 0.001$) and comparable rates of dyslipidaemia (0.2% in twins vs. 0.1% in singleton, $p = 0.059$). However, women with twin pregnancies were less frequently smokers than women with singleton pregnancies (4.0% vs. 5.6%, $p < 0.001$).

Among women with twin pregnancies, 14,785 (92.67%) were normoglycaemic, 1088 (6.82%) were diagnosed with GDM and 83 (0.52%) had pre-existing diabetes. Women with pre-existing diabetes included 63 (0.39%) with "type 2 diabetes mellitus and other pre-existing diabetes" and 20 (0.13%) with type 1 diabetes mellitus. The prevalence of GDM was higher in twin vs. singleton pregnancies whereas no differences were observed in pre-existing diabetes (Figure 1).

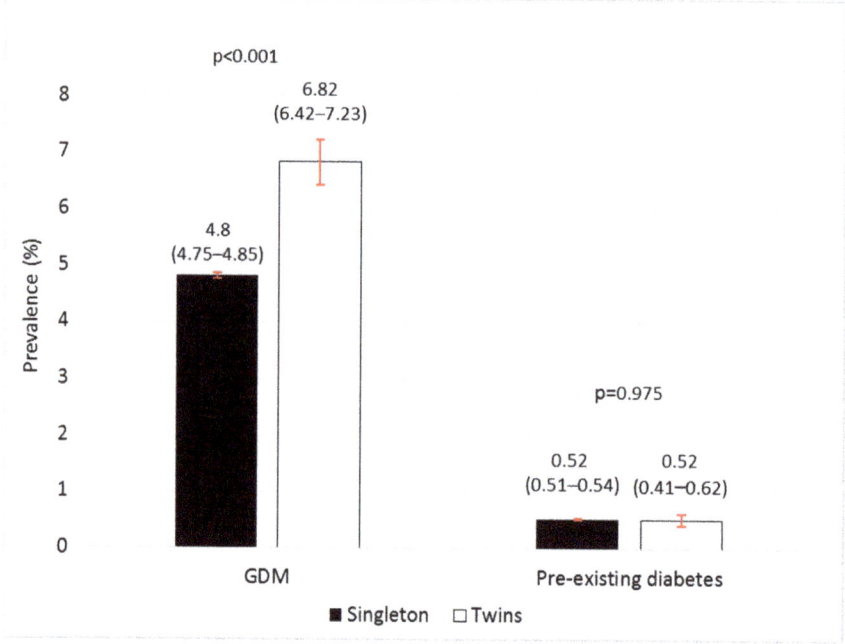

Figure 1. Prevalence (95% CI) of gestational diabetes mellitus (GDM) and pre-existing diabetes in twin and singleton pregnancies in Catalonia between 2006 and 2015.

The prevalence of GDM increased among twin pregnancies during the study period (from 6.01% to 8.48%, $p < 0.001$). The prevalence of pre-existing diabetes in twin pregnancies remained stable ($p = 0.416$) (Figure 2).

3.1. Pregnancy Outcomes of Twin Pregnancies According to Glycaemic Status

Maternal characteristics and perinatal outcomes of twin pregnancies by maternal diabetes status are shown in Table 1.

In twin pregnancies, diabetes (either pre-existing or GDM) was associated with older mean maternal age and higher rates of pre-existing hypertension compared to non-diabetic pregnancies. The risk of pre-eclampsia was greater in twin pregnancies with pre-existing diabetes (15.66%) and GDM (11.39%) compared to normoglycaemic twin pregnancies (7.55%). By contrast, diabetes did not increase the risk of caesarean section; in particular, the caesarean section rate of GDM women was lower than non-diabetic women (65.63% vs. 68.12%, $p = 0.002$). The risk of preterm birth was higher in women with pre-existing diabetes compared with normoglycaemic women, although no statistically-significant differences were observed for women with GDM. The risk of stillbirth was not increased in women with diabetes (both pre-gestational and GDM) compared to normoglycaemic twin gestations.

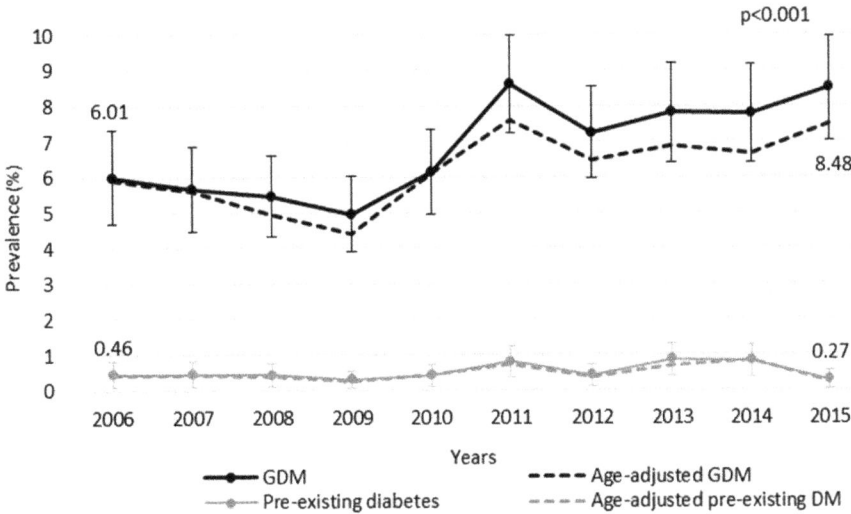

Figure 2. Trends in crude and age-adjusted prevalence (95% CI) of GDM and other pre-existing diabetes in twin pregnancies in Catalonia between 2006 and 2015.

Regarding birth weight outcomes in twin pregnancies, newborns of mothers with pre-existing diabetes were at increased risk of LGA (OR: 1.98) compared to those of non-diabetic mothers, while no statistically significant differences were observed in those of women with GDM. Moreover, no differences were found in rates of SGA, mean birthweight and macrosomia in neonates of women with diabetes (either pre-existing or GDM) compared to those of normoglycemic mothers.

3.2. Interaction between Twin Gestations and Glycaemic Status in Relation to Adverse Perinatal Outcomes

The effect of twin gestations, glycaemic status and the interaction of both conditions on adverse perinatal outcomes are shown in Table 2. Data on prevalence of diabetes and rates of perinatal outcomes in women according to their glycaemic status in singleton pregnancies have been published elsewhere [3,4].

The risk of pre-eclampsia was strongly increased in twin gestations (OR 5.38) and to a lesser extent in singleton pregnancies with pre-existing DM (OR 3.95) and GDM (OR 1.70). An attenuating effect of the interaction between twin pregnancies and pre-existing diabetes was observed (B coefficient −0.63, p = 0.045); however, women with pre-existing diabetes and twin pregnancies continued to have an increased risk of pre-eclampsia compared to non-DM. No significant interaction was detected between twin pregnancies and GDM.

In reference to preterm birth, the risk was increased in twin pregnancies compared to singleton (OR:16.8) and in singleton gestations with pre-existing diabetes (OR 3.17) or GDM (OR 1.2). A negative interaction between twin gestations and GDM was detected; as a result, their risk of preterm birth was not increased compared to non-DM twin pregnancies.

The risk of caesarean section was increased in twin pregnancies (OR 5.4) and in singleton gestations with pre-existing diabetes (OR 3.17) and GDM (OR 1.2). Moreover, an attenuating effect in caesarean section risk was observed between twin gestations and pre-existing DM and GDM. This attenuating effect translated into similar risks for pre-existing diabetes and normoglycemic twin pregnancies whereas GDM women had a lower risk.

Table 1. Maternal characteristics, obstetric and perinatal outcomes of twin pregnancies.

	Normoglycaemic n = 14,785	GDM n = 1088	OR, GDM vs. Non-DM	Pre-Existing DM n = 83	OR, Pre-Existing DM vs. Non-DM	ANOVA p Value
Age (years)	33.6 ± 5.1	35.3 ± 5.0		35.1 ± 6.1		p < 0.001
Chronic hypertension, n (%)	127 (0.86)	18 (1.65)	1.81 (1.10–2.99) p = 0.020	3 (3.61)	4.09 (1.27–13.14) p = 0.018	
Dyslipidaemia, n (%)	26 (0.18)	2 (0.18)	1.05 (0.25–4.44) p = 0.949	1 (1.20)	7.06 (0.94–52.78) p = 0.057	
Smoking, n (%)	583 (3.94)	54 (4.96)	1.40 (1.05–1.87) p = 0.002	3 (3.61)	0.98 (0.31–3.11) p = 0.969	
Pre-eclampsia, n (%)	1116 (7.55)	124 (11.39)	1.43 (1.17–1.74) p < 0.001	13 (15.66)	2.04 (1.12–3.72) p = 0.020	
Preterm birth, n (%)	7373 (51.84)	566 (53.04)	1.06 (0.94–1.21) p = 0.327	55 (69.62)	2.15 (1.33–3.48) p = 0.002	
Caesarean section, n (%)	10,072 (68.12)	714 (65.63)	0.82 (0.71–0.93) p = 0.002	61 (73.49)	1.20 (0.73–1.97) p = 0.468	
Stillbirth, n (%)	473 (3.20)	26 (2.39)	0.76 (0.51–1.14) p = 0.189	2 (2.41)	0.77 (0.18–3.31) p = 0.712	
Macrosomia, n (%)	22 (0.08)	1 (0.05)	0.595 (0.08–4.43) p = 0.612	0 (0)	0 p = 0.966	
LGA (>90th), n (%)	3247 (11.63)	273 (12.95)	1.12 (0.98–1.28) p = 0.09	33 (20.89)	1.98 (1.35–2.91) p = 0.001	
SGA (<10th), n (%)	2339 (8.37)	202 (9.58)	1.15 (0.99–1.34) p = 0.078	8 (5.06)	0.58 (0.28–1.19) p = 0.134	
Mean birth weight (g)	2333 ± 503	2336 ± 486		2295 ± 616		p = 0.304

GDM, gestational diabetes; DM, diabetes mellitus; Non-DM, non-diabetic; LGA, large for gestational age; SGA, small for gestational age. ANOVA was used to compare age and mean birthweight among the three groups. Hypertension and dyslipidaemia OR were adjusted for maternal age and smoking habit. Pre-eclampsia, preterm birth, caesarean section, stillbirth, macrosomia, LGA and SGA OR were adjusted for maternal age, chronic hypertension, dyslipidaemia, year of delivery and smoking status. Birthweight outcomes were calculated using the total number of living newborns with weight data (27,931 normoglycaemic, 2108 GDM and 158 pre-existing DM). Preterm birth was calculated considering the cases with gestational age at delivery data (14,222 normoglycaemic, 1067 GDM, 79 pre-existing DM). The other outcomes were calculated using the total number of deliveries in each group.

Table 2. Interaction between twin pregnancies and glycaemic status on adverse perinatal outcomes.

	Twins vs. Singleton			Gestational Diabetes				Pre-Existing Diabetes			
	B Coefficient Normoglycaemic Pregnancies p Value	OR Twins vs. Singleton p Value	B Coefficient Singleton Pregnancies p Value	OR GDM vs. Non-DM (Singleton) p Value	OR GDM vs. Non-DM (Twins) p Value	Interaction GDM and Twins B Coefficient p Value	Beta Coefficient Singleton Pregnancies p Value	OR Pre-Existing DM vs. Non-DM (Singleton) p Value	OR Pre-Existing DM vs. Non-DM (Twins) p Value	Interaction Pre-Existing DM and Twins B Coefficient p Value
Pre-eclampsia	1.68 p < 0.001	5.38 (5.04–5.74) p < 0.001	0.532 p < 0.001	1.70 (1.59–1.82) p < 0.001	1.43 (1.17–1.74) p < 0.001	−0.12 p = 0.275	1.37 p < 0.001	3.95 (3.44–4.51) p < 0.001	2.04 (1.12–3.72) p = 0.020	−0.63 p = 0.045
Preterm birth	2.82 p < 0.001	16.8 (16.26–17.43) p < 0.001	0.18 p < 0.001	1.20 (1.15–1.25) p < 0.001	1.06 (0.94–1.21) p = 0.327	−0.15 p = 0.028	1.15 p < 0.001	3.17 (2.91–3.44) p < 0.001	2.15 (1.33–3.48) p = 0.002	−0.429 p = 0.085
Caesarean section	1.73 p < 0.001	5.64 (5.44–5.84) p < 0.001	0.086 p < 0.001	1.09 (1.06–1.12) p < 0.001	0.82 (0.71–0.93) p = 0.002	−0.30 p < 0.001	0.791 p < 0.001	2.20 (2.07–2.35) p < 0.001	1.20 (0.73–1.97) p = 0.468	−0.621 p = 0.015
Stillbirth	1.92 p < 0.001	6.85 (6.21–7.57) p < 0.001	−0.305 p < 0.001	0.74 (0.62–0.88) p < 0.001	0.76 (0.51–1.14) p = 0.189	−0.025 p = 0.912	0.73 p < 0.001	2.08 (1.52–2.83) p < 0.001	0.77 (0.18–3.31) p = 0.712	−1.072 p = 0.145
Macrosomia	−4.406 p = 0.012	0.012 (0.008–0.019) p < 0.001	0.414 p < 0.001	1.51 (1.45–1.57) p < 0.001	0.595 (0.08–4.43) p = 0.612	−0.905 p = 0.376	0.99 p < 0.001	2.68 (2.45–2.94) p < 0.001	0 p = 0.966	−15.037 p = 0.996
LGA	−0.14 p < 0.001	0.87 (0.84–0.90) p < 0.001	0.43 p < 0.001	1.53 (1.49–1.58) p < 0.001	1.12 (0.98–1.28) p = 0.09	−0.302 p < 0.001	1.31 p < 0.001	3.69 (3.46–3.95) p < 0.001	1.98 (1.35–2.91) p = 0.001	−0.610 p = 0.002
SGA	−0.07 p = 0.001	0.93 (0.89–0.97) p < 0.001	−0.137 p < 0.001	0.87 (0.83–0.91) p < 0.001	1.15 (0.99–1.34) p = 0.078	0.27 p = 0.001	−0.55 p < 0.001	0.58 (0.50–0.60) p < 0.001	0.58 (0.28–1.19) p = 0.134	−0.01 p = 0.98

GDM, gestational diabetes; Non-DM, non-diabetic; LGA, large for gestational age; SGA, small for gestational age. OR were adjusted for maternal age, chronic hypertension, dyslipidaemia, year of delivery and smoking status.

The risk of LGA was reduced in twin pregnancies (OR 0.87) and increased in singleton pregnancies with pre-existing diabetes (OR 3.69) and GDM (OR 1.53). The attenuating effect observed between twin pregnancies and pre-existing DM and GDM resulted in similar rates of LGA in GDM and normoglycemic women although women with pre-existing diabetes and twin pregnancies continued to have an increased risk of LGA compared to non-DM.

The risk of SGA was decreased in twin pregnancies (OR 0.93) and to a greater extent in singleton pregnancies with GDM (OR 0.87) and pre-existing DM (OR 0.58). We detected an enhancing effect between twin gestations and GDM; therefore, no differences were observed in SGA rates between twins with GDM and without DM.

No interaction was detected between twin pregnancies and glycaemic status for macrosomia and stillbirth.

4. Discussion

This large, population-based study revealed a 27% rise in twin pregnancies and a 41% increase in GDM prevalence among twin gestations in Catalonia from 2006 to 2015. The prevalence of GDM in twin pregnancies was 6.82%, clearly higher than the prevalence of GDM in singleton gestations (4.80%). Regarding obstetric and perinatal outcomes in twin pregnancies, diabetes, both pre-existing and GDM, were associated with an increased risk of pre-eclampsia compared to normoglycaemic women. Prematurity and LGA were more frequent in women with pre-existing diabetes than in non-diabetic mothers. However, the impact of both, pre-existing diabetes and GDM, on twin pregnancy outcomes was attenuated when compared with its impact on singleton gestations. To our knowledge, no previous study has analysed the interaction of both, twin pregnancy and diabetic conditions, on pregnancy outcomes.

The twin pregnancy rate observed in our study was consistent with the 1.4–3% rates reported in previous studies [12,17–20]. The increasing rate of twin pregnancies observed has also been described worldwide over recent decades [12]. In particular, a multi-centre-based study conducted in Spain reported an increase in the rate of twin gestations from 1.69% in 2000 to 2.06% in 2004 [17]. The principal factors related to this trend are delayed childbearing and the rise in ART. Advanced maternal age is a known risk factor for spontaneous twin pregnancies [12]. In this respect, it has been proposed that, under equal ovarian feedback, premenopausal mothers of dizygotic twins have hyper-stimulation by endogenous follicle-stimulating hormones [21]. The use of ART treatments steadily increased in Spain over the study period. A change in embryo transference policies in the recent decades, with a change from multiple to single embryo transferences, has led to a lower rate of multiple pregnancies among women receiving ART treatments [22]. However, the overall number of ART treatments and twin pregnancies has continued to rise which, together with older mean maternal age, might account for the trend in twin pregnancy rates observed in our study.

Previous studies described GDM prevalences in twin pregnancies ranging from 3.0% to 9.0% [13,18,19,23–26]. Lai et al. conducted a population-based study in Alberta, Canada between 2003–2014 and found a 7.3% prevalence of GDM among twin pregnancies, slightly higher than the 6.8% prevalence observed in our study [18]. Furthermore, Gonzalez et al. reported a 7.7% prevalence in a multi-centre-based study in Spain where medical reports between 2004 and 2008 were reviewed. Data from two hospitals in Catalonia were included and the same GDM diagnostic approach as in our study was used [27].

The prevalence of GDM was higher in twin than in singleton pregnancies in the present study. This finding is in line with most previous studies [13,18,28–30] although some authors reported conflicting results on the subject [31,32]. Although factors associated with twin pregnancies such as maternal age, obesity, increased weight gain and the use of ART might have played a role in the higher prevalence observed, a study by Rauh-Hain et al. found twin pregnancy to be associated with a two-fold increase in the risk of GDM, after adjusting for maternal age, ethnicity, body mass index, high blood pressure, smoking and parity, suggesting that twin pregnancy itself might be an independent risk factor for GDM [33]. In this respect, it has been suggested that larger placental mass and higher levels of human placenta lactogen, oestrogen and progesterone in twin pregnancies might increase the risk of GDM [34,35].

A growing trend of GDM among twin pregnancies has also been described in previous studies. In a population-based study conducted in Finland which analysed > 23,000 twin pregnancies, the prevalence of GDM in twin pregnancies rose from 3.3% in 1987 to 20.7% in 2014 [20] and a three-fold higher prevalence was observed in a single-centre Australian study between 2003 and 2012 [24]. This increasing trend is in line with the rise in GDM prevalence observed worldwide [6] and in particular with that observed in our population study in Catalonia [3].

Few studies assessed the prevalence of pre-existing diabetes in twin pregnancies. Lai et al. reported an 0.8% prevalence of pre-existing diabetes in twin pregnancies and an 0.9% prevalence in singleton gestations [18]. However, Gonzalez et al. found a lower prevalence of pre-existing diabetes in twins of 0.025% [36]. To our knowledge, the present study is the first one to report the trend in prevalence of pre-existing diabetes among twin pregnancies, and the results show no change overtime during the study period.

Regarding hypertensive complications in twin pregnancies, women with a diabetic condition were found to have higher rates of pre-eclampsia; 15% for those with pre-existing diabetes (odds ratio: 2.11) and 11% for those with GDM (odds ratio: 1.45). This finding is in line with several previous studies [18,24,27]; however, evidence on the effect of diabetes on hypertensive disorders in twin pregnancies is mixed. Dinham et al. found a 19.8% prevalence of hypertensive disorders in GDM compared to the 11.6% rate observed in normoglycaemic twin gestations [24]. Lai et al. also observed an increased risk of pre-eclampsia in women with GDM, but no significant differences in pre-existing diabetes [18]. Okby et al. reported an increase in mild pre-eclampsia in GDM (10.7% vs. 5.2%, $p < 0.001$), but not in severe pre-eclampsia (4.6% vs. 3.3%, $p = 0.18$) in their cohort of twin pregnancies [19]. On the other hand, Mourad et al. observed that the increased risk of hypertensive disorders in twin gestations with GDM lost significance after adjustment for maternal age, in vitro fertilisation treatment and pre-pregnancy BMI [37]. Furthermore, Hiersch et al. concluded that, unlike in singleton pregnancies, GDM in twins was not associated with hypertensive complications [13]. In the present study, we found an attenuation in the impact of pre-existing diabetes in the rate of pre-eclampsia in twin pregnancies, not observed in women with GDM.

In our study, diabetes did not raise the risk of caesarean section in twin pregnancies. While some previous studies reported an increased risk of caesarean section in women with diabetes and twin pregnancies [13,33,37], others found no significant differences [23,26,27,38]. In a retrospective population-based study conducted from 1998 to 2010 in Israel, Okby et al. observed a higher risk of caesarean section for GDM twin pregnancies; however, GDM was not found to be an independent risk factor for caesarean section in a multivariable analysis (controlling for maternal age, fertility treatments and hypertensive disorders) [19]. The similar rate of caesarean section observed in twin pregnancies with diabetes contrasts with the findings in singleton pregnancies. In this respect, twin pregnancies have a high base line risk of caesarean section and thus the effect of diabetes might be less relevant. Moreover, the increased risk of caesarean section in singleton pregnancies with diabetic conditions might be partly driven by high rates of macrosomia. In this respect, as described in the present study, macrosomia very rarely complicates twin pregnancies. It has been suggested that this might explain the similar rates of caesarean section in GDM and normoglycaemic twin gestations [19].

In the present study, the risk of preterm birth in twin pregnancies was increased in women with pre-existing diabetes. Previous studies have yielded consistent results [18,36,39]. However, in contrast with the results in singleton pregnancies, no differences in prematurity rates were observed in twin pregnancies with GDM. Previous studies evaluating GDM reported mixed results. Gonzalez et al. found an increased risk of preterm birth in women with GDM and twin pregnancies, although after adjusting for potential confounders, the presence of diabetes did not appear to significantly influence prematurity [27]. Hiersch et al. and Luo et al. reported higher prematurity rates in women with GDM and twin pregnancies, but the increased risk was less marked compared to the results observed in singleton [13,30]. In line with our findings, other previous studies did not report an increased risk of prematurity in women with twin pregnancies with GDM [18,19,24]. Women with twin pregnancies, regardless of glycaemic status, had a very high rate of prematurity (almost 50%). The fact that GDM increases the risk of prematurity in singleton pregnancies might be related, at least in part, with excessive foetal growth, a situation that does not occur in GDM twin pregnancies.

In the present study cohort, diabetes was not associated with an increased risk of stillbirth in twin pregnancies, a finding which is consistent with prior evidence [18,19,24,27,33,39]. However, it contrasts with the results observed in singleton pregnancies, with increased risk of stillbirth in women with pre-existing diabetes and a reduction in the risk in women with GDM. While the increased risk of stillbirth in women with pre-existing diabetes is widely accepted, prior evidence related to stillbirth and GDM in singleton pregnancies is conflicting. Nevertheless, other population-based studies similarly described a reduction in risk of stillbirth in these women [11,18].

Our results show that twin gestations with pre-existing diabetes were at increased risk of LGA compared to non-diabetic twin gestations. This finding is consistent with previous studies [18,30,39]. The increasing effect of pre-existing diabetes on LGA was attenuated in our cohort of twins. In this respect, Luo et al. consistently reported a higher risk of LGA in women with diabetes mellitus and singleton pregnancies (OR 1.89) than in twin gestations (OR 1.21) [30].

In regard to the effect of GDM on birthweight outcomes, previous evidence is conflicting. In our study, we observed no effect of GDM in the risk of LGA and SGA. These findings are in line with prior evidence on the risk of LGA [24,27,38] and SGA [13,18,24,26] and contrast with the results observed in singleton pregnancies. In this context, it has been suggested that gestational diabetes might not have a large impact on foetal overgrowth [38]. These findings, together with the fact that macrosomia is very rare in twin pregnancies, has led some authors to propose potential benefits of mildly-elevated glucose levels on foetal growth, compensating for other growth restricting circumstances observed in twin pregnancies [13,30,38]. In fact, a meta-analysis conducted by McGrath et al. found no association between GDM in twin pregnancies and serious adverse perinatal outcomes [25]. Moreover, Luo et al. reported a reduced risk of low 5-min Apgar score and neonatal death in women with DM and twin pregnancies [30]. The reduction in risk of low 5-min Apgar score and perinatal mortality was also observed by Okby et al. [19]. Nevertheless, other authors alert to the potential harm of hyperglycaemia regarding other maternal and perinatal outcomes as well as potential long-term metabolic complications [13,27]. In this respect, it might be hypothesized that these improved results are related to a more intensive follow-up and care in women with GDM and twin gestations. The higher maternal age in the GDM group could be associated with higher ART treatment rates, which in turn, might contribute to the compliance with pregnancy follow-up.

Evidence on the impact of GDM treatment in twin pregnancies is scant and shows mixed results. Fox et al. reported that improved glycaemic control in twin pregnancies with GDM was not related to improved outcomes and was associated with a higher risk of SGA [23]. Unfortunately, recommendations on the diagnosis and treatment of gestational diabetes are based on randomised controlled trials that excluded twin pregnancies or only included a small number of them [9,40,41]. Therefore, prospective studies on twin gestations are needed to assess a specific diagnostic approach, glycaemic control targets and management guidelines in twin pregnancies with DM.

The main strengths of our study lie in the population-based design, using a validated and widely-used database, and the large sample size. We analysed data from >750,000 deliveries and >15,000 twin deliveries over a ten-year period. It should be outlined that, unlike other previous studies, we were able to distinguish between gestational diabetes and pre-existing diabetes and we innovatively analysed the interaction between twin gestation and glycaemic status. Moreover, no changes were made in the diagnostic GDM protocol over the study period, allowing us to assess trends in the prevalence of GDM in twin pregnancies. However, this study did have several limitations. First, we conducted a retrospective analysis of an administrative database and diagnoses were based on ICD-9-CM codes with potential bias related to validity and accuracy of coding. Unfortunately, this study lacked data on maternal BMI, ethnicity, ART rates, level of glycaemic control and chorionicity. Furthermore, we were not able to analyse major perinatal outcomes such as neonatal and perinatal mortality, congenital anomalies and newborn intensive care unit admission since linked maternal and neonatal data were not available. Moreover, we were unable to control for unmeasured confounders such as increased maternal BMI, ethnicity and other socioeconomic factors Finally, although universal screening for GDM is recommended in Spain, published data on actual screening rates are lacking.

In conclusion, prevalence of GDM in twin pregnancies increased between 2006 and 2015 in Catalonia whereas the prevalence of pre-existing diabetes remained stable. In our study cohort, both GDM and pre-gestational diabetes entailed an additional risk of pre-eclampsia and the latter also increased the risk of prematurity and LGA. However, the effect of diabetes on adverse perinatal outcomes was attenuated in twin gestations when compared with singleton pregnancies. In the light of these results, it should be questioned if women with twin pregnancies should receive the same treatment for their diabetic condition as those with singleton pregnancies. Population-based data provide helpful information on risk of perinatal outcomes; however, randomised studies evaluating the treatment of these conditions in twin pregnancies are required to help guide the management of diabetes in these women.

Author Contributions: Conceptualization, L.G., J.A.F.-L.R., D.B., E.S. and A.G.; Data curation, L.G., D.B., E.S. and A.G.; Formal analysis, L.G., J.A.F.-L.R., D.B., E.S. and A.G.; Methodology, L.G., J.A.F.-L.R., D.B., E.S., A.P. and A.G.; Supervision, J.A.F.-L.R., D.B. and A.G.; Writing—original draft, L.G. and D.B.; Writing—review & editing, J.A.F.-L.R., D.B., E.S., H.N., A.P., L.M., J.P.-B. and A.G. All authors have read and agreed to the published version of the manuscript.

Funding: This research received no external funding.

Institutional Review Board Statement: The study was conducted according to the principles of the Declaration of Helsinki and approved by the clinical research ethics committee of our institution (CEIC-Parc de Salut MAR, number 2017/7209/I).

Informed Consent Statement: Data from all delivery reports remained anonymous and therefore informed consent was not recorded.

Data Availability Statement: Data are available upon request from the authors.

Acknowledgments: We thank Christine O'Hara for review of the English version of the manuscript, Montse Clèries from Unitat d'Informació i Coneixement, Servei Català de la Salut (CatSalut), Marta Albacar from Divisió d'anàlisi de la demanda i l'activitat, Servei Català de la Salut (CatSalut), and Conxa Castell from Public Health Agency of Catalonia, Department of Health.

Conflicts of Interest: The authors declare no conflict of interest.

References

1. Eades, C.E.; Cameron, D.M.; Evans, J.M.M. Prevalence of gestational diabetes mellitus in Europe: A meta-analysis. *Diabetes Res. Clin. Pract.* **2017**, *129*, 173–181. [CrossRef]
2. Buckley, B.S.; Harreiter, J.; Damm, P.; Corcoy, R.; Chico, A.; Simmons, D.; Vellinga, A.; Dunne, F. Gestational diabetes mellitus in Europe: Prevalence, current screening practice and barriers to screening. A review. *Diabet. Med.* **2012**, *29*, 844–854. [CrossRef] [PubMed]
3. Gortazar, L.; Flores-Le Roux, J.A.; Benaiges, D.; Sarsanedas, E.; Payà, A.; Mañé, L.; Pedro-Botet, J.; Goday, A. Trends in prevalence of gestational diabetes and perinatal outcomes in Catalonia, Spain, 2006 to 2015: The Diagestcat Study. *Diabetes Metab. Res. Rev.* **2019**, *35*, e3151. [CrossRef]

4. Gortazar, L.; Goday, A.; Flores-Le Roux, J.A.; Sarsanedas, E.; Payà, A.; Mañé, L.; Pedro-Botet, J.; Benaiges, D. Trends in prevalence of pre-existing diabetes and perinatal outcomes: A large, population-based study in Catalonia, Spain, 2006–2015. *BMJ Open Diabetes Res. Care* **2020**, *8*, e001254. [CrossRef] [PubMed]
5. Mackin, S.T.; Nelson, S.M.; Kerssens, J.J.; Wood, R.; Wild, S.; Colhoun, H.M.; Leese, G.P.; Philip, S.; Lindsay, R.S. Diabetes and pregnancy: National trends over a 15 Year Period. *Diabetologia* **2018**, *61*, 1081–1088. [CrossRef] [PubMed]
6. Ferrara, A. Increasing prevalence of gestational diabetes mellitus: A public health perspective. *Diabetes Care* **2007**, *30* (Suppl. 2), S141–S146. [CrossRef]
7. Getahun, D.; Nath, C.; Ananth, C.V.; Chavez, M.R.; Smulian, J.C. Gestational diabetes in the United States: Temporal trends 1989 through 2004. *Am. J. Obstet. Gynecol.* **2008**, *198*, 525.e1–525.e5. [CrossRef]
8. Bell, R.; Bailey, K.; Cresswell, T.; Hawthorne, G.; Critchley, J.; Lewis-Barned, N. Trends in prevalence and outcomes of pregnancy in women with pre-existing type I and type II diabetes. *BJOG* **2008**, *115*, 445–452. [CrossRef]
9. Metzger, B.E.; Gabbe, S.G.; Persson, B.; Buchanan, T.A.; Catalano, P.M.; Damm, P. Hyperglycemia and Adverse Pregnancy Outcomes. *N. Engl. J. Med.* **2008**, *358*, 1991–2002. [CrossRef] [PubMed]
10. Billionnet, C.; Mitanchez, D.; Weill, A.; Nizard, J.; Alla, F.; Hartemann, A.; Jacqueminet, S. Gestational diabetes and adverse perinatal outcomes from 716,152 births in France in 2012. *Diabetologia* **2017**, *60*, 636–644. [CrossRef]
11. Jovanovič, L.; Liang, Y.; Weng, W.; Hamilton, M.; Chen, L.; Wintfeld, N. Trends in the incidence of diabetes, its clinical sequelae, and associated costs in pregnancy. *Diabetes Metab. Res. Rev.* **2015**, *31*, 707–716. [CrossRef] [PubMed]
12. Ananth, C.V.; Chauhan, S.P. Epidemiology of twinning in developed countries. *Semin. Perinatol.* **2012**, *36*, 156–161. [CrossRef]
13. Hiersch, L.; Berger, H.; Okby, R.; Ray, J.G.; Geary, M.; McDonald, S.D.; Murray-Davis, B.; Riddell, C.; Halperin, I.; Hasan, H.; et al. Gestational diabetes mellitus is associated with adverse outcomes in twin pregnancies. *Am. J. Obstet. Gynecol.* **2019**, *220*, 102.e1–102.e8. [CrossRef]
14. Institut d'Estadistica de Catalunya. IDESCAT. Available online: http://www.idescat.net (accessed on 1 December 2020).
15. GEDE (Grupo Español de Diabetes y Embarazo). Asistencia a la gestante con diabetes. Guía de práctica clínica actualizada En 2014. *Av. Diabetol.* **2015**, *31*, 45–59. [CrossRef]
16. Departament de Salut. *Corbes de Referencia de Pes, Perímetre Cranial i Longitud en Néixer de Nounats D'embarassos Únics, de Bessons i de Trigèmins a Catalunya*; Departament de Salut: Barcelona, Spain, 2008.
17. González-González, N.L.; Medina, V.; Ruano, A.; Perales, A.; Pérez-Mendaña, J.M.; Melchor, J.C. Base de Datos Perinatales Nacionales 2004 (National Perinatal Data Sets 2004). *Prog. Obstet. Ginecol.* **2005**, *49*, 1084–1089.
18. Lai, F.Y.; Johnson, J.A.; Dover, D.; Kaul, P. Outcomes of singleton and twin pregnancies complicated by pre-existing diabetes and gestational diabetes: A population-based study in Alberta, Canada, 2005–2011. *J. Diabetes* **2016**, *8*, 45–55. [CrossRef]
19. Okby, R.; Weintraub, A.Y.; Sergienko, R.; Eyal, S. Gestational diabetes mellitus in twin pregnancies is not associated with adverse perinatal outcomes. *Arch. Gynecol. Obstet.* **2014**, *290*, 649–654. [CrossRef] [PubMed]
20. Rissanen, A.R.S.; Jernman, R.M.; Gissler, M.; Nupponen, I.; Nuutila, M.E. Maternal complications in twin pregnancies in Finland during 1987–2014: A retrospective study. *BMC Pregnancy Childbirth* **2019**, *19*, 337. [CrossRef]
21. Lambalk, C.B.; Boomsma, D.I.; de Boer, L.; de Koning, C.H.; Schoute, E.; Popp-Snijders, C.; Schoemaker, J. Increased levels and pulsatility of follicle-stimulating hormone in mothers of hereditary dizygotic twins. *JCEM* **1998**, *83*, 481–486. [CrossRef]
22. Comisión Nacional de Reproducción Humana Asistida. Ministerio de Sanidad. Registro Nacional de Actividad y Resultados de los Centros y Servicios de Reproducción Humana Asistida. Available online: https://cnrha.sanidad.gob.es/registros/actividades.htm (accessed on 5 December 2020).
23. Fox, N.S.; Gerber, R.S.; Saltzman, D.H.; Gupta, S.; Fishman, A.Y.; Klauser, C.K.; Rebarber, A. Glycemic control in twin pregnancies with gestational diabetes: Are we improving or worsening outcomes? *J. Matern. Fetal Neonatal Med.* **2016**, *29*, 1041–1045. [CrossRef]
24. Dinham, G.K.; Henry, A.; Lowe, S.A.; Nassar, N.; Lui, K.; Spear, V.; Shand, A.W. Twin pregnancies complicated by gestational diabetes mellitus: A single centre cohort study. *Diabet. Med.* **2016**, *33*, 1659–1667. [CrossRef]
25. McGrath, R.T.; Hocking, S.L.; Scott, E.S.; Seeho, S.K.; Fulcher, G.R.; Glastras, S.J. Outcomes of twin pregnancies complicated by gestational diabetes: A meta-analysis of observational studies. *J. Perinatol.* **2017**, *37*, 360–368. [CrossRef]
26. Simoes, T.; Queiros, A.; Correia, L.; Rocha, T.; Dias, E.; Blickstein, I. Gestational diabetes mellitus complicating twin pregnancies. *J. Perinat. Med.* **2011**, *39*, 437–440. [CrossRef] [PubMed]
27. González, N.L.G.; Goya, M.; Bellart, J.; Lopez, J.; Sancho, M.A.; Mozas, J.; Medina, V.; Padrón, E.; Megia, A.; Pintado, P.; et al. Obstetric and perinatal outcome in women with twin pregnancy and gestational diabetes. *J. Matern. Fetal Neonatal Med.* **2012**, *25*, 1084–1089. [CrossRef]
28. Schwartz, D.B.; Daoud, Y.; Zazula, P.; Goyert, G.; Bronsteen, R.; Wright, D.; Copes, J. Gestational diabetes mellitus: Metabolic and blood glucose parameters in singleton versus twin pregnancies. *Am. J. Obstet. Gynecol.* **1999**, *181*, 912–914. [CrossRef]
29. Retnakaran, R.; Shah, B.R. Impact of twin gestation and fetal sex on maternal risk of diabetes during and after pregnancy. *Diabetes Care* **2016**, *39*, e110–e111. [CrossRef]
30. Luo, Z.C.; Simonet, F.; Wei, S.Q.; Xu, H.; Rey, E.; Fraser, W.D. Diabetes in pregnancy may differentially affect neonatal outcomes for twins and singletons. *Diabet. Med.* **2011**, *28*, 1068–1073. [CrossRef] [PubMed]
31. Corrado, F.; Caputo, F.; Facciola, G.; Mancuso, A. Gestational glucose intolerance in multiple pregnancy. *Diabetes Care* **2003**, *26*, 1646. [CrossRef]

32. Buhling, K.J.; Henrich, W.; Starr, E.; Lubke, M.; Bertram, S.; Siebert, G.; Dudenhausen, J.W. Risk for gestational diabetes and hypertension for women with twin pregnancy compared to singleton pregnancy. *Arch. Gynecol. Obstet.* **2003**, *269*, 33–36. [CrossRef] [PubMed]
33. Rauh-Hain, J.A.; Rana, S.; Tamez, H.; Wang, A.; Cohen, B.; Cohen, A.; Brown, F.; Ecker, J.L.; Karumanchi, S.A.; Thadhani, R. Risk for developing gestational diabetes in women with twin pregnancies. *J. Matern. Fetal Neonatal Med.* **2009**, *22*, 293–299. [CrossRef]
34. Yamashita, H.; Shao, J.; Friedman, J.E. Physiologic and molecular alterations in carbohydrate metabolism during pregnancy and gestational diabetes mellitus. *Clin. Obstet. Gynecol.* **2000**, *43*, 87–98. [CrossRef] [PubMed]
35. Sivan, E.; Maman, E.; Homko, C.J.; Lipitz, S.; Cohen, S.; Schiff, E. Impact of fetal reduction on the incidence of gestational diabetes. *Obstet. Gynecol.* **2002**, *99*, 91–94. [CrossRef] [PubMed]
36. González González, N.L.; González Dávila, E.; Goya, M.; Vega, B.; Hernández Suarez, M.; Bartha, J.L. Twin pregnancy among women with pregestational type 1 or type 2 diabetes mellitus. *Int. J. Gynecol. Obstet.* **2014**, *126*, 83–87. [CrossRef]
37. Mourad, M.; Too, G.; Gyamfi-Bannerman, C.; Zork, N. Hypertensive disorders of pregnancy in twin gestations complicated by gestational diabetes. *J. Matern. Fetal Neonatal Med.* **2019**, *16*, 1–5. [CrossRef] [PubMed]
38. Guillén, M.A.; Herranz, L.; Barquiel, B.; Hillman, N.; Burgos, M.A.; Pallardo, L.F. Influence of gestational diabetes mellitus on neonatal weight outcome in twin pregnancies. *Diabet. Med.* **2014**, *31*, 1651–1656. [CrossRef]
39. Darke, J.; Glinianaia, S.V.; Marsden, P.; Bell, R. Pregestational diabetes is associated with adverse outcomes in twin pregnancies: A regional register-based study. *Acta Obstet. Gynecol. Scand.* **2016**, *95*, 339–346. [CrossRef]
40. Crowther, C.A.; Hiller, J.E.; Moss, J.R.; McPhee, A.J.; Jeffries, W.S.; Robinson, J.S. Effect of treatment of gestational diabetes mellitus on pregnancy outcomes. *N. Engl. J. Med.* **2005**, *352*, 2477–2486. [CrossRef]
41. Landon, M.B.; Spong, C.Y.; Thom, E.; Carpenter, M.W.; Ramin, S.M.; Casey, B.; Wapner, R.J.; Varner, M.W.; Rouse, D.J.; Thorp, J.M.; et al. A multicenter, randomized trial of treatment for mild gestational diabetes. *N. Engl. J. Med.* **2009**, *361*, 1339–1348. [CrossRef] [PubMed]

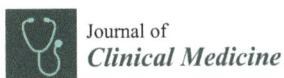

Article

Mobile-Based Lifestyle Intervention in Women with Glucose Intolerance after Gestational Diabetes Mellitus (MELINDA), A Multicenter Randomized Controlled Trial: Methodology and Design

Caro Minschart [1,*], Toon Maes [2], Christophe De Block [3], Inge Van Pottelbergh [4], Nele Myngheer [5], Pascale Abrams [6,7], Wouter Vinck [7], Liesbeth Leuridan [8], Chantal Mathieu [1,9], Jaak Billen [10], Christophe Matthys [1,9], Babs Weyn [11], Annouschka Laenen [12], Annick Bogaerts [13,14] and Katrien Benhalima [1,9]

1. Clinical and Experimental Endocrinology, Department of Chronic Diseases and Metabolism, KU Leuven, 3000 Leuven, Belgium; chantal.mathieu@uzleuven.be (C.M.); christophe.matthys@uzleuven.be (C.M.); katrien.benhalima@uzleuven.be (K.B.)
2. Department of Endocrinology, Imelda Hospital, 2820 Bonheiden, Belgium; Toon.Maes@imelda.be
3. Department of Endocrinology-Diabetology-Metabolism, Antwerp University Hospital, 2650 Edegem, Belgium; Christophe.DeBlock@uza.be
4. Department of Endocrinology, OLV Hospital Aalst, 9300 Aalst, Belgium; Inge.Van.Pottelbergh@olvz-aalst.be
5. Department of Endocrinology, General Hospital Groeninge, 8510 Kortrijk, Belgium; nele.myngheer@azgroeninge.be
6. Department of Endocrinology, GZA Hospital Sint-Vincentius, 2018 Antwerp, Belgium; Pascale.Abrams@gza.be
7. Department of Endocrinology, GZA Hospital Sint-Augustinus, 2610 Wilrijk, Belgium; wouter.vinck@gza.be
8. Department of Endocrinology, General Hospital Klina, 2930 Brasschaat, Belgium; Liesbeth.Leuridan@klina.be
9. Department of Endocrinology, University Hospitals Leuven, 3000 Leuven, Belgium
10. Department of Laboratory Medicine, University Hospitals Leuven, 3000 Leuven, Belgium; jaak.billen@uzleuven.be
11. Department of Electrical Engineering, Processing Speech and Images, KU Leuven, 3000 Leuven, Belgium; barbara.weyn@kuleuven.be
12. Centre of Biostatics and Statistical Bioinformatics, KU Leuven, 3000 Leuven, Belgium; annouschka.laenen@kuleuven.be
13. Department of Development and Regeneration, KU Leuven, 3000 Leuven, Belgium; annick.bogaerts@kuleuven.be
14. Faculty of Medicine and Health Sciences, Centre for Research and Innovation in Care (CRIC), University of Antwerp, 2610 Wilrijk, Belgium
* Correspondence: caro.minschart@kuleuven.be

Received: 22 June 2020; Accepted: 12 August 2020; Published: 13 August 2020

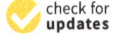

Abstract: The aims of the 'Mobile-based lifestyle intervention in women with glucose intolerance after gestational diabetes mellitus (GDM)' study (MELINDA) are: (1) to evaluate the prevalence and risk factors of glucose intolerance after a recent history of GDM; and (2) to evaluate the efficacy and feasibility of a telephone- and mobile-based lifestyle intervention in women with glucose intolerance after GDM. This is a Belgian multicenter randomized controlled trial (RCT) in seven hospitals with the aim of recruiting 236 women. Women in the intervention group will receive a blended program, based on one face-to-face education session and further follow-up through a mobile application and monthly telephone advice. Women in the control group will receive follow-up as in normal routine with referral to primary care. Participants will receive an oral glucose tolerance test (OGTT) one year after baseline. Primary endpoint is the frequency of weight goal achievement (≥5% weight loss if pre-pregnancy BMI ≥ 25 Kg/m^2 or return to pre-gravid weight if BMI < 25 Kg/m^2). At each visit blood samples are collected, anthropometric measurements are obtained, and self-administered questionnaires are completed. Recruitment began in May 2019.

Keywords: gestational diabetes mellitus; type 2 diabetes mellitus; postpartum; glucose intolerance; lifestyle intervention; mobile-based

1. Introduction

Gestational diabetes mellitus (GDM) is a frequent medical complication during pregnancy and is defined as diabetes diagnosed in the second or third trimester of pregnancy, provided that overt diabetes early in pregnancy has been excluded [1]. The incidence of GDM is rising globally and it represents an important modifiable risk factor for adverse pregnancy outcomes such as macrosomia and preeclampsia [2,3]. Shortly after delivery glucose values generally normalize, but the underlying beta-cell dysfunction often persists [4]. In the long term, women with a history of GDM have a seven-fold increased risk of developing type 2 diabetes mellitus (T2DM) compared to women without previous GDM [5,6]. About 50% of women with a history of GDM will develop T2DM within 10 years after delivery [5]. Moreover, women with a history of GDM progress more rapidly to T2DM compared to women with similarly elevated glucose levels [7]. Women with glucose intolerance (impaired fasting glucose (IFG) and/or impaired glucose tolerance (IGT)) in early postpartum are a particularly high risk group, with about 50% who will develop T2DM within five years after delivery [8].

Lifestyle modifications have been shown to be effective in the prevention or delay of T2DM when offered to high-risk middle-aged individuals. Two landmark trials, the United States Diabetes Prevention Program (DPP) and the Finnish Diabetes Prevention Study (DPS), showed a reduction of 58% in the incidence of T2DM in individuals presenting with IGT after an average of three years of intensive lifestyle interventions, with a weight loss of approximately 5 kg [9,10]. Subgroup analyses of the DPP trial, focusing on women with previous GDM, found a 53% reduction at the end of the trial and a 35% reduction after 10 years [7,11]. However, women in this trial were on average 12 years after index pregnancy, and the lifestyle intervention was very intensive and therefore challenging to implement in normal routine care, for both patient and clinic. In addition, there is limited evidence regarding the efficacy of lifestyle interventions in women with a recent history of GDM. Studies published in this population generally show limited benefits on metabolic outcomes, mostly because of low adherence rates and failure to produce meaningful behavior change due to barriers such as the need for child care, low family support and return to work [12–14]. A recent meta-analysis reviewed the benefits of lifestyle interventions for women with previous GDM and demonstrated moderate weight reductions, but only if the interventions were offered within the first six months after delivery [15]. The benefits shown were smaller than those observed in the large lifestyle intervention trials performed on older subjects.

Lifestyle interventions in women with previous GDM need to be adapted to address their unique barriers to behavior change in order to optimize adherence. A study of 300 women with a recent history of GDM showed that a telephone-delivered diabetes prevention program was associated with greater engagement compared to a group-delivered program (82% vs. 38%) in the postpartum period, and that the greater engagement was associated with greater reduction in weight and waist circumference [16]. Digital health interventions seem to be highly acceptable among postpartum women and should therefore be considered for lifestyle management in this population, provided that they focus on delivering behavior change strategies and addressing practical barriers faced by postpartum women [17]. Several mobile-based lifestyle interventions have shown potential for improved metabolic control in different populations, including women with a history of GDM and overweight or obese patients [18–20]. The B-slim project compared a conventional face-to-face weight loss and weight control program with a standalone mobile program and a combined program for overweight and obese patients [20]. They showed that the weight loss goal of 5% was reached in only 6% of the control group compared to 19% in the standalone mobile program, 28% in the conventional program and 46% in the combined program [20]. These results indicate that the content of a conventional weight loss program could be delivered through a combination of face-to-face coaching and a mobile health program without affecting the effectiveness of the intervention.

2. Objectives of the Melinda Study

Since women with glucose intolerance have a very high risk of developing T2DM, we designed the MELINDA study to investigate the efficacy and feasibility of a telephone- and mobile-based lifestyle intervention in women with glucose intolerance after a recent history of GDM. We also aim to evaluate the prevalence and risk factors of glucose intolerance in early postpartum in women with previous GDM.

Specific objectives are:

1. To evaluate whether a telephone- and mobile-based lifestyle coaching program leads to a higher frequency of weight goal achievement ($\geq$5% weight loss if pre-pregnancy Body Mass Index (BMI) $\geq$ 25 Kg/m^2 or return to pre-gravid weight if BMI < 25 Kg/m^2).
2. To evaluate whether a telephone- and mobile-based lifestyle coaching intervention can reduce the incidence of metabolic syndrome, leading to an improved beta-cell function and lower insulin resistance in women with glucose intolerance after a recent history of GDM.
3. To investigate the prevalence of glucose intolerance and T2DM after a recent diagnosis of GDM based on the 2013 World Health Organization (WHO) criteria and to evaluate the risk factors of developing glucose intolerance postpartum.
4. To investigate factors related to success or failure in diabetes prevention and to develop materials and expertise to assist in the development of diabetes prevention programs in primary care.

3. Materials and Methods

3.1. Study Design and Setting

The MELINDA study is a multicenter randomized controlled trial with the participation of 7 hospitals to test the efficacy of a telephone- and mobile-based lifestyle intervention for one year to stimulate weight loss in women with glucose intolerance after a previous pregnancy with GDM. The Leuven University Hospital is the coordinating center.

In order to maintain uniform criteria for the diagnosis of GDM, all participating centers use the 75 g oral glucose tolerance test (OGTT) with the 'International Association of Diabetes in Pregnancy Study Groups' (IADPSG) criteria, now commonly referred to as the 2013 WHO criteria for GDM [21,22]. As part of normal routine, women with a history of GDM are offered a 75 g OGTT between 6 and 16 weeks after delivery. Data from eligible and consenting women are collected during the postpartum OGTT, including baseline characteristics and data on medical and obstetrical history. Women with glucose intolerance based on the postpartum OGTT are offered participation in the intervention randomized controlled trial (RCT). Participants are randomized with a 1:1 allocation ratio and stratified by center and baseline BMI to the telephone- and mobile-based lifestyle intervention or to the control group. A password-protected, computer-generated, variable block randomization is used to prevent disclosure of the allocation sequence to recruiters. This results in concealed and varying block sizes of two and four patients.

Both women in the intervention and control group receive a 75 g OGTT one year after the postpartum OGTT as part of the trial. The 'Standard Protocol Items: Recommendations for Interventional Trials' (SPIRIT) flow diagram illustrates the design of the study (Figure 1). The study is registered in ClinicalTrials.gov as NCT03559621 and was approved by the Medical Ethical Committees of all participating centers (Belgian number: B322201837047).

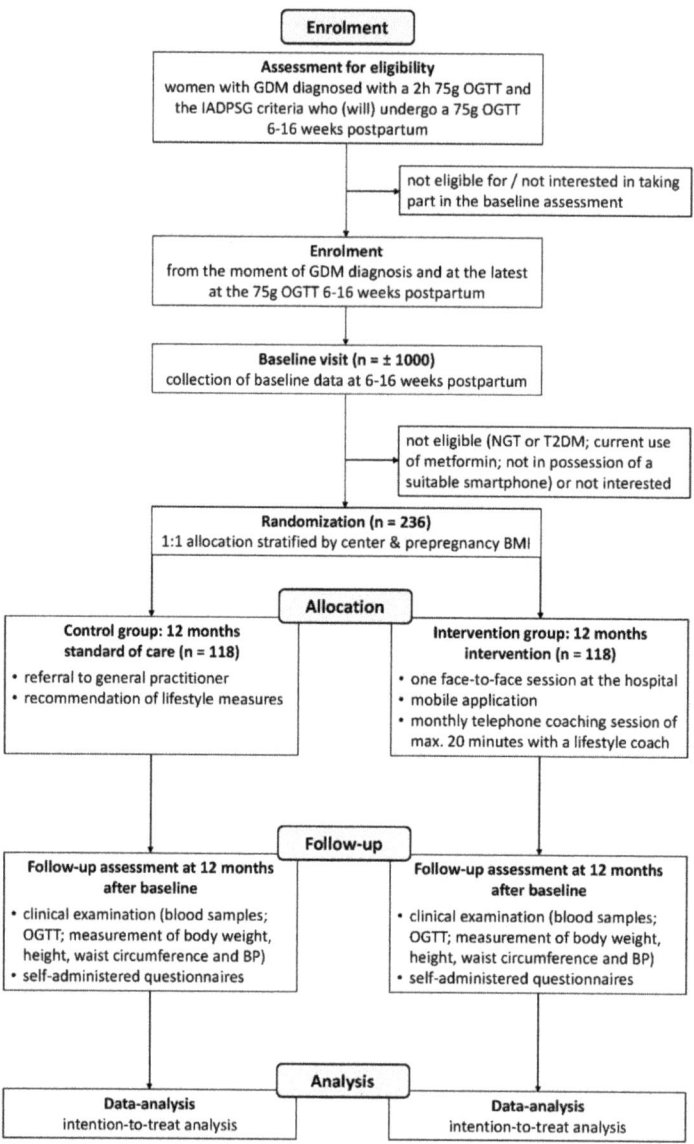

Figure 1. 'Standard Protocol Items: Recommendations for Interventional Trials' (SPIRIT) flow diagram showing the flow of participants through the phases of the Mobile-based lifestyle intervention in women with glucose intolerance after gestational diabetes mellitus (MELINDA) randomized controlled trial. GDM: gestational diabetes mellitus; OGTT: oral glucose tolerance test; IADPSG: The International Association of Diabetes and Pregnancy Study Groups; NGT: normal glucose tolerance; T2DM: type 2 diabetes mellitus; BMI: Body Mass Index; BP: blood pressure.

3.2. Recruitment and Eligibility

The cohort is recruited from two university centers (Leuven University Hospital and Antwerp University Hospital) and six non-university centers (Imelda Hospital, Bonheiden, OLV Hospital, Aalst, General Hospital, Groeninge Kortrijk, GZA Hospital site, Sint-Augustinus, GZA Hospital site,

Sint-Vincentius and General Hospital, Klina Brasschaat). All Dutch, English or French speaking women aged 18 or older with GDM based on the 2013 WHO criteria and presenting at the 75 g OGTT 6–16 weeks after delivery are invited to participate. A first written informed consent is obtained from the participants before any trial-related activities are performed. Women with glucose intolerance based on the 75 g OGTT 6 to 16 weeks after delivery are offered participation in the intervention RCT and a more extensive written informed consent is therefore obtained from this group. Glucose intolerance is defined as IFG [fasting plasma glucose (FPG) 100–125 mg/dL] and/or IGT (2-h glucose value on the OGTT between 140–199 mg/dL) as described by the American Diabetes Association (ADA) [1]. The maximum study duration for participants in the RCT is one year. The planned recruitment period is 2.5 years.

Exclusion criteria for the baseline study:

- current use of medication that can affect glucose values (such as glucocorticoids) or receiving treatment for glucose intolerance (such as metformin)
- women who do not undergo the 75 g OGTT 6–16 weeks at the hospital
- women who are not diagnosed with GDM based on the 2013 WHO criteria
- insufficient Dutch, English or French language skills

Additional exclusion criteria for the RCT:

- diabetes (FPG ≥ 126 mg/dL and/or 2-h glucose value ≥ 200 mg/dL)
- normal glucose tolerance
- current use of metformin
- health limitations or treatments (as assessed by the local investigator according to a standardized protocol) which would restrict participation in the intervention trial
- not in possession of a suitable smartphone (iOS or Android)

3.3. Study Visits

3.3.1. Baseline Measurements during the 75 g OGTT 6–16 Weeks After Delivery

Baseline characteristics are collected for all eligible women through a clinical examination, self-administered questionnaires, collection of blood samples and extraction of data on medical history and pregnancy from the electronic medical records. A standard 75 g OGTT is performed with blood samples taken fasting and at 30, 60 and 120 min. Aliquots of serum and plasma are stored for future measurements.

3.3.2. Enrolment in the Intervention RCT

Women with glucose intolerance are included in the RCT and randomly assigned to one of the two comparison groups with 1:1 allocation, stratified by center and pre-pregnancy BMI. Assignment is allocated automatically and received through a secure, password protected program to guarantee adequate concealment of allocation.

3.3.3. Intervention Group

Women in the intervention group receives a blended lifestyle intervention for one year based on a unique combination of one face-to-face meeting, monthly telephone coaching and the use of a mobile application (MELINDA app) to promote healthy lifestyle behaviors. Within one month after the 75 g OGTT, participants receive an individual face-to-face coaching session at the hospital, given by a health professional trained in motivational interviewing. During this session, participants receives information on the long-term risks associated with GDM, the importance of a healthy lifestyle and how this can be achieved. In addition, information on the coaching program and instructions for using the MELINDA app are provided. After the face-to-face coaching session, participants receive a monthly telephone coaching session of maximum 20 min to allow for personalized feedback and support, focusing on individual needs. After one year, participants undergo a 75 g OGTT with the same examination as during the postpartum visit 6–16 weeks after delivery.

3.3.4. Control Group

At the postpartum visit 6–16 weeks after delivery, women in the control group receive general information from the diabetes educator on the long-term risks associated with GDM and the need for a healthy lifestyle to prevent T2DM. Additionally, they are referred to primary care for further follow-up, in line with normal routine. As part of the study, after one year, participants undergo a 75 g OGTT with the same examination as during the postpartum visit 6–16 weeks after delivery. The Melinda app has not been made publicly available and was therefore not accessible to participants of the control group.

3.4. Key Aspects of the Blended Lifestyle Intervention

The lifestyle program for the MELINDA study has been developed by several research teams of the KU Leuven university. It builds on lifestyle interventions from previous studies by our research group [20,23,24] and is adapted to meet the particular needs of women with a recent history of GDM. This blended approach runs through a specific platform, which consists of three main functionalities: (1) a dashboard for the lifestyle coach; (2) the personalized MELINDA coaching app for the participants; and (3) integration of objective measures obtained via external devices (Xiaomi Mi Band pedometer connected to the MELINDA app).

The MELINDA app has been developed for the purpose of this study after consulting patients and healthcare professionals. The app and dashboard are developed by the Medical image computing department of the KU Leuven. The platform for the application is based on the existing IT framework from the B-Slim project [20]. In a first phase, a small feasibility study was conducted with eighty volunteers with a recent history of GDM to provide feedback on the functioning and usability of the MELINDA app. The app was tested during one month, evaluated through an online questionnaire and adapted according to the comments of the volunteers. After the app was adjusted, it was presented and made available to the lifestyle coaches in a training session. In this phase, some final adjustments were made to the content and functionality of the app, based on the comments of the coaches.

The app consists of a coaching module and a data entry module. The data entry module asks information about dietary intake, food literacy related determinants, weight, waist circumference and motivational status. The coaching module provides a 12-week dietary coaching trajectory interspersed with a 12-week physical activity coaching trajectory. A model of food literacy is used to focus on a broader set of processes, such as food planning, selecting the right foods, food preparation, eating habits and evaluating information about food [25]. The MELINDA app uses a set of limited questions on food literacy to produce tailored goals and tips. Physical activity is automatically monitored via a pedometer connected to the app in order to tailor the physical activity advice and skills training. If goals are achieved within six months, the app will help to maintain and support the current healthy lifestyle. If goals are not achieved, based on the telephone contact and the monitored data new goals and/or recommendations will be formulated in consultation with the participant and new tailored modules will be offered to optimize lifestyle.

During the monthly telephone coaching sessions, the lifestyle coach consults the dashboard that provides an overview of the evolution of weight, waist circumference, physical activity and motivational status of the participant. This information is used to optimize the advice and to zoom in on those areas with most needs and priorities.

3.5. Data Collection

An overview of all data collection procedures is provided in Table 1.

Table 1. Data collection procedures in the MELINDA trial.

Outcomes	Assessments	Baseline	1 Month *	Monthly * (Month 2 to 11)	3 Months *	6 Months *	9 Months *	12 Months **
Outcomes Collected from Medical Records								
Demographic data	Age; date of birth	x						
Medical and obstetric history	Pre-pregnancy weight and BMI; weight at delivery; parity; previous pregnancy outcomes	x						
Patient-Reported Outcomes								
General lifestyle behaviour and socio-economic factors	Self-constructed questionnaire	x						
Medication use	Questioned by study nurse	x	x		x	x	x	x
Diet	Food Frequency Questionnaire (FFQ)	x			x	x	x	x
Physical activity	International Physical Activity Questionnaire Long Form (IPAQ-LF)	x						x
Mental health and well-being	Center for Epidemiologic Studies -Depression (CES-D) questionnaire and Spielberger State-Trait Anxiety Inventory (STAI-6) questionnaire	x						x
Quality of life	36-Item Short Form Health Survey (SF-36)	x						x
Diabetes risk perception	Risk Perception Survey for Developing Diabetes (RPS-DD)	x						x
Motivation for lifestyle change	Treatment Self-Regulation Questionnaire (TSRQ)	x (v2)						x (v3)
Breastfeeding and anticonception	Self-constructed questionnaire	x						x
Sense of coherence	Sense of Coherence (SOC) questionnaire	x						x
Acceptability and subjective quality of the lifestyle intervention	Self-constructed questionnaire							x
Clinical and Biochemical Outcomes								
Anthropometry	Height (only baseline), weight, waist circumference, blood pressure, BMI	x						x
Glucose and insulin	Fasting 75 g OGTT (0, 30, 60 and 120 min)	x				x		x
HbA1c	Fasting	x						x
Lipid profile	Total cholesterol, triglycerides, HDL, LDL (fasting)	x						x
Outcomes Collected from the MELINDA App								
Weight	Self-reported weight in the MELINDA app			x				
Motivational status	Self-reported motivational status in the MELINDA app			x				
Waist circumference	Self-reported waist circumference in the MELINDA app				x	x	x	
Physical activity	Steps collected from pedometer connected to Melinda app							x
Use of the MELINDA app	App-based tracking to evaluate the use of the MELINDA app							x

* Only for participants in the intervention group of the randomized control trial (RCT); ** Only for participants in the intervention group and control group of the RCT.

3.5.1. Blood Collection

A fasting blood test is performed at 6–16 weeks after delivery for all baseline participants and after one year for the participants in the RCT.

At 6–16 weeks after delivery, the fasting blood test consists of HbA1c, lipid profile (total cholesterol, triglycerides, HDL and LDL cholesterol) and a 2-h 75 g OGTT with measurements of glucose and insulin fasting, at 30 min, 60 min and 120 min. For the 2-h 75 g OGTT, participants are instructed to fast for at least 10 h and not to smoke, engage in any physical activity, or give breastfeeding during the test. They are also instructed to drink only water, but no coffee, cola or any drink containing sugar or caffeine. All analyses, except for insulin, are performed locally at each participating center in line with normal routine. The insulin samples are analyzed centrally at the Leuven University Hospital (UZ Leuven).

For participants in the RCT, an additional 2-h 75 g OGTT with the same lab tests as baseline is performed one year. All laboratory tests are analyzed centrally at UZ Leuven to ensure uniformity. Only the analyses of glucose (fasting, 30 min, 60 min and 120 min) are performed locally so that there is no delay in diagnosing diabetes. Every three months, blood samples are collected for longer term storage in a -80 °C freezer at the biobank of UZ Leuven.

3.5.2. Clinical Examinations

Blood pressure (BP), height, weight and waist circumference are measured during the 75 g OGTT at baseline and after 1 year. BP is measured twice with a five min interval using an automated blood pressure monitor (Omron Philips large 34–44 cm). Height is measured to the nearest 0.5 cm using a calibrated wall-mounted stadiometer. Weight is measured using a calibrated portable Tanita HD 382 digital scale, which measures up to 150 Kg. BMI is calculated as Kg/m^2. Waist circumference is measured in centimeters by applying the tape directly on the skin, horizontally at the lateral level that is midway between the iliac crest and the lowest lateral portion of the rib cage.

3.5.3. Self-Administered Questionnaires

Questionnaire on general habits and socio-economic factors: a self-designed questionnaire was previously used in the Belgian Diabetes in Pregnancy Study (BEDIP-N) study [26] to extensively collect information on socio-economic status and habits.

Food Frequency Questionnaire (FFQ) validated for the Belgian population [27]: a questionnaire containing questions on frequency and portion size of consumption of foods and beverages.

International Physical Activity Questionnaire Long Form (IPAQ-LF) validated for use in the Belgian population [26,28]: questionnaire measuring different areas of physical activity such as job-related physical activity, transportation, house work and caring for family, recreation and time spent sitting. We added a question on time watching television or playing computer games to better assess sedentary behavior.

Center for Epidemiologic Studies-Depression (CES-D) questionnaire: widely used in pregnant and postpartum women to asses symptoms of clinical depression over the past seven days [29].

Questionnaire on breastfeeding and contraception: a self-designed questionnaire as previously used in the BEDIP-N study to extensively collect information on the duration and frequency of breastfeeding as well as on the type of contraception used [26].

36-Item Short Form Health Survey (SF-36): a set of generic, coherent, and easily administered quality-of-life measures that is validated for use in the maternity context [30]. Data from this questionnaire will be used to calculate Quality-Adjusted Life Years (QUALY's) to explore the cost-effectiveness of the lifestyle intervention.

Risk Perception Survey For Developing Diabetes (RPS-DD): since it has been shown that women with a history of GDM often underestimate their risk of developing T2DM, a validated questionnaire to evaluate their perception of the development of diabetes is used [31].

Treatment Self-Regulation Questionnaire (TSRQ): a validated questionnaire that is widely used in the study of behavior change in healthcare settings to evaluate motivation for lifestyle change [32,33].

Spielberger State-Trait Anxiety Inventory (STAI-6) questionnaire: the validated short version STAI-6 is used to measure levels of anxiety state [34,35].

Sense of Coherence (SOC) questionnaire: a 13-item questionnaire to assess comprehensibility, manageability, and meaningfulness of one's life [36].

General questionnaire on the acceptability and subjective quality of the MELINDA lifestyle intervention: a self-designed questionnaire evaluating the coaching system, the use and user-friendliness of the MELINDA app, and the monthly telephone coaching.

3.5.4. Melinda App

The following data are collected for participants in the intervention group from the MELINDA app: self-reported weight and motivational status at least once a month; self-reported waist circumference at least once every three months; steps collected from the pedometer connected to the Melinda app; and app-based tracking to evaluate the use of the MELINDA app.

3.6. Outcomes of the Study

3.6.1. Primary Outcome

The primary outcome of the RCT is the number of women reaching the weight-loss goal ≥5% of body weight when BMI ≥ 25 Kg/m^2 or returning to pre-gravid weight if BMI < 25 Kg/m^2 (based on pre-pregnancy BMI or, if not available, based on BMI in early pregnancy).

3.6.2. Secondary Outcomes

- frequency of T2DM based on the ADA criteria after one year [37] and risk factors for the development of T2DM after one year
- frequency of glucose intolerance and the risk factors of glucose intolerance in early postpartum
- frequency of the metabolic syndrome based on the WHO criteria [38]
- insulin resistance and beta-cell function. The insulin sensitivity will be measured using the Matsuda index and the reciprocal of the homeostasis model assessment of insulin resistance (1/HOMA-IR) [39,40]. Beta-cell function will be assessed by HOMA-B, the insulinogenic index divided by HOMA-IR, and by the insulin secretion sensitivity index [41,42]. All these measures have been validated for use in women with GDM [26].
- mean weight loss
- duration of breastfeeding and rate of exclusive breastfeeding
- quality of life, symptoms of depression and anxiety
- motivation for behavior change and perceived risk of developing diabetes
- dietary quality
- intensity and duration of physical activity
- process outcome: the percentage of women adhering to the protocol of intervention, by monitoring the use of the MELINDA app and the number of telephone coaching sessions.

3.6.3. Pregnancy and Delivery Outcome Data (Collected from the Electronical Medical Record)

Maternal data: parity; pre-pregnancy weight; gestational week of GDM diagnosis; results of the 50 g glucose challenge test (GCT) and 75 g OGTT during pregnancy; treatment of GDM during pregnancy; pregnancy complications such as preeclampsia (de novo BP ≥ 140/90 mmHg > 20 weeks with proteinuria or signs of end-organ dysfunction), eclampsia, gestational hypertension (de novo BP ≥ 140/90 mmHg > 20 weeks), preexisting hypertension and pregnancy-induced cholestasis.

Delivery data: pregnancy duration; type of labor (spontaneous, induced or caesarean before labor) and indications; type of delivery (spontaneous vaginal, forceps or vacuum, caesarean section during labor or planned caesarean section) and indications.

Neonatal data: macrosomia (>4 Kg), large for gestational age (LGA)(birth weight > 90 percentile according to standardized Flemish birth charts adjusted for sex of the baby and parity) [43], small for gestational age (SGA)(birth weight < 10 percentile according to standardized Flemish birth charts adjusted for sex of the baby and parity) [43], preterm delivery (<37 completed weeks), 10 min Apgar score, shoulder dystocia, birth trauma, neonatal respiratory distress syndrome, neonatal hypoglycemia (defined as glycemia < 40 mg/dL or need for intravenous dextrose), neonatal jaundice, duration and indication for admission on the neonatal intensive care unit (admission defined as >24 h).

3.7. Power Calculation and Statistical Analysis

3.7.1. Sample Size

Based on the results of the B-slim project, we assume that 20% of women in the control group will reach the weight-loss goal compared to 40% in the intervention group [20]. The sample size is calculated to show with 80% power and 5% significance level a difference in the proportion reaching the weight-loss goal after 1 year. The sample size calculation is based on a two-sided Chi-square test. Assuming a drop-out rate of 30%, a total sample size of 236 for the RCT is needed.

Data from our research group at UZ Leuven show that 44% of women with a recent history of GDM based on the two-step screening strategy and the 2013 WHO criteria have glucose intolerance three months after delivery [44]. Since UZ Leuven attends to a higher risk population than many other centers in Belgium, a lower overall rate of 30% of glucose intolerance in early postpartum across all participating centers is estimated. We further estimate that 30–50% of women with glucose intolerance postpartum will agree to participate in the trial. In order to enroll 236 women with glucose intolerance in the RCT, we estimate that about 1000 participants will have to be recruited baseline in early postpartum.

3.7.2. Data Analysis

Descriptive statistics will be presented as frequencies and percentages for categorical variables and means with standard deviations or medians with interquartile range for continuous variables. Comparison of the outcomes in the intervention groups will be based on logistic regression analyses for binary outcomes, proportional odds models for ordinal data, or linear models for continuous outcomes. The principle of intention-to-treat will be adopted for all outcomes. Inferential analyses will be performed for the following secondary endpoints: frequency of normal glucose tolerance, frequency of the metabolic syndrome, insulin resistance and beta-cell function, weight loss and motivation for behavior change. The remaining secondary endpoints will be analyzed using descriptive statistics. The number of patients with missing data will be statistically compared across intervention arms to check for any imbalance. The method of multiple imputation will be adopted for all outcome variables, in case of evidence of such imbalance ($p < 0.20$). Logistic regression models will be used for binary outcomes, or linear models for continuous outcomes. Imputation models will include the study group and patient characteristics. 10 imputations will be performed. All analyses will be performed as two-sided tests at 5% significance level.

3.8. Quality Control Procedures

Every participating site is opened after a first initiation visit. Monitoring visits are conducted every four months to check adherence of the participating sites to the protocol and completeness of data collection forms. Each participant gets a subject identification number to ensure confidentiality of the data. All data collected in this study are referred to by subject identification number only. All obtained data are entered in the Good Clinical Practice (GCP) compliant Electronic Data Capture (EDC) platform 'Castor EDC' [45].

4. Discussion

Lifestyle modifications need to be adapted for women with previous GDM to address their unique barriers to behavior change in order to optimize adherence. Digital health interventions seem to be highly acceptable among postpartum women and should therefore be considered for lifestyle management in this population, provided that they focus on delivering behavior change strategies and addressing practical barriers faced by postpartum women. Mobile interventions should therefore be evaluated so that the intervention can be adapted to the time demands of young mothers, be less resource intensive and be more suited for implementation in primary care. A limitation in previous studies is the inclusion of women with normal glucose tolerance, which might explain the difficult engagement of participants since they might perceive themselves to be at low risk of diabetes.

To our knowledge, this is the first RCT to investigate the efficacy of a blended telephone- and mobile-based lifestyle intervention in women with glucose intolerance shortly after a pregnancy with GDM. The intervention consists of a novel combination of one face-to-face meeting, coaching by telephone and mobile support through the MELINDA app. Moreover, the coaching program is based on the new concepts of precision public health prevention and food literacy. The MELINDA app is made available in Dutch, French and English, so that ethnic minorities and non-native Dutch speaking women (often a higher risk group) can also participate. By collaboration with seven hospitals (both university and non-university centers), a multi-ethnic population can be recruited, representative for the background population with GDM in the Northern part of Belgium (Flanders). Additionally, this study will provide accurate data on the prevalence of glucose intolerance and T2DM in early postpartum across Flanders and will therefore allow the evaluation of the extent to which the newer 2013 WHO criteria for GDM will affect the demand for diabetes prevention services postpartum.

While this RCT has many strengths, it might also have some potential limitations. A potential limitation is that the study is not powered to detect a difference in T2DM risk as a primary outcome. However, our primary outcome—based on weight-loss goals—is a strong predictor of T2DM development, as different studies have shown that moderate weight loss is effective in reducing risk of T2DM [9,10,46]. Although we have taken as many measures as possible to include a broad population, some exclusion bias might occur unintentionally, especially from foreign-speaking immigrants or women who do not have the appropriate smartphone at their disposal.

In conclusion, lifestyle interventions in women with a recent history of GDM need to be adapted to address their unique barriers to behavior change. The MELINDA study investigates a novel telephone- and mobile-based lifestyle intervention to promote a healthy lifestyle in women with glucose intolerance after a recent history of GDM.

Author Contributions: Conceptualization, C.M. (Caro Minschart), C.M. (Chantal Mathieu) and K.B.; Writing—Original draft, C.M. (Caro Minschart) and K.B.; Writing—Review & editing, C.M. (Caro Minschart), T.M., C.D.B., I.V.P., N.M., P.A., W.V., L.L., C.M. (Chantal Mathieu), J.B., C.M. (Christophe Matthys), B.W., A.L., A.B. and K.B. All authors have read and agreed to the published version of the manuscript.

Funding: Funding for this investigator-initiated study was provided by the research fund of UZ Leuven and by an unrestricted grant of Novo Nordisk. The following companies provided limited research grants: Sanofi, AstraZeneca, Boehringer-Ingelheim and Lilly. The sponsors have no role in the design of the study, in writing of the manuscript or the collection and analysis of data.

Acknowledgments: Caro Minschart has a PhD Fellowship Strategic Basic Research of the Research Foundation—Flanders (FWO). Katrien Benhalima is the recipient of a Senior Clinical Research grant of 'FWO Vlaanderen'.

Conflicts of Interest: The authors declare no conflict of interest.

References

1. American Diabetes Association. Standards of Medical Care in Diabetes-2017. *Diabetes Care* **2017**, *40* (Suppl. 1), S11–S24.
2. Crowther, C.A.; Hiller, J.E.; Moss, J.R.; Mcphee, A.J.; Jeffries, W.S.; Robinson, J.S. Effect of Treatment of Gestational Diabetes Mellitus on Pregnancy Outcomes. *N. Engl. J. Med.* **2005**, *352*, 2477–2486. [CrossRef] [PubMed]
3. Landon, M.B.; Spong, C.Y.; Thom, E.; Carpenter, M.W.; Ramin, S.M.; Casey, B.; Wapner, R.J.; Varner, M.W.; Rouse, D.J.; Thorp, J.M., Jr.; et al. A multicenter, randomized trial of treatment for mild gestational diabetes. *N. Engl. J. Med.* **2009**, *361*, 1339–1348. [CrossRef] [PubMed]
4. Buchanan, T.A. Pancreatic B-Cell Defects in Gestational Diabetes: Implications for the Pathogenesis and Prevention of Type 2 Diabetes. *J. Clin. Endocrinol. Metab.* **2001**, *86*, 989–993. [CrossRef] [PubMed]
5. Bellamy, L.; Casas, J.-P.; Hingorani, A.D.; Williams, D. Type 2 diabetes mellitus after gestational diabetes: A systematic review and meta-analysis. *Lancet* **2009**, *373*, 1773–1779. [CrossRef]
6. Benhalima, K.; Lens, K.; Bosteels, J.; Chantal, M. The Risk for Glucose Intolerance after Gestational Diabetes Mellitus since the Introduction of the IADPSG Criteria: A Systematic Review and Meta-Analysis. *J. Clin. Med.* **2019**, *8*, 1431. [CrossRef]
7. Ratner, R.E.; Christophi, C.A.; Metzger, B.E.; Dabelea, D.; Bennett, P.H.; Pi-Sunyer, X.; Fowler, S.; Kahn, S.E. The Diabetes Prevention Program Research Group. Prevention of Diabetes in Women with a History of Gestational Diabetes: Effects of Metformin and Lifestyle Interventions. *J. Clin. Endocrinol. Metab.* **2008**, *93*, 4774–4779. [CrossRef]
8. Gerstein, H.C.; Santaguida, P.; Raina, P.; Morrison, K.M.; Balion, C.; Hunt, D.; Yazdi, H.; Booker, L. Annual incidence and relative risk of diabetes in people with various categories of dysglycemia: A systematic overview and meta-analysis of prospective studies. *Diabetes Res. Clin. Pract.* **2007**, *78*, 305–312. [CrossRef]
9. Tuomilehto, J.; Lindstrom, J.; Eriksson, J.G.; Valle, T.T. Prevention of type 2 diabetes mellitus by changes in lifestyle among subjects with impaired glucose tolerance. *N. Engl. J. Med.* **2001**, *344*, 1343–1350. [CrossRef]
10. Diabetes Prevention Program Research Group. Reduction in the incidence of type 2 diabetes with lifestyle intervention or metformin. *N. Engl. J. Med.* **2002**, *346*, 393–403. [CrossRef]
11. Aroda, V.R.; Christophi, C.A.; Edelstein, S.L.; Zhang, P.; Herman, W.H.; Barrett-Connor, E.; Delahanty, L.M.; Montez, M.G.; Ackermann, R.T.; Zhuo, X.; et al. The effect of lifestyle intervention and metformin on preventing or delaying diabetes among women with and without gestational diabetes: The Diabetes Prevention Program outcomes study 10-year follow-up. *J. Clin. Endocrinol. Metab.* **2015**, *100*, 1646–1653. [CrossRef] [PubMed]
12. Cheung, N.W.; Smith, B.J.; Henriksen, H.; Tapsell, L.C.; McLean, M.; Bauman, A. A group-based healthy lifestyle program for women with previous gestational diabetes. *Diabetes Res. Clin. Pract.* **2007**, *77*, 333–334. [CrossRef] [PubMed]
13. Kim, C.; Draska, M.; Hess, M.L.; Wilson, E.J.; Richardson, C.R. A web-based pedometer programme in women with a recent history of gestational diabetes. *Diabet. Med.* **2012**, *29*, 278–283. [CrossRef] [PubMed]
14. Ferrara, A.; Hedderson, M.; Albright, C.; Ehrlich, S.; Quesenberry, C.; Peng, T.; Feng, J.; Ching, J.; Crites, Y. A pregnancy and postpartum lifestyle intervention in women with gestational diabetes mellitus reduces diabetes risk factors: A feasibility randomized control trial. *Diabetes Care* **2011**, *34*, 1519–1525. [CrossRef]
15. Goveia, P.; Cañon-Montañez, W.; De Paula Santos, D.; Lopes, G.W.; Ma, R.C.W.; Duncan, B.B.; Ziegelman, P.K.; Schmidt, M.I. Lifestyle intervention for the prevention of diabetes in women with previous gestational diabetes mellitus: A systematic review and meta-analysis. *Front. Endocrinol.* **2018**, *9*, 583. [CrossRef]
16. Lim, S.; Dunbar, J.A.; Versace, V.L.; Janus, E.; Wildey, C.; Skinner, T.; O'Reilly, S. Comparing a telephone- and a group-delivered diabetes prevention program: Characteristics of engaged and non-engaged postpartum mothers with a history of gestational diabetes. *Diabetes Res. Clin. Pract.* **2017**, *126*, 254–262. [CrossRef]
17. Lim, S.; Tan, A.; Madden, S.; Hill, B. Health professionals' and postpartum women's perspectives on digital health interventions for lifestyle management in the postpartum period: A systematic review of qualitative studies. *Front. Endocrinol.* **2019**, *10*, 767. [CrossRef]
18. Nicklas, J.M.; Zera, C.A.; England, L.J.; Rosner, B.A.; Horton, E.; Levkoff, S.E.; Seely, E.W. A web-based lifestyle intervention for women with recent gestational diabetes mellitus: A randomized controlled trial. *Obs. Gynecol.* **2014**, *124*, 563–570. [CrossRef]

19. Appel, L.J.; Clark, J.M.; Yeh, H.-C.; Wang, N.-Y.; Coughlin, J.W.; Daumit, G.; Miller, E.R., III; Dalcin, A.; Jerome, G.J.; Geller, S.; et al. Comparative effectiveness of weight-loss interventions in clinical practice. *N. Engl. J. Med.* **2011**, *365*, 1959–1968. [CrossRef]
20. Hurkmans, E.; Matthys, C.; Bogaerts, A.; Scheys, L.; Devloo, K.; Seghers, J. Face-to-Face Versus Mobile Versus Blended Weight Loss Program: Randomized Clinical Trial. *JMIR mHealth uHealth* **2018**, *6*, e14. [CrossRef]
21. International Association of Diabetes and Pregnancy Study Groups Consensus Panel. International association of diabetes and pregnancy study groups recommendations on the diagnosis and classification of hyperglycemia in pregnancy. *Diabetes Care* **2010**, *33*, 676–682. [CrossRef] [PubMed]
22. World Health Organization (WHO). *Diagnostic Criteria and Classification of Hyperglycaemia First Detected in Pregnancy*; WHO: Geneva, Switzerland, 2013.
23. Boedt, T.; Dancet, E.; Lie Fong, S.; Peeraer, K.; De Neubourg, D.; Pelckmans, S.; van de Vijver, A.; Seghers, J.; Van der Gucht, K.; Van Calster, B.; et al. Effectiveness of a mobile preconception lifestyle programme in couples undergoing in vitro fertilisation (IVF): The protocol for the PreLiFe randomised controlled trial (PreLiFe-RCT). *BMJ Open* **2019**, *9*, e029665. [CrossRef] [PubMed]
24. Bogaerts, A.; Bijlholt, M.; Mertens, L.; Braeken, M.; Jacobs, B.; Vandenberghe, B.; Ameye, L.; Devlieger, R. Development and Field Evaluation of the INTER-ACT App, a Pregnancy and Interpregnancy Coaching App to Reduce Maternal Overweight and Obesity: Mixed Methods Design. *JMIR Form. Res.* **2020**, *4*, e16090. [CrossRef] [PubMed]
25. Vidgen, H.A.; Gallegos, D. Defining food literacy and its components. *Appetite* **2014**, *76*, 50–59. [CrossRef]
26. Benhalima, K.; Van Crombrugge, P.; Verhaeghe, J.; Vandeginste, S.; Verlaenen, H.; Vercammen, C.; Dufraimont, E.; De Block, C.; Jacquemyn, Y.; Mekahli, F.; et al. The Belgian Diabetes in Pregnancy Study (BEDIP-N), a multi-centric prospective cohort study on screening for diabetes in pregnancy and gestational diabetes: Methodology and design. *BMC Pregnancy Childbirth* **2014**, *14*, 226. [CrossRef] [PubMed]
27. Matthys, C.; Meulemans, A. Development and validation of general FFQ for use in clinical practice. *Nutr. Metab.* **2015**, *67*, 239.
28. Harrison, C.; Thompson, R.; Teede, H.; Lombard, C. Measuring physical activity during pregnancy. *Int. J. Behav. Nutr. Phys. Act.* **2011**, *8*, 19. [CrossRef]
29. Dalfrà, M.G.; Nicolucci, A.; Bisson, T.; Bonsembiante, B.; Lapolla, A. Quality of life in pregnancy and post-partum: A study in diabetic patients. *Qual. Life Res.* **2012**, *21*, 291–298. [CrossRef]
30. Petrou, S.; Morrell, J.; Spiby, H. Assessing the empirical validity of alternative multi-attribute utility measures in the maternity context. *Health Qual. Life Outcomes* **2009**, *7*, 40–52. [CrossRef]
31. Kim, C.; Mcewen, L.N.; Piette, J.D.; Goewey, J.; Ferrara, A.; Walker, E.A. Risk Perception for Diabetes among Women with Histories of Gestational Diabetes Mellitus. *Diabetes Care* **2007**, *30*, 2281–2286. [CrossRef]
32. Shigaki, C.; Kruse, R.L.; Mehr, D.; Sheldon, K.M.; Bin, G.; Moore, C.; Lemaster, J. Motivation and diabetes self-management. *Chronic Illn.* **2010**, *6*, 202–214. [CrossRef] [PubMed]
33. Levesque, C.S.; Williams, G.C.; Elliot, D.; Pickering, M.A.; Bodenhamer, B.; Finley, P.J. Validating the theoretical structure of the Treatment Self-Regulation Questionnaire (TSRQ) across three different health behaviors. *Health Educ. Res.* **2007**, *22*, 691–702. [CrossRef] [PubMed]
34. Marteau, T.M.; Bekker, H. The development of a six-item short-form of the state scale of the Spielberger State—Trait Anxiety Inventory (STAI). *Br. J. Clin. Psychol.* **1992**, *31*, 301–306. [CrossRef] [PubMed]
35. Van der Bij, A.K.; de Weerd, S.; Cikot, R.J.L.M.; Steegers, E.A.P.; Braspenning, J.C.C. Validation of the Dutch Short Form of the State Scale of the Spielberger State-Trait Anxiety Inventory: Considerations for Usage in Screening Outcomes. *Community Genet.* **2003**, *6*, 84–87. [CrossRef] [PubMed]
36. Eriksson, M.; Lindström, B. Antonovsky's sense of coherence scale and its relation with quality of life: A systematic review. *J. Epidemiol. Community Health.* **2007**, *61*, 938–944. [CrossRef]
37. American Diabetes Association. 2. Classification and diagnosis of diabetes. *Diabetes Care* **2016**, *39*, S13–S22. [CrossRef]
38. Grundy, S.M.; Brewer, H.B.; Cleeman, J.I.; Smith, S.C.; Lenfant, C. Definition of metabolic syndrome: Report of the National Heart, Lung, and Blood Institute/American Heart Association conference on scientific issues related to definition. *Circulation* **2004**, *109*, 433–438. [CrossRef]
39. Matsuda, M.; DeFronzo, R.A. Insulin sensitivity indices obtained from oral glucose tolerance testing: Comparison with the euglycemic insulin clamp. *Diabetes Care* **1999**, *22*, 1462–1470. [CrossRef]

40. Matthews, D.R.; Hosker, J.P.; Rudenski, A.S.; Naylor, B.A.; Treacher, D.F.; Turner, R.C. Homeostasis model assessment: Insulin resistance and β-cell function from fasting plasma glucose and insulin concentrations in man. *Diabetologia* **1985**, *28*, 412–419. [CrossRef]
41. Kahn, S.E. The relative contributions of insulin resistance and beta-cell dysfunction to the pathophysiology of Type 2 diabetes. *Diabetologia* **2003**, *46*, 3–19. [CrossRef]
42. Retnakaran, R.; Qi, Y.; Goran, M.I.; Hamilton, J.K. Evaluation of proposed oral disposition index measures in relation to the actual disposition index. *Diabet. Med.* **2009**, *26*, 1198–1203. [CrossRef] [PubMed]
43. Devlieger, H.; Martens, G.; Bekaert, A.; Eeckels, R. Standaarden van geboortegewicht-voor-zwangerschapsduur voor de vlaamse boreling. *Tijdschr Geneeskd* **2000**, *56*, 1–14. [CrossRef]
44. Benhalima, K.; Jegers, K.; Devlieger, R.; Verhaeghe, J.; Mathieu, C. Glucose intolerance after a recent history of gestational diabetes based on the 2013 WHO criteria. *PLoS ONE* **2016**, *10*, e0157272. [CrossRef] [PubMed]
45. Ciwit B.V. *Castor Electronic Data Capture*; Ciwit B.V.: Amsterdam, The Netherlands, 2018.
46. Saaristo, T.; Moilanen, L.; Korpi-Hyövälti, E.; Vanhala, M.; Saltevo, J.; Niskanen, L.; Jokelainen, J.; Peltonen, M.; Oksa, H.; Tuomilheto, J.; et al. Lifestyle intervention for prevention of type 2 diabetes in primary health care: One-year follow-up of the finnish national diabetes prevention program (FIN-D2D). *Diabetes Care* **2010**, *33*, 2146–2151. [CrossRef]

© 2020 by the authors. Licensee MDPI, Basel, Switzerland. This article is an open access article distributed under the terms and conditions of the Creative Commons Attribution (CC BY) license (http://creativecommons.org/licenses/by/4.0/).

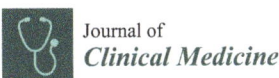

Article

Benefits of Adhering to a Mediterranean Diet Supplemented with Extra Virgin Olive Oil and Pistachios in Pregnancy on the Health of Offspring at 2 Years of Age. Results of the San Carlos Gestational Diabetes Mellitus Prevention Study

Verónica Melero [1,2,†], Carla Assaf-Balut [1,2,†], Nuria García de la Torre [1,3], Inés Jiménez [1], Elena Bordiú [1,2], Laura del Valle [1], Johanna Valerio [1], Cristina Familiar [1], Alejandra Durán [1,2], Isabelle Runkle [1,2], María Paz de Miguel [1,2], Carmen Montañez [1], Ana Barabash [1,3], Martín Cuesta [1,3], Miguel A. Herraiz [2,4], Nuria Izquierdo [2,4], Miguel A. Rubio [1,2] and Alfonso L. Calle-Pascual [1,2,3,*]

1. Endocrinology and Nutrition Department, Hospital Clínico Universitario San Carlos and Instituto de Investigación Sanitaria del Hospital Clínico San Carlos (IdISSC), 28040 Madrid, Spain; veronica.meleroalvarez10@gmail.com (V.M.); carlaassafbalut90@hotmail.co.uk (C.A.-B.); nurialobo@hotmail.com (N.G.d.l.T.); i.jimenez.varas@gmail.com (I.J.); elena.bordiu@salud.madrid.org (E.B.); lauradel_valle@hotmail.com (L.d.V.); valeriojohanna@gmail.com (J.V.); cristinafamiliarcasado@gmail.com (C.F.); aduranrh@hotmail.com (A.D.); irunkledelavega@gmail.com (I.R.); pazdemiguel@telefonica.net (M.P.d.M.); mcmnita@hotmail.com (C.M.); ana.barabash@gmail.com (A.B.); cuestamartintutor@gmail.com (M.C.); marubioh@gmail.com (M.A.R.)
2. Facultad de Medicina. Medicina II Department, Universidad Complutense de Madrid, 28040 Madrid, Spain; maherraizm@gmail.com (M.A.H.); nuriaizquierdo4@gmail.com (N.I.)
3. Centro de Investigación Biomédica en Red de Diabetes y Enfermedades Metabólicas Asociadas (CIBERDEM), 28029 Madrid, Spain
4. Gynecology and Obstetrics Department, Hospital Clínico Universitario San Carlos and Instituto de Investigación Sanitaria del Hospital Clínico San Carlos (IdISSC), 28040 Madrid, Spain
* Correspondence: acalle.edu@gmail.com
† These authors have contributed equally to this work.

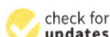

Received: 16 April 2020; Accepted: 11 May 2020; Published: 13 May 2020

Abstract: The intrauterine environment may be related to the future development of chronic diseases in the offspring. The St. Carlos gestational diabetes mellitus (GDM) prevention study, is a randomized controlled trial that evaluated the influence of the early (before 12th gestational week) Mediterranean diet (MedDiet) on the onset of GDM and adverse gestational outcomes. Out of 874 women assessed after delivery (440 control group (CG)/434 intervention group (IG)), 703 children were followed (365/338; CG/IG), with the aim to assess whether the adherence to a MedDiet during pregnancy induces health benefits for the offspring during the first two years of life. Logistic regression analysis showed that the IG in children of mothers with pre-gestational body mass index (BMI) < 25 kg/m^2 and normal glucose tolerance (NGT), was associated with a lower risk (RR(95% CI)) of suffering from severe events requiring hospitalization due to bronchiolitis/asthma (0.75(0.58–0.98) and 0.77(0.59–0.99), respectively) or other diseases that required either antibiotic (0.80(0.65–0.98) and 0.80(0.65–0.99), respectively), corticosteroid treatment (0.73(0.59–0.90) and 0.79(0.62–1.00) respectively) or both (all $p < 0.05$). A nutritional intervention based on the MedDiet during pregnancy is associated with a reduction in offspring's hospital admissions, especially in women with pre-gestational BMI < 25 kg/m^2 and NGT.

Keywords: glucose tolerance; Mediterranean diet; nutritional intervention; obesity; offspring; pregnancy nutrition

1. Introduction

Adherence to healthy eating patterns in pregnancy, such as the Mediterranean diet (MedDiet), is being widely studied. There seems to be associations between the development of certain diseases that can affect pregnancy, such as gestational diabetes mellitus (GDM), and the onset of immune and metabolic diseases in the offspring later in life [1–21].

Evidence suggests a possible beneficial effect of following appropriate eating habits during pregnancy in terms of disease development. Indeed, the MedDiet seems to have a protective role against diseases such as bronchiolitis and also in diseases of an autoimmune nature such as asthma, wheezing, allergic rhinitis, atopic dermatitis and food allergies in childhood [1,2,13,15–18]. Conversely, a western diet can have the opposite effects [3,19,20]. Furthermore, recent findings point out that pregnancy could be an optimal time to establish suitable eating patterns in the mother, thus guaranteeing the offspring's health [4].

The adverse intrauterine environment provided by either GDM or obesity is linked to epigenetic changes that predispose the offspring to develop a metabolic disease later in life. In turn, these can be transmitted to the following generation, thereby perpetuating the vicious cycle of metabolic diseases [5–10]. In fact, several studies have shown how maternal obesity and GDM during pregnancy are associated with an increase in the risk of asthma in early childhood. This has been observed even in women without a history of asthma [11]. Moreover, having GDM and obesity are associated with a higher risk for the offspring of developing respiratory diseases and of having poorer health [12,14,21].

Recently, it has been shown that adherence to a MedDiet can reduce the risk of GDM [22]. In fact, our group has shown that an early adherence to a MedDiet-supplemented with extra virgin olive oil (EVOO) and nuts-in pregnancy can reduce the risk of GDM and other adverse materno-fetal outcomes [23,24]. It has also been associated with a better postpartum metabolic profile in the mother [25]. Whether these benefits are conveyed to the offspring, remains to be known.

While the current evidence suggests a possible association between diet and the development of diseases in children, few have evaluated the effect of an intervention based on a Mediterranean diet in the development of metabolic and immune diseases in the offspring. In addition, the results of these studies are heterogeneous and have not been developed as a randomized controlled trial (RCT), so they are not conclusive.

This study aims to assess whether the MedDiet supplemented with EVOO and pistachios during pregnancy induces benefits to the offspring's health during the first two years of life.

2. Materials and Methods

2.1. Study Design

This is a prospective analysis of the St. Carlos GDM prevention study [23]. This paper includes offspring of women who attended the postpartum follow-up between 2017 and 2018.

Concisely, this RCT evaluated whether an early nutritional intervention based on a MedDiet (supplemented with EVOO and pistachios) could reduce the incidence of GDM. Women in the intervention group (IG) were told to enhance the consumption of EVOO and pistachios while those in the control group (CG) were told to restrict all kinds of fats.

After the delivery, women received the same dietary recommendation.

The study was approved by the Ethics Committee of Hospital Clínico San Carlos (full protocol approved 17 July 2013 (CI 13/296-E)) and conducted according to the Helsinki Declaration. All women signed a letter of informed consent.

This trial was registered on 4 December 2013, at http://www.isrctn.com/ with the number ISRCTN84389045 (DOI 10.1186/ISRCTN84389045). The authors confirm that all ongoing and related trials for this intervention are registered.

2.2. Study Population

To obtain children's data, the 874 women who were analyzed in the St. Carlos GDM prevention study were invited to participate in the follow-up at 2 years postpartum.

A total of 171 (75 from CG and 96 from IG) did not attend the 2-year follow-up. Of these, it was not possible to access the children's data because of changes in the place of residence to outside of the community of Madrid, making it impossible to contact the mothers and to access their children's medical records. Thus, the total of children assessed was 703 (80.5%), 365 from CG and 338 from IG (Figure 1).

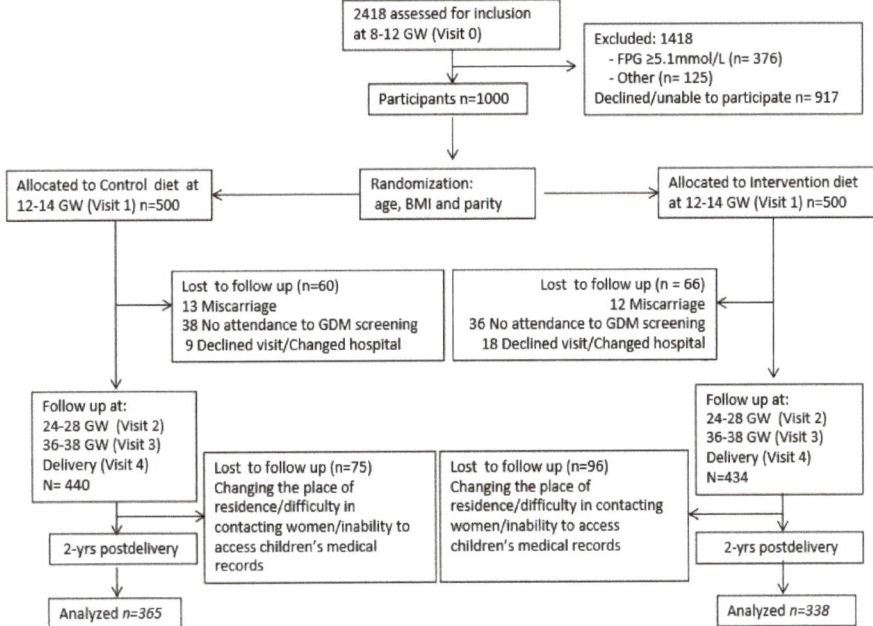

Figure 1. The CONSORT 2010 flow diagram for scope.

2.3. Outcomes

Primary outcome: to assess the incidence of bronchiolitis/asthma, atopic dermatitis and food allergies as well as the number and duration of all-cause hospital admissions in children at 2 years of age. Secondary outcomes: to evaluate the rates of hospital admissions due to severe episodes of bronchiolitis/asthma and other diseases requiring pharmacological treatment with antibiotics, corticosteroids or both.

2.4. Data Collection

The hospital Clínico San Carlos is a hospital within the public health system that provides health care services for a population of about 380,000 habitants of the central area of Madrid. The public health system covers health care at pediatric age, including medical and nursing consultations, and provides free access to the mandatory vaccination program. It also facilitates access to optional vaccines. At the first visit with the pediatrician and nurse after birth, usually before the first month, the child receives a health card. This card includes data about their anthropometric development, the vaccines received and the introduction of different foods. The medication prescribed by the pediatrician is recorded in the electronic history and dispensed in the pharmacy after being included in the unique prescription module (MUP). When hospital admission is required, the diagnosis and treatment received are recorded in the discharge report and can be accessed through the HORUS program (Historia Clínica Digital del Sistema Nacional de Salud).

2.4.1. Clinical Data: Mothers

The maternal data referred to in this study belong to mothers whose children were evaluated in this study. These data were obtained during their gestational period.

This information included family history of metabolic disorders such as type 2 diabetes, obstetric history (miscarriages and GDM), educational level, employment status, number of prior pregnancies, smoking habits (registering whether they are currently smoking, or they smoked until they found out they were pregnant) and gestational age at entry concurring to the first ultrasound.

The mother's lifestyle during and after pregnancy was registered. The adherence to a healthy lifestyle (including physical activity) was evaluated with the Diabetes Nutrition and Complication Trial (DNCT) questionnaire and provided the nutrition score and physical activity score. The adherence to the MedDiet was assessed with the 14-point Mediterranean diet Adherence Screener (MEDAS) questionnaire and was used to obtain the MEDAS score. A more detailed description has been previously published [23].

2.4.2. Clinical Data: Children

Children's data were obtained at 2 years of age after a face to face interview with the mother. The interview was conducted by a dietician. It was carried out in the hospital and its duration was about 30 min. They brought the mandatory pediatric health registry (primary source) to this visit. Anthropometric data (weight and height taken at different time points), vaccination schedule (compulsory and optional vaccination) and food introduction during the first two years were obtained from this mandatory pediatric health registry. Other data about the children's health had to be obtained from a secondary data source. If the mothers did not attend this visit, these data were recovered by contacting them via telephone calls. All information provided by the mother was later verified with the data found in the secondary sources.

Secondary data source: Information about prescription of pharmacological treatments, including antibiotics and corticosteroids and number of episodes requiring pharmacological treatment, was obtained from MUP. Information about the number of hospital admissions and their cause was obtained from the hospital discharge registry. The number of minor diseases (requiring only outpatient treatment) and their treatment were obtained from the electronic medical history system (through the HORUS application) and SERMAS (Servicio Madrileño de Salud) where all information related to children's health is registered. This includes attendance to emergency room, hospitalization (cause, duration and discharge are registered), diseases diagnoses, allergies and the pharmacological treatment received.

Moreover, the vaccination schedule can also be accessed through the electronic medical history, and includes the moment of reception and the dose of the vaccine received. All this information could be retrieved as long as the child was attended to within the Community of Madrid. Access to the electronic medical history system outside of this area was not possible.

The following variables were extracted: (1) Food allergy or intolerance, bronchiolitis/asthma and atopic eczema. It was recorded at the time of diagnosis along with the number of episodes in which their pediatrician prescribed antibiotic treatment, corticosteroids or both. (2) Vaccination schedule: this includes the mandatory vaccines in Spain (chickenpox, diphtheria, hemophilus influenza type B, hepatitis B, measles, meningococcus C, mumps, pertussis, pneumococcus 13 V, polio, rubella and tetanus) and the optional ones (meningococcus B and rotavirus). It was considered complete when they received all the recommended doses. (3). The total number of all-cause hospital admissions and their durations. Additionally, the number of hospitalizations due to severe episodes of bronchiolitis/asthma, as well as the number and duration of hospital admissions in which the children required antibiotic or corticosteroids treatment, or both. This information had to be recorded in the hospital discharge report and was accessed through the HORUS program.

The following additional data were also registered: (1) Breastfeeding: recorded as either exclusive lactation; mixed, which includes any product (artificial lactation) or complementary feeding; registering the moment the children started consuming cereals (both with and without gluten). (2) Kindergarten attendance: whether they attended and the age they started (measured in months).

2.5. Statistical Analysis

The categorical variables are expressed numerically (%) and continuous variables are expressed as mean (SD). The comparison of frequencies between groups of the categorical variable was evaluated by the χ^2 test. For continuous variables, values were compared with Student's t test or the Mann–Whitney U test if distribution of continuous variables was not normal, as verified by the Shapiro–Wilk test. Logistic regression analysis was used to assess the adjusted effect of the intervention on the risk for adverse offspring outcomes that were significantly different in the binary analysis. The magnitude of association was evaluated using the relative risk (RR) and 95% confidence interval (CI) adjusted for age, ethnicity and parity and categorized by BMI and glucose tolerance, were estimated. The reason for adjusting age, ethnicity and parity was because advanced maternal age, parity and ethnicity are associated with worse health in the offspring [26–29]

All p values are 2-tailed at less than 0.05. Analyses were performed using SPSS, version 21 (SPSS, Chicago, IL, USA).

3. Results

A total of 703/874 (80.5%) children of women who completed the St. Carlos GDM prevention study were evaluated: 365 of the CG and 338 of the IG. Compared to women in the CG, women of the IG were similar in relation to the baseline characteristics at 12 weeks of gestation (GW). However, they maintained a greater adherence to the nutritional intervention (as reflected by the MEDAS and nutrition score), lower rates of GDM, lower fasting glucose levels and less weight gain at 24–28 GW. The mothers' baseline characteristics are shown in Table 1.

A non-significant reduction in the rates of all-cause hospital admissions and in the number of children who required it was observed in the IG versus the CG. In total, there were 51 (15.1%) and 65 (17.8%) hospital admissions, respectively, and 46 (13.6%) and 54 (14.9%) children hospitalized respectively, both $p > 0.05$. However, the length of stay was significantly shorter in IG than in the CG (6.8 ± 9.1 vs. 11.9 ± 25.2 days; $p = 0.02$). Data of the children of mothers from the CG and IG at 23 ± 2.5 months of age are shown in Table 2

The supplementary tables show the data of the children according to the maternal pre-pregnancy body mass index (BMI) and by glucose tolerance, comparing the IG versus the CG. When evaluating children born to women with pre-gestational BMI < 25 kg/m^2, a significantly lower hospital admissions rate due to bronchiolitis/asthma, antibiotic treatment and corticosteroid treatment, was observed in the IG (all $p < 0.05$) (Table S1). There were no significant results found when comparing the children of mothers with BMI ≥ 25 kg/m^2. Similar results were observed when analyzing the children of women who had normal glucose tolerance (NGT), where a significantly lower number of hospital admissions due to bronchiolitis/asthma, antibiotic treatment and corticosteroid treatment was also observed in the IG (all $p < 0.05$). These results were not found when making these same comparisons between children of mothers who developed GDM (Table S2).

Table 1. Baseline characteristics of mothers whose children were analyzed.

	CONTROL GROUP n = 365	INTERVENTION GROUP n = 338	p
Age (years)	32.8 ± 5.3	33.2 ± 5.0	0.316
Race/Ethnicity			
Caucasian	237 (64.9)	222 (65.6)	
Hispanic	114 (31.2)	109 (32.2)	
Others	14 (3.9)	7 (2.2)	0.804
Family history of			
Type 2 Diabetes	82 (23.5)	92 (27.7)	
MetS (>2 components)	65 (17.8)	76 (22.5)	0.154
Previous history of			
GDM	11 (3.0)	11 (3.3)	
Miscarriages	117 (32.0)	117 (34.6)	0.688
Educational status			
Elementary education	41 (11.2)	21 (6.2)	
Secondary School	145 (39.7)	146 (43.2)	
University Degree	174 (47.7)	168 (49.7)	
UNK	5 (1.4)	3 (0.9)	0.467
Employment	276 (75.6)	266 (78.7)	0.950
Number of pregnancies			
Primiparous	144 (39.5)	142 (42.1)	
Second pregnancy	119 (32.6)	115 (34.1)	
>2 pregnancies	102 (27.9)	81 (22.8)	0.622
Smoker			
Never	202 (55.3)	184 (54.1)	
Current	26 (7.1)	26 (7.7)	0.994
Gestational Age (weeks) at baseline	12.1 ± 0.6	12.0 ± 0.3	0.899
Pre-pregnancy Body Weight (kg)	61.5 ± 11.1	60.3 ± 9.9	0.131
Weight gain at:			
24–28 GW	7.73 ± 4.22	7.04 ± 3.71	0.022
36–38 GW	11.02 ± 6.71	11.49 ± 6.87	0.452
Pre-pregnancy BMI (kg/m^2)	23.3 ± 3.9	23.1 ± 3.5	0.354
BMI ≥ 25 kg/m^2	107 (29.3)	86 (25.4)	0.486
Systolic BP/Diastolic BP (mm Hg)			
12 GW	107 ± 11/64 ± 9	107 ± 10/66 ± 9	0.957/0.061
24 GW	105 ± 11/63 ± 9	105 ± 11/63 ± 8	0.370/0.747
36 GW	113 ± 13/72 ± 9	113 ± 13/73 ± 9	0.319/0.303
Fasting Blood Glucose (mg/dl)			
12 GW	81.4 ± 6.1	81.2 ± 6.0	0.687
24 GW	85.8 ± 6.7	84.0 ± 6.5	0.001
36 GW	77.1 ± 7.7	75.0 ± 7.7	0.007
GDM at 24–28 GW n (%)	91 (24.9)	58 (17.2)	0.036
Caesarean Section n (%)	56 (15.3)	54 (16.0)	0.111
TSH mcUI/mL			
12 GW	1.9 ± 1.2	2.1 ± 1.4	0.223
24 GW	2.0 ± 1.2	2.1 ± 1.1	0.464
36 GW	1.7 ± 1.3	1.6 ± 0.9	0.890
MEDAS Score			
12 GW	4.1 ± 1.7	4.4 ± 1.6	0.090
24 GW	4.5 ± 1.7	6.3 ± 1.7	0.001
36 GW	5.5 ± 1.9	6.6 ± 2.1	0.001
Nutrition Score			
12 GW	0.6 ± 3.3	0.2 ± 3.1	0.078
24 GW	1.2 ± 3.4	4.2 ± 3.2	0.001
36 GW	3.6 ± 3.7	5.3 ± 3.6	0.001
Physical Activity Score			
12 GW	−1.7 ± 1.0	−1.9 ± 1.0	0.059
24 GW	−1.8 ± 0.9	−1.8 ± 0.9	0.482
36 GW	−1.8 ± 0.7	−1.6 ± 0.9	0.055

Data are mean ± SD or number (%). MetS, metabolic syndrome; UNK, unknown; BMI, body mass index; GW, gestational weeks; GDM, gestational diabetes mellitus; BP, blood pressure; MEDAS Score, 14-point Mediterranean diet Adherence Screener (MEDAS); nutrition score, Diabetes Nutrition and Complications Trial (DNCT); physical activity score, (walking daily (>5 days/week) Score 0: At least 30 min. Score+1, if >60 min. Score−1, if <30 min. Climbing stairs (floors/day, >5 days a week): Score 0, between 4 and 16; Score+1, >16; Score−1: <4). p differences between groups analyzed with the χ^2 test (categorical variable); Student's t test (continuous variables) or the Mann–Whitney U test (not-normal distribution in continuous variables). Verified by the Shapiro–Wilk test.

Table 2. Children's data at 2 years follow-up according to whether their mothers belonged to the intervention (IG) or control group (CG).

	CG	IG	p
Number (n)	365	338	
Born, n (%)			
Preterm (<37 GW)	14 (3.8)	5 (1.5)	0.477
Small for gestational age (SGA)	23 (6.3)	5 (1.5)	0.002
Large for gestational age (LGA)	10 (2.7)	4 (1.2)	0.049
Age (months)	23.13 ± 2.55	23.29 ± 2.51	0.433
Body Weight (kg)	12.11 ± 1.48	12.17 ± 1.54	0.555
Percentile	47.7 ± 27.0	49.2 ± 27.4	0.483
Height (cm)	86.26 ± 3.96	86.16 ± 4.01	0.759
Percentile	39.3 ± 27.0	39.7 ± 28.6	0.867
Breastfeeding n (%)	340 (94.4%)	314 (93.5%)	0.703
Exclusive (months)	5.20 ± 1.50	5.36 ± 1.47	0.194
Mixed (months)	10.34 ± 7.74	10.60 ± 7.55	0.705
Cereal Introduction (months)			
Gluten-free cereal	4.77 ± 0.81	4.74 ± 0.81	0.702
Gluten cereal	6.58 ± 1.28	6.62 ± 2.02	0.787
Nursery			
n (%)	247 (67.7)	237 (70.7)	0.213
Age (months)	15.8 ± 6.0	14.8 ± 6.8	0.139
Vaccinations n (%)			
Compulsory	359 (99.4%)	338 (100%)	0.270
Recommended n (%)			
Meningitis	210 (58.2)	214 (64.3)	0.059
Rotavirus	251 (69.5)	240 (72.1)	0.257
Outpatient diseases n (%)			
Treatment with antibiotics	251 (68.8%)	234 (69.4%)	0.456
Treatment with corticosteroids	187 (51.2%)	166 (49.3%)	0.327
Diagnoses n (%)			
Food allergies	29 (8.0%)	21 (6.2%)	0.225
Asthma	7 (1.9%)	11 (3.3%)	0.189
Bronchiolitis/respiratory problems	74 (20.3%)	75 (22.3%)	0.298
Atopic dermatitis	101 (27.7%)	106 (31.5%)	0.161
Severe Diseases inpatients treatment			
All-cause hospital stays n (%)	65 (17.8%)	51 (15.1%)	0.193
Children n (%)	54 (14.9%)	46 (13.6%)	0.079
Duration (days)	11.9 ± 25.2	6.8 ± 9.1	0.020
Asthma/bronchiolitis disease	27 (7.4%)	18 (5.3%)	0.167
Treatment with antibiotics	59 (16.2%)	40 (11.9%)	0.063
Treatment with corticosteroids	41 (11.2%)	25 (7.4%)	0.054
Treatment with antibiotics and corticosteroids	36 (9.9%)	25 (7.4%)	0.155

Results expressed as mean ± SD or n (%). p differences between groups analyzed with the χ^2 test (categorical variable); Student's t test (continuous variables) or the Mann–Whitney U test (not-normal distribution in continuous variables). Verified by the Shapiro–Wilk test.

When analyzing children of mothers with pre-gestational BMI < 25 kg/m² of the IG, the RR (95% CI) in the IG of having a severe event requiring hospital admission due to bronchiolitis/asthma, due to any disease requiring antibiotic treatment, either any disease requiring corticosteroid treatment or both, were 0.75 (0.58–0.98), 0.80 (0.65–0.98), 0.73 (0.59–0.90) and 0.78 (0.61–0.99), respectively. In children of mothers with NGT, the RRs were 0.77 (0.59–0.99), 0.80 (0.65–0.99), 0.75 (0.60–0.93) and 0.79 (0.62–1.00), respectively, for children of mothers with NGT, respectively. These data are shown in Figure 2.

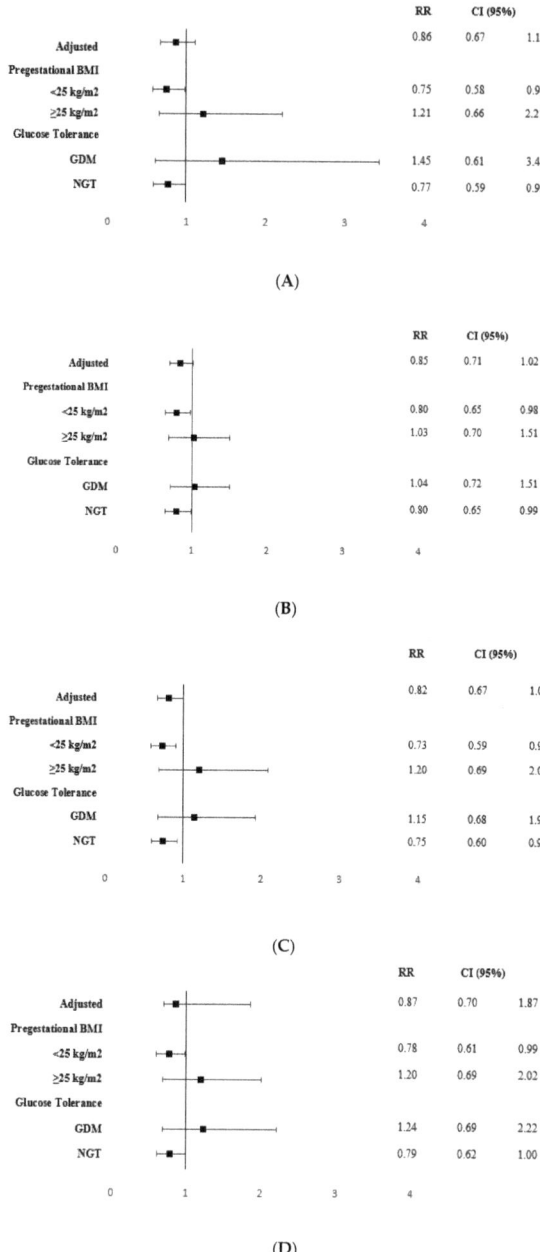

Figure 2. Relative risk (RR) and 95% confidence interval (CI) of suffering severe adverse events that require hospitalization adjusted for age, parity and ethnicity, and categorized by BMI and glucose tolerance. (**A**) Bronchiolitis/asthma in hospitalized children; (**B**) antibiotic treatment in hospitalized children; (**C**) corticosteroid treatment in hospitalized children; (**D**) antibiotic and corticosteroid treatment in hospitalized children. BMI, body mass index; RR, relative risk; CI, confidence interval; GDM, gestational diabetes mellitus; NGT, normal glucose tolerance. Regression analysis was assessed with SPSS, version 21 (reference group = control group).

4. Discussion

This study shows that the adherence to the MedDiet enriched with EVOO and pistachios during pregnancy seems to be associated with a lower risk of hospitalization in children at two years of age. This was especially observed in women who had a pre-gestational BMI < 25 kg/m^2 and in those with NGT. To our knowledge, this is the first RCT study that analyses the influence of a nutritional intervention based on a MedDiet in pregnancy on the offspring's health.

The MedDiet enriched with EVOO and pistachios has been associated with health benefits in the mother [25,30,31]. There are also suggestions that these benefits can be transferred to postnatal life [32]. In fact, recent published studies seem to indicate that the MedDiet decreases the incidence of wheezing, asthma and allergies [1,2,18]. A confounding factor could be the caesarean section rates since it has been shown that the immune system of children born by caesarean section matures later and therefore they have a higher risk of developing allergies in the future [33]. The results showed similar data in both groups. Thus, a reduction in infectious and allergic events would be expected. However, we have not found differences between the IG and CG in relation to rates of bronchiolitis/asthma, diseases of autoimmune origin (food allergies and dermatitis eczema) and infectious illness that did not require hospital admission. Adherence to childhood vaccination programs is associated with a reduction of these diseases during the first years of life [34]. Considering this, the vaccination program was completed by more than 99% of children in both groups. That is to say, it could overcome the benefit of food during pregnancy. On the other hand, it is known that breastfeeding is the greatest protective factor in offspring during the early years of life, preventing early childhood diseases and several infectious diseases [35,36]. The present study revealed that more than 90% of women (from both the IG and CG) performed exclusive breastfeeding at least during the first five months of life. In many cases, mothers continued combining breastfeeding with complementary feeding during at least 10 months. This could be the reason why we have not found more significant differences between children at two years of age. In fact, some studies have found certain differences in older children [37]. Therefore, it would be interesting to evaluate these children at an older age.

Nevertheless, our study shows significant differences between the IG and CG in relation to the reduction of severe events requiring hospitalization in children whose mothers had a pre-gestational BMI < 25 kg/m^2 and NGT. These are considered low-risk women, who make up most of our studied population.

Indeed, according to the results, the rates of corticosteroid treatment in children would be higher in the IG, but these are not statistically significant. On the other hand, the reduction in the hospitalized rate due to severe adverse effects is highly significant.

GDM and obesity have negative effects on the offspring, and when both coexist these effects are enhanced [7,8,10,38]. In our study, no significant differences were observed between women from the IG and CG in those with a BMI ≥ 25 kg/m^2 or with GDM. This could suggest that the nutritional intervention used in our study may not be strong enough to decrease the incidence of severe events in children, of high-risk mothers, at this age. A longer follow-up period may clarify whether these benefits can be observed in those born to high-risk mothers.

EVOO and pistachios, rich in phenolic components, are associated with a better anti-inflammatory, immunomodulatory and microbiota profile. In pregnancy, changes occur in the mother's immune system, affecting normal gut function and composition of the microbiota. These changes, which could also be affected by the mother's diet, could enhance the long-term health of the mother and her offspring [39–42].

Several limitations were found in our study. First, differences in diet between groups may have not been wide enough to induce changes in offspring health. Both groups (IG and CG) received recommendations based on the Mediterranean diet, reinforced or restricted in the consumption of fats. The differences obtained in the score of the questionnaires used between both groups were over two points during pregnancy, a difference that can be considered insufficient to detect statistically significant differences.

Secondly, a major limitation is that some data had to be completed through the register. This does not allow all data to be extracted in the same way. However, these data were always recorded by the same person, thus avoiding differences in data collection; therefore, it is unlikely that this could affect our results.

Lastly, breastfeeding, vaccination and other relevant factors within the first two years of life could have influenced the results. For instance, the rate of SGA and LGA newborns, although it is significantly lower in the IG, the number is small enough to affect our results. However, its effect in a wider cohort, or an older age, cannot be ruled out. Therefore, a follow-up at two-years of age may be insufficient to detect statistically significant differences in non-serious diseases at this age. Consequently, a study evaluating children at 5–6 years of age is ongoing.

Our results strengthen the recommendation to implement the MedDiet-reinforced with EVOO and pistachios-during pregnancy, since it also seems to provide health benefits for the offspring, at least in those born to low-risk women. Whether these results are sustained over the time, remains to be known.

5. Conclusions

A nutritional intervention based on the MedDiet during pregnancy seems to be associated with a reduction in the offspring's hospital admissions requiring antibiotic and corticosteroid treatment, and admissions related to asthma/bronchiolitis, especially in women who have pre-gestational BMI <25 kg/m^2 and NGT.

Supplementary Materials: The following are available online: http://www.mdpi.com/2077-0383/9/5/1454/s1. Table S1: Children's data at 2 years follow-up according to whether their mothers belonged to the intervention or control group, and subdivided according to glucose tolerance (GDM or NGT). Table S2: Children's data at 2 years follow-up according to whether their mothers belonged to the intervention or control group, and subdivided according to BMI (<25 kg/m^2 or ≥25 kg/m^2).

Author Contributions: V.M. and C.A.-B. contributed equally to this work; conceptualization: V.M., C.A.-B., N.G.d.l.T., E.B., A.D., I.R., M.P.d.M., C.M., A.B., M.C., M.A.H., M.A.R. and A.L.C.-P.; data curation: V.M., C.A.-B., I.J., L.d.V., J.V., C.F., A.B., M.A.H., N.I. and A.L.C.-P.; formal analysis: V.M., C.A.-B., N.G.d.l.T., I.J., E.B., A.B., M.A.R. and A.L.C.-P.; funding acquisition: N.G.d.l.T. and A.L.C.-P.; investigation: I.J., L.d.V., J.V., C.F., I.R., M.P.d.M., C.M., A.B., M.A.H., N.I. and A.L.C.-P.; methodology: I.J., L.d.V., J.V., C.F., I.R., M.P.d.M., C.M., A.B., M.A.H. and N.I.; supervision: M.C., M.A.R. and A.L.C.-P.; validation: A.L.C.-P.; visualization: A.L.C.-P.; writing—original draft: V.M., C.A.-B., N.G.d.l.T., A.D. and A.L.C.-P.; writing—review and editing: V.M., C.A.-B., N.G.d.l.T., A.D., M.A.R. and A.L.C.-P. A.L.C.-P. is the guarantor of this work and as such had full access to all the data in the study and takes responsibility for the integrity of the data and the accuracy of the data analysis. All authors have read and agreed to the published version of the manuscript.

Funding: This research was funded by grants from Fundación para Estudios Endocrinometabolicos, IdISSC Hospital Clínico San Carlos, Universidad Complutense of Madrid, Medicine Department; the Instituto de Salud Carlos III of Spain under grant number PI17/01442; (Plan Nacional de I + D + I, AES 2013–2016 subvencionado por el ISCIII y cofinanciado and Fondo Europeo de Desarrollo Regional (FEDER)). The design and conduct of the study; collection, management, analysis, and interpretation of the data; preparation, review, and approval of the manuscript; and decision to submit the manuscript for publication are the responsibilities of the authors alone and independent of the funders.

Acknowledgments: We wish to acknowledge our deep appreciation to the administrative personnel and nurses and dieticians from the Laboratory Department (Marisol Sanchez Orta, María Dolores Hermoso Martín, María Victoria Saez de Parayuelo, Luzdivina Fernandez Muñoz) and the Pregnancy and Diabetes Unit (Maria Luisa Santos Pesquera, and Georgina Cutillas Dominguez).

Conflicts of Interest: The authors declare no conflict of interest.

References

1. Zhang, Y.; Lin, J.; Fu, W.; Liu, S.; Gong, C.; Dai, J. Mediterranean diet during pregnancy and childhood for asthma in children: A systematic review and meta-analysis of observational studies. *Pediatr. Pulmonol.* **2019**, *54*, 949–961. [CrossRef] [PubMed]
2. Castro-Rodriguez, J.A.; Garcia-Marcos, L. What are the effects of a mediterranean diet on allergies and asthma in children? *Front. Pediatr.* **2017**, *5*, 72. [CrossRef] [PubMed]

3. Saunders, C.M.; Rehbinder, E.M.; Lødrup Carlsen, K.C.; Gudbrandsgard, M.; Carlsen, K.H.; Haugen, G.; Hedlin, G.; Jonassen, C.M.; Sjøborg, K.D.; Landrø, L.; et al. Food and nutrient intake and adherence to dietary recommendations during pregnancy: A nordic mother–child population-based cohort. *Food Nutr. Res.* **2019**, *63*. [CrossRef] [PubMed]
4. Hillesund, E.R.; Bere, E.; Sagedal, L.R.; Vistad, I.; Seiler, H.L.; Torstveit, M.K.; Øverby, N.C. Pre-pregnancy and early pregnancy dietary behavior in relation to maternal and newborn health in the norwegian fit for delivery study—A post hoc observational analysis. *Food Nutr. Res.* **2018**, *62*. [CrossRef]
5. Koletzko, B.; Brands, B.; Chourdakis, M.; Cramer, S.; Grote, V.; Hellmuth, C.; Kirchberg, F.; Prell, C.; Rzehak, P.; Uhl, O.; et al. The Power of Programming and the EarlyNutrition project: Opportunities for health promotion by nutrition during the first thousand days of life and beyond. *Ann. Nutr. Metab.* **2014**, *64*, 187–196. [CrossRef] [PubMed]
6. El Hajj, N.; Schneider, E.; Lehnen, H.; Haaf, T. Epigenetics and life-long consequences of an adverse nutritional and diabetic intrauterine environment. *Reproduction* **2014**, *148*, R111–R120. [CrossRef] [PubMed]
7. Lowe, W.L.; Scholtens, D.M.; Kuang, A.; Linder, B.; Lawrence, J.M.; Lebenthal, Y.; McCance, D.; Hamilton, J.; Nodzenski, M.; Talbot, O.; et al. Hyperglycemia and adverse Pregnancy Outcome follow-up study (HAPO FUS): Maternal gestational diabetes mellitus and childhood glucose metabolism. *Diabetes Care* **2019**, *42*, 372–380. [CrossRef]
8. Brown, F.M.; Isganaitis, E.; James-Todd, T. Much to HAPO FUS About: Increasing Maternal Glycemia in Pregnancy Is Associated With Worsening Childhood Glucose Metabolism. *Diabetes Care* **2019**, *42*, 393–395. [CrossRef]
9. Moses, R.G.; Cefalu, W.T. Considerations in theManagement of Gestational Diabetes Mellitus: "You Are What Your Mother Ate!". *Diabetes Care* **2016**, *39*, 13–15. [CrossRef]
10. Langer, O. Obesity or diabetes: Which is more hazardous to the health of the offspring? *J. Matern. Neonatal Med.* **2016**, *29*, 186–190. [CrossRef]
11. Forno, E.; Young, O.M.; Kumar, R.; Simhan, H.; Celedón, J.C. Maternal obesity in pregnancy, gestational weight gain, and risk of childhood asthma. *Pediatrics* **2014**, *134*, e5354–e5356. [CrossRef] [PubMed]
12. Polinski, K.J.; Liu, J.; Boghossian, N.S.; McLain, A.C. Maternal obesity, gestational weight gain, and asthma in offspring. *Prev. Chronic Dis.* **2017**, *14*, e109. [CrossRef] [PubMed]
13. Netting, M.J.; Middleton, P.F.; Makrides, M. Does maternal diet during pregnancy and lactation affect outcomes in offspring? A systematic review of food-based approaches. *Nutrition* **2014**, *30*, 1225–1241. [CrossRef] [PubMed]
14. Dumas, O.; Varraso, R.; Gillman, M.W.; Field, A.E.; Camargo, C.A. Longitudinal study of maternal body mass index, gestational weight gain, and offspring asthma. *Allergy Eur. J. Allergy Clin. Immunol.* **2016**, *71*, 1295–1304. [CrossRef] [PubMed]
15. Venter, C.; Brown, K.R.; Maslin, K.; Palmer, D.J. Maternal dietary intake in pregnancy and lactation and allergic disease outcomes in offspring. *Pediatr. Allergy Immunol.* **2017**, *28*, 135–143. [CrossRef] [PubMed]
16. Baïz, N.; Just, J.; Chastang, J.; Forhan, A.; De Lauzon-Guillain, B.; Magnier, A.M.; Annesi-Maesano, I. Maternal diet before and during pregnancy and risk of asthma and allergic rhinitis in children. *Allergy Asthma Clin. Immunol.* **2019**, *15*, 40. [CrossRef]
17. Tuokkola, J.; Luukkainen, P.; Tapanainen, H.; Kaila, M.; Vaarala, O.; Kenward, M.G.; Virta, L.J.; Veijola, R.; Simell, O.; Ilonen, J.; et al. Maternal diet during pregnancy and lactation and cow's milk allergy in offspring. *Eur. J. Clin. Nutr.* **2016**, *70*, 554–559. [CrossRef]
18. Rice, J.L.; Romero, K.M.; Galvez Davila, R.M.; Meza, C.T.; Bilderback, A.; Williams, D.L.; Breysse, P.N.; Bose, S.; Checkley, W.; Hansel, N.N.; et al. Association Between Adherence to the Mediterranean Diet and Asthma in Peruvian Children. *Lung* **2015**, *193*, 893–899. [CrossRef]
19. Griffiths, P.S.; Walton, C.; Samsell, L.; Perez, M.K.; Piedimonte, G. Maternal high-fat hypercaloric diet during pregnancy results in persistent metabolic and respiratory abnormalities in offspring. *Pediatr. Res.* **2016**, *79*, 278–286. [CrossRef]
20. Bédard, A.; Northstone, K.; Henderson, A.J.; Shaheen, S.O. Maternal intake of sugar during pregnancy and childhood respiratory and atopic outcomes. *Eur. Respir. J.* **2017**, *50*, 1700073. [CrossRef]
21. Azad, M.B.; Moyce, B.L.; Guillemette, L.; Pascoe, C.D.; Wicklow, B.; McGavock, J.M.; Halayko, A.J.; Dolinsky, V.W. Diabetes in pregnancy and lung health in offspring: Developmental origins of respiratory disease. *Paediatr. Respir. Rev.* **2017**, *21*, 19–26. [CrossRef] [PubMed]

22. H Al Wattar, B.; Dodds, J.; Placzek, A.; Beresford, L.; Spyreli, E.; Moore, A.; Gonzalez Carreras, F.J.; Austin, F.; Murugesu, N.; Roseboom, T.J.; et al. Mediterranean-style diet in pregnant women with metabolic risk factors (ESTEEM): A pragmatic multicentre randomised trial. *PLoS Med.* **2019**, *16*, e1002857. [CrossRef] [PubMed]
23. Assaf-Balut, C.; García De La Torre, N.; Durán, A.; Fuentes, M.; Bordiú, E.; Del Valle, L.; Familiar, C.; Ortolá, A.; Jiménez, I.; Herraiz, M.A.; et al. A Mediterranean diet with additional extra virgin olive oil and pistachios reduces the incidence of gestational diabetes mellitus (GDM): A randomized controlled trial: The St. Carlos GDM prevention study. *PLoS ONE* **2017**, *12*, e0185873. [CrossRef] [PubMed]
24. De La Torre, N.G.; Assaf-Balut, C.; Varas, I.J.; Del Valle, L.; Durán, A.; Fuentes, M.; Del Prado, N.; Bordiú, E.; Valerio, J.J.; Herraiz, M.A.; et al. Effectiveness of following mediterranean diet recommendations in the real world in the incidence of gestational diabetes mellitus (GDM) and adverse maternal-foetal outcomes: A prospective, universal, interventional study with a single group. the st carlos study. *Nutrients* **2019**, *11*, 1210. [CrossRef]
25. Assaf-Balut, C.; Garcia de la Torre, N.; Durán, A.; Bordiu, E.; del Valle, L.; Familiar, C.; Valerio, J.; Jimenez, I.; Herraiz, M.A.; Izquierdo, N.; et al. An Early, Universal Mediterranean Diet-Based Intervention in Pregnancy Reduces Cardiovascular Risk Factors in the "Fourth Trimester". *J. Clin. Med.* **2019**, *8*, 1499. [CrossRef]
26. Myrskylä, M.; Fenelon, A. Maternal Age and Offspring Adult Health: Evidence from the Health and Retirement Study. *Demography* **2012**, *49*, 1231–1257. [CrossRef]
27. Hinkle, S.N.; Albert, P.S.; Mendola, P.; Sjaarda, L.A.; Yeung, E.; Boghossian, N.S.; Laughon, S.K. The association between parity and birthweight in a longitudinal consecutive pregnancy cohort. *Paediatr. Perinat. Epidemiol.* **2014**, *28*, 106–115. [CrossRef]
28. Sonneveldt, E.; Decormier Plosky, W.; Stover, J. Linking high parity and maternal and child mortality: What is the impact of lower health services coverage among higher order births? *BMC Public Health* **2013**, *13*, S7. [CrossRef]
29. Moore Simas, T.A.; Waring, M.E.; Callaghan, K.; Leung, K.; Ward Harvey, M.; Buabbud, A.; Chasan-Taber, L. Weight gain in early pregnancy and risk of gestational diabetes mellitus among Latinas. *Diabetes Metab.* **2019**, *45*, 26–31. [CrossRef]
30. Assaf-Balut, C.; Familiar, C.; García de la Torre, N.; Rubio, M.A.; Bordiú, E.; Del Valle, L.; Lara, M.; Ruiz, T.; Ortolá, A.; Crespo, I.; et al. Gestational diabetes mellitus treatment reduces obesity-induced adverse pregnancy and neonatal outcomes: The St. Carlos gestational study. *BMJ Open Diabetes Res. Care* **2016**, *4*, e000314. [CrossRef]
31. Assaf-Balut, C.; García de la Torre, N.; Duran, A.; Fuentes, M.; Bordiú, E.; Del Valle, L.; Familiar, C.; Valerio, J.; Jiménez, I.; Herraiz, M.A.; et al. A Mediterranean Diet with an Enhanced Consumption of Extra Virgin Olive Oil and Pistachios Improves Pregnancy Outcomes in Women Without Gestational Diabetes Mellitus: A Sub-Analysis of the St. Carlos Gestational Diabetes Mellitus Prevention Study. *Ann. Nutr. Metab.* **2019**, *74*, 69–79. [CrossRef]
32. Amati, F.; Hassounah, S.; Swaka, A. The impact of mediterranean dietary patterns during pregnancy on maternal and offspring health. *Nutrients* **2019**, *11*, 1098. [CrossRef] [PubMed]
33. Gu, L.; Zhang, W.; Yang, W.; Liu, H. Systematic review and meta-analysis of whether cesarean section contributes to the incidence of allergic diseases in children: A protocol for systematic review and meta analysis. *Medicine* **2019**, *98*, e18394. [CrossRef] [PubMed]
34. Bozzola, E.; Bozzola, M.; Calcaterra, V.; Barberi, S.; Villani, A. Infectious diseases and vaccination strategies: How to protect the "unprotectable"? *ISRN Prev. Med.* **2013**, *2013*, e765354. [CrossRef] [PubMed]
35. Greer, F.R.; Sicherer, S.H.; Wesley Burks, A.; Abrams, S.A.; Fuchs, G.J.; Kim, J.H.; Wesley Lindsey, C.; Magge, S.N.; Rome, E.S.; Schwarzenberg, S.J. The effects of early nutritional interventions on the development of atopic disease in infants and children: The role of maternal dietary restriction, breastfeeding, hydrolyzed formulas, and timing of introduction of allergenic complementary foods. *Pediatrics* **2019**, *143*, e20190281. [CrossRef] [PubMed]
36. Gunderson, E.P.; Greenspan, L.C.; Faith, M.S.; Hurston, S.R.; Quesenberry, C.P. Breastfeeding and growth during infancy among offspring of mothers with gestational diabetes mellitus: A prospective cohort study. *Pediatr. Obes.* **2018**, *13*, 492–504. [CrossRef]

37. Fernández-Barrés, S.; Romaguera, D.; Valvi, D.; Martínez, D.; Vioque, J.; Navarrete-Muñoz, E.M.; Amiano, P.; Gonzalez-Palacios, S.; Guxens, M.; Pereda, E.; et al. Mediterranean dietary pattern in pregnant women and offspring risk of overweight and abdominal obesity in early childhood: The INMA birth cohort study. *Pediatr. Obes.* **2016**, *11*, 491–499. [CrossRef]
38. Lahti-Pulkkinen, M.; Bhattacharya, S.; Wild, S.H.; Lindsay, R.S.; Räikkönen, K.; Norman, J.E.; Bhattacharya, S.; Reynolds, R.M. Consequences of being overweight or obese during pregnancy on diabetes in the offspring: A record linkage study in Aberdeen, Scotland. *Diabetologia* **2019**, *62*, 1412–1419. [CrossRef]
39. Martín-Peláez, S.; Mosele, J.I.; Pizarro, N.; Farràs, M.; de la Torre, R.; Subirana, I.; Pérez-Cano, F.J.; Castañer, O.; Solà, R.; Fernandez-Castillejo, S.; et al. Effect of virgin olive oil and thyme phenolic compounds on blood lipid profile: Implications of human gut microbiota. *Eur. J. Nutr.* **2017**, *56*, 119–131. [CrossRef]
40. Hernández-Alonso, P.; Cañueto, D.; Giardina, S.; Salas-Salvadó, J.; Cañellas, N.; Correig, X.; Bulló, M. Effect of pistachio consumption on the modulation of urinary gut microbiota-related metabolites in prediabetic subjects. *J. Nutr. Biochem.* **2017**, *45*, 48–53. [CrossRef]
41. Edwards, S.M.; Cunningham, S.A.; Dunlop, A.L.; Corwin, E.J. The Maternal Gut Microbiome during Pregnancy. *Mcn Am. J. Matern. Nurs.* **2017**, *42*, 310–317. [CrossRef] [PubMed]
42. Dunlop, A.L.; Mulle, J.G.; Ferranti, E.P.; Edwards, S.; Dunn, A.B.; Corwin, E.J. Maternal Microbiome and Pregnancy Outcomes That Impact Infant Health: A Review. *Adv. Neonatal Care* **2015**, *15*, 377–385. [CrossRef] [PubMed]

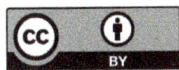

© 2020 by the authors. Licensee MDPI, Basel, Switzerland. This article is an open access article distributed under the terms and conditions of the Creative Commons Attribution (CC BY) license (http://creativecommons.org/licenses/by/4.0/).

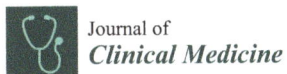

Review

Gestational Diabetes Mellitus and the Long-Term Risk for Glucose Intolerance and Overweight in the Offspring: A Narrative Review

Hannah Nijs [1] and Katrien Benhalima [2,*]

1. Medical school, University Hospital Gasthuisberg, KU Leuven, Herestraat 49, 3000 Leuven, Belgium; hannah.nijs@student.kuleuven.be
2. Department of Endocrinology, University Hospital Gasthuisberg, KU Leuven, Herestraat 49, 3000 Leuven, Belgium
* Correspondence: katrien.benhalima@uzleuven.be

Received: 7 January 2020; Accepted: 18 February 2020; Published: 22 February 2020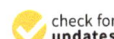

Abstract: Gestational diabetes mellitus (GDM) is a common condition with increasing prevalence worldwide. GDM is associated with an increased risk for maternal and neonatal complications. In this review we provide an overview of the most recent evidence on the long-term metabolic risk associated with GDM in the offspring. We conducted an extensive literature search on PubMed and Embase between February 2019 and December 2019. We performed a narrative review including 20 cohort studies, one cross-sectional study, and two randomized controlled trials. Our review shows that the prevalence of overweight/obesity and glucose intolerance is higher in children exposed to GDM compared to unexposed children. Maternal overweight is an important confounding factor, but recent studies show that in general the association remains significant after correction for maternal overweight. There is limited evidence suggesting that the association between GDM and adverse metabolic profile in the offspring becomes more significant with increasing offspring age and is also more pronounced in female offspring than in male offspring. More research is needed to evaluate whether treatment of GDM can prevent the long-term metabolic complications in the offspring.

Keywords: gestational diabetes mellitus; long-term metabolic outcome; offspring; overweight; obesity; adiposity; glucose intolerance; abnormal glucose tolerance; insulin resistance

1. Introduction

Gestational diabetes mellitus (GDM) is a worldwide public health problem. The prevalence is increasing due to delayed motherhood, the rising prevalence of obesity, and unhealthy lifestyles. The prevalence of GDM ranges from 1.8–31.5%, depending on the used diagnostic criteria and the population studied [1]. Since glucose crosses the placenta, GDM leads to fetal hyperglycemia, which in turn causes hyperinsulinemia. Since insulin acts as a growth hormone during pregnancy, this will induce macrosomia-related perinatal adverse outcomes [2]. In recent years, there is increasing evidence that intrauterine exposure to hyperglycemia also influences the long-term outcome of the offspring [3]. Many studies have shown that GDM increases the risk of glucose intolerance and overweight in the offspring [4]. However, it is less clear whether these associations are based on a direct relationship or are mediated by confounding factors such as maternal obesity. The use of different diagnostic criteria for GDM and the fact that not all studies have corrected for potential confounding factors, could partially explain the inconsistent results. In addition, the susceptibility to a potential effect of GDM may vary by age and gender of offspring. Further clarification is needed, since the prevalence of overweight and obesity in children is increasing [5,6]. These children are likely to become obese as adults and have an increased risk for diabetes and cardiovascular diseases [6–8]. It is therefore important to evaluate whether GDM is an independent risk factor and whether treatment of GDM can reduce the long-term metabolic risk in the offspring. We performed a review to evaluate whether GDM is an independent risk factor for glucose intolerance and overweight in the offspring. We included therefore studies evaluating the long-term metabolic risk in offspring from mothers with GDM compared to offspring of mothers with normal glucose tolerance. In addition, we determined whether the risk varied according to gender and age of the offspring.

2. Methods

2.1. Data Sources and Search Strategies

Between February 2019 and December 2019, a literature search was conducted on PubMed and Embase. We included studies published from 2000 onward. Cross-sectional studies, case-control studies, cohort studies, and randomized controlled trials (RCT) were considered for this review. This is a narrative review. We did not perform a systematic review and could therefore not perform a meta-analysis.

We used the following inclusion criteria:

1. The study population were offspring born to mothers with GDM (OGDM).
2. The control group could either be offspring of mothers with normal glucose tolerance (NGDM) or offspring of mothers with intensive (with insulin or other pharmacological treatment) treated GDM.
3. The following comparisons were made: the OGDM group was compared to the NGDM group or children of mothers with untreated GDM were compared to children of mothers with intensive treated GDM.
4. The different outcomes studied related to adiposity were overweight and obesity (defined by sex- and age-specific reference values according to the International Obesity Task Force, Centers of Disease Control and Prevention, World Health Organization, or local criteria), body fat percentage (BF%), waist circumference (WC), and body mass index (BMI). The outcomes studied related to glucose intolerance were abnormal glucose tolerance (AGT) and indices of insulin sensitivity and beta-cell function. AGT was defined as pre-diabetes or type 2 diabetes mellitus (T2DM). Pre-diabetes was defined as the presence of impaired fasting glucose (IFG) and/or impaired glucose tolerance (IGT). Insulin sensitivity was defined using the Matsuda index, a measurement of whole-body insulin sensitivity [9] or homeostatic model assessment of insulin sensitivity (HOMA-S), a measure of largely hepatic insulin sensitivity [10]. HOMA-S is defined as the reciprocal of insulin resistance (1/HOMA-IR) [10]. As measures of beta-cell function, the insulinogenic index and the disposition index (DI), were used [11,12]. DI was calculated by combining measurements of insulin secretion and sensitivity according to different formulas used in the included articles.

We excluded animal studies, descriptive designs (case series and case reports), studies that made no distinction between the different types of diabetes, studies with a low quality (no method section, no *p*-values mentioned, less than 100 participants), and articles written in a language other than English or French. We did not limit our search to a specific population or ethnicity or to a specific age category. We used the following search strategies:

1. PubMed: ("Diabetes, Gestational"[Mesh]) AND ("Child, Preschool"[Mesh] OR "Child"[Mesh] OR "Adolescent"[Mesh] OR "Adult Children"[Mesh]) AND (("Diabetes Mellitus, Type 2"[Mesh] OR "Blood Glucose"[Mesh] OR "Insulin/blood"[Mesh] OR "Insulin Resistance"[Mesh] OR "Hyperglycemia/blood"[Mesh] OR "Glucose Intolerance"[Mesh] OR "Prediabetic State"[Mesh]) OR ("Adiposity"[Mesh] OR "Body Mass Index"[Mesh] OR "Obesity"[Mesh] OR "Overweight"[Mesh]))
2. Embase: 'pregnancy diabetes mellitus'/exp AND 'progeny'/exp AND ('obesity'/exp OR 'body mass'/exp OR 'non insulin dependent diabetes mellitus'/exp OR 'glucose intolerance'/exp OR

'glucose blood level'/exp OR 'hyperglycaemia'/exp OR 'insulin resistance'/exp OR 'impaired glucose tolerance'/exp). We limited our search results by using the mapping option "Limit to terms indexed in article as major focus".

In addition to this, we hand-searched the reference lists of the selected articles and relevant reviews.

2.2. Data Synthesis and Analysis

The extracted data included the study design, location, age of follow-up, number of study participants, the GDM diagnosis criteria, adjustments that were made, and offspring outcomes. We reported our results in a descriptive manner. A *p*-value <0.05 was considered to be significant.

3. Results

3.1. Search Results

We identified 783 articles of which 123 articles were selected as possibly relevant. After examination of the full text, 23 studies were included in the current review (Figure 1).

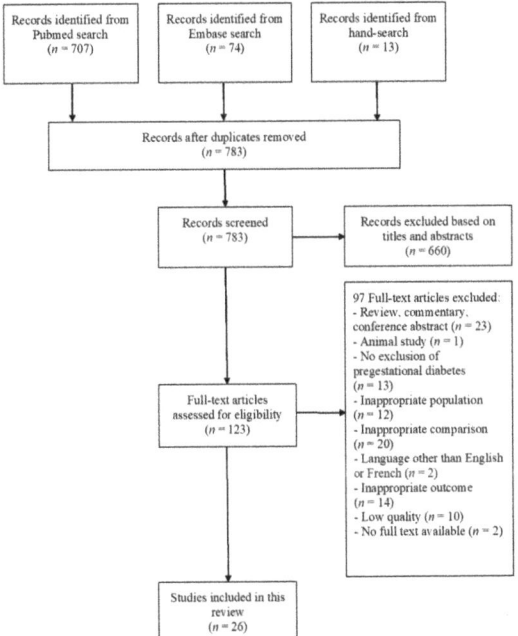

Figure 1. The literature search and selection process.

3.2. Study Characteristics

The study characteristics are shown in Table 1. In total, there were 15 prospective cohorts (65%), five retrospective cohorts (22%), one cross-sectional study (4%), and two RCTs (9%). Three studies were performed in Asia (13%), six studies in North America (26%), 11 in Europe (48%), one was performed in Oceania (4%), and two studies were multinational (9%). All 23 studies were published between 2003 and 2019, of which 19 studies (83%) were published from 2010 onward. The follow-up ranged from one to 27 years. In 13 studies (57%), the offspring was older than ten years. Only three studies (13%) evaluated the impact on adult offspring (>18 years). The sample size varied between 129 and 14,881 participants. Eighteen studies (78%) evaluated more than 500 children. Two studies used the

'International Association of Diabetes and Pregnancy Study Group' (IADPSG) criteria (9%), five studies used the Coustan and Carpenter criteria (22%), two studies the American Diabetes Association criteria (9%), three studies the Finnish Diabetes Association criteria (13%), one study the German Diabetes Association criteria (4%), three studies used local standards (13%), and three studies used multiple criteria for GDM (13%). In four studies (17%), no information was available about the diagnostic criteria used for GDM. Appendix A Table A1 gives an overview of the most commonly used diagnostic criteria for GDM across the different studies.

Table 1. The characteristics of included studies.

Author, Year	Design	Country	Subjects (N)	Age	GDM Criteria	Comparison
Lowe, 2019 [13] (HAPO cohort)	Prospective cohort study	Multinational	4775	10–14 y	IADPSG	Continuous measures of maternal glucose levels
Lowe, 2019 [14] (HAPO cohort)	Prospective cohort study	Multinational	4775	10–14 y	IADPSG	OGDM vs. NGDM
Scholtens, 2019 [15] (HAPO cohort)	Prospective cohort study	Multinational	4160	10–14 y	IADPSG	Continuous measures of maternal glucose levels
Lowe, 2018 [16] (HAPO cohort)	Prospective cohort study	Multi-national	4832	10–14 y	IADPSG	OGDM vs. NGDM
Kaseva, 2018 [8] (ESTER and AYLS cohort)	Prospective cohort study	Finland	700	22–25 y	Finnish Diabetes Association	OGDM vs. NGDM
Le Moullec, 2018 [17] (OBEGEST cohort)	Prospective cohort study	France	1251	5–7 y	C&C	OGDM vs. NGDM
Grunnet, 2017 [18] (Danish National Birth Cohort)	Prospective cohort study	Denmark	1158	9–16 y	Self-report and the Danish National Patient Register	OGDM vs. NGDM
Tam, 2017 [19] (HAPO cohort)	Prospective cohort study	China	926	7 y	IADPSG	OGDM vs. NGDM
Bider-Canfield, 2017 [20]	Retrospective cohort study	US	15,170	2 y	C&C	OGDM vs. NGDM
Zhao, 2016 [21]	Cross-sectional	Multi-national	4740	9–11 y	WHO 1999 and ADA	OGDM vs. NGDM
Landon, 2015 [22]	Randomized controlled trial	US	500	5–10 y	C&C	Treated OGDM vs. untreated OGDM
Kelstrup, 2013 [12]	Prospective cohort study	Denmark	295	18–27 y	Local (Denmark)*	OGDM vs. NGDM
Nehring, 2013 [23] (German Perinatal Prevention of Obesity cohort)	Retrospective cohort study	Germany	7355	5–6 y	ADA	OGDM vs. NGDM
Regnault, 2013 [24] (Viva cohort)	Prospective cohort study	US	839	7–9 y	C&C	OGDM vs. NGDM
Pham, 2013 [25]	Retrospective cohort study	US	2093	2–4 y	Until April 2007: NDDG After April 2007: C&C	OGDM vs. NGDM
Patel, 2012 [26]	Prospective cohort study	Great Britain	4861	15–16 y	Questionnaire	OGDM vs. NGDM
Boerschmann, 2010 [27]	Prospective cohort study	Germany	663	2 y, 8 y, 11 y	German Diabetes Association	OGDM vs. NGDM
Tam, 2010 [28]	Prospective cohort study	China	129	15 y	ADA	OGDM vs. NGDM
Pirkola, 2010 [29] (Northern Finland Birth Cohort)	Prospective cohort study	Finland	4168	7 y, 16 y	Finnish Diabetes Association	OGDM vs. NGDM
Gillman, 2010 [30] (ACHOIS cohort)	Randomized controlled trial	Australia	199	4–5 y	Local (Australia)**	Routine care control group vs. intervention group
Krishnaveni, 2010 [31]	Prospective cohort study	India	416	5 y, 9 y	C&C	OGDM vs. NGDM
Lawlor, 2010 [32] (ALSPAC cohort)	Prospective cohort study	Great Britain	6516	9–11 y	Medical records	OGDM vs. NGDM
Clausen, 2009 [33]	Retrospective cohort study	Denmark	296	18–27 y	Local (Denmark)*	OGDM vs. NGDM
Vääräsmäki, 2009 [34] (Northern Finland Birth cohort)	Prospective cohort study	Finland	4004	16 y	Finnish Diabetes Association	OGDM vs. NGDM
Hillier, 2007 [35]	Prospective cohort study	US	8152	5–7 y	C&C and NDDG	OGDM according to C&C criteria and OGDM according to NDGG criteria vs. NGDM
Gillman, 2003 [7]	Retrospective cohort study	US	14,881	9–14 y	Interview	OGDM vs. NGDM

GDM: gestational diabetes mellitus; OGDM: offspring of mothers with gestational diabetes; NGDM: offspring of mothers with normal glucose tolerance during pregnancy; HAPO: Hyperglycemia and Adverse Pregancy Outcome; ESTER: Maternal Pregnancy Disorders and Early-Life Programming of Adult Health and Disease; AYLS: Arvo Ylppö Longitudinal Study; OBEGEST: South Reunion Island cohort; ACHOIS: Australian Carbohydrate Intolerance Study in Pregnant Women; ALSPAC: Avon Longitudinal Study of Parents and Children; IADPSG: International Association of the Diabetes and Pregnancy Study Group; C&C: Carpenter and Coustan; WHO: World Health Organization; ADA: American Diabetes Association; NDDG: National Diabetes Data Group. * Local (Denmark): Two of seven values exceeded the mean + 3SD values for a reference group of normal-weight nonpregnant women without a family history of diabetes [36]. ** Local (Australia): Fasting plasma glucose <7.8 mmoL/L (<140 mg/dL) and 2 h plasma glucose between 7.8 mmoL/L (140 mg/dL) and 11 mmoL/L (198 mg/dL) after a 2 h 75 g oral glucose tolerance test; VS: versus.

3.3. Overweight and Obesity

The prevalence of overweight and obesity was higher in children exposed to GDM compared to the control group (Table 2). In the OGDM group, 21–40% of the children were overweight (including obesity) compared to 10.4–30% in the NGDM group, and 6.4–20.2% of the children were obese compared to 1.9–12.2% in the NGDM group.

Nine studies reported an odds ratio (OR) for overweight. Four studies showed a significantly increased OR of 1.44–2.29 for overweight in the OGDM group [16,19,23,33]. These four studies adjusted for maternal BMI, but after this adjustment, the result remained significant in only two studies [23,33]. Pirkola et al. showed a higher risk of overweight in the offspring of overweight GDM mothers, but not in the offspring of normal-weight mothers [29]. In contrast, Grunnet et al. demonstrated a significant higher BMI in the offspring of normal-weight GDM mothers (mean difference 5%, 95% CI 3–7%) but not in the offspring of underweight or overweight GDM mothers [18]. Hillier et al. demonstrated a significant increased OR of overweight in the offspring of mothers diagnosed with GDM based on the Carpenter and Coustan criteria (untreated women) but not in the offspring of mothers diagnosed with GDM based on the National Diabetes Data Group (treated women) criteria [35].

Five studies reported an OR for obesity. Four showed a significantly increased OR of 1.53–3.59 in the OGDM group. Three of these studies adjusted for maternal BMI and after adjustment the result remained significant in two studies [16,23]. Hillier et al. only showed a significant increased OR in the offspring of untreated women [35].

Seven studies evaluated the impact of GDM on the waist circumference. Four of them showed a significantly increased waist circumference in the OGDM group [16,21,23,34], of which three studies corrected for maternal BMI [16,21,23].

The Hyperglycemia and Adverse Pregnancy Outcome (HAPO) follow-up study evaluated 4832 children of untreated women (defined post hoc by the 2013 WHO criteria) 10–14 years after delivery. This study showed a continuous association between maternal glucose levels during pregnancy and a higher risk of adiposity [13]. Each standard deviation (SD) increase in maternal fasting plasma glucose (FPG) was associated with an increased risk of obesity and body fat percentage >85th percentile, but not with an increased risk of overweight or a high waist circumference. A higher maternal plasma glycemia level 60 and 120 min after an OGTT was related to an increased risk of all these adiposity outcomes. These results were independent of maternal BMI.

3.4. Glucose Intolerance

We included seven studies that investigated the impact of GDM on AGT and insulin resistance (IR) in the offspring (Table 3). Four of these studies did not correct for any confounding factor. Five studies evaluated AGT as a whole (IFG and/or IGT and/or T2DM). Three of these demonstrated an increased incidence of AGT in the OGDM group, with a total AGT prevalence of 21–41% in the OGDM group compared to 4–15.3% in the NGDM group [12,33,34]. This relationship seems linear related to rising glycemic values in pregnancy since Tam et al. demonstrated an OR for offspring's AGT of 1.85–2.00 for each SD increase in maternal glycemic level (adjusted for confounding factors including maternal weight and neonatal weight) [19].

Five studies investigated FPG separately. Only one study showed a significant higher FPG level in the OGDM group compared to the NGDM group (mean difference 4%, 95% CI 2–5%) [18]. In addition, the HAPO follow-up study showed an increased risk for IGT (OR 1.96, 95% CI 1.41–2.73) in the OGDM group and demonstrated that this increased risk was linear across the spectrum of maternal glucose levels during pregnancy [14,15]. This association was independent of maternal BMI, child BMI, and child's family history of diabetes.

Five studies evaluated indices of IR in the offspring. Four studies showed an increased IR in the OGDM group, defined by HOMA or the Matsuda index [12,14,18,34]. GDM was not associated with a decreased insulinogenic index in the offspring, although there was a significant decreased DI in the OGDM group [12,14,19]. The HAPO follow-up study showed an inverse continuous relationship between maternal pregnancy glucose levels and child insulin sensitivity and DI [15]. This association was attenuated, but remained significant, after adjustment for maternal BMI and/or child BMI.

Table 2. The impact of GDM on overweight and adiposity in the offspring.

Article	Age	Outcome	OR for One SD Increase in Maternal Glucose Value	p-Value	Adjusted for
Lowe, 2019 [13]	10–14 y	FPG	Overweight or obesity [a]		Field center, child pubertal status, maternal variables during pregnancy OGTT (age, height, any family history of diabetes, mean arterial pressure, parity, smoking, alcohol, gestational age, maternal BMI).
			1.05 (0.98, 1.14)	0.19	
		2 h glucose	1.09 (1.01, 1.17)	0.019	
			Obesity [a]		
		FPG	1.16 (1.05, 1.29)	0.005	
		2 h glucose	1.21 (1.09, 1.34)	<0.001	
			BF% >85th percentile		
		FPG	1.15 (1.05, 1.26)	0.002	
		2 h glucose	1.15 (1.06, 1.26)	0.001	
			WC >85th percentile		
		FPG	1.09 (0.99, 1.19)	0.067	
		2 h glucose	1.17 (1.07, 1.27)	0.003	

Article	Age	Outcome	OGDM	NGDM	p-Value[d]	Adjusted for
Lowe, 2018 [16]	10–14 y	Overweight or obesity [a]	39.50%	28.60%	0.05	Field center, child pubertal status, maternal variables during pregnancy OGTT (age, height, any family history of diabetes, mean arterial pressure, parity, smoking, alcohol, gestational age, maternal BMI).
		Obesity [a]	1.21 (1.00, 1.46)			
			19.10%	9.90%	<0.001	
		BF% >85th percentile	1.58 (1.24, 2.01)		0.68	
		WC >85th percentile	1.35 (1.08, 1.68)		0.009	
			1.34 (1.08, 1.67)			
Bider-Canfield, 2017 [20]	2 y	Overweight or obesity [b]	0.96 (0.83, 1.11)		NS	Pre-pregnancy BMI, excessive gestational weight gain.
Grunnet, 2017 [18]	9–16 y	Mean difference BMI (%)	4% (2, 6)		<0.0001	Offspring age, sex, maternal pre-pregnancy BMI
		Mean difference WC (cm)	0.52 (−0.06, 1.08)		0.08	
		Mean difference BF%	0.72% (−0.17, 1.61)		NS	
Tam, 2017 [19]	7 y	Overweight or obesity [b]	22.70%	15.30%	NS	Maternal age, parity, BMI before pregnancy, children's exercise level, current maternal and paternal DM status and children's age and/or sex.
		Obesity [b]	1.59 (0.97, 2.59)			
		Obesity [c]	8.40%	6.80%		
			18.40%	12%		
Zhao, 2016 [21]	9–11 y	WC ≥90th percentile	1.37 (0.92, 2.04)		0.13	Child age, education, infant feeding mode, gestational age, number of younger siblings, child unhealthy diet pattern scores, moderate-to-vigorous physical activity, sleeping time, sedentary time, sex, birth weight, current maternal BMI.
		BF% ≥90th percentile	1.54 (1.01, 2.35)		0.046	
			1.30 (0.81, 2.06)		0.29	
Nehring, 2013 [23]	5–6 y	Overweight or obesity [a]	1.81 (1.23, 2.65)	10.40%	<0.05	Maternal pre-pregnancy BMI, Large for gestational age maternal age, gestational weight gain, breastfeeding, socio-economic status, child's physical activity score, child's television viewing.
		Obesity [a]	8.20%	2.40%	<0.05	
		WC ≥90th percentile	2.80 (1.58, 4.99)		<0.05	
			1.64 (1.16, 2.33)			
Pham, 2013 [25]	2–4 y	Overweight or obesity [b]	23.90%		NS	Maternal age, height, race or ethnicity, child age.
			0.9 (0.7, 1.3)			

Table 2. Cont.

Article	Age	Outcome	OGDM	NGDM	p-Valued	Adjusted for
Patel, 2012 [26]	15–16 y	Overweight or obesity [a]	29.60% 0.54 (0.10, 3.03)	16.40%	NS	Sex, age, maternal age, manual social class, maternal smoking during pregnancy, parity, maternal pre-pregnancy BMI, gestational age, birth weight, mode of delivery.
		WC 90th percentile	0.90 (0.32, 2.52)		NS	
Lawlor, 2010 [32]	9–11 y	Overweight or obesity [a]	30% 0.62 (0.32, 1.23)	23%	NS	Sex, age, gestational age, height and height squared in models with fat mass as outcome, maternal age, social class, parity, smoking during pregnancy, mode of delivery, maternal pre-pregnancy BMI.
		WC ≥90th percentile	48% 1.00 (0.55, 1.85)	38%	NS	
Pirkola, 2010 [29]	16 y	Overweight or obesity [a]	Overweight mother: 4.05 (1.09, 8.62)		<0.001	Maternal overweight, maternal smoking status, paternal overweight, paternal smoking status, sex, birth weight.
			Normal weight mother: 0.73 (0.26, 2.08)		NS	
Clausen, 2009 [33]	18–27 y	Overweight or obesity [d]	40% 1.79 (1.00, 3.24)	24%	<0.05	Maternal age at delivery, maternal pregestational BMI, offspring age, family occupational social class, maternal hypertension at first visit.
		Overweight [e]	18.80%	8.40%		
		Obesity [e]	6.40%	1.90%		
Väärasmäki, 2009 [34]	16 y	WC ≥94 cm in men and ≥80 cm in women	3.10 (1.28, 7.52)		<0.05	Birth weight, gestational age and sex.
		C&C	2.71 (1.52, 4.82)		<0.05	
		Overweight [b]	34.70% 1.89 (1.30, 2.76)	23.50%	<0.05	
		Obesity [b]	20.20% 1.82 (1.15, 2.88)	12.20%	<0.05	
Hillier, 2007 [35]	5–7 y	NDDG				Maternal age, parity, weight gain during pregnancy, ethnicity, macrosomia at birth (>4,000 g), sex.
		Overweight [b]	27.80% 1.29 (0.85, 1.97)	23.50%	NS	
		Obesity [b]	17.30% 1.38 (0.84, 2.27)	12.20%	NS	
Gillman, 2003 [7]	9–14 y	Overweight [b]	17.10% 1.0 (0.7, 1.3)	14.20%	NS	Age, gender, tanner stage, television watching, physical activity, energy intake, breastfeeding duration, birth order, household income, mother's smoking, dietary restraint, weight cycling, weight concerns, birth weight, mother's current BMI.
		Obesity [b]	9.70% 1.2 (0.8, 1.7)	6.60%	NS	

Data are expressed as prevalence (%), odds ratio or mean differences (SD). We only mentioned the most adjusted data of each study. OGDM: offspring of mothers with gestational diabetes; NGDM: offspring of mothers with normal glucose tolerance during pregnancy; FPG: fasting plasma glucose; 2 h glucose: maternal glucose values 2 h after a 75 g OGTT; BF%: Body Fat Percentage; WC: waist circumference; BMI: Body Mass Index; C&C: Carpenter and Coustan; NDDG: National Diabetes Data Group; NS: not significant; OGTT: oral glucose tolerance test. a: According to sex- and age specific cut-offs based on the International Obesity Task Force. b: According to sex- and age specific BMI percentiles based on the Centers of Disease Control and Prevention. c: According to sex- and age specific BMI z-score based on the WHO growth reference. d: BMI ≥ 25 kg/m^2. e: BMI ≥ 30 kg/m^2. f: BMI ≥ 90th percentile adjusted for age and sex according to German reference data.

Table 3. The impact of GDM on glucose intolerance and insulin resistance in the offspring.

Article	Age	Outcome	OGDM	NGDM	p-Value	Adjusted for
Lowe, 2019 [14]	10–14 y	FPG (mmol/L)	5.1 (4.7, 5.5)	5.0 (4.6, 5.4)	NS	Field center, child age, child sex, pubertal status, maternal variables at pregnancy OGTT (age, height, mean arterial pressure, parity, smoking, drinking, gestational age), child's family history of diabetes in first-degree relatives, maternal BMI at pregnancy OGTT, child's BMI z-score.
		IFG [a]	9.20%	7.40%	NS	
		IGT [a]	1.09 (0.78, 1.52)		0.61	
			10.60%	5.00%		
		RC Matsuda index [d]	1.96 (1.41, 2.73)		<0.001	
		RC Insulinogenic index [f]	−76.3 (−130.3, −22.4)		0.0063	
		RC Disposition index [g]	−0.06 (−0.12, 0.003)		0.061	
		FPG (mmol/L)	−0.12 (−0.17, −0.064)		<0.0001	
Grunnet, 2017 [18]	9–16 y	Mean difference FPG (%)	5.0 (4.2, 5.8)	4.8 (4.2, 5.4)	<0.001	Age, sex, offspring BMI, maternal pre-pregnancy BMI.
		HOMA-IR [h]	4% (2, 5)			
		Mean difference HOMA-IR (%)	2.2 (0.6, 3.8)	1.9 (0.8, 3)	0.02	
			8% (1, 16%)			
Tam, 2017 [19]	7 y	FPG (mmol/L)	4.57 (4.22, 4.92)	4.64 (4.15, 5.13)	0.12	No adjustments made
		IFG and/or IGT [a]	3.90%	1.70%	0.04	
		DM type II [a]	0.80%	0%	0.04	
		Matsuda index [c]	15.0 (6.7, 23.3)	16.2 (7.3, 25.1)	0.14	
		Insulinogenic index [e]	67.8 (2.8, 132.8)	81 (−13.2, 175.2)	0.05	
		Oral disposition index [i]	6.6 (0.7, 12.6)	7.9 (−1.5, 17.4)	0.04	
		IFG [b] and/or IGT [b] and/or DM type II [b]	21%	4%	<0.0001	
Kelstrup, 2013 [12]	18–27 y	HOMA-IR [h]	10.53 (9.58, 11.57)	8.47 (7.71, 9.31)	<0.05	No adjustments made
		Insulinogenic index [e]	86.9 (76.6, 96.4)	90.3 (80.1, 101.9)	NS	
		Disposition index [j]	15,743 (13877, 17861)	24,820 (22197, 27752)	<0.05	
Tam, 2010 [28]	15 y	FPG (mmol/L)	4.6 (4.3, 4.9)	4.7 (4.4, 5.0)	0.51	No adjustments made
		IFG [a] and/or IGT [a] and/or DM type II [a]	11.90%	10.30%	0.77	
Vääräsmäki, 2009 [34]	16 y	FPG (mmol/L)	5.30 (5.00, 5.50)	5.10 (4.90, 5.40)	NS	Birth weight, gestational age, sex, current BMI
		IFG [a] and/or IGT [a] and/or DM type II [a]	23.60%	15.30%		
		HOMA-S [h]	1.63 (0.97, 2.74)		<0.05	
Clausen, 2009 [33]	18–27 y	IFG [a] and/or IGT [a] and/or DM type II [a]	74.7 (54.1, 91.2)	82.3 (64.0, 104.7)	NS	No adjustments made
			41%	10%	<0.05	

The outcomes "Impaired Fasting Glucose", "Impaired Glucose Tolerance" and "Diabetes Mellitus Type II" are expressed as prevalence (%) or odds ratio's. The other data are mean (SD), unless specified otherwise. OGDM: offspring of mothers with gestational diabetes; NGDM: offspring of mothers with normal glucose tolerance during pregnancy; FPG: Fasting Plasma Glucose; OGTT: oral glucose tolerance test; IFG: Impaired Fasting Glucose; IGT: Impaired Glucose Tolerance; RC: Regression Coefficient; HOMA-IR: Homeostatic Model Assessment of Insulin Resistance; DM type II: Diabetes Mellitus type II; HOMA-S: Homeostatic Model Assessment of Insulin Sensitivity; NS: not significant. a: According to the American Diabetes Association diagnostic criteria. b: According to the World Health Organization criteria of 1999. c: According to the formula described by Matsuda [9]. d: Modified Matsuda index [14]. e: According to the formula described by Phillips [11]. f: Modified Insulinogenic index [14]. g: Log transformed: Matsuda index x insulinogenic index [14]. h: According to the formula described by Matthews [10]. i: Insulinogenic index x Matsuda index [19]. j: Corrected insulin response x Matsuda index [12].

3.5. Age

Only two studies examined different age categories. One study observed an increased incidence of overweight in 8- and 11-year-old OGDM but not in 2-year-old OGDM, while the other study showed an increased HOMA-IR in 9.5-year-old OGDM but not in 5-year-old OGDM [27,31]. Of all five studies evaluating young children, only one study showed an increased risk of overweight or obesity in OGDM <10 years. In contrast, of all nine studies evaluating older children, five studies showed an increased risk of overweight or obesity in OGDM ≥10 years. Only one study examined the impact on glucose intolerance in offspring <10 years and showed a significant increased risk of AGT in the OGDM group [19].

3.6. Sex Differences

Of all studies, only seven studies evaluated possible sex differences. Four studies showed a significant increase in adiposity measures in 7–25-year-old girls, but not in boys, when exposed to intrauterine GDM. Girls from mothers with GDM had a significantly higher prevalence of overweight (22.7% vs. 13.0%, $p = 0.03$) [19], higher BMI (16.4 kg/m^2 vs. 14.3 kg/m^2, $p <0.001$) [31], and higher waist circumference [8,21]. In contrast, only one study showed an OR for overweight of 2.34 (95% CI 1.26–4.34) in 5–7-year-old male OGDM and no increased risk in females [17]. Another study showed no difference in both waist circumference and BMI, irrespective of gender [24]. Only one study examined the differences in sex with regard to glucose intolerance and insulin resistance [31]. This study showed a significant increased IR and plasma glucose levels 30 min after OGTT in 9.5-year-old female OGDM but not in males.

3.7. Can Treatment of GDM Reduce the Long-Term Metabolic Complications in the Offspring?

Two RCT's have shown that treatment of GDM lowers the risk of perinatal adverse outcomes [37,38]. The 'Australian Carbohydrate Intolerance Study in Pregnant Women' (ACHOIS) was an RCT in women with GDM based on the 1999 WHO criteria [38]. The Landon RCT was a multicenter study that randomly assigned 958 American woman who met the criteria for mild GDM (FPG <5.3 mmol/L; two abnormal values after a 100 g OGTT according to the Carpenter and Coustan criteria) into a treatment group and a control group and compared the infants of both groups [37]. The follow-up study of ACHOIS was conducted in 4–5-year-old offspring of women who lived in the state of South Australia and were checked by a health care program at kindergartens and preschools (resulting in 199 children, 19% of the original cohort) [30]. Treatment of GDM did not result in a change in BMI. The Landon follow-up study evaluated the treatment effect of GDM on BMI in 500 children (52% of the original cohort), aged 5–10 years [22]. Treatment was also not associated with a reduction in childhood obesity. However, a subanalysis showed higher rates of IFG in girls of mothers in the control group compared to the treatment group (12.1% vs. 2.9%, $p = 0.02$). In addition, treatment of GDM was associated with a decreased frequency of HOMA-IR in female offspring (1.05 vs. 1.30, $p = 0.04$). These results were adjusted for race/ethnicity and maternal baseline BMI.

4. Discussion

4.1. Summary of Findings

In the current review, we show that there is increasing evidence that offspring of mothers with GDM are at increased risk for overweight and glucose intolerance and that this risk is independent of maternal overweight. In addition, recent studies, such as the HAPO follow-up study, also demonstrated a linear relationship between rising maternal glucose levels during pregnancy and the risk for overweight and AGT in the offspring.

4.2. Results in Relation to What We Already Know

In recent years, there is increasing evidence that GDM is associated with an increased risk for overweight and AGT in the offspring [4]. However, it remained less clear whether these associations are based on a direct relationship or whether they are mediated by confounding factors. Maternal overweight is a well-known confounding factor, likely due to shared genes and environment [39]. In this review, we aimed to investigate whether GDM is a risk factor independent of maternal BMI.

We showed that the association between GDM and offspring overweight or obesity is frequently attenuated after adjustment for maternal BMI, but that the association remained significant in recent, large studies. The HAPO follow-up study even showed a continuous relationship between maternal glycemia levels during pregnancy and childhood adiposity outcomes [14]. This study was not confounded by treatment of maternal hyperglycemia, since only women with glucose levels below those diagnostic of diabetes were included. In line with these results, the Hillier study showed an increased OR for overweight and obesity in the offspring of women with untreated GDM and no increased OR in the offspring of women with treated GDM [35]. Previous studies have shown that the combination of maternal overweight and maternal GDM has a greater impact on adverse pregnancy outcomes than either one alone [40]. In this review, we found evidence for a comparable result concerning the impact on childhood overweight. One study showed that prenatal exposure to maternal overweight combined with GDM conveyed a greater risk of childhood overweight than exposure to one of these alone [29]. Therefore, adjustment for maternal overweight may mask this potential synergistic relationship [21]. Additional adjustment for birth weight, smoking during pregnancy, prolonged breastfeeding, and socioeconomic variables did not significantly change the results. The mechanisms by which GDM might influence childhood overweight are not fully known. Fetal hyperinsulinemia during critical periods may induce leptin resistance (leptin is a hormone that reduces food intake and increases energy expenditure) [39]. Furthermore, intrauterine exposure to GDM may influence the expression of genes that direct the accumulation of body fat through epigenetic changes [21].

Of all 23 studies included in our review, only seven studies investigated the long-term risk for AGT in the offspring after GDM. Most studies confirmed that GDM was associated with an increased prevalence of AGT in the OGDM group. Only two studies showed no effect, of which one was most likely underpowered [28]. The HAPO follow-up study demonstrated an increased childhood prevalence of IGT, but not of IFG, independent of maternal BMI and childhood BMI. This finding is in line with a recent large meta-analysis [41]. It indicates that IFG and IGT may need to be considered as two distinct pathophysiologic conditions [42,43]. In addition, our review showed that GDM is associated with an increased IR and a low DI in the offspring of GDM mothers [12,14,18,34]. A low DI suggests that there is insufficient beta-cell compensation for the higher IR, and this is seen in children with a high risk to progress to T2DM [12,14].

Studies suggested that the long-term effect of GDM may not become apparent until early adolescence [44]. In this review, we confirm that the risk of childhood overweight seems higher in children >10 years, however, only two studies specifically examined different age categories.

There is limited evidence from subgroup analysis that the risk of childhood overweight and AGT is higher in female offspring compared to male offspring, but only seven studies evaluated possible sex differences. Previous research has shown that women carrying a male fetus have a 4% increased risk of developing GDM compared to women carrying a female fetus. Women developing GDM with a female fetus, therefore probably have more underlying IR and/or impaired insulin secretion, which might lead to an increased risk for long-term metabolic complications [45].

The intervention RCTs in pregnancy have shown that treatment of GDM reduces the risk for adverse pregnancy outcomes. However, follow-up studies of both RCTs showed no significant difference in the risk of childhood obesity in offspring of women who were treated for GDM compared to the untreated group. Therefore, there is currently no evidence that treatment of GDM can prevent the long-term metabolic complications in the offspring. However, the follow-up of these studies was limited to a maximum of ten years, only a subgroup of the offspring was evaluated, and the impact might also be more pronounced in offspring of mothers with more severe GDM.

4.3. Novelty and Practical Implications

Our review provides an updated extensive overview on the impact of GDM on the long-term metabolic risks in the offspring. In contrast to other recent reviews [46,47], we specifically assessed the impact of different confounders such as maternal BMI and the impact of age and sex of the offspring on the associated risk of GDM with overweight and AGT. Our review has several implications for clinical practice. First, we show that there is now increasing evidence that GDM is associated with an increased risk for overweight, IR, and AGT in the offspring, independent of maternal BMI. This highlights the importance to start early after delivery with follow-up in offspring of mothers with GDM to prevent and timely detect metabolic complications in this high-risk group. In addition, there is some evidence suggesting that girls have a higher risk for these long-term metabolic complications than boys. As childhood overweight is associated with a higher risk of being overweight as an adult, and an increased IR and low DI are early expressions of ATG, timely detection and treatment of GDM might reduce these long-term metabolic complications in the offspring [12]. However, larger and longer follow-up studies are needed to evaluate a potential treatment benefit. Increased awareness is needed to stimulate a sustained healthy lifestyle for the whole family starting early after delivery.

4.4. Strengths and Limitations

We provide an extensive narrative review on the long-term metabolic risk in offspring associated with GDM. We specifically assessed the impact of different confounders such as maternal BMI and the impact of age and sex of the offspring on the associated risk of GDM with overweight and AGT. However, our review had several limitations. We did not perform a systematic review and could not perform a meta-analysis because of the heterogeneity of studies. We did not asses the risk of bias of individual studies and did not contact the authors for obtaining missing and unpublished data. Most studies used definitions for overweight and obesity based on BMI and more detailed parameters on adiposity were often lacking. In addition, some studies corrected for current maternal BMI instead of pre-gestational maternal BMI. However, an acceptable correlation between these two BMI values has been reported [48]. Only two studies corrected for paternal diabetes, ten studies corrected for socioeconomic variables, and four studies corrected for lifestyle behaviors. Most studies investigating the impact on AGT did not correct for any confounding factor. Due to the small prevalence of T2DM in the offspring, AGT was reported instead of T2DM alone. Since the majority of included studies were cohort studies (with only two RCTs), we could not determine a causal relationship of the reported associations.

5. Conclusions

Our review shows that intrauterine exposure to GDM increases the risk of overweight and AGT in the offspring, independent of maternal BMI. Screening for GDM might therefore also offer a window of opportunity to prevent or reduce the risk for long-term metabolic complications in the offspring by increasing the awareness for a healthy lifestyle in this high-risk group. It remains unclear whether treatment of GDM can reduce the long-term risk of adverse metabolic complications in the offspring.

Author Contributions: H.N. and K.B. wrote the manuscript. All authors agree to the published version of the manuscript.

Acknowledgments: K.B. is the recipient of a "Fundamenteel Klinisch Navorserschap FWO Vlaanderen".

Conflicts of Interest: The authors declare no conflict of interest.

Appendix A

Table A1. This list gives an overview of the most commonly used gestational diabetes mellitus diagnosis criteria.

Criteria	OGTT	FPG	1 h	2 h	3 h	Number of Abnormal Values
C&C	100 g	≥5.3 mmol/L (=95 mg/dL)	≥10 mmol/L (=180 mg/dL)	≥8.6 mmol/L (=155 mg/dL)	≥7.8 mmol/L (=140 mg/dL)	≥2
NDDG	100 g	≥5.8 mmol/L (=105 mg/dL)	≥10.5 mmol/L (=190 mg/dL)	≥9 mmol/L (=165 mg/dL)	≥8 mmol/L (=145 mg/dL)	≥2
IADPSG, WHO 2013	75 g	≥5.1 mmol/L (=92 mg/dL)	≥10 mmol/L (=180 mg/dL)	≥8.5 mmol/L (=153 mg/dL)		≥1
ADA	100 g	≥5.3 mmol/L (=95 mg/dL)	≥10 mmol/L (=180 mg/dL)	≥8.6 mmol/L (=155 mg/dL)	≥7.8 mmol/L (=140 mg/dL)	≥2
WHO 1999	75 g	≥7 mmol/L (=126 mg/dL)		≥7.8 mmol/L (=140 mg/dL)		≥1
German Diabetes Association	75 g	>5 mmol/L (=90 mg/dL)	>10 mmol/L (=180 mg/dL)	>8.6 mmol/L (=155 mg/dL)		≥2
Finnish Diabetes Association	75 g	>5.5 mmol/L (=99 mg/dL)	>11.0 mmol/L (=198 mg/dL)	>8.0 mmol/L (=144 mg/dL)		≥1

OGTT: oral glucose tolerance test; FPG: fasting plasma glucose; C&C: Carpenter and Coustan; NDDG: National Diabetes Data Group; IADPSG: International Association of the Diabetes and Pregnancy Study Groups; ADA: American Diabetes Association; WHO: World Health Organization.

References

1. Zhu, Y.; Zhang, C. Prevalence of Gestational Diabetes and Risk of Progression to Type 2 Diabetes: A Global Perspective. *Curr. Diab. Rep.* **2016**, *16*, 7. [CrossRef] [PubMed]
2. Kc, K.; Shakya, S.; Zhang, H. Gestational Diabetes Mellitus and Macrosomia: A Literature Review. *Ann. Nutr. Metab.* **2015**, *66*, 14–20. [CrossRef] [PubMed]
3. Damm, P. Future Risk of Diabetes in Mother and Child after Gestational Diabetes Mellitus. *Int. J. Gynecol. Obstet.* **2009**, *104*, 2008–2009. [CrossRef]
4. Dabelea, D. The Predisposition to Obesity and Diabetes in Offspring of Diabetic Mothers. *Diabetes Care* **2007**, *30* Suppl. 2, S169–S174. [CrossRef]
5. Wu, J.F. Childhood Obesity: A Growing Global Health Hazard Extending to Adulthood. *Pediatr. Neonatol.* **2013**, *54*, 71–72. [CrossRef] [PubMed]
6. Ng, M.; Fleming, T.; Robinson, M.; Thomson, B.; Graetz, N.; Margono, C.; Mullany, E.C.; Biryukov, S.; Abbafati, C.; Abera, S.F.; et al. Global, Regional, and National Prevalence of Overweight and Obesity in Children and Adults during 1980–2013: A Systematic Analysis for the Global Burden of Disease Study 2013. *Lancet* **2014**, *384*, 766–781. [CrossRef]
7. Gillman, M.W.; Rifas-Shiman, S.; Berkey, C.S.; Field, A.E.; Colditz, G.A. Maternal Gestational Diabetes, Birth Weight, and Adolescent Obesity. *Pediatrics* **2003**, *111*, e221–e226. [CrossRef]
8. Kaseva, N.; Vääräsmäki, M.; Matinolli, H.M.; Sipola-Leppänen, M.; Tikanmäki, M.; Heinonen, K.; Lano, A.; Wolke, D.; Andersson, S.; Järvelin, M.R.; et al. Pre-Pregnancy Overweight or Obesity and Gestational Diabetes as Predictors of Body Composition in Offspring Twenty Years Later: Evidence from Two Birth Cohort Studies. *Int. J. Obes.* **2018**, *42*, 872–879. [CrossRef]
9. Matsuda, M.; DeFronzo, R.A. Insulin Sensitivity Indices Obtained from Oral Glucose Tolerance Testing: Comparison with the Euglycemic Insulin Clamp. *Diabetes Care* **1999**, *22*, 1462–1470. [CrossRef]
10. Matthews, D.R.; Hosker, J.P.; Rudenski, A.S.; Naylor, B.A.; Treacher, D.F.; Turner, R.C. Homeostasis Model Assessment: Insulin Resistance and β-Cell Function from Fasting Plasma Glucose and Insulin Concentrations in Man. *Diabetologia* **1985**, *28*, 412–419. [CrossRef]
11. Phillips, D.I.W.; Clark, P.M.; Hales, C.N.; Osmond, C. Understanding Oral Glucose Tolerance: Comparison of Glucose or Insulin Measurements During the Oral Glucose Tolerance Test with Specific Measurements of Insulin Resistance and Insulin Secretion. *Diabet. Med.* **1994**, *11*, 286–292. [CrossRef] [PubMed]
12. Kelstrup, L.; Damm, P.; Mathiesen, E.R.; Hansen, T.; Vaag, A.A.; Pedersen, O.; Clausen, T.D. Insulin Resistance and Impaired Pancreatic β-Cell Function in Adult Offspring of Women with Diabetes in Pregnancy. *J. Clin. Endocrinol. Metab.* **2013**, *98*, 3793–3801. [CrossRef] [PubMed]
13. Lowe, W.L.; Lowe, L.P.; Kuang, A.; Catalano, P.M.; Nodzenski, M.; Talbot, O.; Tam, W.H.; Sacks, D.A.; McCance, D.; Linder, B.; et al. Maternal Glucose Levels during Pregnancy and Childhood Adiposity in the Hyperglycemia and Adverse Pregnancy Outcome Follow-up Study. *Diabetologia* **2019**, *62*, 598–610. [CrossRef] [PubMed]
14. Lowe, W.L.; Scholtens, D.M.; Kuang, A.; Linder, B.; Lawrence, J.M.; Lebenthal, Y.; McCance, D.; Hamilton, J.; Nodzenski, M.; Talbot, O.; et al. Hyperglycemia and Adverse Pregnancy Outcome Follow-up Study (HAPO FUS): Maternal Gestational Diabetes Mellitus and Childhood Glucose Metabolism. *Diabetes Care* **2019**, *42*, 372–380. [CrossRef]
15. Scholtens, D.M.; Kuang, A.; Lowe, L.P.; Hamilton, J.; Lawrence, J.M.; Lebenthal, Y.; Brickman, W.J.; Clayton, P.; Ma, R.C.; McCance, D.; et al. Hyperglycemia and Adverse Pregnancy Outcome Follow-up Study (HAPO FUS): Maternal Glycemia and Childhood Glucose Metabolism. *Diabetes Care* **2019**, *42*, 381–392. [CrossRef]
16. Lowe, W.L.; Scholtens, D.M.; Lowe, L.P.; Kuang, A.; Nodzenski, M.; Talbot, O.; Catalano, P.M.; Linder, B.; Brickman, W.J.; Clayton, P.; et al. Association of Gestational Diabetes with Maternal Disorders of Glucose Metabolism and Childhood Adiposity. *JAMA* **2018**, *320*, 1005–1016. [CrossRef]
17. Le Moullec, N.; Fianu, A.; Maillard, O.; Chazelle, E.; Naty, N.; Schneebeli, C.; Gérardin, P.; Huiart, L.; Charles, M.A.; Favier, F. Sexual Dimorphism in the Association between Gestational Diabetes Mellitus and Overweight in Offspring at 5–7 Years: The OBEGEST Cohort Study. *PLoS ONE* **2018**, *13*, 1–14. [CrossRef]

18. Grunnet, L.G.; Hansen, S.; Hjort, L.; Madsen, C.M.; Kampmann, F.B.; Thuesen, A.C.B.; Granstrømi, C.; Strøm, M.; Maslova, E.; Frikke-Schmidt, R.; et al. Adiposity, Dysmetabolic Traits, and Earlier Onset of Female Puberty in Adolescent Offspring of Women with Gestational Diabetes Mellitus: A Clinical Study within the Danish National Birth Cohort. *Diabetes Care* **2017**, *40*, 1746–1755. [CrossRef]
19. Tam, W.H.; Ma, R.C.W.; Ozaki, R.; Li, A.M.; Chan, M.H.M.; Yuen, L.Y.; Lao, T.T.H.; Yang, X.; Ho, C.S.; Tutino, G.E.; et al. In Utero Exposure to Maternal Hyperglycemia Increases Childhood Cardiometabolic Risk in Offspring. *Diabetes Care* **2017**, *40*, 679–686. [CrossRef]
20. Bider-Canfield, Z.; Martinez, M.P.; Wang, X.; Yu, W.; Bautista, M.P.; Brookey, J.; Page, K.A.; Buchanan, T.A.; Xiang, A.H. Maternal Obesity, Gestational Diabetes, Breastfeeding and Childhood Overweight at Age 2 Years. *Pediatr. Obes.* **2017**, *12*, 171–178. [CrossRef]
21. Zhao, P.; Liu, E.; Qiao, Y.; Katzmarzyk, P.T.; Chaput, J.P.; Fogelholm, M.; Johnson, W.D.; Kuriyan, R.; Kurpad, A.; Lambert, E.V.; et al. Maternal Gestational Diabetes and Childhood Obesity at Age 9–11: Results of a Multinational Study. *Diabetologia* **2016**, *59*, 2339–2348. [CrossRef] [PubMed]
22. Landon, M.B.; Rice, M.M.; Varner, M.W.; Casey, B.M.; Reddy, U.M.; Wapner, R.J.; Rouse, D.J.; Biggio, J.R.; Thorp, J.M.; Chien, E.K.; et al. Mild Gestational Diabetes Mellitus and Long-Term Child Health. *Diabetes Care* **2015**, *38*, 445–452. [CrossRef] [PubMed]
23. Nehring, I.; Chmitorz, A.; Reulen, H.; von Kries, R.; Ensenauer, R. Gestational Diabetes Predicts the Risk of Childhood Overweight and Abdominal Circumference Independent of Maternal Obesity. *Diabet. Med.* **2013**, *30*, 1449–1456. [CrossRef] [PubMed]
24. Regnault, N.; Gillman, M.W.; Rifas-Shiman, S.L.; Eggleston, E.; Oken, E. Sex-Specific Associations of Gestational Glucose Tolerance with Childhood Body Composition. *Diabetes Care* **2013**, *36*, 3045–3053. [CrossRef]
25. Pham, M.T.; Brubaker, K.; Pruett, K.; Caughey, A.B. Risk of Childhood Obesity in the Toddler Offspring of Mothers with Gestational Diabetes. *Obstet. Gynecol.* **2013**, *121*, 976–982. [CrossRef]
26. Patel, S.; Fraser, A.; Smith, G.D.; Lindsay, R.S.; Sattar, N.; Nelson, S.M.; Lawlor, D.A. Associations of Gestational Diabetes, Existing Diabetes, and Glycosuria with Offspring Obesity and Cardiometabolic Outcomes. *Diabetes Care* **2012**, *35*, 63–71. [CrossRef]
27. Boerschmann, H.; Pflüger, M.; Henneberger, L.; Ziegler, A.G.; Hummel, S. Prevalence and Predictors of Overweight and Insulin Resistance in Offspring of Mothers with Gestational Diabetes Mellitus. *Diabetes Care* **2010**, *33*, 1845–1849. [CrossRef]
28. Tam, W.H.; Ma, R.C.W.; Yang, X.; Li, A.M.; Ko, G.T.C.; Kong, A.P.S.; Lao, T.T.H.; Chan, M.H.M.; Lam, C.W.K.; Chan, J.C.N. Glucose Intolerance and Cardiometabolic Risk in Adolescents Exposed to Maternal Gestational Diabetes: A 15-Year Follow-up Study. *Diabetes Care* **2010**, *33*, 1382–1384. [CrossRef]
29. Pirkola, J.; Pouta, A.; Bloigu, A.; Hartikainen, A.L.; Laitinen, J.; Järvelin, M.R.; Vääräsmäki, M. Risks of Overweight and Abdominal Obesity at Age 16 Years Associated with Prenatal Exposures to Maternal Prepregnancy Overweight and Gestational Diabetes Mellitus. *Diabetes Care* **2010**, *33*, 1115–1121. [CrossRef]
30. Gillman, M.W.; Oakey, H.; Baghurst, P.A.; Volkmer, R.E.; Robinson, J.S.; Crowther, C.A. Effect of Treatment of Gestational Diabetes Mellitus on Obesity in the next Generation. *Diabetes Care* **2010**, *33*, 964–968. [CrossRef]
31. Krishnaveni, G.V.; Veena, S.R.; Hill, J.C.; Kehoe, S.; Karat, S.C.; Fall, C.H.D. Intrauterine Exposure to Maternal Diabetes Is Associated With Higher Adiposity and Insulin Resistance and Clustering of Cardiovascular Risk Markers in Indian Children. *Diabetes Care* **2010**, *33*, 402–404. [CrossRef] [PubMed]
32. Lawlor, D.A.; Fraser, A.; Lindsay, R.S.; Ness, A.; Dabelea, D.; Catalano, P.; Davey Smith, G.; Sattar, N.; Nelson, S.M. Association of Existing Diabetes, Gestational Diabetes and Glycosuria in Pregnancy with Macrosomia and Offspring Body Mass Index, Waist and Fat Mass in Later Childhood: Findings from a Prospective Pregnancy Cohort. *Diabetologia* **2010**, *53*, 89–97. [CrossRef] [PubMed]
33. Clausen, T.D.; Mathiesen, E.R.; Hansen, T.; Pedersen, O.; Jensen, D.M.; Lauenborg, J.; Schmidt, L.; Damm, P. Overweight and the Metabolic Syndrome in Adult Offspring of Women with Diet-Treated Gestational Diabetes Mellitus or Type 1 Diabetes. *J. Clin. Endocrinol. Metab.* **2009**, *94*, 2464–2470. [CrossRef] [PubMed]
34. Vääräsmäki, M.; Pouta, A.; Elliot, P.; Tapanainen, P.; Sovio, U.; Ruokonen, A.; Hartikainen, A.-L.; McCarthy, M.; Järvelin, M.-R. Adolescent Manifestations of Metabolic Syndrome Among Children Born to Women With Gestational Diabetes in a General-Population Birth Cohort. *Am. J. Epidemiol.* **2009**, *169*, 1209–1215. [CrossRef] [PubMed]

35. Hillier, T.A.; Pedula, K.L.; Schmidt, M.M.; Mullen, J.A.; Charles, M.-A.; Pettitt, D.J. Childhood Obesity and Metabolic Imprinting. *Diabetes Care* **2007**, *30*, 2287–2292. [CrossRef] [PubMed]
36. Damm, P. Gestational Diabetes Mellitus and Subsequent Development of Overt Diabetes Mellitus. *Dan. Med. Bull.* **1998**, *45*, 495–509. [PubMed]
37. Landon, M.B.; Spong, C.Y.; Thom, E.; Carpenter, M.W.; Ramin, S.M.; Casey, B.; Wapner, R.J.; Varner, M.W.; Rouse, D.J.; Thorp, J.M.; et al. A Multicenter, Randomized Trial of Treatment for Mild Gestational Diabetes. *N. Engl. J. Med.* **2009**, *361*, 1339–1348. [CrossRef]
38. Crowther, C.A.; Hiller, J.E.; Moss, J.R.; McPhee, A.J.; Jeffries, W.S.; Robinson, J.S. Effect of Treatment of Gestational Diabetes Mellitus on Pregnancy Outcomes. *N. Engl. J. Med.* **2005**, *352*, 2477–2486. [CrossRef]
39. Kim, S.Y.; Sharma, A.J.; Callaghan, W.M. Gestational Diabetes and Childhood Obesity: What Is the Link? *Curr. Opin. Obstet. Gynecol.* **2012**, *24*, 376–381. [CrossRef]
40. Catalano, P.M.; McIntyre, H.D.; Cruickshank, J.K.; McCance, D.R.; Dyer, A.R.; Metzger, B.E.; Lowe, L.P.; Trimble, E.R.; Coustan, D.R.; Hadden, D.R.; et al. The Hyperglycemia and Adverse Pregnancy Outcome Study: Associations of GDM and Obesity with Pregnancy Outcomes. *Diabetes Care* **2012**, *35*, 780–786. [CrossRef]
41. Kawasaki, M.; Arata, N.; Miyazaki, C.; Mori, R.; Kikuchi, T.; Ogawa, Y.; Ota, E. Obesity and Abnormal Glucose Tolerance in Offspring of Diabetic Mothers: A Systematic Review and Meta-Analysis. *PLoS ONE* **2018**, *13*, 1–19. [CrossRef] [PubMed]
42. Weiss, R.; Santoro, N.; Giannini, C.; Galderisi, A.; Umano, G.R.; Caprio, S. Prediabetes in Youths: Mechanisms and Biomarkers. *Lancet Child Adolesc. Health* **2017**, *1*, 240–248. [CrossRef]
43. Tabák, A.G.; Herder, C.; Rathmann, W.; Brunner, E.J.; Kivimäki, M. Prediabetes: A High-Risk State for Diabetes Development. *Lancet* **2012**, *379*, 2279–2290. [CrossRef]
44. Crume, T.L.; Ogden, L.; West, N.A.; Vehik, K.S.; Scherzinger, A.; Daniels, S.; McDuffie, R.; Bischoff, K.; Hamman, R.F.; Norris, J.M.; et al. Association of Exposure to Diabetes in Utero with Adiposity and Fat Distribution in a Multiethnic Population of Youth: The Exploring Perinatal Outcomes among Children (EPOCH) Study. *Diabetologia* **2011**, *54*, 87–92. [CrossRef] [PubMed]
45. Jaskolka, D.; Retnakaran, R.; Zinman, B.; Kramer, C.K. Sex of the Baby and Risk of Gestational Diabetes Mellitus in the Mother: A Systematic Review and Meta-Analysis. *Diabetologia* **2015**, *58*, 2469–2475. [CrossRef]
46. Catalano, P.M. The Impact of Gestational Diabetes and Maternal Obesity on the Mother and Her Offspring. *J. Dev. Orig. Health Dis.* **2010**, *1*, 208–215. [CrossRef]
47. Damm, P.; Houshmand-Oeregaard, A.; Kelstrup, L.; Lauenborg, J.; Mathiesen, E.R.; Clausen, T.D. Gestational Diabetes Mellitus and Long-Term Consequences for Mother and Offspring: A View from Denmark. *Diabetologia* **2016**, *59*, 1396–1399. [CrossRef]
48. Hu, G.; Tian, H.; Zhang, F.; Liu, H.; Zhang, C.; Zhang, S.; Wang, L.; Liu, G.; Yu, Z.; Yang, X.; et al. Tianjin Gestational Diabetes Mellitus Prevention Program: Study Design, Methods, and 1-Year Interim Report on the Feasibility of Lifestyle Intervention Program. *Diabetes Res. Clin. Pract.* **2012**, *98*, 508–517. [CrossRef]

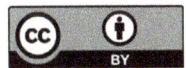 © 2020 by the authors. Licensee MDPI, Basel, Switzerland. This article is an open access article distributed under the terms and conditions of the Creative Commons Attribution (CC BY) license (http://creativecommons.org/licenses/by/4.0/).

MDPI
St. Alban-Anlage 66
4052 Basel
Switzerland
Tel. +41 61 683 77 34
Fax +41 61 302 89 18
www.mdpi.com

Journal of Clinical Medicine Editorial Office
E-mail: jcm@mdpi.com
www.mdpi.com/journal/jcm

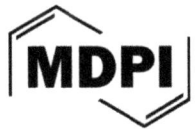

www.ingramcontent.com/pod-product-compliance
Lightning Source LLC
LaVergne TN
LVHW070140100526
838202LV00015B/1861